JJZ
To Judi, Robbie, Michael, Julia, and Sarah

ERA
With love and thanks to Michael, Ava, and Talia

LB
To Naomi and the next generation of pediatricians

KL
To my mother Joan

BM
To Judi, Max, Zachary, and Grace

CM
To Thom, Anna, Claire and my parents, Bill and Janet Johnson

LR
To Frank and Hannah

Schwartz's

Clinical Handbook
of Pediatrics

Fourth Edition

Schwartz's Clinical Handbook of

Pediatrics

Fourth Edition

EDITOR

Joseph J. Zorc

Associate Editors

Elizabeth R. Alpern

Lawrence W. Brown

Kathleen M. Loomes

Bradley S. Marino

Cynthia J. Mollen

Leslie J. Raffini

 Wolters Kluwer | Lippincott Williams & Wilkins
Health

Philadelphia • Baltimore • New York • London
Buenos Aires • Hong Kong • Sydney • Tokyo

Acquisitions Editor: Charles W. Mitchell
Managing Editors: Stacey Sebring, Jennifer Verbiar
Marketing Manager: Emilie J. Moyer
Production Editor: Beth Martz
Design Coordinator: Holly Reid McLaughlin
Compositor: International Typesetting and Composition

Fourth Edition

Copyright © 2009 Lippincott Williams & Wilkins, a Wolters Kluwer business.

351 West Camden Street   530 Walnut Street
Baltimore, MD 21201   Philadelphia, PA 19106

Printed in the People's Republic of China

First Edition, 1996   Second Edition, 1999   Third Edition, 2003

9 8 7 6 5 4 3 2 1

Library of Congress Cataloging-in-Publication Data

Schwartz's clinical handbook of pediatrics / editor, Joseph J. Zorc ;
associate editors, Elizabeth R. Alpern ... [et al.]. — 4th ed.
   p. ; cm.
  Rev. ed. of: Clinical handbook of pediatrics / editor, M. William Schwartz;
associate editors, Lawrence W. Brown ... [et al.]. 3rd ed. c2003.
  Includes bibliographical references and index.
  ISBN-13: 978-0-7817-7013-2
  ISBN-10: 0-7817-7013-0
  1. Pediatrics—Handbooks, manuals, etc.   I. Zorc, Joseph J.   II. Schwartz,
M. William, 1935–   III. Clinical handbook of pediatrics.   IV. Title: Clinical
handbook of pediatrics.
  [DNLM: 1. Pediatrics—Handbooks.   WS 39 S399 2008]
  RJ48.C55 2008
  618.92—dc22

                2008018514

DISCLAIMER

Care has been taken to confirm the accuracy of the information present and to describe generally accepted practices. However, the authors, editors, and publisher are not responsible for errors or omissions or for any consequences from application of the information in this book and make no warranty, expressed or implied, with respect to the currency, completeness, or accuracy of the contents of the publication. Application of this information in a particular situation remains the professional responsibility of the practitioner; the clinical treatments described and recommended may not be considered absolute and universal recommendations.

The authors, editors, and publisher have exerted every effort to ensure that drug selection and dosage set forth in this text are in accordance with the current recommendations and practice at the time of publication. However, in view of ongoing research, changes in government regulations, and the constant flow of information relating to drug therapy and drug reactions, the reader is urged to check the package insert for each drug for any change in indications and dosage and for added warnings and precautions. This is particularly important when the recommended agent is a new or infrequently employed drug.

Some drugs and medical devices presented in this publication have Food and Drug Administration (FDA) clearance for limited use in restricted research settings. It is the responsibility of the health care provider to ascertain the FDA status of each drug or device planned for use in their clinical practice.

To purchase additional copies of this book, call our customer service department at **(800) 638-3030** or fax orders to **(301) 223-2320**. International customers should call (301) 223-2300.

Visit Lippincott Williams & Wilkins on the Internet: http://www.lww.com. Lippincott Williams & Wilkins customer service representatives are available from 8:30 am to 6:00 pm, EST.

Preface

For this fourth edition of the *Clinical Handbook of Pediatrics,* I've taken over the editorial role from Dr. M. William Schwartz. In recognition of Dr. Schwartz's lifelong contribution to improving knowledge and education in pediatrics, we've retitled the book in his honor. We've tried to continue the pragmatic approach to assessment, differential diagnosis, and management of pediatric illness exemplified in prior editions while updating it to reflect the rapidly changing world of 21st-century medicine. We've also responded to recommendations from readers to streamline and reduce the size of the book to make it easier to bring to the bedside. I hope that we've succeeded in those goals and look forward to receiving suggestions for the design of future editions.

Special thanks go to the associate editors, Elizabeth R. Alpern, Lawrence W. Brown, Kathleen M. Loomes, Bradley S. Marino, Cynthia J. Mollen, and Leslie J. Raffini, who worked closely with the authors and added much to the quality of this text. Thanks go to all of the authors who updated the evidence in their area and often brought on junior colleagues to add a fresh perspective. I'd also like to thank the team at Lippincott/Wolters Kluwer, including Jenn Verbiar and Stacey Sebring. A book such as this resembles a quilt representing the efforts of many individuals, and I hope that we've successfully woven it together into a whole that will benefit the clinicians and children for whom it was intended.

Contributors

Nicholas S. Abend, MD
Fellow in Neurology
Department of Neurology
The Children's Hospital of Philadelphia
Philadelphia, Pennsylvania

Paula Agosto, RN, MHA
Director of Nursing
Departments of Emergency Care, Critical Care,
    Trauma, and Transport Medicine
The Children's Hospital of Philadelphia
Philadelphia, Pennsylvania

Sabreen Akhter, DO
Instructor of Pediatrics
Pediatric Emergency Medicine
Medical College of Wisconsin
Milwaukee, Wisconsin
Fellow
Department of Pediatric Emergency
    Medicine
Children's Hospital of Wisconsin
Milwaukee, Wisconsin

Elizabeth R. Alpern, MD, MSCE
Associate Professor
Department of Pediatrics
University of Pennsylvania
Philadelphia, Pennsylvania
Attending Physician
Department of Pediatrics, Division of
    Emergency Medicine
The Children's Hospital of Philadelphia
Philadelphia, Pennsylvania

Craig Alter, MD
Associate Professor of Pediatrics
University of Pennsylvania School
    of Medicine
Philadelphia, Pennsylvania
Attending Physician
Department of Pediatrics Endocrinology
The Children's Hospital of Philadelphia
Philadelphia, Pennsylvania

Oluwakemi B. Badaki-Makun, MD CM
Instructor in Pediatrics
Department of Pediatrics
University of Pennsylvania School
    of Medicine
Philadelphia, Pennsylvania
Pediatric Emergency Medicine Fellow
Division of Emergency Medicine
The Children's Hospital of Philadelphia
Philadelphia, Pennsylvania

Robert N. Baldassano, MD
Associate Professor of Pediatrics
University of Pennsylvania School
    of Medicine
Director
Center for Pediatric Inflammatory Bowel
    Disease
The Children's Hospital of Philadelphia
Philadelphia, Pennsylvania

Jill Baren, MD
Associate Professor of Pediatrics
    and Emergency Medicine
University of Pennsylvania School
    of Medicine
Philadelphia, Pennsylvania
Attending Physician
Emergency Department
Hospital of the University of Pennsylvania
    and The Children's Hospital
    of Philadelphia
Philadelphia, Pennsylvania

Louis M. Bell, MD
Professor of Pediatrics
University of Pennsylvania School
    of Medicine
Philadelphia, Pennsylvania
Chief
Department of General Pediatrics
The Children's Hospital of Philadelphia
Philadelphia, Pennsylvania

Mercedes M. Blackstone, MD
Clinical Instructor
Department of Pediatrics
University of Pennsylvania School
    of Medicine
Philadelphia, Pennsylvania
Fellow
Division of Emergency Medicine
The Children's Hospital of Philadelphia
Philadelphia, Pennsylvania

Nathan J. Blum, MD
Associate Professor of Pediatrics
Department of Pediatrics
University of Pennsylvania School
    of Medicine
Philadelphia, Pennsylvania
Director, Section of Behavioral Pediatrics
Division of Child Development, Rehabilitation,
    and Metabolic Disease
The Children's Hospital of Philadelphia
Philadelphia, Pennsylvania

William L. Border, MBChB
Assistant Professor of Pediatrics
University of Cincinnati
Cincinnati, Ohio
Attending Physician
Pediatric Cardiology
Cincinnati Children's Medical Center
Cincinnati, Ohio

John T. Boyle, MD
Academic Clinical Professor
    of Pediatrics
University of Pennsylvania School
    of Medicine
Philadelphia, Pennsylvania
Attending Physician
Division of Gastroenterology, Hepatology
    and Nutrition
The Children's Hospital of Philadelphia
Philadelphia, Pennsylvania

Amy R. Brooks-Kayal, MD
Assistant Professor of Pediatrics
    and Neurology
University of Pennsylvania School
    of Medicine
Philadelphia, Pennsylvania
Attending Physician
Department of Child Neurology
The Children's Hospital of Philadelphia
Philadelphia, Pennsylvania

Lawrence W. Brown, MD
Associate Professor of Neurology and Pediatrics
University of Pennsylvania School of Medicine
Director, Pediatric Neuropsychiatry Program
The Children's Hospital of Philadelphia
Philadelphia, Pennsylvania

James M. Callahan, MD
Associate Professor of Clinical Pediatrics
Department of Pediatrics
University of Pennsylvania School of Medicine
Philadelphia, Pennsylvania
Director, Medical Education
Division of Emergency Medicine
The Children's Hospital of Philadelphia
Philadelphia, Pennsylvania

Cynthia Campen, MD
Fellow
Department of Child Neurology
The Children's Hospital of Philadelphia
Philadelphia, Pennsylvania

Christine S. Cho, MD, MPH
Assistant Clinical Professor
Department of Pediatrics
UCSF School of Medicine
San Francisco, California
Attending
Department of Emergency Medicine
Children's Hospital & Research Center
    in Oakland
Oakland, California

Cindy W. Christian, MD
Associate Professor of Pediatrics
University of Pennsylvania School of Medicine
Philadelphia, Pennsylvania
Director, Child Abuse Services
Department of General Pediatrics
The Children's Hospital of Philadelphia
Philadelphia, Pennsylvania

Esther K. Chung, MD, MPH
Associate Professor
Department of Pediatrics
Jefferson Medical College
Philadelphia, Pennsylvania
Attending Physician
Department of Pediatrics
Alfred I. duPont Hospital for Children
Wilmington, Delaware

Mitchell I. Cohen, MD
Pediatric Cardiologist
Phoenix, Arizona

Jenell Coleman, MD, MPH
Assistant Professor
Department of Obstetrics and Gynecology
University of Pennsylvania
Philadelphia, Pennsylvania
Clinical Affiliate
Department of Adolescent Medicine
The Children's Hospital of Philadelphia
Philadelphia, Pennsylvania

Michelle Denburg, MD
Fellow
Department of Nephrology
The Children's Hospital of Philadelphia
Philadelphia, Pennsylvania
Fellow
Department of Nephrology
The Children's Hospital of Philadelphia
Philadelphia, Pennsylvania

Joel A. Fein, MD, MPH
Associate Professor of Pediatrics
    and Emergency Medicine
University of Pennsylvania School
    of Medicine
Philadelphia, Pennsylvania
Attending Physician
Emergency Department
The Children's Hospital of Philadelphia
Philadelphia, Pennsylvania

Alexander G. Fiks, MD, MSCE
Assistant Professor of Pediatrics
Department of Pediatrics
University of Pennsylvania School
    of Medicine
Philadelphia, Pennsylvania
Attending Physician
Department of General Pediatrics/
    Primary Care
The Children's Hospital of Philadelphia
Philadelphia, Pennsylvania

Kristin N. Fiorino, MD
Fellow
Department of Gastroenterology
The Children's Hospital of Philadelphia
Philadelphia, Pennsylvania

Jonathan D. Fish, MD
Instructor
Department of Pediatrics
University of Pennsylvania
Philadelphia, Pennsylvania
Attending Physician
Department of Oncology and Blood & Marrow
    Transplantation
The Children's Hospital of Philadelphia
Philadelphia, Pennsylvania

Susan A. Friedman, MD
Clinical Associate Professor
Department of Pediatrics, Division of
    General Pediatrics
University of Pennsylvania School
    of Medicine
Philadelphia, Pennsylvania
Department of Pediatrics
The Children's Hospital of Philadelphia
Philadelphia, Pennsylvania

Janet H. Friday, MD
Associate Clinical Professor
Department of Pediatrics
University of California, San Diego
La Jolla, California
Attending Physician
Department of Pediatrics
Rady Children's Hospital
San Diego, California

Marc H. Gorelick, MD
Professor of Pediatrics and Population
    Health
Medical College of Wisconsin
Milwaukee, Wisconsin
Chief
Department of Pediatrics Emergency
    Medicine
Children's Hospital of Wisconsin
Milwaukee, Wisconsin

Monika Goyal, MD
Instructor
Department of Pediatrics
University of Pennsylvania School
    of Medicine
Philadelphia, Pennsylvania
Fellow
Department of Emergency Medicine
The Children's Hospital of Philadelphia
Philadelphia, Pennsylvania

Adda Grimberg, MD, FAAP

Assistant Professor
Department of Pediatrics
University of Pennsylvania School
    of Medicine
Philadelphia, Pennsylvania
Attending Physician
Division of Pediatric Endocrinology
The Children's Hospital of Philadelphia
Philadelphia, Pennsylvania

Toni Gross, MD, MPH

Assistant Professor
Department of Pediatrics
University of Pennsylvania School
    of Medicine
Philadelphia, Pennsylvania
Attending Physician
Department of Pediatric Emergency Medicine
The Children's Hospital of Philadelphia
Philadelphia, Pennsylvania

Andrew Grossman, MD

Department of Pediatrics
University of Pennsylvania School
    of Medicine
Philadelphia, Pennsylvania
Fellow
Department of Pediatrics, Division of
    GI/Nutrition
The Children's Hospital of Philadelphia
Philadelphia, Pennsylvania

Timothy M. Hoffman, MD

Associate Professor
Department of Pediatrics
The Ohio State University College of Medicine
Columbus, Ohio
Medical Director, Heart Transplant and Heart
    Failure Program
The Heart Center
Nationwide Children's Hospital
Columbus, Ohio

Andrew Hashikawa, MD

Instructor of Pediatrics
Department of Pediatrics, Division of
    Emergency Medicine
Medical College of Wisconsin
Milwaukee, Wisconsin
Fellow
Department of Pediatric Emergency Medicine
Children's Hospital of Wisconsin
Milwaukee, Wisconsin

Kan N. Hor, MD

Assistant Professor of Pediatrics
Department of Pediatrics
University of Cincinnati
Cincinnati, Ohio
Assistant Professor of Pediatrics
Department of Pediatrics
Cincinnati Children's Hospital Medical Center
Cincinnati, Ohio

Patty Huang, MD

Fellow in Developmental and Behavioral
    Pediatrics
Department of Pediatrics
The Children's Hospital of Philadelphia
Philadelphia, Pennsylvania

Paul Ishimine, MD

Associate Professor
Departments of Medicine and Pediatrics
University of California, San Diego School
    of Medicine
San Diego, California
Director, Pediatric Emergency Medicine
Department of Emergency Medicine
University of California, San Diego Medical Center
San Diego, California

Binita M. Kamath, MBBChir

Assistant Professor
Department of Pediatrics
University of Pennsylvania
Philadelphia, Pennsylvania
Attending Physician
Division of Gastroenterology, Hepatology
    and Nutrition
The Children's Hospital of Philadelphia
Philadelphia, Pennsylvania

Thomas L. Kennedy, MD

Clinical Professor of Pediatrics
Department of Pediatrics
Yale University
New Haven, Connecticut
Chairman
Department of Pediatrics
Bridgeport Hospital
Bridgeport, Connecticut

Dorit Koren, MD

Fellow
Division of Endocrinology and Diabetes
The Children's Hospital of Philadelphia
Philadelphia, Pennsylvania

Richard M. Kravitz, MD
Assistant Professor
Department of Pediatrics
Duke University
Durham, North Carolina
Attending, Pediatric Pulmonology
Department of Pediatrics; Division of Pediatrics
    Pulmonary and Sleep Medicine
Duke University Medical Center
Durham, North Carolina

Mary B. Leonard, MD, MSCE
Associate Professor
Department of Pediatrics
University of Pennsylvania School of Medicine
Philadelphia, Pennsylvania
Attending Physician
Department of Pediatrics
The Children's Hospital of Philadelphia
Philadelphia, Pennsylvania

Lorraine E. Levitt Katz, MD
Associate Professor
Department of Pediatric
    Endocrinology/Diabetes
University of Pennsylvania School of Medicine
Philadelphia, Pennsylvania
Associate Professor
Division of Pediatric Endocrinology/Diabetes
The Children's Hospital of Philadelphia
Philadelphia, Pennsylvania

Valerie Lewis, MD, MPH
Fellow Physician
Craig-Dalsimer Division of Adolescent
    Medicine
The Children's Hospital of Philadelphia
Philadelphia, Pennsylvania
Fellow Physician
Craig-Dalsimer Division of Adolescent
    Medicine
The Children's Hospital of Philadelphia
Philadelphia, Pennsylvania

Chris A. Liacouras, MD
Professor of Pediatrics
Department of Pediatrics
University of Pennsylvania School of Medicine
Philadelphia, Pennsylvania
Attending Physician
Division of Gastroenterology, Hepatology
    and Nutrition
The Children's Hospital of Philadelphia
Philadelphia, Pennsylvania

Kathleen M. Loomes, MD
Assistant Professor
Department of Pediatrics
University of Pennsylvania
Attending Physician
Division of Gastroenterology, Hepatology,
    and Nutrition
The Children's Hospital of Philadelphia
Philadelphia, Pennsylvania

Katherine MacRae Dell, MD
Assistant Professor
Department of Pediatrics
Case Western Reserve University
Cleveland, Ohio
Attending Pediatric Nephrologist
Division of Pediatric Nephrology
Rainbow Babies and Children's Hospital
Cleveland, Ohio

Bradley S. Marino, MD, MPP, MSCE
Associate Professor of Pediatrics
Department of Pediatrics
University of Cincinnati College
    of Medicine
Cincinnati, Ohio
Associate Professor of Pediatrics
Department of Pediatrics, Divisions of
    Cardiology and Critical Care Medicine
Cincinnati Children's Hospital
    Medical Center
Cincinnati, Ohio

Shoshana Melman, MD
Associate Professor
Department of Pediatrics
University of Medicine and Dentistry
    of New Jersey School of Medicine
Stratford, New Jersey
Medical Director
Foster Care Program
CARES Institute
Stratford, New Jersey

Kevin E.C. Meyers, MB, BCh
Assistant Professor
Division of Nephrology, Pediatric
    Department
University of Pennsylvania
Philadelphia, Pennsylvania
Attending
Pediatric Department/Nephrology
The Children's Hospital
    of Philadelphia
Philadelphia, Pennsylvania

Okeoma Mmeje, MD, MPH
Medical Resident
Department of Obstetrics
    and Gynecology
Philadelphia, Pennsylvania
Medical Resident
Department of Obstetrics
    and Gynecology
Hospital of University of Pennsylvania
Philadelphia, Pennsylvania

Cynthia J. Mollen, MD, MSCE
Assistant Professor of Pediatrics
    and Emergency Medicine
University of Pennsylvania
Attending Physician
Division of Emergency Medicine
The Children's Hospital
    of Philadelphia
Philadelphia, Pennsylvania

Thomas Mollen, MD
Clinical Associate
Department of Pediatrics
University of Pennsylvania School
    of Medicine
Philadelphia, Pennsylvania
Associate Medical Director
Intensive Care Nursery
Pennsylvania Hospital
Philadelphia, Pennsylvania

Laura Mulreany, MD
Assistant Clinical Professor
Department of Pediatrics
Uniformed Services University of the Health
    Sciences
Bethesda, MD
Staff Pediatric Pulmonologist
Department of Pediatrics
Walter Reed Army Medical Center
Washington, DC

Frances M. Nadel, MD, MSCE
Associate Professor
Department of Pediatrics
University of Pennsylvania School
    of Medicine
Philadelphia, Pennsylvania
Attending Physician
Emergency Medicine
The Children's Hospital
    of Philadelphia
Philadelphia, Pennsylvania

Cynthia Norris, MD
Clinical Associate
Department of Pediatrics
University of Pennsylvania
Philadelphia, Pennsylvania
Medical Director
Department of Hematology, Acute
    Care Unit
The Children's Hospital of Philadelphia
Philadelphia, Pennsylvania

Michael A. Posencheg, MD
Assistant Professor of Clinical Pediatrics
Department of Pediatrics
University of Pennsylvania School
    of Medicine
Philadelphia, Pennsylvania
Associate Medical Director, Intensive
    Care Nursery
Division of Neonatology
    and Newborn Services
Hospital of the University
    of Pennsylvania
Philadelphia, Pennsylvania

Madhura Pradhan, MD
Assistant Professor of Clinical Pediatrics
Department of Pediatrics
University of Pennsylvania School
    of Medicine
Philadelphia, Pennsylvania
Assistant Professor of Clinical Pediatrics
Division of Nephrology
The Children's Hospital of Philadelphia
Philadelphia, Pennsylvania

Jill C. Posner, MD, MSCE
Assistant Professor of Pediatrics
Department of Pediatrics
University of Pennsylvania School
    of Medicine
Philadelphia, Pennsylvania
Attending Physician
Department of Pediatrics
The Children's Hospital of Philadelphia
Philadelphia, Pennsylvania

Ryan Raffaelli, MD
Department of Pediatrics
University of Pennsylvania
Philadelphia, Pennsylvania
Fellow
Division of Nephrology
The Children's Hospital of Philadelphia
Philadelphia, Pennsylvania

Leslie J. Raffini, MD
Assistant Professor of Pediatrics
University of Pennsylvania School
    of Medicine
Philadelphia, Pennsylvania
Attending Physician
Division of Hematology
The Children's Hospital of Philadelphia
Philadelphia, Pennsylvania

Claudio Ramaciotti, MD
Professor of Pediatrics
UT Southwestern Medical Center
Dallas, Texas
Director of Echocardiography Laboratory
Children's Hospital Center of Dallas
Dallas, Texas

Erin Rebele, MD
Resident
Department of Obstetrics and Gynecology
Philadelphia, Pennsylvania
Medical Resident
Department of Obstetrics and Gynecology
Hospital of University of Pennsylvania
Philadelphia, Pennsylvania

Jack Rychik, MD
Director, Echocardiography Laboratory
Pediatric Cardiology
The Children's Hospital of Philadelphia
Philadelphia, Pennsylvania

Matthew Sampson, MD
Instructor
Department of Pediatrics
University of Pennsylvania
Philadelphia, Pennsylvania
Pediatrics Resident
Department of Pediatrics
The Children's Hospital of Philadelphia
Philadelphia, Pennsylvania

Marta Satin-Smith, MD
Assistant Professor
Department of Pediatrics
Eastern Virginia Medical School
Norfolk, Virginia
Medical Director, CHKD Diabetes
    Program
Department of Pediatrics
Children's Hospital of the Kings
    Daughters
Norfolk, Virginia

Amy H. Schultz, MD, MSCE
Assistant Professor
Department of Pediatrics
University of Washington School
    of Medicine
Seattle, Washington
Attending Physician
Children's Heart Center
Children's Hospital and Regional
    Medical Center
Seattle, Washington

Charles Schwartz, MD, FAAP
Assistant Clinical Professor of Pediatrics
University of Pennsylvania School
    of Medicine
Philadelphia, Pennsylvania

Jeffrey A. Seiden, MD
Clinical Instructor
Department of Pediatrics
University of Pennsylvania
Philadelphia, Pennsylvania
Fellow
Department of Emergency Medicine
The Children's Hospital
    of Philadelphia
Philadelphia, Pennsylvania

Christine B. Sethna, MD, EdM
Fellow (Lecturer)
Department of Pediatrics, Division
    of Nephrology
University of Pennsylvania
Philadelphia, Pennsylvania
Fellow
Department of Pediatrics, Division
    of Nephrology
The Children's Hospital
    of Philadelphia
Philadelphia, Pennsylvania

Kara Shah, MD, PhD
Assistant Professor
Department of Pediatrics
University of Pennsylvania
Philadelphia, Pennsylvania
Attending Physician
Department of General Pediatrics, Section
    of Pediatric Dermatology
The Children's Hospital
    of Philadelphia
Philadelphia, Pennsylvania

Samir S. Shah, MD, MSCE
Assistant Professor
Department of Pediatrics and Biostatistics
   and Epidemiology
University of Pennsylvania School of Medicine
Philadelphia, Pennsylvania
Attending Physician
Infectious Diseases
The Children's Hospital of Philadelphia
Philadelphia, Pennsylvania

Kathy N. Shaw, MD, MSCE
Professor
Department of Pediatrics
University of Pennsylvania School of Medicine
Philadelphia, Pennsylvania
Division Chief
Department of Emergency Medicine
The Children's Hospital of Philadelphia
Philadelphia, Pennsylvania

Laura N. Sinai, MD, MSCE, FAAP
Pediatrician
Department of Pediatrics
Gaston Memorial Hospital
Gastonia, North Carolina

Kim Smith-Whitley, MD
Associate Professor
Department of Pediatrics
University of Pennsylvania School of Medicine
Philadelphia, Pennsylvania
Clinical Director
Division of Hematology
The Children's Hospital of Philadelphia
Philadelphia, Pennsylvania

Philip R. Spandorfer, MD, MSCE
Attending
Department of Pediatric Emergency Medicine
Children's Healthcare of Atlanta
   at Scottish Rite
Atlanta, Georgia

Karena L. Swan, MD
Associate Research Scientist
Department of Pediatrics
Yale University
New Haven, Connecticut
Attending Physician
Department of Pediatrics
Yale New Haven Hospital
New Haven, Connecticut

Nicholas Tsarouhas, MD
Associate Professor of Clinical
   Pediatrics
Department of Pediatrics
University of Pennsylvania School
   of Medicine
Philadelphia, Pennsylvania
Medical Director, Emergency
   Transport Team
Division of Emergency Medicine
The Children's Hospital
   of Philadelphia
Philadelphia, Pennsylvania

Lisa K. Tuchman
Assistant Professor
Department of Pediatrics
University of Pennsylvania
Philadelphia, Pennsylvania
Assistant Professor/Adolescent Medicine
   Physician Specialist
Craig-Dalsimer Division of Adolescent
   Medicine
The Children's Hospital
   of Philadelphia
Philadelphia, Pennsylvania

Brenda Waber RD, CSP, CNSD, LDN
Neonatal Dietitian
Department of Clinical Nutrition
The Children's Hospital
   of Philadelphia
Philadelphia, Pennsylvania

Stuart A. Weinzimer, MD
Associate Professor
Department of Pediatrics
Yale University
New Haven, Connecticut
Attending Physician
Department of Pediatrics
Yale-New Haven Medical Center
New Haven, Connecticut

Catherine C. Wiley, MD
Associate Professor
Department of Pediatrics
University of Connecticut School of Medicine
Farmington, Connecticut
Clinical Director
Primary Care Center
Connecticut Children's Medical Center
Hartford, Connecticut

James F. Wiley II, MD, MPH
Professor
Department of Pediatrics and Emergency
    Medicine/Traumatology
University of Connecticut School of Medicine
Farmington, Connecticut
Attending, Pediatrics Emergency Medicine
Department of Pediatrics
Connecticut Children's Medical Center
Hartford, Connecticut

Clyde J. Wright, MD
Instructor
Department of Pediatrics
University of Pennsylvania School of Medicine
Philadelphia, Pennsylvania
Fellow, Division of Neonatology
Department of Pediatrics
The Children's Hospital of Philadelphia
Philadelphia, Pennsylvania

Courtney J. Wusthoff, MD
Child Neurology Fellow
Division of Neurology
The Children's Hospital of Philadelphia
Philadelphia, Pennsylvania

Joseph Zorc, MD, MSCE
Associate Professor of Pediatrics
    and Emergency Medicine
University of Pennsylvania
Attending Physician
The Children's Hospital of Philadelphia
Philadelphia, Pennsylvania

Kathy Zsolway, DO
Attending Physician
Department of General Pediatrics
The Children's Hospital of Philadelphia
Philadelphia, Pennsylvania

Contents

chapter

1

Obtaining and Presenting a Patient History

Joseph J. Zorc
M. William Schwartz (Third edition)

This chapter presents a guide to obtaining a history for a pediatric patient and presenting a case on rounds or to an audience. Not every item described in this chapter is necessary in every write-up or presentation. The goal is to communicate key information about a patient; the reader should not be overwhelmed with details that do not tell the patient's story.

HISTORY

Chief Complaint

Always ask the patient or parent to describe their concerns, and record their actual words. The age and sex of the patient, as well as the duration of the problem, should be noted when presenting the chief complaint.

> **HINT:** Experienced pediatric clinicians state that most of the key evidence leading to a diagnosis is obtained through the history. Often the physical examination and laboratory tests serve to confirm what the history suggests.

History of Present Illness

Indicate who the person was that provided the history (e.g., patient, parent, guardian). Provide a clear, concise chronology of important events surrounding the problem. When did the problem start? How has it changed over time? What tests and treatments were performed? Include key negative findings that may contribute to the differential diagnosis.

Medical History

- **Prenatal history**—mother's age and number of pregnancies; length of pregnancy; prenatal care, abnormal bleeding, illness, or exposure to illness; medications or substance use (alcohol, drugs, tobacco) during pregnancy.

- **Birth history**—birthweight; duration of labor; mode of delivery, use of induction, anesthesia, or forceps; complications, Apgar scores if known.
- **Neonatal history**—length of stay, location (nursery versus intensive care); complications such as jaundice, respiratory problems; feeding history.

HINT: Details about birth history are included in a write-up when they are relevant but generally should be included for all children younger than 2 years.

- **Developmental history**—milestones for smiling, rolling over, sitting, standing, speaking, and toilet training; growth landmarks for weight gain and length. If delays are present, determine the approximate age at which the child functions for motor, verbal, and social skills.
- **Behavioral history**—Proceed from less to more sensitive areas. The mnemonic SHADSSS can help structure the interview with an adolescent:

School: grades, likes/dislikes, plans for the future
Home: others present, relationship with family
Activities: friends, hobbies
Depression: emotions, confidants, suicidal thoughts/acts
Substance abuse: exposure or use of drugs, tobacco, alcohol
Sexuality: partners, contraception use, history of sexually transmitted diseases (STDs)
Safety: violence, access to weapons

- **Immunization history**—immunizations by type and date, dates of recent boosters, recent tuberculosis testing results.

HINT: A statement in the patient's write-up that the patient's immunizations are "up to date" does not indicate whether recent changes in the recommendations were followed. Specific information should be provided when possible.

- **Past medical history**—childhood illnesses, estimated frequency of infections, hospitalizations.
- **Surgical history**—procedures, complications, dates of each.

Review of Systems

Do not duplicate the history of the present illness in this section of the write-up.

- **Head**—injuries, headaches, hair loss, scalp infections.
- **Eyes**—acuity of vision; use of glasses; history of discharges, abnormal tearing, or injuries; prior surgery.
- **Ears**—acuity of hearing; history of otitis, discharges, or foreign bodies.
- **Nose**—breathing difficulties, discharges, bleeding, sinus infections.
- **Oral cavity and throat**—frequency of sore throats, dental problems, bleeding gums, herpes infections, ulcers.
- **Lungs**—exercise tolerance (ability to keep up with peers during exercise), breathing difficulties, cough (day or night), history of pneumonia, wheezing, pains, hemoptysis, exposure to tuberculosis, previous chest radiographs.
- **Heart**—exercise tolerance; history of murmurs; history of rheumatic fever in patient or family; history of Lyme disease or other infections that may affect the heart; feeling of heart racing, dyspnea, orthopnea, palpitations or chest pain; cyanosis; edema.
- **Gastrointestinal system**—appetite, weight changes, problems with food (e.g., allergy, intolerance), abdominal pain (location, intensity, precipitating events), bowel movements (number and character), jaundice, rectal bleeding.
- **Genitourinary system**—history of infection, frequency of urination, dysuria, hematuria, character of the urine stream, bedwetting, urethral or vaginal discharge, age of menarche.
- **Extremities**—joint or muscle pain, muscle strength, swelling, limitation of movement.
- **Neurologic system**—seizures, weakness, headaches, tremors, abnormal movements, development, school achievement, hyperactivity.
- **Skin**—rashes, type of soap and detergent used.

Family History

- Ages of Parents and Siblings
- **Family history of illness**—seizures, asthma, cancer, behavior problems, allergies, cardiac disease, unexplained deaths, lipid disorders
- **Deaths in family**—causes of, age of family member at the time
- **Social history**—other household members, sleeping arrangements, marital status of the parents, parents' employment status, health insurance status

> **HINT:** In a patient with a suspected metabolic disorder, the most important question concerns early deaths of the patient's siblings or cousins. In a patient with a suspected infectious disease problem, the most important question concerns the patient's contact with others who are ill.

HINTS FOR PATIENT PRESENTATIONS

One of my images of hell is to be forced to spend a day listening to medical students' case presentations on rounds—both of them.   Burt Sloane

Consider the Audience and Setting

The group members often have short attention spans, are usually standing, and often have other obligations. Make a **brief presentation,** no longer than 2 minutes, that offers highlights of the problem and leads the audience to the diagnosis. This is not the time to demonstrate your thoroughness or compulsive nature.

Also **consider the style** of the preceptor and those attending. Some may prefer a Socratic dialogue; others want a more detailed presentation. Keep in mind that the Socratic style leads to interactive questions and answers. It is important, however, to appreciate the time pressures of audiences in inpatient rounds or clinics.

In contrast, **grand rounds** or formal case presentations may last as long as 10 minutes. These presentations focus on a diagnostic dilemma with many differential diagnoses, provide data for someone else to discuss with regard to findings and reaching a diagnosis or treatment, and include detailed histories, many negative findings, and most laboratory test results.

Decide What Information Is Important to Include

It is important to **decide what negative information to include** in the presentation and what to rule out. The negative information should help exclude one or two of the major differential diagnoses. For example, you should mention respiratory distress in a case of cardiac failure but not in a case of urinary tract infection. Likewise, you should mention family history in a case of asthma or mental retardation but not in leg trauma.

After gathering information about the patient's problem, **select the highlights,** arranging them in an interesting and logical manner to lead to the diagnosis.

Organize the Presentation

The following format is suggested.

Chief Complaint

State in the patient's or parent's words the reason for referral or admission. Mention the patient's age and the source of the referral. Avoid starting with a list of descriptors (e.g., "product of a gravida 1, para 1 full-term pregnancy" or "was well until 2 days before admission, when the following events occurred").

History of Present Illness

Give a summary of the pertinent events preceding admission and the changes in the patient's condition that precipitated the visit.

Review of the Patient History

Include only information that suggests the diagnosis or rules out major differential diagnoses. Consider the patient's developmental history, immunization history, past medical history, and family and social history.

Physical Examination Findings

Discuss how the child looked, but include only pertinent positive findings and the few negative findings that help eliminate major differential diagnoses or lead to the diagnosis.

Summary

Summarize the key facts that lead to the suspected diagnosis. Review other diagnoses that are in the differential. Outline your plan to complete the workup. Always think through your diagnosis and plan prior to a presentation, even if you are unsure, because this is the way to strengthen diagnostic skills.

Audience Questions

Be prepared for questions. They are compliments and mean that the audience was listening and thinking about the problem and the information you discussed. Questions are not criticisms of an incomplete presentation.

The Physical Examination

GENERAL CONSIDERATIONS

Performing the Physical Examination

The physical examination of a child is as much an art as a scientific procedure. The goal is to make the examination as productive and non-traumatic as possible.

To **minimize fear** in young children, conduct most of the physical examination with the child sitting on the parent's lap or nestled against his or her shoulder. If the child appears fearful, talk with the parent first, so the child has a chance to study you. Speak quietly, using a friendly tone of voice. Move gently and slowly, avoiding loud, sudden movements.

The physical examination is routinely presented and written in standard (adult) order, although it may not be carried out in that sequence. Children about 8 years and older can usually be examined easily in standard adult order, but with younger patients it is important to **examine the most critical areas first,** before the child cries. Always start with observation. Next, in a young child with a specific presenting complaint, it is often helpful to examine the corresponding organ system. In a young child with no specific complaints, palpate the fontanelles, and then auscultate the heart and lungs. Wait until the end of the examination to check the most threatening areas (e.g., the ears and oral cavity).

Special Concerns

Mental Status

Because children often cannot vocalize their symptoms, their overall mental status is an essential clue to their degree of illness. Will the child smile or play? Observe interactions with parents or siblings. Be careful to differentiate a child who is simply tired from one who is lethargic (difficult to arouse). Similarly, distinguish the cranky child who comforts easily from one who is truly irritable and inconsolable.

> **HINT:** Cranky, febrile young children are often much more pleasant after their fevers are brought down. Children with meningitis are not easily comforted by being held; in fact, when picked up they may cry more.

Hydration Status

Physical findings consistent with dehydration include an increased pulse, decreased blood pressure, sunken fontanelles, dry mucous membranes, decreased skin turgor, and increased capillary refill time (>2 seconds).

VITAL SIGNS AND STATISTICS

Temperature

Body temperatures are more labile in children than in adults and can be raised depending on the time of day (e.g., in the late afternoon) or following vigorous activity, excitement, or even eating.

A child's **normal oral temperature** is similar to an adult's, typically about **98.6°F.** The rectal temperature is typically approximately 1° higher than the oral equivalent, and an axillary temperature (the least accurate method) is typically about 1° lower. Study results regarding the reliability of tympanic thermometers have been mixed; they are often used in low-risk older children.

> **HINT:** An infant or young child can have a temperature of 103°F to 105°F, even with a minor infection. In contrast, a sick newborn may have a lower than normal temperature.

Pulse Rate

In an infant, palpate for pulse rate over the brachial artery. In an older child or adult, the wrist is generally the optimal location. Pulse rate is usually **120 to 160 beats per minute in the newborn** and steadily **declines as the child grows.** A typical teenager's pulse rate would be 70 to 80 beats per minute.

> **HINT:** In infants and children, the pulse rate responds much more distinctly to disease, exercise, or stress than it does in adults.

Respiration Rate

The most accurate measurements are obtained while the patient is asleep. In infants and young children, breathing is mostly diaphragmatic; the respiratory rate can be determined by **counting movements** of the abdomen. In older children and adolescents, chest movement should be **directly observed.** Table 2-1 summarizes the normal pediatric respiratory rates.

> **HINT:** Infants typically exhibit "periodic breathing," short periods of rapid breathing followed by several seconds without a breath. Pauses of 10 seconds or more are abnormal.

TABLE 2-1 Normal Pediatric Respiratory Rates (Respirations/Min)

Newborns	Toddlers	School-Age Children	Adolescents
30–50	20–40	15–25	12

Blood Pressure

To obtain an accurate blood pressure measurement, **patient relaxation** is especially critical. Explain to a young child that the "balloon" will squeeze his arm, and encourage him to watch the display.

Cuff width is also important. Choose a cuff width that covers 50% to 75% of the upper arm length. A too-narrow cuff may artificially increase the blood pressure reading.

If you are concerned about the possibility of heart disease, check blood pressure in **all four extremities.** Compare blood pressure measurements with standard norms for age and sex.

Length (Height)

To obtain a length measurement, place the infant on a firm table. Hold the baby's feet against a stationary board, keeping the knees straight, and bring a movable upright firmly against the baby's head to measure the infant's recumbent length.

Children >2 years can be measured with the child standing erect. The child should be positioned with feet flat, eyes looking straight ahead, and occiput, shoulders, buttocks, and heels against a vertical measuring board.

Figure 2-1 shows the National Center for Health Statistics percentiles for physical growth in girls and boys from birth through the age of 20 years.

Weight

Routinely **weigh infants unclothed.** For patients in whom small variations in weight are important, it is helpful to consistently use a single scale, preferably at the same time of day.

The growth charts in Figure 2-1 include **body mass index, or BMI** (wt/ht^2). This number is used in patients ≥2 years of age to determine if weight is appropriate for height. By plotting BMI for age, health care providers can achieve early identification of patients at risk for being overweight/obese.

HEAD

Head Circumference

Start your examination of the head by measuring the head circumference at the maximum point of the occipital protuberance posteriorly and at

A.

Figure 2-1 ■ National Center for Health Statistics (NCHS). Clinical Growth Charts.
(A) Girls, birth–36 months: Length-for-age and weight-for-age. *(B)* Girls, 2–20 years: Stature-for-age and weight-for-age. *(C)* Girls, BMI-for-age. *(D)* Boys, birth–36 months: Length-for-age and weight-for-age. *(E)* Boys, 2–20 years: Stature-for-age and weight-for-age. *(F)* Boys, BMI-for-age. *(Centers for Disease Control and Prevention. January 11, 2007. http://www.cdc.gov/nchs/about/major/nhanes/growthcharts/clinical_charts.htm September 2, 2007)*

B.

2 to 20 years: Girls
Stature-for-age and Weight-for-age percentiles

Published May 30, 2000 (modified 11/21/00).
SOURCE: Developed by the National Center for Health Statistics in collaboration with the National Center for Chronic Disease Prevention and Health Promotion (2000).
http://www.cdc.gov/growthcharts

Figure 2-1 ■ (*Continued*)

the midforehead anteriorly. **Microcephaly** (small head size) could result from abnormalities such as craniosynostosis (premature fusion of the sutures) or congenital TORCH (toxoplasmosis, other infections, rubella, cytomegalovirus, and herpes simplex) infection. **Macrocephaly** (large head size) could be caused by problems such as hydrocephalus or an intracranial mass. Figure 2-2 presents normal head circumferences.

C.

2 to 20 years: Girls
Body mass index-for-age percentiles

NAME _____

RECORD # _____

*To Calculate BMI: Weight (kg) ÷ Stature (cm) ÷ Stature (cm) x 10,000
or Weight (lb) ÷ Stature (in) ÷ Stature (in) x 703

Published May 30, 2000 (modified 10/16/00).
SOURCE: Developed by the National Center for Health Statistics in collaboration with
the National Center for Chronic Disease Prevention and Health Promotion (2000).
http://www.cdc.gov/growthcharts

Figure 2-1 ■ (*Continued*)

Skull Depressions

Depressions of the skull may represent fractures but are most commonly **sutures** (i.e., membranous tissue spaces that separate the skull bones) and **fontanelles** (i.e., areas where the major sutures intersect; also known as "soft spots"). The cranial sutures usually overlap in the newborn because of intrauterine pressure. Sutures that are widely palpable after 5 to 6 months of age may indicate hydrocephalus.

D.

Birth to 36 months: Boys
Length-for-age and Weight-for-age percentiles

NAME _____

RECORD # _____

Published May 30, 2000 (modified 4/20/01).
SOURCE: Developed by the National Center for Health Statistics in collaboration with
the National Center for Chronic Disease Prevention and Health Promotion (2000).
http://www.cdc.gov/growthcharts

Figure 2-1 ■ (*Continued*)

The anterior fontanelle is 4 to 6 centimeters in diameter at birth and usually closes between the ages of 4 and 26 months. The posterior fontanelle is usually 0 to 2 centimeters at birth and generally closes by 2 months of age. When describing fontanelles, mention their status (open or closed), size, and fullness. If palpated while the baby is sitting, a tense

E.

Figure 2-1 ▪ (*Continued*)

or elevated fontanelle may reflect increased intracranial pressure. A depressed fontanelle can be a sign of dehydration.

> **HINT:** At birth, the anterior fontanelle may appear closed as a result of overriding sutures from molding of the head during parturition.

F.

2 to 20 years: Boys
Body mass index-for-age percentiles

NAME _____

RECORD # _____

*To Calculate BMI: Weight (kg) ÷ Stature (cm) ÷ Stature (cm) x 10,000
or Weight (lb) ÷ Stature (in) ÷ Stature (in) x 703

Published May 30, 2000 (modified 10/16/00).
SOURCE: Developed by the National Center for Health Statistics in collaboration with
the National Center for Chronic Disease Prevention and Health Promotion (2000).
http://www.cdc.gov/growthcharts

Figure 2-1 ■ (*Continued*)

> **HINT:** Try to examine the anterior fontanelle with the child calm and sitting upright.

Head Shape

Observe the shape of the child's head. Areas of **flatness,** especially in the occipital or parietal regions, may be caused by lying too long in one

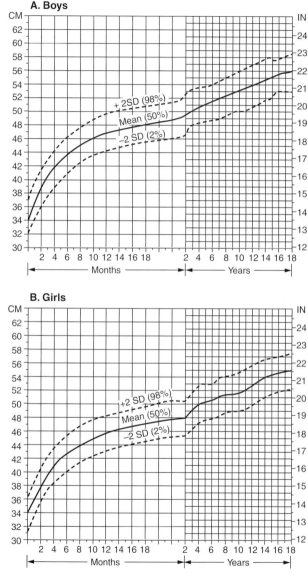

Figure 2-2 ■ Head circumferences in boys (A) and girls (B).
CM = centimeters; IN = inches; SD = standard deviations.
(Redrawn with permission from Horan MJ, Nelhaus G: Head circumference from birth to eighteen years. Pediatrics 79:1–25, 1987.)

position and may occur in an infant suffering from neglect, prematurity, or mental retardation. **Frontal bossing** may be a sign of rickets. Areas of **localized head swelling** could be caused by neoplastic, infectious, or traumatic processes.

Newborns often have **caput succedaneum** (a soft swelling of the occipitoparietal scalp) caused by injury during birth. **Cephalohematoma**, another birth injury, is a swelling caused by subperiosteal hemorrhage involving one of the cranial bones. In cephalohematoma, the swelling does not cross the suture lines as it does in caput succedaneum.

Percussion and Auscultation of the Head

Percussion of the head may reveal **Macewen sign** (a resonant sound in children with closed fontanelles that indicates increased intracranial pressure [ICP] or **Chvostek sign** (contraction of the facial muscles in response to percussion just below the zygomatic [cheek] bone). Chvostek sign can be found in normal newborns as well as in children with hypocalcemic tetany. Percussion over the parietal bone may produce a **"cracked-pot sound,"** a normal finding prior to suture closure.

Auscultation of the head for **bruits** is not particularly useful until late childhood. Systolic or continuous bruits may be heard in the temporal area until age 5. Abnormal conditions that may be associated with bruits include arteriovenous malformation (AVM), cerebral vessel aneurysms, brain tumors, and coarctation of the aorta.

Inspection of the Hair and Scalp

The child's hair should be assessed for quantity, color, texture, and infestations. Causes of **alopecia** include fungal infections (tinea capitis), stress (telogen effluvium), and excessive hair pulling (trichotillomania). **Dry, coarse hair** may be a sign of hypothyroidism, and **fine, thin hair** may be seen in children with homocystinuria. In children with **pediculosis capitis** (head lice), close inspection reveals small adherent nits (eggs).

EYES

The eye examination is very important, providing information about the eyes and, in many cases, systemic problems. It is usually counterproductive (not to mention unkind) to try to pry a child's eye open. Instead, **distract the patient** with a toy or other object whenever possible to gain cooperation. A recalcitrant newborn can be encouraged to open his eyes by having an assistant gently rotate the baby from side to side while supporting him vertically (i.e., under the arms).

Assessment of the Eyes

Range of Motion and Orientation

Check for full range of motion by attracting the child's attention with a toy or piece of equipment. **Strabismus** (a condition in which the eyes do not move in a parallel manner) can manifest as **esotropia** (turning in of an eye) or **exotropia** (turning out of an eye). The following tests can be used to test for strabismus:

- **Corneal light reflection**. Have the child focus on a small light. When the child is looking at the light, the reflection of the light from each cornea should be symmetrically placed. Asymmetries suggest the presence of strabismus.
- **Cover–uncover test**. The child focuses on a light, and one eye is covered and then uncovered. If either eye moves, strabismus may be present.

> **HINT:** Intermittent esotropia or exotropia in a young infant may be normal, but deviations beyond 6 months of age can cause permanent vision loss.

Distance Between the Eyes

Observe the distance between the eyes, which can be documented as either the inner canthal distance or the interpupillary distance. **Hypotelorism** (abnormal closeness of eyes) is frequently found with holoprosencephaly sequence, maternal phenylketonuria, trisomy 13, and trisomy 20p. **Hypertelorism** (increased distance between the eyes) is frequently associated with a wide number of syndromes, including Apert syndrome, DiGeorge sequence, fetal hydantoin effects, Noonan syndrome, trisomies 8 and 9p, and absence of the corpus callosum.

Nystagmus and "Setting Sun" Sign

Observe for nystagmus (rhythmical movements of the eyeballs) and "setting sun" sign (in which the eyes constantly appear to be looking downward). Nystagmus may be physiologic or it may be found with early loss of central vision, labyrinthitis, multiple sclerosis (MS), intracranial tumors, or drug toxicity. "Setting sun" sign may be seen with hydrocephalus or intracranial tumor, but it also may be transiently noted in some healthy infants.

General Appearance

Check for an abnormal upward, outward **eye slant** and for **epicanthal folds** (vertical folds of skin over the medial portions of the eyes). Both can be associated with Down syndrome.

Assessment of the Individual Eyes

Visual Inspection

The following should be noted:

- Pupil size and reaction to light—both direct and consensual
- Condition of the eyelids—potential abnormalities include edema (swelling), erythema (redness), drooping, or the presence of masses
- Hazy corneas—causes include glaucoma and inborn errors of metabolism
- Injected or inflamed conjunctivae
- Icteric sclerae

> **HINT:** A jaundiced child has icteric sclerae, but a child with carotenemia (e.g., from too much enthusiasm for carrots or sweet potatoes) has clear sclerae.

- Brushfield spots on the irises—small white spots frequently associated with Down syndrome
- Excess tearing—often caused by congenital obstruction of the nasolacrimal duct

Funduscopic Examination

In infants, a minimal funduscopic evaluation consists of evaluation of the **red reflex:** the ophthalmoscope is set at 0 diopters. At a distance of approximately 1 foot away from the patient, a reddish orange color (generally brightest in Caucasians) should be visible through the pupil. Leukocoria, a **white pupillary reflex,** can indicate serious disease, including cataracts, retinal detachment, or retinoblastoma. Inflammation or opacity of the **cornea** should be noted. Finally, if possible, the **optic disc and vessels** should be examined, ruling out fundal lesions and papilledema.

Vision Screening

The infant's vision should be screened using a brightly colored object. Note the infant's response and ability to track an object. Formal vision testing (often using the Snellen E Chart) can usually start at about 3 years of age (see Chapter 3, "Developmental Surveillance").

> **HINT:** Normal newborns typically have about 20/400 vision, improving to about 20/100 by 6 months of age.

HINT: Newborns often do not produce visible tears in the first few days of life.

EARS

External Examination

Rashes that favor the postauricular area include seborrheic dermatitis, measles, and rubella. **Pain** on gentle traction of the pinna or tragus can signal external otitis.

Otoscopic Examination

Before examining the tympanic membrane, ensure that any uncooperative child is **well restrained.** One simple method is to have the parent firmly hold the supine child's raised arms against either side of the head. This also allows easy access for the oral examination that follows.

 HINT: In an uncooperative child, press your otoscope hand against the patient's face. If the child suddenly moves despite proper restraint, the otoscope will move in tandem, decreasing the likelihood of injury.

It is also critical to **position the child's ear properly.** For an infant, pull the pinna down and back. For a school-age child, pull straight back. For an adolescent, pull up and back.

- Check the tympanic membrane for **continuity.** Is it intact or perforated? Are there myringotomy tubes in place?
- Note the **color** and **degree of lucency.** Redness can indicate inflammation or merely be caused by a child's crying. A dull, purulent appearance indicates infection.
- Observe for **bulging** of the tympanic membrane, which suggests the presence of pus and fluid in the middle ear.
- Check for **visibility** of the bony landmarks and the cone of light reflex (which is absent with inflammation).
- Assess **mobility,** using a squeeze bulb. Poor movement can indicate the presence of fluid or purulent material in the middle ear.

Determining Hearing Acuity

Determining hearing acuity clinically is difficult in babies and young children. Watch the child's face as you make noise with a rattle or rustle paper behind each ear. Check to see if the child is **startled** by the sound (usually by age 1 month) or **looks toward the source** of the sound (by about age 5 months).

 HINT: One helpful approach to determining hearing acuity in infants and young children is simply to ask the parents.

NOSE

Check the **nasal mucosae.** Pale, boggy mucosae with a watery discharge suggest allergy, whereas hyperemic mucosae with a mucopurulent discharge suggest infection. Be alert for the possibility of nasal **foreign bodies,** which often present with a unilateral, malodorous rhinorrhea. Examine the **nasal septum** for deviation, ulcerations, perforation, or bleeding. Check the **nasal turbinates** for bogginess or polyps.

HINT: A newborn that is cyanotic when calm but pink when crying may have pulmonary disease with collapsed alveoli. Another possible diagnosis is choanal atresia (a congenital failure to develop openings between the nose and the nasopharynx).

ORAL CAVITY

Lips and Buccal Mucosa

Examine the lips for **asymmetry, fissures, clefts, lesions,** and **color.** Gray or purple lips may reflect cyanosis. Vigorous sucking can produce a callus on the lips. Small vesicles on an erythematous base can indicate herpes simplex infection.

Assess the buccal mucosae for **moistness,** and check for **lesions.** For example, tiny blue-white dots on an erythematous base may be Koplik spots, an early sign of measles. Small white adherent plaques may be oral thrush (*Candida* infection). Note any **strange odors** to the breath (e.g., sweet [acetone], ammoniac [uremia]).

Tongue

Examine the tongue, checking for color, size, coating, and dryness. A bluish color to the tongue indicates central cyanosis, which reflects the presence of unsaturated hemoglobin. A **"strawberry" tongue** (characterized by large red papillae) may be seen with scarlet fever or Kawasaki disease.

Teeth and Oropharynx

Examine the **teeth** for number and condition. Observe the **tonsils** for color or exudate. Check the **palate** for a high arch, cleft, or mucosal lesions. The palates of newborns often have small whitish epithelial masses known as Epstein pearls. Examine the **posterior pharynx** for exudate, vesicles, or bifid uvula.

NECK

Torticollis

Check for torticollis (fixed position of the head to one side), which may be **congenital** or **acquired.** Congenital torticollis may be caused by injury to the sternomastoid muscle. Acquired torticollis has many causes, including cervical spine disease, gastroesophageal reflux disease (GRD), posterior fossa or brainstem tumors, and infections within the head or neck.

Range of Motion

Have the child touch the chin to the chest (to test the inferior cervical spine), look up and move the head side to side (to test the atlantoaxial joint), and bend the neck laterally ear to shoulder (to test the lower cervical spine). Always examine ill children for the presence of nuchal rigidity, which can signal the possibility of meningitis. To help rule out **nuchal rigidity** in a young child, encourage him to look up and down by shining a bright light or shaking noisy objects (e.g., keys).

> **HINT:** Children <2 years do not consistently develop nuchal rigidity with meningitis.

Palpation, Auscultation, and Visual Inspection of the Neck

Palpate the **thyroid gland,** evaluating both lobes for swelling, symmetry, consistency, and surface characteristics (e.g., smooth versus nodular).

> **HINT:** Lymph nodes are relatively more prominent in children than in adults. Shotty cervical (as well as axillary and femoral) lymph nodes (up to 1 cm in diameter) are normal in children <10 years.

Auscultation may reveal a bruit, suggestive of thyrotoxicosis.

Examine the **neck** for other swellings or defects, including dermoid cysts, branchial cysts, and thyroglossal duct cysts. A thyroglossal duct cyst arises from a remnant of the embryonic thyroglossal duct. It is usually located in the midline, anywhere between the tongue and hyoid bone. It should move up when the patient sticks out her tongue or swallows.

NEUROLOGIC SYSTEM

Assessment of Developmental Milestones

Assessment of a young child's developmental milestones is critical to the overall neurologic examination. Therefore, a **screening developmental examination,** such as the Denver II (see Chapter 3, "Developmental Surveillance," Figure 3-1), should be a part of every well-child neurologic assessment.

Assessment of Reflexes

Table 2-2 describes the examination of the infantile reflexes.

Test **deep tendon reflexes** using your finger, a reflex hammer, or the side of a stethoscope bell. Check for ankle or knee clonus (quick, repetitive muscle contractions). Bilateral clonus may be normal in an infant but can also reflect exaggerated muscle tone and deep tendon reflexes.

Assessment of Cranial Nerve Function

Table 2-3 describes the examination of the cranial nerves.

TABLE 2-2 Infantile Reflexes			
Reflex	Usual Infant Age	Method of Elicitation	Description of Reflex
Moro (startle) reflex	Birth to 4–6 months	Lift the baby's head 15°, and then let it fall gently into your hands	Arms suddenly extend then flex; various movements of legs
Asymmetric tonic neck reflex	Birth to 4 months	Place the baby supine, head turned to one side	Isolateral arm and leg extend; contralateral arm contracts, like a fencer
Babinski reflex	Birth to 18 months	Stroke the dorsum of the baby's foot	Toe dorsiflexion, fanning
Palmar grasp reflex	Birth to 4 months	Place finger on the baby's palm	Involuntary grasping motion
Rooting reflex	Birth to 4 months	Touch corner of the baby's mouth	Head turns to side, baby opens mouth
Parachute reflex	6–7 months	Hold baby prone, move carefully downward	Extension of arms (to break fall)

TABLE 2-3 Examination of the Cranial Nerves

Cranial Nerve	Function	Elicitation Technique	Potential Abnormalities
I: Olfactory nerve	Smell	Cannot assess until child can speak	Absent responses
II: Optic nerve	Vision	In newborns, note response to objects brought from behind (peripheral vision) and ability to track objects in front (central vision) Children ≥4 years can undergo formal vision testing	Deviation from typical visual acuity (newborn = 20/400, improving to about 20/100 by age 6 months)
III: Oculomotor nerve	Elevation of upper eyelid, upward and downward gaze	Observe ocular movements and pupillary reflexes	Ptosis, pupil dilation, nystagmus
IV: Trochlear nerve	Upward gaze		
V: Trigeminal nerve	Chewing, sensation on face, forehead, lips, and tongue	Evaluate corneal reflexes; check facial sensation with a piece of gauze	Absent responses
VI: Abducens nerve	Lateral gaze		
VII: Facial nerve	Facial muscle control (eyelid closure, forehead wrinkling, asymmetry of face), taste (anterior two thirds of tongue)	Check for facial symmetry at rest and when the child is smiling or crying	Asymmetry
VIII: Vestibulocochlear nerve	Hearing	In newborns, check for acoustic blink (in response to a loud noise); by age 4 months, baby should turn to sound	Absent responses
IX: Glossopharyngeal nerve	Taste (posterior two thirds of tongue), elevation of palate, sensory gag reflex	Observe ability to handle secretions or beverages	Difficulty swallowing
X: Vagus nerve	Swallowing, movement of pharynx		
XI: Accessory nerve	Turning head, shrugging shoulders	Assess the child's posture	Head tilt or shoulder drop
XII: Hypoglossal nerve	Protrusion of tongue	Ask cooperative child to stick out her tongue	Fasciculations or deviations from midline (tongue moves to side of lesion)

23

Sensory Examination

Assess an infant's general sensation by checking for a response to light touch.

Assessment of Coordination

Assess the child's coordination as he reaches for a toy, crawls, or walks. Check for unusual muscle movements:

- **Fasciculations**—twitchings of groups of muscle fibers
- **Tremors**—trembling movements of the extremities
- **Chorea**—irregular, spastic, involuntary movements
- **Athetosis**—constant, slow, writhing movements, sometimes found in normal infants and in children with cerebral palsy (CP) and tuberous sclerosis
- **Spasmus nutans**—periodic head nodding, sometimes associated with GRD, decreased intelligence quotient (IQ), or neuroblastoma, and often combined with nystagmus and head tilt

> **HINT:** The most critical part of the routine neurologic examination is your impression of the child's developmental abilities and general responsiveness. A reluctant toddler will often walk if her parent moves several steps away from her and offers encouragement. Entice the child to play with an interesting toy or object.

CHEST AND LUNGS

Shape of the Chest

A **barrel-shaped chest** in a child >6 years can be associated with acute asthma or a chronic pulmonary disease such as cystic fibrosis. **Pectus excavatum** (a funnel-shaped chest) is caused by a congenitally depressed sternum and costal cartilages. **Pectus carinatum** ("pigeon chest") is characterized by protrusion of the sternum and costal cartilages. Although this is often an idiopathic problem that is not associated with actual medical difficulties, pectus carinatum is sometimes caused by rickets or osteoporosis.

Assessment of Breathing

Check carefully for signs of **respiratory distress,** including nasal flaring, retractions, or grunting. Nasal flaring refers to a widening of the nostrils, which often occurs with each inspiration in respiratory distress. Retractions are movements of the spaces between the ribs, occurring with each breath in a child with respiratory distress. Grunting is an end-expiratory sound, most often heard in the newborn or infant with respiratory distress.

Percussion of the Lungs

Hyperresonance is usually caused by an increased amount of air in the chest (e.g., as in patients with asthma). Dullness is normally heard over the scapulae, liver, heart, and diaphragm.

Auscultation of the Lungs

In an infant, press the diaphragm of a small stethoscope firmly to the chest wall. Position the head in the midline, facing forward. Do not be reluctant to examine the lungs of a crying baby. Inspiratory sounds are actually enhanced by the deep inspiration.

> **HINT:** Warm your stethoscope before auscultation.
>
>

Breath Sounds and Air Movement

Listen carefully for breath sounds, **comparing air movement** in the two lungs. Decreased breath sounds suggest decreased air exchange. It is important to evaluate air movement because a patient with severe asthma can have such overwhelming obstruction that no wheezing is heard. The patient with severe asthma but no wheezing may be in impending respiratory failure!

> **HINT:** Breath sounds tend to be harsher sounding (more bronchial) in children (as compared with adults) because the thinner chest wall of the child does not muffle the breath sounds as much.

Chest Sounds

Identify adventitious chest sounds:

- **Rales** are fine crackles, usually heard best at the end of inspiration, that generally reflect the presence of fluid or exudate in the alveoli. In patients with rales, consider bronchopneumonia, atelectasis, and congestive heart failure.
- **Rhonchi** are coarse inspiratory and expiratory sounds, caused by secretions in the upper airway. They are often caused by crying or upper respiratory infection.
- **Wheezes** are palpable and audible vibrations, often musical in character, produced when airflow is restricted. Expiratory wheezes are most common and typically reflect lower airway obstruction. Wheezes are most commonly found with asthma and bronchiolitis. Other causes include congestive heart failure and foreign body aspiration.

Extraneous Sounds

- **Peristalsis,** if heard in the pulmonary examination, can suggest a diagnosis of diaphragmatic hernia (an abnormal opening of the diaphragm that allows the protrusion of abdominal contents into the chest).
- **A pleural friction rub** (a coarse grating sound with each breath) is occasionally present with pneumonia, lung abscess, or tuberculosis.

> **HINT:** Young children cannot cooperate as well as older children with a lung examination. Therefore, auscultation is not as reliable as in an older child, and a chest radiograph should be ordered more readily.

CIRCULATORY SYSTEM

Many general physical examination clues can signal a child with cardiac disease. Typical observations include poor growth (weight affected more than length), developmental delay, cyanosis, clubbing of the fingers or toes, tachypnea, tachycardia, and peripheral edema. Routinely compare right-arm pulse strength with femoral pulse strength, which can be decreased in patients with coarctation of the aorta.

When examining the heart, first observe for **chest deformities** and **cardiac pulsations.** Palpate for the **point of maximum impulse (PMI).** In children <7 years, the heart's general horizontal position usually results in a PMI in the fourth intercostal space, to the left of the midclavicular line. In children >7 years, the PMI is usually in the fifth to sixth intercostal space within the midclavicular line. A PMI displaced down or lateral to these sites can indicate congestive heart failure.

The PMI may feel prominent in a thin child, in a child who has just finished exercising, or in a child who is anxious, febrile, in impending heart failure, or hyperthyroid. It is decreased in patients with pericardial or pleural effusions or pneumomediastinum (presence of gas or air in the mediastinal tissues). Thrills and pericardial friction rubs manifest as fine or coarse vibrations.

Listen with the child in both the **supine** and **sitting positions.** Listen over the whole precordium, especially at the apex, the pulmonic area (second interspace, left of the sternum), the aortic area (second interspace, right of the sternum), and the tricuspid valve (fourth interspace over the sternum). Listen for a split second heart sound (S_2), heard best over the pulmonic area during inspiration. (This finding is more obvious in school-age children than in adults. It is usually only a potential problem if there is a large fixed split, such as that found with atrial septal defect [ASD].)

- **Are the heart sounds clear?** Distant sounds can suggest pericardial fluid.

- Is there a third heart sound (S_3)? (Usually heard at the apex, an S_3 may indicate mitral valve prolapse or ASD.)
- Is there a gallop rhythm and other physical signs consistent with congestive heart failure?

Rhythms

Sinus arrhythmia refers to the normal variation in pulse rate found with respiration. It is particularly prominent in young teenagers. Pulse rate increases with inspiration and decreases with expiration. **Premature ventricular contractions** are fairly common in the pediatric population. Generally, they should number less than six per minute at rest and decrease with exertion.

Murmurs

Description

Murmurs are described as follows:

- **Loudness**—reported as grade I to grade VI
- **Timing in the cardiac cycle**—described as diastolic or systolic, early or late
- **Pitch**—high or low
- **Quality**—blowing, musical, or rough
- **Location**—for example, apex, left lower sternal border
- **Transmission across the chest**—for example, radiating to the right lower sternal border

Innocent Murmurs

Nonpathologic murmurs typically heard in childhood include Still murmur and venous hum. **Still murmur** is the most common murmur in children between the ages of 2 years and adolescence. It is typically described as musical or vibratory, short, high pitched, early systolic, and grade I to III. It is usually heard best in the apical region. A **venous hum** is a continuous, low-pitched murmur heard under the clavicle and in the neck. It is caused by blood draining down the jugular vein. See Chapter 53, "Murmurs."

> **HINT:** The most important first step in assessing a murmur is to distinguish innocent from pathologic. Innocent murmurs are typically grade III or less, systolic in timing, and with no accompanying signs of cardiovascular disease.

ABDOMEN

A successful abdominal examination is especially reliant on having the **patient relaxed**. Position the patient in a supine position, with her knees bent and her arms at her sides. Warm your stethoscope and hands and then allow your hand to rest quietly for a moment on the patient's abdomen before making initial probing movements. To reduce ticklishness, place the child's hand on yours. Talking with the child about her siblings, friends, or school can be a useful distraction. It can also be helpful to allow children to examine your stethoscope while you examine them.

Abdominal Contour

Examine the abdominal contour. Is the abdomen flat, protuberant (common in toddlers), scaphoid (depressed, sometimes found with diaphragmatic hernia), or distended? Check for diastasis recti (vertical separation of the rectus abdominis muscles).

Abdominal Wall Motion

Respirations are generally abdominal in children <6 to 7 years. In young children, absence of abdominal wall motion may be caused by peritonitis, diaphragmatic paralysis, or large amounts of fluid or air in the abdomen. In older children, respirations that are mostly abdominal can indicate pneumonia or other pulmonary disorders.

Auscultation

Auscultation of the abdomen should be done **before palpation** to avoid altering the sounds of peristalsis. **Normal sounds** are short and metallic, occurring every 10 to 30 seconds. **Excessively frequent and high-pitched sounds** can indicate early peritonitis, gastroenteritis, or intestinal obstruction. **Absence of sounds** for >3 minutes can occur with paralytic ileus or peritonitis. Vascular obstruction may be indicated by a murmur over the aorta or renal arteries. It is especially important to check for vascular obstructions in any child with hypertension.

Percussion

Percussion can be useful to assess the liver (and occasionally the spleen) and to identify ascites, abdominal masses, or air in the gastrointestinal tract. Babies often have more swallowed air in their gastrointestinal tracts than adults do.

Percuss lightly in all **four quadrants** to assess general distribution of tympany and dullness. Tympany is generally the predominant sound. A distended abdomen with little tympany may contain fluid or solid masses. Dullness is typically found over the liver, over a full urinary bladder, or over masses.

To determine **liver span,** percuss the upper and lower borders in the right midclavicular line, and measure the vertical distance. Normal spans are approximately 2 centimeters at 6 months, 4 centimeters at

3 years, 6 centimeters at 10 years, and 8 centimeters in adults. Causes of hepatomegaly include passive congestion, hepatitis, and tumor.

Palpation

> **HINT:** For crying children, palpate immediately on inspiration. The child often will relax his abdominal musculature for a moment.

Abdomen

Palpation of the abdomen is best done **on inspiration and on deep expiration.** Place one hand on the patient's back and the other on the abdomen. First palpate lightly, then deeply. Start in the left lower quadrant and continue in a clockwise manner. If any area seems tender, palpate that area last.

Rigidity (a tense abdomen) can indicate a surgical condition but is sometimes caused by voluntary muscle tightening in a frightened child.

Check for **tenderness,** trying to localize the point of maximum pain. The location of the tenderness can offer clues regarding the cause (Table 2-4). Rebound tenderness is associated with peritoneal inflammation.

> **HINT:** When checking for abdominal tenderness, ask a young child, "Does this feel OK?" Toddlers and preschoolers will often nod yes indiscriminately when asked if something hurts. Facial expression is the most reliable sign of true tenderness.

Spleen

The spleen is often normally palpated in the first few years of life. It can be enlarged with infection (especially infectious mononucleosis),

TABLE 2-4 Suggested Causes of Abdominal Tenderness According to Location

Location of Abdominal Tenderness	Possible Causes
Right upper quadrant	Acute hepatomegaly, hepatitis, intussusception
Left upper quadrant	Intussusception, splenic enlargement or rupture
Midline upper abdomen	Gastroenteritis, gastric or duodenal ulcer
Right lower quadrant	Appendicitis, abscess
Left lower quadrant	Constipation
Midline suprapubic area	Cystitis
Lower abdomen in general	Gastroenteritis, tumor, Meckel diverticulum, ovarian or testicular torsion
Poorly localized	Pneumonia, mesenteric adenitis, peritonitis, sickle cell crisis

sickle cell or other hemolytic anemias, or leukemia. See Chapter 73, "Splenomegaly."

Liver

The liver generally can be palpated 1 to 2 centimeters below the right costal margin. Its edge is usually sharp and soft. A pathologically enlarged liver usually extends >2 centimeters below the right costal margin and has a rounded, firm edge. See Chapter 42, "Hepatomegaly."

Kidneys

In newborns, the kidneys can be gently trapped between the examiner's hands, allowing examination for masses. In all children, percussing gently over the costovertebral angles bilaterally can reveal tenderness over the kidneys.

GENITALIA

In infants, first assess the genitals for **ambiguity.** Is the baby "boy" really a virilized female with clitoromegaly and fused labial folds? Is the baby "girl" a male with a micropenis?

When examining children and teenagers, always respect the **patient's modesty.** Provide a gown and be sure to have a chaperone present.

Boys

- **Examine the glans penis and locate the meatus.** Is it ventrally displaced (hypospadias) or dorsally displaced (epispadias)? Observe for inflammation of the glans penis (balanitis) or of the prepuce (posthitis). Is there a penile discharge?
- **Note whether the child has been circumcised.** In an uncircumcised boy, is there phimosis (i.e., an inability to retract the foreskin)? Normally the foreskin is not retractable until age 2 years.
- **Observe for scrotal masses.** Hydrocele is caused by an accumulation of fluid in the tunica vaginalis. You may demonstrate the fluid by shining a light to the scrotum. (Unlike inguinal hernias, hydroceles do not reduce.) Palpate for the testicles and note their location. In determining the presence of a retractile testis, it is helpful to have the boy sit cross-legged; the testes can then be "milked down" from the inguinal canal. Check for testicular masses.

Table 2-5 describes the Tanner staging of penis, testes, scrotum, and pubic hair development.

Girls

- **Observe the labia majora and minora.** Are the labia minora fused? Is the fusion complete? (Sometimes a thin membrane can be gently opened with a cotton swab.)

Tanner Stage	Penis	Testes	Scrotum	Pubic Hair
TABLE 2-5 Tanner Staging of the Penis, Testes, Scrotum, and Pubic Hair				
1	Immature	Small	Immature	None present
2	Immature	Initial enlargement	Initial rugae, reddening	Small amount near penile base
3	Initial enlargement	Continued enlargement	Increased rugae, reddening	Increased amount, distribution, coarseness, curl
4	Continued enlargement	Continued enlargement	Increased rugae, reddening	Increasing as above
5	Full adult	Full adult	Full adult	Adult amount and distribution (pubic area and medial thighs)

TABLE 2-6 Tanner Staging of Female Breasts

Tanner Stage	Breast	Areola
1	Prepubertal	Prepubertal
2	Small breast bud	Beginning enlargement
3	Continued development	Developing, continuous with breast
4	Continued development	Projection separate from breast
5	Full adult breasts	Flattened areola and protruding nipple

- **Check for enlargement of the clitoris.** Examine the introitus (vaginal opening) for size, discharge, excoriation, or scarring. Pseudomenstruation (i.e., a usually minimal, bloody vaginal discharge caused by placental transfer of maternal hormones) may be noted in newborn girls. Infections, bleeding, or bruising may be an indication of sexual abuse. Is the hymen intact? Lack of a hymen does not necessarily imply sexual contact; participation in active games and sports can also rupture it.
- A **pelvic examination** is usually performed on sexually active teenagers or if a specific problem is suspected. In adolescent girls, the possibility of pregnancy should always be considered, even if the patient denies sexual experience.

Tanner staging of pubic hair in females is the same as in males (Table 2-5). Table 2-6 describes the Tanner staging of breasts.

RECTUM AND ANUS

Rule out fissures or anal prolapse. Check newborns for anal patency. A digital rectal examination is usually only performed if there are abdominal or rectal symptoms, a pelvic mass, or malformation. Check for sphincter tone, masses, and tenderness.

SKIN

- First, assess overall **skin color.** General erythema can reflect fever, sun exposure, or atropine toxicity. Pallor may be found in children with shock, anemia, or poor local circulation. Peripheral cyanosis (evidenced by bluish discoloration of the nail beds) can be caused by cold stress, local venous obstruction, or shock.

HINT: In normal newborns, it is common for the hands and feet to be cyanotic, especially when they have been exposed to cold surroundings.

- Check for **skin pigmentation** (areas of generalized or localized color change). Hypopigmented lesions can be caused by tinea versicolor, vitiligo, tuberous sclerosis, or albinism. Bluish black lesions, especially over the lower back and buttocks in infants, are often Mongolian spots.
- **Vascular nevi** are commonly found in infants and children. Nevus flammeus lesions occur as flat, irregular pink patches. Strawberry hemangiomas are typically soft, compressible lesions. Port wine stains are flat markings embedded in the skin.
- **Burns** are classified as first degree (erythema only), second degree (erythema plus blister formation), and third degree (involving the subcutaneous tissue).
- **Skin puffiness** from edema (excess extracellular water and sodium) may be associated with renal, cardiac, or hepatic disease.

MUSCULOSKELETAL SYSTEM

Gross Deformities and Congenital Anomalies

Deformities are most commonly caused by **fractures** but can also be **congenital** (e.g., polydactyly [extra fingers or toes] or syndactyly [webbed or fused digits]).

> **HINT:** In evaluating injuries, consider child abuse if the damage is worse than accounted for by the history, if the child has multiple bruises, if there is a mixture of old and new injuries, or if there is a delay in seeking medical care.

Fingers and Toes

Observe the fingers and toes for **clubbing** (broadening and thickening of the terminal phalanges). Clubbing can be associated with many different systemic diseases, including congenital heart disease, pulmonary disease (e.g., cystic fibrosis), chronic hepatic disease, and gastrointestinal disorders (e.g., Crohn disease, ulcerative colitis).

Legs

Examine the shape of the leg bones:

- **Genu varum (bowleggedness)** develops routinely in infants until about 18 months of age. Severe genu varum may be an indication of rickets or Blount disease (a growth disorder of the tibia).
- **Genu valgum (knock-knees)** is most often seen in children >2 years and often persists until adolescence.

- **Tibial torsion** is a twisting of the tibia thought to be caused by uterine pressure on the developing fetus. It often resolves spontaneously once the child begins walking.

Feet

In metatarsus adductus (inversion of the forefoot), the lateral border of the foot is "C" shaped instead of straight. The most serious congenital foot deformity is **clubfoot** (talipes equinovarus). This condition involves three major abnormalities: metatarsus adductus, fixed foot inversion, and equinus (or downward positioning of the foot).

> **HINT:** It is important to distinguish *rigid deformities,* which are more serious, from *flexible deformities.* With a flexible deformity, the foot can be brought to a normal position with gentle pressure.

Gait and Stance

Infants starting to walk typically have a wide-based gait that persists until approximately age 2 years.

- **Joints.** The joints should be examined for range of motion, warmth, redness, tenderness, and presence of effusion. In infants <6 months, always check for congenital hip dislocation using the Ortolani maneuver (Figure 2-3). Other useful signs of congenital hip dislocation are unequal leg length and asymmetric thigh skin folds.
- **Muscles.** Examine the muscles for tone by grasping the muscle and estimating its firmness during passive range of motion. Assess muscle strength, observing for weakness or paralysis. Look for contractures (fixed deformities that often have accompanying muscle atrophy). Check muscle mass, observing for atrophy or hypertrophy.
- **Spine.** Inspect the spine, observing for tufts of hair, dimples, abnormal coloration, masses, or cysts. Any of these can indicate spina bifida (a limited defect in the spinal column through which spinal membranes and spinal cord tissue may protrude). A small dimple anywhere in the midline can indicate a dermoid sinus (an epidermis-lined tract leading from the skin to the spinal cord that presents a risk of central nervous system [CNS] infection). Check for spinal masses, including meningoceles, teratomas, or lipomas.
- **Posture.** Observe the child's posture, checking for abnormal spinal curvatures. In lumbar lordosis, the curve is anteroposterior, with the convexity anterior. Lumbar lordosis is usually normal for children but if severe can be a sign of rickets or abdominal wall weakness. In kyphosis, the anteroposterior curve of the spine has a posterior convexity. Scoliosis refers to a lateral curvature of the spine. All school-age children

Figure 2-3 ▪ Ortolani maneuver to check for dislocated hip.
With your index finger over the greater trochanter and your thumb over
the inner thigh, flex the hip 90° and slowly abduct it from the midline.
Feel for an abnormal "clunk" as a dislocated femoral head slips into the
acetabulum.

and adolescents should be examined for scoliosis. Have the child bend forward, and look for unilateral elevation of the rib cage and hip.

> **HINT:** The posture of the newborn often reflects the newborn's intrauterine position. For example, babies born breech often have very flexed hips and extended knees.

Suggested Readings

Barness LA: *Manual of Pediatric Physical Diagnosis*, 6th ed. St. Louis, Mosby, 1991.

Jones KL (ed): *Smith's Recognizable Patterns of Human Malformation*, 6th ed. Philadelphia, Saunders, 2005.

Zitelli BJ, Davis HW (eds): *Atlas of Pediatric Physical Diagnosis*, 5th ed. Philadelphia, Elsevier, 2007.

Developmental Surveillance

Patty Huang and Nathan J. Blum

Primary care physicians play a vital role in identifying children at risk for developmental disabilities and in referring them for appropriate early intervention services. Developmental surveillance involves using information obtained from the history, physical examination, and developmental screening tests to assess development on an ongoing basis. This ongoing monitoring of development is critical for two reasons. First, **new circumstances** (e.g., medical illness, family or environmental disruption, injuries) may interfere with development. Second, as children develop, they gain **new categories of skills** that are difficult to assess at earlier points (e.g., one cannot usually detect isolated language delays in children younger than 18 to 24 months, the point at which children begin to develop a good repertoire of language skills). In 2006, the American Academy of Pediatrics published guidelines recommending developmental surveillance at every well-child visit, as well as additional periodic developmental screening using a standardized test at the 9-, 18-, and 30-month-old visits.

HISTORY

The following information should be elicited:

- **Parental concerns regarding the child's development.** In most cases, parental concerns regarding the child's language development, articulation, fine motor skills, or global development are likely to be associated with true developmental delays. Parental concerns about behavior or personal-social skills are associated with developmental delays in some cases.
- **Risk factors for developmental disabilities** (Table 3-1).
- **Attainment of developmental milestones** (Table 3-2).

PHYSICAL EXAMINATION

Head Circumference

Brain growth is the principal stimulus for increasing head circumference. Therefore, a small head circumference may indicate abnormalities in brain growth that place a child at risk for developmental disabilities. A large head circumference may be a sign of hydrocephalus, a genetic syndrome, or a metabolic storage disease (see Chapter 51, "Macrocephaly"). However, before assuming pathology in a child, one should measure the parents' head sizes because a small or large head circumference may be a family trait.

TABLE 3-1 Risk Factors for Developmental Disabilities
Prenatal
Maternal illness, infection, or malnutrition Maternal exposure to toxins, teratogens, alcohol, illicit drugs, anticonvulsants, antineoplastics, or anticoagulants Decreased fetal movements Intrauterine growth retardation Family history of deafness, blindness, or mental retardation Chromosomal abnormalities
Perinatal
Asphyxia: Apgar scores of 0–3 at 5 min Prematurity, low birthweight Abnormal presentation
Postnatal
Meningitis, encephalitis Seizure disorder Hyperbilirubinemia: bilirubin >25 mg/dL in full-term infant Severe chronic illness Central nervous system trauma Child abuse and neglect

> **HINT:** Microcephaly is defined as a head circumference <3rd percentile; macrocephaly is defined as a head circumference >97th percentile.

Congenital Anomalies or Dysmorphic Features

Congenital anomalies or dysmorphic features are associated with many genetic syndromes that may cause mental retardation or learning disabilities. Although a karyotype is a good initial screen, syndromes associated with small deletions (e.g., Williams syndrome, Prader-Willi syndrome, velocardiofacial syndrome) are not detected by a routine karyotype. Detecting these disorders requires the use of fluorescent in situ hybridization (FISH) technology, using a probe for the specific region of the chromosome to be investigated. Genetics consultation is indicated when considering these tests.

Dermal Lesions of Neurocutaneous Syndromes

- **Ash leaf spots** are hypomelanotic macules found in 90% of patients with tuberous sclerosis. Ultraviolet light may be necessary to visualize the spots. One or two hypopigmented lesions may be seen in normal individuals. Approximately 50% of patients with tuberous sclerosis have mental retardation.

TABLE 3-2	Developmental Milestones from Birth to 5 Years of Age			
Age (Months)	Adaptive/Fine Motor	Language	Gross Motor	Personal–Social
1	Grasp reflex (hands fisted)	Facial response to sounds	Lifts head in prone position	Stares at face
2	Follows object with eyes past midline	Coos (vowel sounds)	Lifts head in prone position to 45°	Smiles in response to others
4	Hands open	Laughs and squeals	Sits: head steady	Smiles spontaneously
		Turns toward voice	Rolls to supine	
6	Brings objects to mouth	Babbles (consonant sounds)	Sits independently	Reaches for toys
	Palmar grasp of objects		Stands, hands held	Recognizes strangers
9	Pincer grasp	Says "mama," "dada" nonspecifically; compre- hends "no"	Pulls to stand	Feeds self
				Waves bye-bye
12	Helps turn pages of book	2–4 words	Stands independently	Points to indicate wants
		Follows command with gesture	Walks, one hand held	
15	Scribbles	4–6 words	Walks independently	Drinks from cup
		Follows command no gesture		Imitates activities
18	Turns pages of book	10–20 words	Walks up steps	Feeds self with spoon
		Points to 4 body parts		
24	Solves single-piece puzzles	Combines 2–3 words	Jumps	Removes coat
		Uses "I" and "you"	Kicks ball	Verbalizes wants
30	Imitates horizontal and vertical lines	Names all body parts	Rides tricycle using pedals	Pulls up pants
				washes, dries hands
36	Copies circle	Gives full name, age, and sex	Throws ball overhand	Toilet trained

(Continued)

TABLE 3-2 Developmental Milestones from Birth to 5 Years of Age *(continued)*

Age (Months)	Adaptive/Fine Motor	Language	Gross Motor	Personal–Social
	Draws person with 3 parts	Names 2 colors	Walks up stairs (alternating feet)	Puts on shirt, knows front from back
42	Copies cross	Understands "cold," "tired," "hungry"	Stands on one foot for 2–3 sec	Engages in associative play
48	Counts 4 objects	Understands prepositions (under, on, behind, in front of)	Hops on one foot	Dresses with little assistance
	Identifies some numbers and letters	Asks "how" and "why"		Shoes on correct feet
54	Copies square	Understands opposites	Broad-jumps 24 inches	Bosses and criticizes
	Draws person with 6 parts			Shows off
60	Prints first name	Asks meaning of words	Skips (alternating feet)	Ties shoes
	Counts 10 objects			

Figure 3-1 ▪ Patient with multiple café-au-lait spots.
(Reprinted with permission from: McMillan JA., ed., et al. Oski's Pediatrics: Principles and Practice. Philadelphia, Lippincott Williams & Wilkins, 1999.)

- **Café-au-lait spots** are light brown flat macules seen in patients with neurofibromatosis but also seen in 10% of the population (Figure 3-1). They are more common on the trunk than on the extremities. Six or more lesions, >5 mm before puberty or >15 mm after puberty, should lead to investigation for other signs of neurofibromatosis. Patients with neurofibromatosis are at risk for hearing loss and learning disabilities.
- **Port wine nevus.** Ten percent of children with cutaneous angioma involving the upper face (forehead and eye) have an intracranial angioma (Sturge-Weber syndrome). Approximately 50% of patients with Sturge-Weber syndrome have mental retardation (Figure 3-2).

Figure 3-2 ▪ Patient with port wine nevus.
(Reprinted with permission from: McMillan JA., ed., et al. Oski's Pediatrics: Principles and Practice. Philadelphia, Lippincott Williams & Wilkins, 1999.)

Muscle Tone

- **Hypertonia** (i.e., increased resistance of muscle groups to movement) may be a sign of cerebral palsy [CP], but in the first year of life children with isolated increases in muscle tone should not be diagnosed with CP because they may outgrow the problem.

- **Hypotonia** (i.e., decreased resistance of muscle groups to movement) occurs in infants with neuromuscular disorders or injury to the brain or spinal cord. Rarely, hypotonia is the only sign of a metabolic disorder (e.g., peroxisomal disorders, acid maltase deficiency). Hypotonia also occurs in some chromosomal disorders, such as Down syndrome, so obtaining a karyotype should be considered if the child is dysmorphic and hypotonic.

Primitive Reflexes

Asymmetries of primitive reflexes may help identify hemiplegias or other nerve injuries. Persistence of primitive reflexes beyond the time of usual disappearance (Table 3-3) or an obligate response may be signs of CP.

HEARING ASSESSMENT

Screening

Universal hearing screening during the newborn period is recommended because screening limited to infants with risk factors for hearing loss (Table 3-4) identifies only half of infants with significant hearing impairment. Approximately three quarters of the 50 states mandate this screening. The most cost-effective screening method is still the subject of some debate, but the currently available methods include otoacoustic emissions and auditory brainstem responses.

- **Otoacoustic emissions (OAEs).** Otoacoustic emissions refers to sounds that are thought to originate from the hair cells of the cochlea. Auditory threshold refers to the decibel (dB) level at which the response is no longer detected. In individuals with an auditory threshold of ≥ 20 dB, OAEs can be evoked by presenting clicking sounds to the ear. If the auditory threshold is above 30 to 40 dB, the evoked OAEs are absent. The test takes 2 to 5 minutes to administer and is relatively inexpensive. However, fluid in the middle ear or debris in the auditory canal may interfere with the test, leading to a false-positive rate as high as 10% in the newborn period.

- **Auditory brainstem response (ABR).** Electroencephalogram (EEG) electrodes attached to the forehead and behind the ears detect brain activity in response to 30 to 40 dB clicks presented to an ear. Absence of the expected brain activity suggests an abnormality of hearing. The test takes 5 to 15 minutes to perform and is significantly more expensive than OAE testing, but the false-positive rate is lower (2% to 3%).

TABLE 3-3 Primitive Reflexes

Primitive Reflex	Age at Disappearance (Months)	Description
Palmar grasp	3–4	Pressing against the palmar surface of the infant's hand results in flexion of all fingers.
Rooting	3–4	Stroking the perioral skin at the corners of the mouth causes the mouth to open and turn to stimulated side.
Galant	2–3	Stroking along the paravertebral area causes lateral flexion of the trunk with the concavity toward the stimulated side.
Moro	4–6	Sudden movement of the head causes symmetric abduction and extension of the arms followed by gradual adduction and flexion of the arms over the body.
Asymmetric tonic neck	4–6	Turning the head to one side leads to extension of extremities on that side and flexion on the contralateral side, putting the infant in the "fencing" position.
Tonic labyrinthine	2–3	In the supine position, neck extension leads to shoulder retraction and trunk and lower extremity extension that is reduced by neck flexion.
Positive support	2–3	Stimulation of the ball of the foot leads to cocontraction of opposing muscle groups, allowing weight to be borne.
Placing/stepping	Variable	When the dorsal surface of one foot touches the underside of a table, the infant places the foot on the tabletop.

43

TABLE 3-4 Risk Factors for Hearing Impairment
Family history of deafness
Congenital toxoplasmosis, other infections, rubella, cytomegalovirus, and herpes simple, (TORCH) infection
Congenital malformation of the head and neck
Prematurity (<1,500 g at birth)
Extended stay in neonatal intensive care unit (>48 hr)
Hyperbilirubinemia requiring exchange transfusion
Meningitis or encephalitis
Anoxia

In some locations a two-step screening process is applied in which those who fail OAEs are then screened by ABRs, and only those who fail both screens are referred for further evaluation. This two-step process may have the lowest false-positive rate.

HINT: Expressive language milestones (e.g., laughing, cooing, babbling) can be misleading because deaf infants also exhibit these milestones in the first 4 to 6 months. By approximately 12 months of age, babbling decreases in deaf infants, but in hearing infants it continues to increase and sounds more like the infant is talking.

Formal Hearing Testing

- **0–6 months: Auditory evoked responses (AERs).** The use of AERs as a screening test was described earlier. When the test is done by an audiologist, the intensity of the sound can be varied so the auditory threshold can be obtained. This test is highly sensitive (false-negative results are rare), but a false-positive result is possible. Therefore, positive test results should be confirmed by audiometry when the child is old enough.
- **6–24 months: Visual reinforcement audiometry.** A sound is paired with a visual event (e.g., a doll's eyes light up). Once the child has learned the association, she looks toward the doll in anticipation of the visual event when a sound is heard.
- **2–5 years: Conditioned play audiometry.** The child is asked to engage in a play task every time a sound is heard.
- **Older than 6 years: Standard audiometry.**

VISION ASSESSMENT

The **detection of amblyopia** is the most important reason for early vision screening because early detection can prevent vision loss in the "neglected" eye. The most common causes of amblyopia are **strabismus** (see Chapter 2, "The Physical Examination") and **anisometropia** (an eye with a refractive error ≥1.5 diopters than its pair).

Visual acuity improves with age. Newborns should be able to fixate on a face; by 1 to 2 months of age, infants should be able to follow an object horizontally across their visual field. By 6 months of age, visual acuity is about 20/100, and at 3 years it is 20/30 to 20/40. By 5 to 6 years of age, children should have 20/20 vision.

Office vision screening using the Snellen chart can be performed with children who know the letters of the alphabet. Variations of this test, such as the tumbling "E" chart and the Allen chart, have been developed for younger children. When using the tumbling "E" chart, the child is asked to point in the direction of the "legs" of the letter. The Allen chart contains pictures of toys, animals, and other familiar objects.

DEVELOPMENTAL SCREENING TESTS

General Development

Ages 0–5 Years: Ages and Stages Questionnaires

The Ages and Stages Questionnaires is a series of parent-completed questionnaires that assess the domains of communication, gross motor, fine motor, problem-solving, and personal adaptive skills. Norms are based on test administration to 2,008 children from diverse ethnic and socioeconomic backgrounds. Responses generate a pass/fail score; failing scores indicating possible need for further evaluation. Additional information about this questionnaire is available at http://www.brookespublishing.com/store/books/bricker-asq/.

Ages 0–8 Years: Parents' Evaluation of Developmental Status (PEDS)

This parent-completed questionnaire elicits parental concerns about aspects of the child's development and behavior. Based on parent response to questions, an algorithm guides the clinician in determining whether the child needs referral, additional screening, or continued surveillance. Additional information on this test is available at http://www.pedstest.com/.

Autism Screening

Ages 16–30 Months: Modified Checklist for Autism in Toddlers (M-CHAT)

This parent-completed questionnaire is designed to identify children at risk of autism spectrum disorder. The screen is considered positive if the parent answers "no" to any 3 of the 23 items or 2 out of 6 critical items. Additional information on this test is available at www.firstsigns.org.

Language Development

Age >2 Years 6 months: Peabody Picture Vocabulary Test-IV (PPVT-IV)

The PPVT-IV tests receptive language skills. From a group of four pictures, the patient must select the one picture that best illustrates a specific word. A progressively more difficult sequence of words and pictures is administered until the patient is no longer identifying the correct picture at a frequency higher than chance. Scores tend to correlate well with the verbal IQ. Additional information on this test is available at http://ags.pearsonassessments.com/.

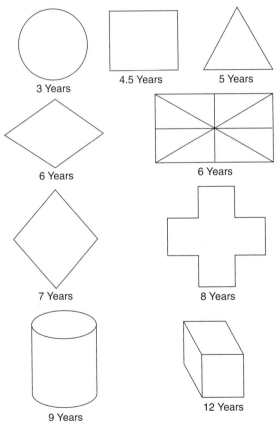

Figure 3-3 ▪ Gesell figures used to assess visual-motor skills. Children are capable of drawing progressively more complex shapes.

Visual-Motor Skills

Ages 3–12 Years: Gesell Figures

Children develop the ability to draw progressively more complex figures in a predictable manner (Figure 3-3).

LABORATORY EVALUATION

Genetic Testing

In the etiologic workup of children with developmental delay or mental retardation, a **comparative genomic hybridization (CGH)** array analysis and **Fragile X** testing should be performed. If CGH testing is normal, then **routine karyotyping** to detect balanced translocations should be considered. Additional genetic testing includes testing for the **MECP2** mutation in girls with severe delays (see Chapter 4, "Developmental Disabilities"). Approximately 5% to 10% of children with global developmental delays have abnormal genetic testing, even in the absence of dysmorphic features.

Neurologic Studies

Neuroimaging should be considered if microcephaly or focal neurologic signs are present. Compared with computed tomography scans, **magnetic resonance imaging** scans are more sensitive in detecting brain abnormalities related to developmental delay.

Metabolic Studies

Metabolic testing (e.g., urine organic acids, serum amino acids, lactate, pyruvate, ammonia, very long chain fatty acids) should be performed in children with a positive family history of metabolic disorders, parental consanguinity, regression of developmental skills, or for whom newborn screening results are unavailable.

Additional Studies

Additional laboratory testing includes **creatine phosphokinase (CPK)** when low muscle tone is present; **thyroid function studies** if signs or symptoms of hypothyroidism are present or if newborn screening tests are unavailable; **lead,** for in addition to being a causative agent, children with developmental delays have increased mouthing behaviors, thereby increasing their risk for lead toxicity; and **iron,** to detect iron-deficiency anemia. An **EEG** is indicated when seizures are suspected.

References

American Academy of Pediatrics, Council on Children with Disabilities, Section on Developmental Behavioral Pediatrics, Bright Futures

Steering Committee, and Medical Home Initiatives for Children with Special Needs Project Advisory Committee: Identifying infants and young children with developmental disorders in the medical home: an algorithm for developmental surveillance and screening. *Pediatrics* 118(1):405–420, 2006.

Friendly DS: Development of vision in infants and young children. *Pediatr Clin North Am* 40:693–703, 1993.

Garganta C, Seashore MR: Universal screening for congenital hearing loss. *Pediatr Ann* 29:302–308, 2000.

Glascoe FP: Early detection of developmental and behavioral problems. *Pediatr Rev* 21:272–280, 2000.

Jones KL: *Smith's Recognizable Patterns of Human Malformation.* Philadelphia, WB Saunders, 1997.

Liptak GS: The pediatrician's role in caring for the developmentally disabled child. *Pediatr Rev* 17:203–210, 1996.

4 *Developmental Disabilities*

Nathan J. Blum and Patty Huang

When caring for children with developmental disabilities, the physician must consider **possible causes** for the disorder, **screening** for problems associated with the disorder, and **interventions** to minimize functional impairment and prevent long-term complications.

CEREBRAL PALSY

Definition and Etiology

Cerebral palsy (CP) is a nonprogressive disorder of motion and posture that results from injury to the developing central nervous system (CNS). It occurs in 1.5 to 2.5 children per 1,000 live births. **Prematurity** is the single most significant risk factor; approximately 8% to 10% of infants with a birthweight <1,500 g develop CP. Although **perinatal asphyxia** was once thought to be a major cause of CP, it is now thought to cause <10% of cases. A genetic abnormality can be identified in about 10% of cases and is more likely to be found in a term infant with CP than a preterm infant. In approximately 15% to 20% of patients, **no cause** can be identified.

Classification

- **Spastic.** This form of CP is characterized by increased deep tendon reflexes and increased muscle tone with a "clasp knife" quality (i.e., initially, resistance to movement is strong but then the muscle gives way suddenly). It can be further subclassified based on the limbs that are involved:
  - Hemiplegia: Involves both the arm and leg on either the left or the right side of the body
  - Quadriplegia: Significant impairment in all four extremities
  - Diplegia: Bilateral leg involvement; Arms may have mild impairment

- **Extrapyramidal.** The most common form of extrapyramidal CP is choreoathetoid CP, which is characterized by sudden involuntary movements of the extremities. Muscle tone is variable within the individual over time. The resistance to movement is described as "lead pipe" rigidity (i.e., persistent pressure results in slow movement of the limb).
- **Mixed.** Components of both spastic and choreoathetoid CP are present.

Associated Problems

- **Cognitive deficits**—mental retardation (50%), learning disabilities
- **Speech and language deficits**—communication disorders, dysarthria

- Sensory deficits—visual impairment, strabismus, hearing impairment
- Gastrointestinal problems—oral-motor dysfunction, gastroesophageal reflex disease, constipation
- Urinary tract problems—spastic bladder, recurrent urinary tract infection (UTI)
- Neurologic problems—spasticity, seizures
- Musculoskeletal problems—joint contractures, dislocated hips, scoliosis
- Psychosocial and behavioral problems

HINT: **Multiple methods are available for managing spasticity and preventing or managing contractures for individuals with spastic cerebral palsy, including physical therapy and positioning, oral medications (e.g., baclofen, dantrolene, diazepam), botulinum toxin injections, intrathecal baclofen, and surgery (e.g., tendon lengthening, dorsal rhizotomy).**

MYELOMENINGOCELE

Definition and Etiology

A myelomeningocele is a sac containing meninges and a malformed spinal cord that protrudes through defective vertebrae. (In contrast, a meningocele is a sac containing only meninges; the spinal cord is normal.)

Myelomeningoceles develop approximately 28 days after conception if the neural tube fails to close. The incidence varies with ethnicity and geography and ranges from one to five per 1,000 live births. The cause of this defect is not known, but both environmental exposures and genetic factors are important. **Maternal oral folic acid supplementation** prior to conception and throughout the first trimester reduces the risk of myelomeningocele by 50% to 70%. The risk of recurrence in the family of a child with a myelomeningocele is 15 to 30 times higher than in the general population; myelomeningocele may also occur in association with a chromosomal abnormality.

Classification

The level of the lesion is predictive of the degree of functional impairment. Difficulties with bowel and bladder function occur with virtually all lesions.

- **Thoracic lesions**—flaccid paralysis of both lower extremities with weakness of the trunk musculature
- **L1 to L2 lesions**—flaccid paralysis of the knees, ankles, and feet with voluntary hip flexion and adduction

- L3 lesions—same as L1 to L2 lesions, but knee flexion is present as well
- L4 to L5 lesions—knee flexion and extension and ankle dorsiflexion are present, but plantar flexion and hip extension are weak or absent
- Sacral lesions—mild weakness of ankles and toes

Associated Problems

The degree and type of associated problems are also related to the level of the lesion.

- Cognitive deficits—mental retardation (33%), learning disabilities
- Neurologic problems—hydrocephalus (70% to 80%), Arnold-Chiari deformity (type II)
- Urinary tract problems—incontinence, recurrent UTI, vesicoureteral reflex, kidney damage
- Bowel dysfunction—incontinence, constipation
- Musculoskeletal disorders—scoliosis, hip dislocation
- Sexual dysfunction—partial erection, retrograde ejaculation
- Ophthalmologic disorders—strabismus
- Dermatologic disorders—decubitus ulcers

> **HINT:** At a few centers, fetal surgery to close the myelomeningocele is being done late in the second or early in the third trimester of the pregnancy. Although results are preliminary, this type of surgery seems to have the potential to decrease the neurologic impairment.

MENTAL RETARDATION

Definition and Etiology

"Mental retardation is a disability characterized by significant limitations both in intellectual functioning and in adaptive behavior as expressed in conceptual, social, and practical adaptive skills. This disability originates before age 18." (American Association on Mental Retardation, Washington, DC, 2002).

> **HINT:** Mental retardation cannot be diagnosed from an intelligence test alone. The individual must also have a deficit in adaptive behavior.

Because of the stigma associated with the diagnosis of mental retardation (MR), some are recommending that the name be changed to intellectual disability. In 2007, the American Association on Mental Retardation changed its name to the American Association on Intellectual and Developmental Disabilities (AAIDD).

The likelihood of identifying the cause of a patient's MR depends on the severity of the retardation. A cause can be identified in approximately 50% of patients with mild MR, and in >80% of patients with severe or profound MR. **Chromosomal abnormalities** (e.g., Down syndrome, fragile X syndrome) are the most commonly identified causes of MR. Other causes of MR include perinatal or postnatal injury, teratogens (e.g., fetal alcohol syndrome), intrauterine infection, and inborn errors of metabolism.

Classification

Descriptions of an individual's strengths, weaknesses, and the level of support needed (intermittent, limited, extensive, pervasive) are most helpful in planning for educational/vocational, social/recreational, and daily living needs. IQ-based subclassifications are often used but are not as helpful for intervention planning.

- Mild MR: IQ 50–55 to approximately 70
- Moderate MR: IQ 35–40 to 50–55
- Severe MR: IQ 20–25 to 35–40
- Profound MR: IQ below 20–25

> **HINT:** For IQ scores in the ranges that overlap between subclassifications, the individual's adaptive functioning should be used to determine the appropriate subclassification.

> **HINT:** Developmental testing results in the toddler and preschool years are often described as a development quotient (DQ) as opposed to an IQ. A DQ equals the mental age divided by the chronological age, multiplied by 100. For example, a 4-year-old functioning at a 2-year-old level would have a DQ of 50.

Associated Problems

For children with a specific syndrome, the associated problems are related to the syndrome. In general, children with MR are at increased risk for **hearing or visual deficits,** which occur in up to 25% of children with mild MR and in >50% of children with severe MR. **Seizures** and **behavior problems** ranging from hyperactivity to self-injury occur with increased frequency in this population.

> **HINT:** Physicians tend to underestimate the capabilities of children with MR. Many children diagnosed with mild MR function independently in the community as adults.

PERVASIVE DEVELOPMENTAL DISORDER

Definition and Etiology

Pervasive developmental disorder (PDD) encompasses a variety of disorders (e.g., autistic disorder, Asperger syndrome, Rett disorder) characterized by impairments in **reciprocal social interactions, communication skills,** and **a restricted range of interests and behaviors.** Many children engage in stereotyped behaviors and adhere inflexibly to nonfunctional routines. PDD is sometimes referred to as an "autism spectrum disorder" (ASD).

The prevalence of ASD has been rising over the past two decades and is currently estimated to be about 1 in 150 children with a male-to-female ratio of approximately 4:1. It is unclear whether this rise in prevalence is because of changing diagnostic criteria, a true increase in incidence, or a combination of both. These disorders are likely caused by damage to the brain or abnormal development of the brain. There is a strong genetic contribution; the incidence of PDD in siblings of affected children is 5 to 15 times higher than in the general population. Evidence does not support an association between immunizations and PDD.

Most cases of classic Rett syndrome have recently been discovered to be caused by mutations in a gene on the X chromosome that codes for methyl-CpG-binding protein 2 (MECP2). Interestingly, not all females with this mutation have Rett syndrome (perhaps related to X chromosome inactivation patterns). It was previously thought that this mutation was almost always lethal in males, but recent studies have described varying phenotypes of MECP2 mutations in males to include severe encephalopathies (leading to early infant death), a Rett-like syndrome, developmental delay with seizures, and nonspecific MR.

Classification

- **Autistic disorder**—severe impairments in reciprocal social interactions, communication skills, and restricted or repetitive interests and behaviors
- **Asperger syndrome**—severe impairments in social interactions, frequent repetitive behaviors, and a restricted range of interests or activities but no significant delays in language skills or global cognitive skills
- **PDD-not otherwise specified (PDD-NOS)**—problems such as those described for autistic disorder and Asperger syndrome but not of sufficient severity to meet criteria for one of these diagnoses
- **Rett disorder**—characterized by loss of speech, loss of purposeful hand movements, acquired microcephaly, and atypical breathing patterns

■ Childhood disintegrative disorder—characterized by the loss of skills in multiple areas of functioning after at least 2 years of normal development; a diagnosis of exclusion after metabolic and neurodegenerative disorders are ruled out

> **HINT:** Children with autistic disorder may learn a few words and then stop using them between 12 and 24 months of age. However, they should not lose more complex language skills or skills in other areas.

Associated Problems

■ Cognitive deficits—mental retardation (60% to 70% of patients with autistic disorder), learning disabilities
■ Neurologic problems—seizure disorder
■ Psychosocial and behavioral problems—hyperactivity, unusual responses to sensory input, self-injurious behaviors, schizophrenia

HEARING IMPAIRMENT

Definition and Etiology

Table 4-1 summarizes the causes of hearing loss.

■ Conductive hearing loss is caused by damage to the external or middle ear. Hearing is decreased for sound conducted by air, but sounds conducted by bone are heard normally.
■ Sensorineural hearing loss is caused by damage to the cochlea or auditory nerve. Both bone and air conduction of sound is abnormal.
■ Central hearing loss is characterized by absent or distorted auditory brainstem response, with intact otoacoustic and cochlear function.
■ Anacusis is total hearing loss.

TABLE 4-1 Causes of Hearing Loss

Congenital

Genetic syndromes (e.g., Waardenburg, Usher, craniofacial)
Familial deafness (70%–80% autosomal recessive)
Congenital toxoplasmosis, other infections, rubella, cytomegalovirus, and herpes simplex (TORCH) infection
Ototoxic drugs taken during first trimester

Acquired

Genetic syndromes (e.g., Alport syndrome, Alström syndrome, neurofibromatosis)
Meningitis or encephalitis
Prematurity
Hyperbilirubinemia requiring exchange transfusion
Birth anoxia (Apgar score 0–3 at 5 min)
Ototoxic medications
Trauma

TABLE 4-2 Classification of Hearing Loss

Degree of Hearing Loss	Decibel Level at Which Sounds Become Inaudible
Slight	16–25
Mild	26–40
Moderate	41–65
Severe	66–95
Profound	≥96

Classification

Table 4-2 summarizes the degrees of hearing loss. Individuals with moderate hearing loss miss most speech sounds at normal conversational levels.

Associated Problems

Associated problems largely depend on the cause of the hearing impairment and when the impairment develops. Difficulty with reading skills and behavioral disturbances are more common than in the general population.

VISION IMPAIRMENT

Definition and Etiology

Most classification schemes would consider an individual visually impaired if the corrected visual acuity in the best eye was 20/60 or worse. In the United States, the legal definition of blindness is a best corrected visual acuity of 20/200 or a peripheral visual field restricted to 20° or less. Table 4-3 summarizes the causes of vision impairment.

TABLE 4-3 Causes of Vision Impairment

Congenital

Congenital toxoplasmosis, other infections, rubella, cytomegalovirus, and herpes simplex (TORCH) infections
Malformations of visual system (coloboma, aniridia, retinal dysplasia)
Cataracts
Glaucoma

Acquired

Retinopathy of prematurity
Strabismus
Genetic syndromes (may be associated with either congenital and acquired vision loss)
Macular disease
Tumors (e.g., retinoblastoma)
Trauma
Infection
Anoxia (associated with cortical visual impairment)

Associated Problems

- Cognitive deficits—mental retardation (20% to 25% of blind children)
- Speech and language deficits—developmental delays (imitation of mouth movements is an important component of speech development)
- Psychosocial and behavioral problems—stereotypic behaviors, self-injurious behavior

HINT: Blind children with normal intelligence have developmental delays. Gross motor skills (e.g., sitting) develop about 2 months later in blind children than in sighted children, and a blind child may begin to walk 3 to 7 months later than a sighted child. Signs of attachment may also occur at different times. Stranger anxiety occurs at approximately the same time as it does in sighted children, but separation anxiety does not develop until later.

SPEECH AND LANGUAGE DISORDERS

Definition and Etiology

Speech refers to the sounds used to communicate information, and language refers to the system by which the sounds are given meaning. Language disorders are present when a child's skills at using language are significantly below her nonverbal cognitive skills.

Language disorders may be acquired through a brain injury or they may be congenital. In some cases, differences in the processing of auditory information are thought to be the cause of congenital language disorders.

HINT: Always test the child's hearing.

HINT: Assess verbal and nonverbal skills. For many children with MR, the initial concern is often about the child's language skills.

Classification

- Expressive language disorder—the child's ability to formulate ideas into words is below the ability to understand language and perform nonverbal skills.
- Mixed receptive-expressive language disorder—the child's ability to formulate ideas into words and to understand language is below the nonverbal cognitive skills.

■ Phonological disorder—the child is not able to use speech sounds that are appropriate for age and dialect.

Associated Problems

■ Language-based learning disabilities—for example, reading, spelling, writing disorders
■ Behavioral problems

LEARNING DISABILITIES

Definition and Etiology

The 2004 reauthorization of the Individuals with Disabilities Education Act continues to define a learning disability as "a disorder in one or more of the basic psychological processes involved in understanding language, spoken or written, which may manifest itself in an imperfect ability to listen, speak, read, write, spell, or do mathematical calculations." However, the law no longer requires that children with learning disabilities be identified on the basis of a severe discrepancy between actual and expected achievement. Instead, the law encourages schools to consider how the child responds to evidence-based instructional interventions in determining whether the child has a learning disability.

> **HINT:** One criticism of the discrepancy criteria in identifying learning disabilities is that it required children to be significantly behind peers before they could be diagnosed and receive interventions.

Learning disabilities may occur along with other conditions but are not the direct result of sensory impairments, mental retardation, social-emotional disturbance, cultural differences, or inappropriate instruction. Although the cause of learning disabilities is not known, **genetic factors** appear to play a role. Multiple members of a family often have learning disabilities, although the pattern does not follow classic Mendelian inheritance. In addition, learning disabilities occur with increased frequency in many **genetic syndromes.**

Classification

Reading learning disability (dyslexia) is the most common learning disability. Learning disabilities may also occur in the areas of math, spelling, and written expression. Reading disability is usually related to deficits in phonemic awareness; thus individuals with reading disability often have difficulty with other language-based skills such as spelling. Children with nonverbal learning disability often have problems with math, visual-perceptual, fine motor, organizational, and social skills.

Associated Problems

- **Psychosocial and behavioral problems**—attention deficit hyperactivity disorder (ADHD), low self-esteem, school avoidance

> **HINT:** Having a child repeat a grade is not an appropriate intervention for a learning disability. Physicians should insist that a psychoeducational evaluation be performed on any child having difficulty in school. There are few situations in which repeating a grade is an appropriate intervention.

ATTENTION DEFICIT HYPERACTIVITY DISORDER

Definition and Etiology

ADHD is characterized by developmentally inappropriate levels of **inattention, impulsivity,** and **hyperactivity.** In almost all cases, school functioning is impaired. Many children also have difficulties in meeting expectations at home and in social relationships.

Research suggests that individuals with ADHD may have decreased activity of basal ganglia and frontal lobe neurons involving the dopamine and norepinephrine neurotransmitter systems. Genetics is the strongest predictor of increased risk for ADHD. Other factors that increase the risk for ADHD include prenatal exposure to environmental toxins (e.g., cigarette smoke, alcohol) and postnatal brain injury (e.g., infections, inborn errors of metabolism, trauma).

> **HINT:** "Developmentally inappropriate" levels of inattention or activity are difficult to define. Clinically, standardized parent and teacher questionnaires are used to help make this assessment.

Classification

- **Primarily inattentive type**—the child is inattentive but does not have high levels of activity or impulsivity.
- **Primarily hyperactive-impulsive type**—the child has high levels of activity and impulsivity but not a high level of inattention.
- **Combined type**—the most common form of ADHD; the child has high levels of hyperactivity, impulsivity, and inattention.

> **HINT:** The hyperactive-impulsive subtype is most often diagnosed in children younger than 7 years. Many of these children are diagnosed with the combined type when they get older.

Associated Problems

- Cognitive-learning disabilities
- Neurologic problems—poor fine motor skills
- Psychosocial and behavioral problems—oppositional defiant disorder, conduct disorder, anxiety disorder, depression, low self-esteem, poor social skills

HINT: Some children may appear to have symptoms of ADHD but really have other problems that are affecting their attention span (e.g., a chaotic or stressful home environment; unrecognized learning disabilities, sensory impairments, psychiatric disorders, or absence seizure disorder). However, children with any of these problems can have coexisting ADHD.

Treatment

- Behavioral counseling and stimulant medications are the most effective treatments for ADHD.

Suggested Readings

Batshaw ML, Pellegrino L, Roizen NJ: *Children with Disabilities*, 6th ed. Baltimore, Brookes, 2007.

Levine MD, Carey WB, Crocker AC: *Developmental-Behavioral Pediatrics*. 3rd ed. Philadelphia, Elsevier, 1999.

Parker SJ, Zuckerman BS, Augustyn MC: *Developmental and Behavioral Pediatrics: A Handbook for Primary Care*. Philadelphia, Lippincott, Williams & Wilkins, 2004.

IMMUNIZATION SCHEDULE

Figure 5-1 outlines the recommended childhood immunization schedule. Important points to remember include the following:

- No contraindications exist to the simultaneous administration of multiple vaccines that are routinely recommended for infants and children.
- Live viral vaccines may be contraindicated in children with immune deficiency; specific recommendations exist for HIV-infected children (see Table 5-1).
- A lapse in the immunization schedule does not require reinstituting the initial series. If a dose of vaccine is missed, merely give it at the next visit.
- Increasing numbers of vaccinations are required for teens. It is important to review the vaccine history at both preventive and acute visits.

ADMINISTRATION GUIDELINES

Procedures

Federal law requires that the date, site, and route of administration, the manufacturer and lot number of the vaccine, as well as the name and business address of the person administering the dose be entered into the patient's permanent medical record. It also requires providers to distribute information on vaccines before each vaccination.

Sites

The preferred sites for the subcutaneous (SC) or intramuscular (IM) administration of vaccines are the anterolateral aspect of the upper thigh or the deltoid area of the upper arm. In **children <1 year,** intramuscular injections should be administered in the **anterolateral aspect of the thigh.** For **children >1 year,** the **deltoid muscle** is the preferred site of administration. Ordinarily, the upper outer aspect of the buttocks should not be used for immunizing an infant because the gluteal region consists mainly of fat until the child has been walking for some time. Furthermore, there is a risk of damaging the sciatic nerve.

Diphtheria, Tetanus, and Acellular Pertussis Vaccine (DTaP Vaccine)

IM: 0.5 mL. The Advisory Committee on Immunization Practices (ACIP) and the American Academy of Pediatrics (AAP) recommend four doses for primary immunization, with the first three administered

Recommended immunization schedule for persons aged 0–6 years—United States • 2008

For those who fall behind or start late, see the catch-up schedule

Vaccine ▼ / Age ▶	Birth	1 month	2 months	4 months	6 months	12 months	15 months	18 months	19–23 months	2–3 years	4–6 years
Hepatitis B[1]	HepB	HepB	See footnote 1		HepB						
Rotavirus[2]			Rota	Rota	Rota						
Diphtheria, Tetanus, Pertussis[3]			DTaP	DTaP	DTaP	See footnote 3	DTaP				DTaP
Haemophilus influenzae type b[4]			Hib	Hib	Hib[4]	Hib					
Pneumococcal[5]			PCV	PCV	PCV	PCV				PPV	PPV
Inactivated Poliovirus			IPV	IPV	IPV						IPV
Influenza[6]					Influenza (Yearly)						
Measles, Mumps, Rubella[7]						MMR					MMR
Varicella[8]						Varicella					Varicella
Hepatitis A[9]						HepA (2 doses)				HepA Series	
Meningococcal[10]										MPSV4	MPSV4

Range of recommended ages

Certain high-risk groups

This schedule indicates the recommended ages for routine administration of currently licensed childhood vaccines, as of December 1, 2007, for children aged 0–6 years. Additional information is available at **www.cdc.gov/vaccines/recs/schedules.** Any dose not administered at the recommended age should be administered at any subsequent visit, when indicated and feasible. Additional vaccines may be licensed and recommended during the year. Licensed combination vaccines may be used whenever any components of the combination are indicated and other components of the vaccine are not contraindicated and if approved by the Food and Drug Administration for that dose of the series. Providers should consult the respective Advisory Committee on Immunization Practices statement for detailed recommendations, including for high-risk conditions: **http://www.cdc.gov/vaccines/pubs/ACIP-list.htm.** Clinically significant adverse events that follow immunization should be reported to the Vaccine Adverse Event Reporting System (VAERS). Guidance about how to obtain and complete a VAERS from is available at **www.vaers.hhs.gov** or by telephone, 800-822-7967.

Figure 5-1 ■ Recommended Childhood Immunization Schedule United States, 2007 Immunization schedules courtesy of the Centers for Disease Control and Prevention, Atlanta, GA, 2008.

Recommended immunization schedule for person aged 17–18 years–United States • 2008

For those who fall behind or start late, see the catch-up schedule

Vaccine ▼ / Age ►	7–10 years	11–12 years	13–18 years
Tetanus, Diphtheria, Pertussis[1]	See footnote 1	Tdap	Tdap
Human Papillomavirus[2]	See footnote 2	HPV (3 doses)	HPV Series
Meningococcal[3]	MCV4	MCV4	MCV3
Pneumococcal[4]		PPV	
Influenza[5]		Influenza (Yearly)	
Hepatitis A[6]		HepA Series	
Hepatitis B[7]		HepB Series	
Inactivated poliovirus[8]		IPV Series	
Measles, Mumps, Rubella[9]		MMR Series	
Varicella[10]		Varicella Series	

Range of recommended ages

Catch-up immunization

Certain high-risk groups

This schedule indicates the recommended ages for routine administration of currently licensed childhood vaccines, as of December 1, 2007, for children aged 7–18 years. Additional information is available at **www.cdc.gov/vaccines/recs/schedules.** Any dose not administered at the recommended age should be administered at any subsequent visit, when indicated and feasible. Additional vaccines may be licensed and recommended during the year. Licensed combination vaccines may be used whenever any components of the combination are indicated and other components of the vaccine are not contraindicated and if approved by the Food and Drug Administration for that dose of the series. Providers should consult the respective Advisory Committee on Immunization Practices statement for detailed recommendations, including for high-risk conditions: **http://www.cdc.gov/vaccines/pubs/ACIP-list.htm.** Clinically significant adverse events that follow immunization should be reported to the Vaccine Adverse Event Reporting System (VAERS). Guidance about how to obtain and complete a VAERS from is available at **www.vaers.hhs.gov** or by telephone, 800-822-7967.

Figure 5-1 ■ (*Continued*)

TABLE 5-1 Recommendations for Routine Immunization of HIV-Infected Children in the United States

Vaccine	Known Asymptomatic HIV Infection	Symptomatic HIV Infection
DTaP	Yes	Yes
Hib	Yes	Yes
Hepatitis A	Yes	Yes
Hepatitis B	Yes	Yes
HPV	Yes	Yes
IPV	Yes	Yes
MMR	Yes	Yes[*]
Meningococcal Conjugate and Polysaccharide	Yes	Yes
Pneumococcal Conjugate and Polysaccharide[†]	Yes	Yes
Rotavirus[‡]	Precaution	Precaution
Varicella	Yes[§]	Yes[§]
Influenza[‖]	Yes	Yes

DTaP = diphtheria and tetanus toxoids acellular pertussis vaccine; HPV = human papilloma virus vaccine; IPV = inactivated poliovirus vaccine; MMR = live-virus measles, mumps, and rubella; Hib = *Haemophilus influenzae* type b conjugate. (Originally adapted from the American Academy of Pediatrics. In Peter G, ed. *1997 Red Book: Report of the Committee on Infectious Diseases,* 24th ed. Elk Grove Village, IL, American Academy of Pediatrics, 1997.)
[*]Severely immunocompromised HIV-infected children should not receive MMR vaccine.
[†]Pneumococcal polysaccharide vaccine should be administered at 2 years of age to all HIV-infected children. Children >2 years should receive pneumococcal vaccine at the time of diagnosis. Revaccination after 3 to 5 years is recommended in either circumstance.
[‡]Immunocompromise is listed as a precaution, not a contraindication, to rotavirus vaccination. This is because the vaccine virus does not replicate well at the intestinal mucosal surface and wild-type infection is inevitable.
[§]Varicella vaccine should be considered for asymptomatic or mildly symptomatic children with HIV with CD4+ T-lymphocyte percentages of 15% or more for age and no evidence of immunity.
[‖]Influenza vaccine should be provided each fall and repeated annually for HIV-exposed infants ≥6 months, HIV-infected children and adolescents, and for household contacts of HIV-infected patients.

at 4- to 8-week intervals starting at 2 months of age, and the fourth dose 6 to 12 months after the third dose and after 1 year of age. A fifth dose is recommended before school entry, at age 4 to 6. Subsequent boosters should be administered starting at 11 years of age using Tdap. Td should be used for all subsequent boosters and given at 10-year intervals throughout life.

Tetanus Immune Globulin

IM: 250 U as a single dose for postexposure prophylaxis. The need for prophylaxis depends on wound cleanliness and severity, as well as prior tetanus toxoid vaccination history. Tetanus toxoid is given along with immune globulin. For treatment of tetanus the optimal dose has not been determined, although doses ranging from 500 to 6000 U are recommended.

Contraindications

Contraindications for DTaP include the following:

- An immediate anaphylactic reaction
- Encephalopathy within 7 days

Precautions

- A seizure, with or without fever, occurring within 3 days of immunization with DTP or DTaP vaccine
- Persistent, inconsolable crying or screaming for >3 hours within 48 hours of immunization
- Collapse or shock-like state within 48 hours of the previous dose
- Temperature >104.9°F(40.5°C) unexplained by another cause within 48 hours of the previous dose

Haemophilus influenza Type b Conjugate Vaccine (Hib)

IM: Three or four 0.5-mL doses are administered at 2 months, 4 months, 6 months, and 12 to 15 months of age. If a three-dose product is used, the third dose may be omitted. In situations in which the brand of vaccine used previously is not known, four doses are required. Hib vaccine is not required after 60 months of age.

Hepatitis A Vaccine

IM: Hepatitis A vaccine 25U (VAQTA) or 720 EL.U (HAVRIX) in the deltoid muscle is recommended for the routine vaccine of all children beginning at 12 months of age. The second dose should be given 6 months later.

Hepatitis B Vaccine

IM (anterolateral thigh or deltoid): Different products are available and generally interchangeable. The first dose is generally administered at birth in the neonatal nursery. The next dose is administered 1 to 4 months later, most commonly at 1 to 2 months of age. The third dose is recommended beginning at 6 months of age and must be given 8 weeks after the second dose and 16 weeks after the first dose. Of note, multiple combination vaccines are available that include hepatitis B. It is acceptable to administer a fourth dose of hepatitis B vaccine if these products are used.

Hepatitis B Immune Globulin (HBIG)

Infants born to HBsAg-positive mothers: Both hepatitis B vaccine (0.5 mL) and HBIG are recommended within 12 hours after birth. The second dose of hepatitis B vaccine is then administered at 1 to 2 months of age and the third dose at 6 months of age. Hepatitis B surface antigen and hepatitis B surface antibody should then be checked starting at 9 months of age or the first preventive visit after completion of the series.

Infants born to mothers with HBsAg unknown: Mothers should be tested on admission for delivery. Administer hepatitis B vaccine by 12 hours of age. HBIG should be administered within 7 days of birth if the mother tests HBsAg positive.

Human Papilloma Virus Vaccine (HPV)

IM: 0.5-mL doses should be administered beginning at 11 to 12 years of age. The second dose is given 2 months after the first dose, and the third dose is administered 6 months after the first. The preferred site of administration is the deltoid muscle, and HPV vaccine is recommended **for females only.** Women may receive the vaccine up to 26 years of age if they have not completed the full series.

Measles-Mumps-Rubella Vaccine (MMR)

SC: 0.5 mL at age 12 to 15 months. A booster dose is now recommended at 4 to 6 years of age. Measles-mumps-rubella-varicella (MMRV) vaccination is now available and can be administered on the same schedule.

Contraindications

Contraindications to measles, mumps, and rubella vaccination include pregnancy, anaphylactic reaction to gelatin or neomycin, recent injection of immune globulin, high-dose steroid use for at least 14 days, and compromised immunity (see discussion of HIV later). Autism is **not associated** with receipt of the MMR vaccine.

> **HINT:** In patients who have been exposed to the measles virus, the vaccine may be given within 72 hours of exposure to provide protection. Alternatively, if given within 6 days of exposure, immune globulin (0.25 mL/kg, IM) may prevent or modify measles in a susceptible person. Children and adolescents with symptomatic HIV infections who are exposed to measles should receive immune globulin prophylaxis (0.5 mL/kg) regardless of their immunization status. The maximum dosage for all patients is 15 mL.

Meningococcal Conjugate Vaccine (MCV4)

IM: Meningococcal vaccine is recommended beginning at 11 to 12 years of age for all teens. One 0.5-mL dose is required. The vaccine should be avoided in those with a history of Guillain-Barré syndrome (GBS).

Meningococcal Polysaccharide Vaccine (MPSV4)

SC: 0.5 mL. Recommended for those between 2 and 10 years of age at increased risk of meningococcal disease. In this age group, the primary recipients are children with terminal complement component deficiencies and those who have anatomic or functional asplenia.

Pneumococcal: Pneumococcal Conjugate Vaccine (PCV7)

IM:

Infants: 0.5 mL/dose given at 2, 4, and 6 months of age, with a booster dose given at 12 to 15 months of age

Previously unvaccinated older infants and children:

7–11 months of age: Two doses are given at least 2 months apart. A third dose is given at 1 year of age

12–23 months of age: A total of two doses are given at least 2 months apart

24–59 months with incomplete vaccination: A single dose is given to healthy children. Children at high risk (sickle cell disease, asplenia, HIV, cochlear implants) or presumed high risk (congenital immune deficiency, chronic cardiac disease, chronic pulmonary disease, cerebrospinal fluid leaks, chronic renal insufficiency, diabetes mellitus, or receiving immunosuppressive or radiation therapy) require additional vaccination.

Pneumococcal Vaccine, Polyvalent (PPV23)

SC or IM: 0.5 mL. Recommended for those at high risk or presumed high risk of pneumococcal disease. Should be given at 24 months of age with an additional dose 3 to 5 years after the first. Doses must be given at least 8 weeks after the last dose of pneumococcal conjugate vaccine.

Poliovirus Vaccine (IPV)

SC: Two 0.5-mL doses are administered at least 4 weeks apart, but preferably 8 weeks apart starting at 2 months of age. A third dose is administered at 6 to 18 months of age and a fourth dose should be given at school entry or at about 4 to 6 years of age. Oral poliovirus vaccine is no longer recommended in the United States.

Rotavirus Vaccine (Rota)

Oral: The rotavirus vaccine is recommended in a three-dose schedule at 2, 4, and 6 months of age. The first dose must be given between 6 and 12 weeks of age. If the first dose of rotavirus vaccine is not administered by 12 weeks of age, the series **should not** be initiated. In addition, rotavirus vaccination **must be completed by 32 weeks of age.**

Precautions for rotavirus vaccination include acute moderate to severe gastroenteritis, moderate to severe illness, preexisting chronic gastrointestinal disease, and intussusception. Of note, altered immunocompetence is a precaution not a contraindication to vaccination because the virus vaccine does not replicate well at the intestinal mucosal surface and wild-type virus infection is inevitable.

Varicella Vaccine

SC: Two 0.5-mL per doses are given, the first at 12 to 15 months and the second at 4 to 6 years of age. For children <13 years who are delayed, two doses may be administered at least 3 months apart. For previously unvaccinated teens ≥13 years, two doses are administered at least 4 weeks apart.

Special Note: To be considered immune without vaccination, individuals must have laboratory evidence of immunity or laboratory confirmation of disease, birth in the United States before 1980 (not applicable to health care workers, pregnant women, or those with immunocompromise), diagnosis or verification of a history of varicella disease by a health care provider, or diagnosis or verification of herpes zoster by a health care provider.

Influenza Vaccine

Inactivated Trivalent Influenza Vaccines (TIV)

IM: TIV is recommended for the routine vaccination of all children between 6 and 60 months of age annually. Those >60 months of age who want to reduce their risk of contracting influenza should also be vaccinated. The dose is 0.25 mL for those <36 months of age and 0.5 mL for older children. Children <9 years of age receiving the vaccine for the first time require two doses at least 1 month apart. In addition, the ACIP recommends that children who only received one dose in their first year of vaccination receive two doses during the second season. For other children, only one dose is needed annually.

High-Risk Populations:

- Children receiving long-term aspirin therapy
- Women who will be pregnant during the flu season
- Children with chronic pulmonary disease (including asthma), cardiovascular disease, renal, hepatic, hematological, or metabolic disorders (including diabetes mellitus), immunosuppression (including HIV), and those with any condition (cognitive dysfunction, spinal cord injury, seizure disorder, neuromuscular disorder) that can compromise respiratory function
- Residents of chronic care facilities

Special Note: Severe egg allergy is a contraindication.

Live Attenuated Influenza Vaccine (LAIV)

Intranasal: LAIV may be substituted for TIV for healthy children >2 years of age. Those with high-risk conditions should not receive LAIV.

Vaccine Refusal

Physicians are often the most trusted source of information on childhood immunizations. For parents with concerns about vaccines, it is recommended that clinicians provide information tailored to the concerns of parents or children. For families refusing vaccination, it is recommended that clinicians revisit the topic at future visits. In addition, clinicians may request that parents sign a refusal to vaccinate form documenting vaccines that are accepted or declined. This form can be accessed through the American Academy of Pediatrics website (http://www.cispimmunize.org/pro/doc/RefusaltoVaccinate.doc).

SPECIAL CIRCUMSTANCES

Premature Infants and Infants with Medical Problems

Premature infants should be immunized **at the usual age** with the usual dose. Reducing or dividing doses of vaccines is not recommended.

Infants who have had an **intraventricular hemorrhage** or other neurologic event soon after birth but are **stable at age 2 months** should also be **immunized.** Infants who are still in the hospital at age 2 months can also receive immunizations. If the infant has a history of **chronic respiratory disease,** the **influenza vaccine** (TIV) should be administered at 6 months of age; family members and caretakers should also be vaccinated.

Immunodeficient and Immunosuppressed Children

Patients being **treated with corticosteroids** may need to be considered immunocompromised depending on the dose, route, and duration of treatment. In general, live vaccines **should not be given** to patients with congenital or secondary disorders of immune function. Table 5-1 summarizes recommendations for HIV-infected children.

Asplenic Children

Children who have undergone splenectomy, children with functional asplenia (sickle cell disease), and children with congenital asplenia have an increased risk of fulminant bacteremia, which is associated with a high mortality rate. Important pathogens in asplenic children include *Streptococcus pneumoniae, Neisseria meningitidis, Haemophilus influenzae* type B, *Staphylococcus aureus, Salmonella species,* and *Escherichia coli.*

Polyvalent pneumococcal vaccine and quadrivalent meningococcal polysaccharide vaccine should be given to all asplenic children >2 years. *H. influenzae* type B vaccine should be **initiated in infancy** as for otherwise healthy children. **Daily antimicrobial prophylaxis** is often recommended for asplenic children regardless of their vaccination status.

Children with Personal or Family History of Seizures

A family history of convulsive disorders is neither a contraindication to immunization with DTP or measles vaccine nor a reason to postpone immunization.

Children with Chronic Disease

In general, children with chronic disease should receive the **same immunizations recommended for healthy children.**

In general, children with immunologic disorders should **not receive live vaccines.** However, patients who are **HIV positive** and not severely immunocompromised should receive the measles-mumps-rubella and varicella vaccines. Rotavirus vaccination is a precaution, not a contraindication, for those who are immunocompromised.

Children with certain chronic diseases (e.g., cardiac, pulmonary, hematologic, metabolic, or adrenal disorders; cystic fibrosis) are more **prone to** the complications of pneumococcal, varicella, and influenza infections and should receive the **appropriate vaccines.** Children awaiting transplants should be immunized prior to the start of immunosuppressive therapy.

TABLE 5-2 Guide to Tetanus Prophylaxis in Routine Wound Management

History of Absorbed Tetanus Toxoid (Doses)	Clean, Minor Wounds		All Other Wounds*	
	Td[†]	TIG[‡]	Td[†]	TIG[‡]
Unknown or <3	Yes	No	Yes	Yes
≥3[§]	No[‖]	No	No[#]	No

Adapted from American Academy of Pediatrics. In Pickering LK, Baker CJ, Long SS, McMillan JA, eds. *Red Book: 2006 Report of the Committee on Infectious Diseases,* 27th ed. Elk Grove Village, IL, American Academy of Pediatrics, 2006.
Td = adult-use tetanus and diphtheria toxoids; TIG = tetanus immune globulin (human).
*Such as, but not limited to, wounds contaminated with dirt, feces, soil, or saliva; puncture wounds; avulsions; and wounds resulting from missiles, crushing, burns, or frostbite.
[†]Tdap is preferred to Td for adolescents who never have received Tdap. Td is preferred to tetanus toxoid (TT) for adolescents who received Tdap previously or when Tdap is not available.
[‡]Immune Globulin Intravenous should be used when TIG is not available.
[§]If only 3 doses of fluid toxoid have been received, a fourth dose of toxoid, preferably an absorbed toxoid, should be given.
[‖]Yes, if ≥10 years since the last dose.
[#]Yes, if ≥5 years since the last dose. (More frequent boosters are not needed and can accentuate side effects.)

Children with Wounds

The treatment of a wound depends on the nature of the wound and on the patient's immunization history. Table 5-2 lists the guidelines for tetanus prophylaxis.

COMMON MISCONCEPTIONS REGARDING CONTRAINDICATIONS TO IMMUNIZATION

Many misconceptions exist regarding contraindications to immunization. The following are *not* appropriate contraindications to immunization:

- A mild acute illness characterized by a low-grade fever or mild diarrhea in an otherwise well child
- Antimicrobial therapy or being in the convalescent phase of an illness
- A reaction to a previous dose that involved only soreness, redness, or swelling in the immediate vicinity of the vaccination site or a temperature <105°F (40.5°C)
- A household contact who is pregnant
- Recent exposure to an infectious disease
- Breast-feeding
- A history of nonspecific allergies or relatives with allergies
- Allergies to penicillin (none of the vaccines licensed in the United States contains penicillin)
- Allergies to duck meat or duck feathers (no vaccine available in the United States is produced in substrates containing duck antigens)
- Family history of convulsions (it is permissible to administer pertussis and measles vaccinations to patients with a family history of convulsions)
- Family history of sudden infant death syndrome (DTP vaccination is permissible in these patients)
- Family history of an adverse event, unrelated to immunosuppression, following a vaccination
- Malnutrition

OTHER SOURCES OF INFORMATION

The schedule for the immunization of children is constantly changing. The following publications are excellent sources of up-to-date information:

- *2006 Red Book: Report of the Committee on Infectious Diseases,* 27th ed. This reference is published at 2- to 3-year intervals by the Committee on Infectious Diseases of the AAP.
- *Pediatrics.* Statements of the Committee on Infectious Diseases of the AAP are published in this monthly journal.

- *Morbidity and Mortality Weekly Report* (**MMWR**). http://www.cdc. gov/mmwr/. This report is published weekly by the Centers for Disease Control and Prevention (CDC) and contains current vaccine recommendations and updates.
- *Health Information for International Travel.* Information is available online from the CDC at http://wwwn.cdc.gov/travel/contentVaccinations.aspx.
- **http://www.aap.org.** This is the website for the American Academy of Pediatrics.

Suggested Readings

2006 Red Book: Report of the Committee on Infectious Diseases, 27th ed. Elk Grove Village, IL, American Academy of Pediatrics, 2006.

http://www.cispimmunize.org/. American Academy of Pediatrics.

http://www.cdc.gov/nip/links.htm. CDC National Immunization Program.

http://www.hhs.gov/nvpo/. National Vaccine Program Office.

6 *Feeding Infants*

Susan A. Friedman and Brenda Waber

NUTRITIONAL NEEDS OF HEALTHY FULL-TERM INFANTS

Table 6-1 summarizes the nutritional needs of a healthy full-term infant.

>
> **HINT: Contraindications to both breast- and bottle-feeding:**
> - **Respiratory rate >80 breaths/minute**
> - **An infant with poor suck/swallow**
> - **An absent gag reflex**
> - **Symptoms of sepsis or asphyxia**

BREAST-FEEDING

Breast-feeding is the optimal choice for feeding almost all infants, and breast milk is the gold standard on which most routine infant formulas are based.

Advantages of Breast-Feeding

- Decreased incidence and severity of infectious diseases, including diarrhea, respiratory tract infections, bacterial meningitis, otitis media, urinary tract infections, necrotizing enterocolitis and bacteremia
- Decreased incidence of sudden infant death syndrome (SIDS)
- Decreased incidence of childhood obesity
- Decreased incidence of type 1 and type 2 diabetes mellitus
- Decreased incidence of leukemia, lymphoma, and Hodgkin disease
- Possibly decreased incidence of hypercholesterolemia
- Possibly enhanced cognitive development
- Maternal benefits, including decreased postpartum bleeding, faster return to prepregnancy weight, decreased risk of breast cancer and ovarian cancer, decreased risk of postmenopausal osteoporosis

Contraindications to Breast-Feeding

- Some inborn errors of metabolism (e.g., classic galactosemia).
- Maternal HIV-positive status.
- Active (untreated) tuberculosis.

TABLE 6-1 Nutritional Needs of Healthy, Full-Term Infants

Nutritional Element	Daily Requirement
Calories	Approximately 108–110 kcal/kg/day
Fluids	Approximately 160 mL/kg/day*
Carbohydrates	37%–44% of calories
Protein	10%–12% of calories
Fat	40%–50% of calories; 3% from linoleic acid

*Of formula or breast milk, to provide adequate calories.

- Maternal alcohol abuse and certain maternal illicit drug use. Significant cigarette smoking (more than four cigarettes per day) should be evaluated on a case-by-case basis.
- Herpes simplex lesions on a breast.
- Breast cancer (currently under treatment).
- Maternal prolactinoma (in most cases).
- History of breast reduction surgery involving ligation of the milk ducts (may breast-feed if supplements are provided as needed).
- Maternal use of medications and/or radioactive materials that are contraindicated with breast-feeding, as per the findings of the American Academy of Pediatrics Committee on Drugs, 2001.

> **HINT:** Maternal hepatitis B infection is not a contraindication to breast-feeding, provided the infant receives hepatitis vaccination and hepatitis immunoglobulin shortly after birth. Maternal hepatitis C infection is not a contraindication to breast-feeding.

Patient Counseling

Drug Use During Lactation

The nursing mother should be counseled to **avoid all drugs,** including over-the-counter and herbal medications, **until she has consulted her physician.** The reference by Hale (see Suggested Readings) is an excellent resource for evaluating maternal medication use. Alcohol intake should be avoided. If the mother does have an occasional small drink (up to 6 oz of beer and 4 oz of wine), she should wait at least 2 to 3 hours before breast-feeding. Cigarette smoking should be discouraged but is no longer considered an absolute contraindication to breast-feeding because its benefits outweigh the risks for light smoking. The mother should be counseled regarding the dangers of decreased milk supply and the effects of nicotine on the infant if smoking exceeds four cigarettes per day.

Nutrition and Rest

Nursing mothers need an **extra 500 calories per day** of nutritious foods and **enough fluids** to satisfy thirst, usually several extra glasses per day. **Supplemental calcium** should be obtained by continuing to include high-calcium food in the diet, along with prenatal vitamins. **Adequate rest** is also important (it is ideal if the mother can nap when the infant naps).

Breast-Feeding Technique

It is neither necessary nor desirable to wash the nipples, but **clean hands are important.** The mother should be comfortable—it may be helpful to place extra pillows under her elbows and on her lap. The baby should be positioned on his side in the mother's arms, facing the mother, so the head is in the "neutral" position (i.e., the infant should not have to turn the head to latch on).

The mother should support the breast, taking care to keep her fingers away from the areola. Tickling the baby's lower lip with the nipple will induce him to open his mouth wide, at which point he should be drawn close to the mother's body, encouraging latching on to as much of the alveolar tissue as possible. Both breasts should be offered at each feeding and the infant allowed to remain on each breast as long as suckling continues. One breast may be sufficient, especially during the first few days of life. The starting breast should be alternated. **Nipples should be allowed to air-dry** or be patted dry before covering them at the end of the feeding.

Feeding Frequency and Intake

The healthy infant should be encouraged to latch on within the first hour after birth. Continuous rooming-in facilitates breast-feeding. Feedings for the first few weeks should take place on demand **at least every 2 to 3 hours, ideally 8 to 12 times per 24 hours. No supplemental water or formula** should be given to the baby **during the first 2 weeks,** unless medically indicated. Table 6-2 summarizes nutrition supplementation for full-term breast-fed infants. An adequate latch-on and suckling should be assured and documented prior to hospital discharge.

TABLE 6-2 Nutrition Supplementation for Full-Term, Breast-Fed Infants

Formula	Not recommended during the first 2 weeks unless medically indicated
Fluoride	0.25 mg/day, starting at 6 months (if tap water is not fluoridated). Avoid fluoridated toothpaste until 2 years of age.
Vitamin D	200 IU/day, starting during the first 2 months of life
Iron	Elemental iron or iron-fortified cereal (1 mg/kg/day), starting at 6 months

Management of Problems

Engorgement

Engorgement may occur on the third or fourth postpartum day and can cause significant discomfort for the mother. It is important to reassure the mother that a high level of engorgement typically lasts only 24 to 48 hours. Management strategies include the following:

- Continuing to nurse frequently.
- Application of hot compresses or taking a hot shower before nursing to alleviate discomfort.
- Application of ice packs to the breasts after nursing. Chilled cabbage leaves are also effective.
- Administration of acetaminophen or ibuprofen.
- Pumping only a small amount of milk to avoid increased milk production (if a breast pump is being used).

Sore, Cracked, or Hemorrhagic Nipples

- The infant's position on the nipple should be reevaluated by a medical professional or lactation consultant; an infant that latches on to an inadequate amount of the nipple is the most common cause of sore nipples. The mother should be sure the infant's lower lip is furled outward.
- Exposure of the nipples to air is important. In addition, applying expressed breast milk to cracked nipples and allowing them to air-dry has resulted in dramatic healing in some patients. Lansinoh cream and ComfortGel pads may also be helpful.
- Mothers should be advised to nurse the baby on the least affected side first. Prefeeding with milk that has been manually expressed may appease the overly vigorous nurser. In severe cases, breast-feeding on the affected side should be temporarily discontinued and a breast pump used.
- Administration of acetaminophen 20 minutes before nursing (not to exceed recommended dosing) may alleviate discomfort.

Galactocele

A galactocele (**plugged milk duct**) presents as a persistent hard, round, or linear lump, usually in the lateral and inferior quadrants of the breast. **Warm moist heat** should be applied to the breast for 20 minutes before each nursing, and the **breast should be massaged** from the body toward the nipple, concentrating on the involved area. Mothers should be advised to **nurse the baby frequently** (i.e., every 1 to 2 hours) for at least 10 minutes on each side. The **affected side should be offered first,** and the infant should be positioned with his chin toward the affected area, which will facilitate emptying of the affected quadrant. It may take several nursing sessions to empty the plugged duct. Complete emptying of the breast is advised; this may require the use of a breast pump after nursing.

Mastitis

Lactating mothers with mastitis present with **fever, shaking chills, and malaise,** followed by **localized breast erythema and pain.** Mothers should be advised to continue to nurse frequently. Treatment is with oral ampicillin, the application of warm compresses, rest, and pain medication (if necessary).

Poor Early Weight Gain

Breast-fed full-term infants may **lose as much as 10% of their birthweight** during the first several days of life, but they should regain it by 7 to 10 days of age. Weight loss of $\geq 10\%$ of birthweight should prompt a reevaluation of the infant and breast-feeding technique, with improvement documented prior to discharge.

Follow-Up of the Breast-Fed Infant

An evaluation by a pediatrician or health professional at 3 to 5 days of age is important to catch any problems early. This visit should include an infant weight and physical examination, with emphasis on hydration status and jaundice. The mother should be questioned regarding:

- The frequency and duration of nursing sessions.
- Signs of established lactation (i.e., diminished breast fullness after nursing, leaking, cessation of nipple discomfort after latching on, uterine cramps during nursing).
- Normal infant voiding (minimum of four to six times per day, pale urine). Note: The baby may void twice between diaper changes so the number of voidings may vary.
- Normal infant defecation (three to four loose stools per day on days 3 to 4, four to six loose stools per day on days 4 to 6, eight to ten loose stools per day during weeks 2 to 4).
- Infant response to feeding (e.g., sleepy, satisfied).

According to Lawrence (6th ed., 2005), these are the most common factors associated with poor early weight gain:

- Ineffective breast-feeding technique
- Infrequent or inappropriately short feedings (e.g., excessive nighttime intervals)
- Water supplementation
- Maternal problems that inhibit milk letdown

BOTTLE-FEEDING

Patient Counseling

Bottle-Feeding Technique

The bottle should be held so no air enters the nipple, and the bottle should never be propped. Prop feeding is associated with a significantly higher risk of otitis media.

Feeding Frequency and Intake

Formula can be given **every 3 to 4 hours.** A small-for-gestational-age infant may require small frequent feedings until his gastric capacity increases, whereas a large-for-gestational-age infant of a mother with diabetes should be given early and frequent feedings, and his blood sugar should be monitored carefully to reduce the risk of hypoglycemia.

The typical full-term neonate drinks only 15 to 30 mL (0.5 to 1 oz) per feeding during the first few days of life. The mother should be assured that this is sufficient because of stores acquired in utero. She should be told to expect an **intake of 2 to 4 oz per feeding** (approximately every 3 to 4 hours) **by the end of the first week.**

Formula Types

Tables 6-3 and 6-4 list the specific compositions of many commonly available infant formulas. Whole cow's milk should not be introduced until 1 year of age.

Cow's Milk–Based Formulas

Full-term (standard) formulas, which provide 20 kcal/oz, are generally suitable for infants with **birthweights >2,000 g,** most **full-term small-for-gestational-age** infants.

Soy-Based (Lactose-Free) Formulas

Soy-based formulas are indicated for infants with **temporary or chronic lactose intolerance** and for infants with **galactosemia.** They are also often used when intolerance to cow's milk protein is suspected. However, the use of soy-based formula in this situation is not generally recommended because of a significant antigenic crossover between cow's milk protein and soy protein. Soy-based formulas are **not recommended for prolonged use in preterm infants** because the phytate content may lead to hypophosphatemia and rickets.

Preterm Formulas

The advantages of breast milk are even more significant for preterm infants because of the anti-infectious properties and easy digestibility

TABLE 6-3 Composition of Infant Formulas

A: Term Formulas

Product (Manufacturer)	Kcal/oz	Carbohydrate (g/100 mL)	Protein (g/100 mL)	Fat (g/100 mL)	Fe mg/100 mL	mOsm kg water
Mature human milk	20	Lactose (7.2)	mature human breast milk (casein, whey) (1.1)	mature human breast milk (3.9)	0.3	290
Enfamil Lipil (Mead Johnson)	20	Lactose (7.3)	Whey Nonfat milk (1.5)	Palmolein, coconut, soy, high-oleic sunflower oils <1% DHA/ARA (3.6)	1.26	300
Similac Advance (Ross)	20	Lactose (7.3)	Nonfat milk Whey concentrate (1.4)	Coconut, soy oils, high-oleic safflower oils <1% DHA/ARA (3.7)	1.2	300
Similac Advance Organic (Ross)	20	Lactose Maltodextrin Evaporated cane juice (7.2)	Nonfat milk (whey) (1.4)	Coconut, soy oils, high-oleic safflower oils <1% DHA/ARA (3.6)	1.2	225
Good Start Supreme (Nestle)	20	Lactose 70% Maltodextrin 30% (7.5)	Whey protein concentrate hydrolysate (1.5)	Palmolein, coconut, soy, high-oleic sunflower oils, <1% DHA/ARA (3.4)	1.0	265
Good Start Supreme with probiotics (Nestle)	20	Lactose 70% Maltodextrin 30% (7.5)	Whey protein concentrate hydrolysate (1.5)	Palmolein, coconut, soy, high-oleic sunflower oils <1% DHA/ARA (3.4)	1.0	250
Bright Beginnings (milk based)	20	Lactose (7.1)	Whey concentrate and nonfat milk (1.5)	High-oleic sunflower, safflower, palm olein, and coconut oils (3.5)	1.2	300
Bright Beginnings (organic milk based)	20	Lactose (7.0)	Whey concentrate and nonfat milk (1.5)	High-oleic sunflower, safflower, palm olein, and coconut oils (3.5)	1.2	274

B: Soy Formulas

Product (Manufacturer)	Kcal/oz	Carbohydrate (g/100 mL)	Protein (g/100 mL)	Fat (g/100 mL)	Fe mg/100 mL	mOsm kg water
Isomil Advance (Ross)	20	Corn syrup and sucrose (6.8)	Soy protein isolate, L-methionine (1.7)	High-oleic safflower, coconut, and soy oils <1% DHA/ARA (3.7)	1.22	230
ProSobee Lipil (Mead Johnson)	20	Corn syrup solids (7.3)	Soy protein isolate, L-methionine (1.7)	Palmolein, coconut, soy, and high-oleic sunflower oils <1% DHA/ARA (3.7)	1.28	200
Bright Beginnings Soy	20	Corn syrup and sucrose (6.9)	Soy protein isolate, L-methionine (1.8)	Palmolein, coconut, soy, and high-oleic sunflower oils Source DHA/ARA? (3.5)	1.2	162

C: Additives

Product (Manufacturer)	Kcal/oz	Carbohydrate (g/100 mL)	Protein (g/100 mL)	Fat (g/100 mL)	Fe mg/100 mL	mOsm kg water
Similac Human Milk Fortifier (per 4 packets) (Ross)	Adds 4 cal/oz fortifier	Corn syrup solids (1.8)	Nonfat dry milk and whey protein concentrate (1.0)	MCT oil and lecithin (0.36)	0.35	Adds 90 (385 total)
Prolact Plus 4 (20:80 to maternal BM) (Prolacta)	Adds 4 cal/oz; includes human milk	Lactose (7.0)	Human milk (2.5)	Human milk (4.8)	0.3	331
MCT oil (Novartis)	Adds 7.3 cal/mL	None	None	MCT oil		
Microlipid (Novartis)	Additive 4.5 cal/mL	None	None	Safflower oil emulsion		

(Continued)

TABLE 6-3 Composition of Infant Formulas (*continued*)

C: Additives

Product (Manufacturer)	Kcal/oz	Carbohydrate (g/100 mL)	Protein (g/100 mL)	Fat (g/100 mL)	Fe mg/100 mL	mOsm kg water
Beneprotein (Novartis)	Add 22 cal/r scoop = 1.5 Tbsp	None	Whey protein isolate lecithin (6.0)	None		
Polycose (Ross)	Add 23 cal/Tbsp	Glucose polymers (5.8)	None	None		
Duocal (Nutricia)	Add 42 cal/Tbsp	Hydrolyzed cornstarch (5.8)	None	Corn, coconut, MCT oil (1.8)		
Rice cereal (per Tbsp)	Adds 9 cal/Tbsp	Rice starch (1.9)	None	None		

D: Premature Formulas

Product (Manufacturer)	Kcal/oz	Carbohydrate (g/100 mL)	Protein (g/100 mL)	Fat (g/100 mL)	Fe mg/100 mL	mOsm kg water
Preterm Human Milk	20	Lactose (6.6)	Human milk (1.4)	Human milk (3.9)	1.2	290
Enfamil Premature Lipil 20 (Mead Johnson)	20	Corn syrup solids and lactose (7.5)	Whey and nonfat milk (2.0)	MCT, soy, and coconut oils <1% DHA/ARA (3.5)	1.2	260
Enfamil Premature Lipil 24 (Mead Johnson)	24	Corn syrup solids and lactose (9.0)	Whey and nonfat milk (2.4)	MCT, soy, and coconut oils <1% DHA/ARA (4.1)	1.5	310
Similac Special Care Advance 20 (Ross)	20	Corn syrup solids and lactose (7.0)	Nonfat milk and whey protein concentrate (2.0)	MCT, soy, and coconut oils <1% DHA/ARA (3.7)	1.22	235

Product (Manufacturer)	Kcal/oz	Carbohydrate (g/100 mL)	Protein (g/100 mL)	Fat (g/100 mL)	Fe mg/100 mL	mOsm kg water
Similac Special Care Advance 24 (Ross)	24	Corn syrup solids and lactose (8.4)	Nonfat milk and whey protein concentrate (2.4)	MCT, soy, and coconut oils <1% DHA/ARA (4.4)	1.46	282
Similac Special Care Advance 30 (Ross)	30	Corn syrup solids and lactose (7.8)	Nonfat milk and whey protein concentrate (3.0)	MCT 50%, soy 30%, and coconut oils 18% remainder DHA/ARA (6.7)	1.83	325
Enfacare Lipil (Mead Johnson)	22	Corn syrup solids and lactose (7.9)	Whey concentrate and nonfat milk (2.1)	Soy, high-oleic sunflower, MCT 20%, and coconut oils <1% DHA/ARA (3.9)	1.3	260
Neosure Advance (Ross)	22	Corn syrup solids and lactose (7.5)	Whey concentrate and nonfat milk (2.1)	Soy, high-oleic safflower, MCT 25%, and coconut oils <1% DHA/ARA (4.1)	1.34	250

E: Formulas with Protein Alterations

Product (Manufacturer)	Kcal/oz	Carbohydrate (g/100 mL)	Protein (g/100 mL)	Fat (g/100 mL)	Fe mg/100 mL	mOsm kg water
Alimentum Advance (Ross)	20	Sucrose, modified tapioca starch (6.8)	Casein hydrolysate, L-Cysteine, L-Tyrosine, L-Tryptophan, L-Methionine (1.8)	Safflower, MCT, and soy oils <1% DHA/ARA (3.7)	1.2	370
Nutramigen Lipil (Mead Johnson)	20	Sucrose, modified cornstarch (7.5)	Casein hydrolysate, L-Cysteine, L-Tyrosine, L-Tryptophan (1.9)	Palmolein, soy, coconut, and high-oleic sunflower oils (3.4)	1.22	260
Pregestimil Lipil (Mead Johnson)	20	Sucrose, modified cornstarch, and dextrose (6.9)	Casein hydrolysate, L-Cysteine, L-Tyrosine, L-Tryptophan (1.9)	MCT, corn, and high-oleic oil, soy oil <1% DHA/ARA (3.8)	1.28	340
EleCare (Ross)	20	Corn syrup solids (7.1)	L-Amino acids (2.0)	MCT, high-oleic safflower oil, soy oil (3.2)	1.2	350

(Continued)

TABLE 6-3 Composition of Infant Formulas (*continued*)

E: Formulas with Protein Alterations

Product (Manufacturer)	Kcal/oz	Carbohydrate (g/100 mL)	Protein (g/100 mL)	Fat (g/100 mL)	Fe mg/100 mL	mOsm kg water
Neocate with DHA/ARA (Nutricia)	20	Corn syrup solids (7.8)	L-Amino acids (2.1)	Hybrid safflower oil and refined vegetable (coconut and soya-distilled) oil <1% DHA/ARA (3.1)	1.2	375

F: "Gentle" Formulas

Product (Manufacturer)	Kcal/oz	Carbohydrate (g/100 mL)	Protein (g/100 mL)	Fat (g/100 mL)	Fe mg/100 mL	mOsm kg water
Enfamil Lipil Gentlease (Mead Johnson)	20	Corn syrup solids, lactose 25% (7.2)	Partially hydrolyzed nonfat milk, whey protein concentrate solids (1.5)	Palmolein, coconut, soy, and high-oleic sunflower oils source DHA/ARA (3.5)	1.2	220
Enfamil Lipil AR (Mead Johnson)	20	Rice starch, lactose, and maltodextrin (7.4)	Nonfat milk (1.7)	Palmolein, coconut, soy, and high-oleic sunflower oils source DHA/ARA (3.5)	1.2	230
Enfamil Lipil LactoFree (Mead Johnson)	20	Corn syrup solids (7.3)	Milk-protein isolate (1.4)	Palmolein, coconut, soy, and high-oleic sunflower oils source DHA/ARA (3.5)	1.2	200
Similac Sensitive RS Advance (Ross)	20	Corn syrup solids, rice starch, sucrose (7.1)	Milk-protein isolate (1.4)	Soy oil, coconut oil, high-oleic safflower <1% source DHA/ARA (3.6)	1.2	180

					Fe	mOsm
Similac Sensitive (Ross)	20	Corn maltodextrin, sucrose (7.1)	Milk-protein isolate (1.4)	Soy oil, coconut oil, high-oleic safflower <1% source DHA/ARA (3.6)	1.2	200
Bright Beginnings Gentle (Bright Beginnings)	20	Corn syrup solids, lactose 25% (7.2)	Whey protein hydrolysate nonfat milk 1.5	Palmolein, coconut, soy, and high-oleic sunflower oils source DHA/ARA (3.5)	1.2	184

G: Special Formulas

Product (Manufacturer)	Kcal/oz	Carbohydrate (g/100 mL)	Protein (g/100 mL)	Fat (g/100 mL)	Fe mg/100 mL	mOsm kg water
Monogen (Nutricia)	20	Corn syrup solids (10.8)	Whey concentrate (1.8)	MCT (90%) and LCT (10%) fractionated coconut oil, walnut oil (1.9)	0.7	227
Portagen (Mead Johnson)	20	Corn syrup solids and sucrose (7.7)	Sodium caseinate (2.3)	MCT (85%) and corn oil (3.2)	1.3	230

TABLE 6-4 Indications for Infant Formulas

Maternal breast milk:

- Best choice for most term infants

Term Infants (If Breast Milk Not Used)

Cow's Milk–based Standard Formulas

- Enfamil LIPIL
- Similac Advance or Similac Advance Organic
- Good Start Supreme with or without probiotics
- Bright Beginnings or Bright Beginnings Organic

Lactose-free Cow's Milk–based Formulas

For short-term diarrhea or lactose intolerance:

- Enfamil LIPIL LactoFree
- Similac Sensitive Advance

For term infants sensitive to lactose or fully intact protein:

- Enfamil LIPIL
- Gentlease
- Bright Beginnings Gentle

For term infants with uncomplicated reflux:

- Enfamil LIPIL AR
- Similac Sensitive RS Advance

Soy Formulas

For infants with primary or secondary lactose intolerance or galactosemia:

- Bright Beginnings Soy
- Isomil Advance
- ProSobee LIPIL

Altered Protein Formulas

- Casein hydrolysates

Altered Protein Formulas Without MCT

For infants sensitive to casein and soy protein/milk-protein allergy:

- Nutramigen LIPIL

Altered Protein Formulas with MCT

For infants with abnormal absorption, digestion and transport, intractable diarrhea:

- Pregestimil LIPIL
- Alimentum Advance

Altered Protein Formulas: Elemental

- Amino acid formulas

Altered Protein Formulas: Elemental with Low MCT

For severe allergy:

- Neocate with DHA/ARA

(Continued)

Altered Protein Formulas: Elemental with High MCT

For severe allergy also with abnormal absorption, digestion and transport, intractable diarrhea:

- EleCare

Preterm Formulas

For preterm infants with need for increased protein, calcium, and phosphate needs:

- Enfamil Premature LIPIL 20
- Similac Special Care 20

For preterm infants with need for increased calories, protein, calcium, and phosphate needs:

- Enfamil Premature LIPIL 24
- Similac Special Care 24

Fluid-restricted preterm infants with need for increased calories, protein, calcium, and phosphate:

- Similac Special Care 30

Preterm Transitional Formulas

Nutrient enriched for preterm infants after hospital discharge (22 cal/oz):

- EnfaCare LIPIL
- NeoSure Advance

Preterm Fortifiers

For preterm infants on breast milk with need for increased calories, protein and electrolytes:

- Similac Human Milk Fortifier
- Enfamil Human Milk Fortifier
- Prolact Plus 4

of breast milk. If breast milk is not available, preterm formulas should be used. These formulas, available as 20, 24, or 30 kcal/oz, are specially designed to meet the needs of preterm infants. These can be mixed in different caloric concentrations to meet the nutritional needs of individual infants. They should be used until the infant reaches 40 weeks post-conception (or longer, if the infant's birthweight is <1,000 g). Transitional formulas providing 22 kcal/oz are available and should be used for preterm infants until 9 to 12 months of adjusted age.

Dietary Calorie Supplementation

Caloric supplements are often required for infants with higher-than-usual caloric needs, decreased oral intake, decreased fluid tolerance, or a combination of these factors (e.g., preterm infants, infants with bronchopulmonary dysplasia, infants with congestive heart failure). Care should be taken to maintain the **correct balance of nutrients.** In general, the first step to increase calories should be to increase the concentration of the formula by adding less water to the powder or liquid concentrate. **Careful instructions must be given to the parents to ensure the correct amount of water is added.**

Multinutritional Supplements

These supplements include calories from a combination of sources (e.g., fat and carbohydrate). Examples include Human Milk Fortifier (Mead Johnson, Ross), Duocal, formula concentrates, and Prolact Plus 4 (concentrated human milk that is extremely expensive).

Carbohydrate

Carbohydrate supplements (e.g., Polycose, corn syrup) are **well tolerated** and **inexpensive** but **low in caloric and nutrient density.** Polycose and corn syrup may cause diarrhea if >2 mL/oz of formula are given. Polycose liquid provides 2 kcal/mL. Polycose powder provides 8 kcal/5 mL.

Fat

Fat supplements are **high in caloric density.** The best-tolerated form, **microlipids** (1 mL/oz of formula), is **more expensive** and **lower in caloric density** than inexpensive, less well-tolerated vegetable oil, which may cause diarrhea. Vegetable oil is also harder to keep mixed with the formula. MCT (medium chain triglycerides) oil, another option, should be reserved for specific indications, such as short-bowel syndrome and malabsorption. It is expensive and can cause diarrhea. Microlipids supply 4.5 kcal/mL, MCT oil supplies 7.6 kcal/mL, and vegetable oil supplies 9 kcal/mL. Note that increasing fat in the formula may slow gastric emptying time.

Protein

Protein supplements are usually **well tolerated** but of relatively **low caloric density. They are generally indicated only for patients with specific malabsorption or food allergies.** Casec provides 17 kcal/15 mL.

Vitamin-Mineral Supplements

Vitamins

Vitamin supplementation is **not required** for healthy, full-term formula-fed infants with normal intake (>200 mL/day) of a vitamin-D fortified formula. Formula-fed infants with specific medical problems, such as malabsorption, may require vitamin supplementation. ADEK is often used for this purpose. **It is recommended that breast-fed infants receive 200 IU/day of vitamin D starting within the first 2 months of life.**

An infant multivitamin such as Tri-Vi-Sol (200 IU/0.5 mL) can be used to provide this.

Fluoride

Fluoride supplementation (0.25 mg/day) is indicated **after 6 months** of age for **all breast-fed infants,** as well as for **formula-fed infants** who are given formula that is reconstituted using nonfluoridated water or who are fed ready-to-feed formula. Nonfluoridated toothpaste should be used for children up to 2 years of age to avoid excessive fluoride intake.

Iron

Formula-fed infants (<1 year of age) should be fed an iron-fortified formula. This is also the formula that should be used for the breast-fed infant <1 year needing a milk supplement. Iron supplementation (10 mg daily) is recommended for full-term breast-fed infants after 6 months of age. This can be provided either by iron-fortified infant cereal or by elemental iron (alone or in a multivitamin preparation). Preterm breast-fed infants generally require iron supplements of 2 mg/kg per day until 1 year of age.

SOLID FOODS

Solid foods are typically introduced to the infant's diet at **6 months of age.** Foods can be introduced earlier (4 to 5 months of age) if the infant seems to require >32 oz/day of formula.

Initially, small volumes of solid foods are provided once daily. The volume is gradually increased, and the frequency is increased to three times daily with some snacks. **Formula or breast milk** remains the basis of the infant's diet **throughout the first year of life** and should be maintained at 24 to 32 oz/day.

The order in which foods are introduced varies widely across cultural groups and is based more on tradition than on science. Table 6-5 offers a suggested schedule for introducing solid foods. **Parents who opt to make their own baby food should be counseled to use the food within 24 hours or freeze it to avoid the danger of a high nitrite content. This is particularly relevant for carrots and beets.**

> **HINT:** Certain foods (e.g., raisins, nuts, popcorn, hard candy, hot dogs, raw carrots, hard teething biscuits, and grapes) should be avoided because of the risk of choking. No honey should be given for the first year of life because of the increased risk of infant botulism.

TABLE 6-5 Suggested Schedule for Introducing Solid Foods

Baby's Age	Appropriate Solid Foods
6–8 months	Iron-fortified infant cereal* mixed with breast milk, water, or juice to a mustard-like consistency and offered on a small spoon (not in a bottle); rice, oatmeal, and barley varieties should be introduced before the mixed type. Pureed meats,*† fruits, and vegetables Note: Meats first for breast-fed infants, cereal first for formula-fed infants
7–9 months	Plain yogurt, cottage cheese Well-cooked vegetables and pasta Soft "finger foods" (e.g., banana chunks, pancakes). Cheerios, fruit and veggies "puffs," crackers Tofu, refried beans Introduce cup: water; limit juice to 4 oz/day Eat together as a family
9–12 months	Decrease pureed foods and increase soft table foods
>12 months	Switch from formula to whole cow's milk (do not use low-fat or skim milk until 2 years of age) Can introduce foods with higher allergenic potential (e.g., egg whites, citrus fruits, chocolate, berries); Continue to avoid peanut products until 3 years of age Continue breast-feeding; wean from bottle Avoid soda or sweetened drinks

*The order is not important, as long as there is a 2- to 3-day interval between new foods to identify any food intolerances.
†Most infants dislike plain pureed meats (a good source of iron, protein, and calories) but accept them if mixed with other foods.

SPECIAL CONSIDERATIONS FOR PRETERM INFANTS

Calorie Requirements

Healthy preterm infants usually grow well with a diet that provides 110 to 130 kcal/kg per day. Infants with complications (e.g., pulmonary bronchodysplasia, congestive heart failure) frequently require 130 to 180 kcal/kg per day, titrated to achieve adequate growth.

To increase caloric intake, it is necessary to increase the feeding volume (if fluid restriction is not a concern), the caloric density of the feedings, or both. If it is necessary to increase the feeding volume but the infant is unable to consume the increased volume, supplemental feedings can be provided through a nasogastric or orogastric tube.

Most preterm infants initially require a caloric density of at least 24 kcal/oz (the density of most preterm formulas). Increased caloric density can be achieved by adding water to 30 kcal/oz preterm formula concentrate until it provides 24 to 27 kcal/oz. Additional increases in caloric density can be achieved by adding caloric supplements (see section on Dietary Calorie Supplementation).

Breast Milk

Breast milk provides a low renal solute load and excellent digestibility and absorption. **In smaller preterm infants, supplementation of breast milk is necessary for long-term growth.** Breast-milk fortifiers developed for supplementation include Enfamil Human Milk Fortifier (Mead Johnson) and Similac Human Milk Fortifier (Ross). Both increase the calories, protein, minerals (particularly calcium and phosphorus), and vitamins of human milk to the levels required for preterm infants. These fortifiers are expensive and difficult to obtain outside of the hospital. If bovine fortifier is not tolerated by the infant, ProLact Plus fortifier can be used. This is concentrated, pasteurized human milk. Note that the cost of this fortifier is approximately 50 times that of the bovine fortifiers!

> **HINT:** An inexpensive alternative for the infant who still requires a caloric density of 24 kcal/oz after hospital discharge is to supplement breast milk with full-term formula (1 tsp formula powder to 3 oz of breast milk) or with transitional formula (Neosure or Enfacare) powder (1 tsp powder to 3 oz breast milk). Breast-milk feedings can also be alternated with 24 or 27 kcal/oz formula feedings.

Formula

Preterm infant formulas (see Table 6-3) should be used for **all preterm infants with a birthweight <2,000 g who are not breast-fed** until the infant reaches the 40-week postconception mark. EnfaCare (Mead Johnson) or Neosure, special formulas designed to be consumed by the preterm infant from the time of hospital discharge until the postconceptional (adjusted) age of 9 months to 1 year, provide the extra calories and minerals these infants need.

Solid Foods

Assuming the baby's oral motor skills are normal, solid foods can be introduced to the preterm infant following the **same recommendations as those for full-term infants,** using the postmenstrual (adjusted) age. Abnormal oral motor skills and other feeding disorders are relatively common in the preterm population; therefore, the baby's **feeding skills should be assessed** carefully for both liquid and solid feedings.

References for Breast-Feeding Mothers

Huggins K: *The Nursing Mother's Companion: Revised Edition.* Boston, Harvard Common Press, 2005.

Eiger MS, Olds SW: *The Complete Book of Breast-Feeding: Revised Edition.* New York, Workman, 1999.

Suggested Readings

American Academy of Pediatrics, Committee on Drugs: The transfer of drugs and other chemicals into human breast milk. *Pediatrics* 108(3):776–789, 2001.

American Academy of Pediatrics, Committee on Nutrition: Hypoallergenic infant formulas. *Pediatrics* 106(2):346–349, 2000.

American Academy of Pediatrics, Committee on Nutrition: *Pediatric Nutrition Handbook*, 5th ed. Elk Grove Village, IL, American Academy of Pediatrics, 2004.

American Academy of Pediatrics, Committee on Nutrition: Soy protein based formulas: recommendations for use in infant feeding. *Pediatrics* 101(1):148–153, 1998.

American Academy of Pediatrics, Section on Breastfeeding: Breastfeeding and the use of human milk. *Pediatrics* 115(2): 496–506, 2005.

Bernbaum JC, Hoffman-Williamson M: *Primary Care of the Preterm Infant*. St. Louis, Mosby, 1991.

Gartner LM, Greer FR, Section on Breastfeeding and Committee on Nutrition: Prevention of rickets and vitamin D deficiency: new guidelines for vitamin D intake. *Pediatrics* 111(4):908–910, 2003.

Groh-Wargo S (ed): *Nutritional Care for High Risk Newborns*, 3rd ed. Chicago, Precept Press, 2000.

Hale T: *Medications and Mothers' Milk*, 12th ed. Amarillo, TX, Pharmasoft, 2006.

Lawrence RA: *Breastfeeding: A Guide for the Medical Profession*, 6th ed. St. Louis, Mosby, 2005.

Lemons P, Stuart M, Lemons JA: Breast-feeding the premature infant. *Clin Perinatol* 13:111–122, 1994.

Schanler RJ, Shulman RJ, Lau C: Feeding strategies for premature infants: beneficial outcomes of feeding fortified human milk versus preterm formula. *Pediatrics* 103:1150–1157, 1999.

Useful Websites

http://www.eatright.org (The American Dietetic Association)
http://www.cdc.gov (The Centers for Disease Control and Prevention: growth charts)
http://www.meadjohnson.com
http://www.rosspediatris.com
http://www.nestle.com

7 | *Well-Newborn Care*
Andria Barnes Ruth and Kathleen Wholey Zsolway

INTRODUCTION

The birth of a new baby is a marvelous time for a family, full of excitement as well as some uncertainty as the amazing journey of child-rearing begins. The well-newborn visits are an opportunity for parents to ask questions regarding the health and development of their baby. These visits enable the physician to **assess the baby's health, growth, and development** and offer guidance to parents throughout their baby's early years. Parents are often given **reassurance** about many aspects of normal newborn physical findings and development. This chapter describes the concerns most frequently encountered during the well-newborn visits.

NEWBORN SCREENING TESTS

Capillary blood from a heelstick is obtained from every infant after 24 hours of age and prior to discharge from the hospital, with the ideal age being between 2 and 4 days of age. This blood is sent for newborn screening tests, which look for a variety of **metabolic and genetic disorders.** The specific tests vary by state, but all states test for congenital hypothyroidism, phenylketonuria (PKU), hemoglobinopathies (sickle cell disease, sickle C disease, and thalassemia), and galactosemia. The *majority* of states screen for biotinidase deficiency and congenital adrenal hyperplasia. New techniques in mass spectroscopy have enabled a majority of states to test for fatty acid disorders (such as medium-chain acyl-coenzyme A dehydrogenase deficiency), organic acid disorders (including methylmalonic academia), and amino acid disorders such as tyrosinemia and homocystinuria. Selected states also screen for glucose-6-phosphatase deficiency (G6PD), toxoplasmosis, and cystic fibrosis.

Follow-up of abnormal newborn screening tests, with appropriate and timely confirmatory testing, referral, and care, requires close cooperation among the primary pediatrician and the birth hospital, state newborn screening laboratory, and appropriate subspecialists in endocrinology, metabolism, or hematology.

SKIN

Generalized Rashes

Neonatal rashes are a common cause of concern for parents. A full discussion of rashes occurring in infancy is provided in Chapter 64, "Rashes."

Diaper Dermatitis (Diaper Rash)

Diaper dermatitis is a common problem presenting in infancy. Multiple conditions can predispose an infant to diaper rash, including sensitive skin, moisture trapped by a diaper, and the acid-base balance of stool and urine. Parents should be advised that **prevention is the best cure.** The diaper area should be kept as dry as possible; frequent diaper changes decrease the occurrence of diaper dermatitis. Parents should also be instructed to leave the perineal area open to air as much as possible and apply a barrier cream to protect against local irritation.

Physical examination allows for the diagnosis of some of the more common skin irritations in the diaper area.

- **Irritant contact dermatitis** appears as erythema with shallow ulcerations predominantly located on the buttocks, thighs, abdomen, and perianal area, sparing the creases. The diagnosis is made clinically, and treatment involves elimination of the irritant, use of a barrier cream, and exposure of the area to air as much as possible.
- **Candida diaper dermatitis** can appear at any age and is characterized by beefy red, scaly plaques with satellite lesions, papules, and pustules. Diagnosis is most often made clinically on the basis of the characteristic appearance of the skin; however, a potassium hydroxide (KOH) preparation would demonstrate the presence of yeast. Treatment involves application of a topical antifungal agent (e.g., nystatin or clotrimazole ointment) and exposure of the perineal area to air.

Mongolian Spots (Congenital Dermal Melanocytosis)

Mongolian spots are **blue-gray macules** that are most commonly seen in Asian, Hispanic, and African American infants. They are typically a few centimeters in diameter and located on the buttocks and lumbosacral area; less commonly, they may be much larger or located on the face or extremities. They typically disappear by 7 to 13 years of age, but some lesions (particularly the larger ones) persist into adulthood.

Salmon Patch (Nevus Simplex, Telangiectatic Nevus)

A salmon patch is a congenital vascular abnormality that involves the eyelids, glabella, forehead, or occiput. It consists of **smooth pink or red macular lesions,** often accompanied by telangiectasia. Salmon patches on the glabellar region or upper eyelids usually disappear by 1 year of age, whereas those on the nape of the neck persist approximately 50% of the time.

Café-au-Lait Macules

Café-au-lait macules are **pale brown macules with irregular margins** that range in size from 2 mm to 2 cm. They may appear at birth or in early childhood. Isolated café-au-lait macules occur in 10% to 20% of the normal population. The presence of six or more café-au-lait macules >5 mm prior to puberty in combination with one of the following additional criteria are diagnostic of neurofibromatosis: two or more neurofibromas, axillary or inguinal freckling, optic glioma, Lisch nodules (iris hamartoma), osseous lesions, or a first-degree relative with neurofibromatosis.

CRANIUM

Fontanelles

There are commonly two palpable fontanelles, the **anterior fontanelle** and the **posterior fontanelle.** The anterior fontanelle may minimally increase in size immediately after birth but then gradually decreases in size and is generally closed by 6 to 18 months of age. The posterior fontanelle is generally smaller than the anterior fontanelle and usually closed to palpation by 4 months of age.

Caput Succedaneum

A caput succedaneum is a **diffuse swelling of the soft tissue of the scalp,** usually involving the presenting portion of the head during a vertex delivery. The edema, which is evident during the first few hours of life, crosses suture lines and may cross the midline. In uncomplicated cases of caput succedaneum, no specific treatment is needed; the swelling resolves during the first few days of life. In rare instances, a hemorrhagic caput may occur and cause shock secondary to loss of circulating blood volume. In this instance, blood transfusion and circulatory support are needed. Extensive ecchymoses may result in hyperbilirubinemia, necessitating phototherapy. Molding of the head and overriding of the parietal bones is often associated with a caput succedaneum; however, these conditions resolve during the first few weeks of life.

Cephalohematoma

A cephalohematoma is a **subperiosteal hemorrhage** that results in swelling limited in distribution to one cranial bone (i.e., the swelling does not cross suture lines). Subperiosteal bleeding is a slow process; therefore, the cephalohematoma may not be evident until several hours after birth. A skull fracture, usually linear, may be an associated finding. Most cephalohematomas are resorbed between the ages of 2 weeks and 3 months of age. In some cases, a bony protuberance remains. Despite this residual calcification, no specific treatment is recommended.

Molding

Asymmetry in the appearance of the cranium, known as molding or positional plagiocephaly, results from the gentle application of asymmetric pressure on the cranial bones, which occurs when an infant spends a significant portion of time in the same position. The incidence of this condition has increased markedly since implementation of the recommendation to place infants to sleep in a supine position. Infants with asymmetric plagiocephaly should be examined carefully for the presence of **torticollis,** which manifests as decreased range of motion of the neck and head tilt to one side. Affected infants may have a characteristic mass in the affected sternocleidomastoid muscle. Positional plagiocephaly can be managed by environmental manipulation and repositioning the infant to eliminate asymmetric pressure. In cases where torticollis is present, passive stretching is also recommended. In severe cases, cranial molding helmet therapy may be prescribed to diminish the asymmetry.

Craniosynostosis (premature closure of a suture) is another cause of progressive cranial asymmetry. Positional plagiocephaly can generally be differentiated from craniosynostosis by clinical features. When the diagnosis is not apparent clinically, conventional skull radiographs can be performed. However, computed tomography (including three-dimensional surface reconstruction) is more informative and used to delineate the extent of craniosynostosis as well as to evaluate intracranial structures. In the event of craniosynostosis, neurosurgical intervention is indicated because of the possibility of asymmetric brain growth and compression of intracranial structures.

EYES

Eye Color

Eye color is a frequent question posed by parents. Eye color is usually established by 3 to 6 months of age; however, additional iris pigmentation continues throughout the first year of life. Depth of eye color may not be evident until the first birthday.

Strabismus

During the newborn period, the eyes frequently wander. However, the **wandering should diminish** (until it eventually disappears) within the first 2 to 3 months of life. Intermittent or persistent esotropia or exotropia after the age of 3 months warrants an evaluation by an ophthalmologist.

Nasolacrimal Duct Obstruction

The lacrimal system develops fully over the first 3 to 4 years of life. The lacrimal glands begin to produce tears by week 3 or 4 of life. In approximately 6% of newborns, one or both of the lacrimal ducts is blocked, preventing drainage of tears.

Affected children appear to have **excessive tearing.** Therapy entails gentle massage of the lacrimal duct in a downward direction and the use of a warm wet cloth to wipe the collection of tears and mucus from the eye. Most (approximately 90%) blocked lacrimal ducts open spontaneously by 6 months of age. Of those that are still blocked at 1 year of age, <1% open spontaneously. Thus children with persistent lacrimal duct obstruction beyond 6 to 12 months of age should be evaluated by an ophthalmologist. Parents should be cautioned to call the pediatrician if the conjunctiva becomes red, if the eye discharge becomes purulent, or if the area surrounding the eye or the medial aspect of the nose becomes swollen. These physical findings may indicate conjunctivitis, ophthalmia neonatorum, or dacryocystitis (see Chapter 65, "Red Eye").

EARS

Hearing

Significant bilateral hearing loss (>35 Db) is present in 1 to 3 per 1,000 well newborns and in 2 to 4 per 1,000 infants in the intensive care unit. Because auditory stimulation during the first 6 months of life is very important for the development of speech and language skills, significant hearing loss that goes undetected can impede speech, language, *and* cognitive development. **Universal hearing screening** should occur prior to discharge from the hospital, with appropriate rescreening for those who do not pass the initial test. For infants with significant hearing loss, audiologic and medical evaluations should be performed before 3 months of age, and intensive interventions should be implemented before 6 months of age.

ORAL CAVITY

Teeth

Primary teeth eruption typically occurs at the age of 6 months (range, 3 to 16 months). Natal teeth are teeth present at or shortly after birth. These teeth are generally poorly formed with thin enamel and poor attachments and often located at the end of a stalk of uncalcified tissue. The **natal teeth often are primary teeth that have erupted early.** If removed, spacing of the secondary teeth may be affected; therefore, removal of the natal teeth is recommended only if they are a significant irritant to the tongue, if they present a danger of aspiration secondary to their poor attachment, or if they interfere with feeding.

Dental Lumina Cysts, Bohn Nodules, and Epstein Pearls

Dental lumina cysts are clear or bluish fluid-filled sacs located bilaterally or quadrilaterally on the gum surfaces. These cysts are generally not painful, do not interfere with feeding, and are not associated with surrounding erythema. They disappear within a few weeks and do not require any intervention.

Yellowish white cysts composed of islands of epithelial cells are termed **Bohn nodules** when they are located on the alveolar ridge and **Epstein pearls** when they are located near the midpalatal raphe at the junction of the hard and soft palate. These cysts require no treatment and commonly disappear within a few weeks.

Thrush

White patches in the mouth of an infant may indicate the presence of thrush, a fairly common infection caused by *Candida albicans*. Unlike residual breast milk or formula, these white patches cannot be easily wiped from the oral mucosa or tongue surface. When thrush is removed from the oral mucosa, the exposed mucosa is typically red and raw and may bleed. Treatment consists of the use of a topical antifungal agent (e.g., nystatin oral suspension). Care should be taken to avoid reinfection from nipples and pacifiers by resterilizing or replacing these items.

CHEST

Breast Hypertrophy and Galactorrhea

Breast buds are present in most infants (both male and female) born after 36 weeks of gestation.

- **Breast hypertrophy** results from the passage of maternal hormones across the placenta during gestation.
- **Galactorrhea** occurs in up to 6% of normal-term infants and typically occurs in infants with larger breast nodules. The thin milky discharge may be caused by maternal estrogen or neonatal prolactin.

Generally, both breast hypertrophy and galactorrhea resolve within several weeks, but occasionally they can persist for several months.

Mastitis

Mastitis, which can manifest as cellulitis or an abscess, occurs in newborns when bacteria invade the already hypertrophied breast tissue. *Staphylococcus aureus* is the most frequently involved organism, but 5% to 10% of infections are caused by Gram-negative enteric bacteria.

Typically, the breast bud is erythematous, enlarged, warm, and tender; purulent drainage from the nipple may be present. Infants usually appear well, with only 25% presenting with fever or ill appearance. After obtaining appropriate cultures (including culture of the purulent nipple drainage), the infant should be treated with intravenous antibiotics. Occasionally, a fluctuant abscess forms, requiring surgical drainage.

UMBILICUS

Normal Umbilicus

The umbilical cord is composed of two umbilical arteries and one umbilical vein, which are surrounded by Wharton's jelly, a gelatinous tissue. After birth, the cord is clamped and cut. The trend of dry cord care, without the application of antimicrobial agents, has become common practice in many areas. The remnant of the cord is then left exposed to dry.

The cord generally falls off on its own in 7 to 21 days, but it may take longer. Parents should be reassured that the presence of **oozing, a few drops of blood, or a mild odor are normal.** Indications for concern are significant redness of the skin (especially circumferential), significant malodorous discharge, or bleeding that is not stopped by gentle pressure.

Umbilical Hernia

An umbilical hernia, which is an outpocketing of layers of skin, fascia, and/or peritoneum, is caused by failure of the fascial opening to close completely. This presents as a **bulge at the umbilicus.** Umbilical hernias are more common in African American infants, premature infants, and infants with certain medical conditions: congenital hypothyroidism, Ehlers-Danlos, Beckwith Wiedemann syndrome, trisomy 18, and Down syndrome.

Most defects close spontaneously by the age of 5 years and incarceration or strangulation rarely occurs, so reassurance is most appropriate. Generally, the **likelihood of closure is inversely related to the size of the hernia,** with most small- to moderate-size hernias closing spontaneously. Hernias with a diameter >2 cm are less likely to close spontaneously. Repair is usually indicated if the hernia persists beyond 5 years. Traditional remedies (e.g., umbilical bands, taping coins over the umbilicus) do not hasten closure of the hernia, may irritate the surrounding skin, and are not recommended.

Omphalitis

Omphalitis is an **infection of the umbilical cord and/or surrounding tissues** resulting when bacteria colonize and invade the umbilical cord stump. Once a major cause of neonatal mortality, omphalitis is now **rare in developed countries.**

The condition typically presents with purulent, foul-smelling drainage from the umbilical cord and erythema (frequently circumferential) that progresses to induration and erythema of the abdominal wall. Systemic signs of lethargy, irritability, fever, and poor feeding may suggest more severe infections. Pathogens typically include *Staphylococcus aureus, Streptococcus pyogenes, Escherichia coli, Klebsiella pneumoniae, Proteus mirabilis,* and occasionally anaerobic bacteria. Complications include sepsis, hepatic abscess, peritonitis, and portal vein thrombosis.

Appropriate cultures of the purulent umbilical discharge, as well as blood and cerebrospinal fluid, if indicated, should be obtained before initiating therapy. Treatment consists of the intravenous administration of an antistaphylococcal penicillin or vancomycin and an aminoglycoside agent. Local resistance patterns as well as culture results guide therapy.

Umbilical Granuloma

Umbilical granuloma results when an **excessive amount of granulation tissue,** which is not covered by epithelium, accumulates after the separation of the umbilical cord. A small pink mass with persistent weeping and crusting is found at the base of the umbilicus. It is important to differentiate this relatively common and benign condition from patent omphalomesenteric duct and urachal remnant (see next section).

Treatment consists of the application of silver nitrate to the granulation tissue once or twice per week for several weeks, but generally only a few applications are required. Care should be taken to avoid the normal surrounding skin, which can be burned by the silver nitrate.

Patent Omphalomesenteric Duct and Patent Urachus

The **omphalomesenteric duct** is a connection between the intestinal tract and the yolk sac during fetal development that normally regresses by the ninth week of gestation. If it remains completely patent, a tubular attachment persists between the ileum and the umbilicus through which intestinal contents can drain. A patent omphalomesenteric duct may be demonstrated by inspection and probing of the tract that is visible at the surface of the umbilicus. Varying degrees of persistent patencies may result in umbilical polyp, Meckel's diverticulum, or omphalomesenteric duct cyst. These require further evaluation and surgical referral.

If the **urachus** persists with complete patency after birth, there is a free connection between the urinary bladder and the abdominal wall through which urine may pass. The patient with this condition may present with a constantly wet umbilicus or with a urinary tract infection. Incomplete patency and persistent tissues may result in an umbilical polyp, bladder diverticulum, or urachal cyst. For these conditions, the treatment is prompt evaluation and surgical repair as indicated.

GENITALIA

Boys

Normal Care of the Penis

In **uncircumcised** boys, the foreskin is generally not retractable at birth. Parents should attempt to keep the foreskin clean, avoiding attempts at forcible retraction of the prepuce, which may result in scarring and in true surgical phimosis. The foreskin gradually becomes retractable over time with growth and with the gentle stretching involved with washing. In newborn **circumcised** boys, the exposed glans should be coated with petroleum jelly with each diaper change until it is epithelialized.

Hypospadias and Epispadias

In **hypospadias,** the urethral meatus is abnormally located ventral to the tip of the glans. Classification of the type of hypospadias is based on the anatomic location of the urethral meatus (i.e., glanular, coronal, midshaft, distal shaft, penoscrotal, or perineal). There is frequently an associated abnormality of the foreskin (absence of the ventral portion of the foreskin) as well as associated chordee (ventral curvature of the penis). The abnormality of the foreskin is usually a clue that hypospadias or chordee may be present. In patients with suspected hypospadias, circumcision should be deferred because the presence of the foreskin facilitates the subsequent repair of hypospadias.

Epispadias, in which the urethra opens on the dorsum of the penis, is a more severe but far less common abnormality that is part of a spectrum of anomalies that includes, in its most severe form, bladder exstrophy. Incontinence is a commonly associated finding.

Cryptorchidism (Undescended Testicle)

Cryptorchidism is found in 3.4% to 5.8% of full-term boys and may be unilateral or bilateral. Most testes that are not descended at birth spontaneously descend during the first 3 to 6 months; few testes descend after this time. The incidence of cryptorchidism at the age of 1 year is approximately 0.8%.

The treatment for cryptorchidism is **orchiopexy,** which can be performed at any age after 4 months and is optimally performed before 1 year of age to decrease the risk of infertility, malignancy, and testicular torsion. Because timing is very important, all infants with unilateral or bilateral undescended testes at the 4- or 6-month visit should be referred to a urologist for evaluation.

Inguinal Hernia and Hydrocele

Both hernias and hydroceles result from failure of the processus vaginalis to undergo fusion and obliteration during fetal life.

- **Inguinal hernia** occurs in 1% to 5% of children, is ten times more common in boys than in girls, and may occur in up to 30% of premature infants born before 36 weeks of gestation.
- **Indirect inguinal hernia** presents as a bulge in the inguinal canal that may be present at rest or may only be appreciated during straining or crying as a loop of intestine descends into the hernia sac. Appropriate

therapy consists of referral for surgical repair within a short time of diagnosis to minimize the risk of incarceration or strangulation.

- A **hydrocele** represents persistence of the processus vaginalis with partial closure proximally, which allows fluid to pass into the scrotal sac. The condition is evidenced by the presence of scrotal swelling, which transilluminates in the absence of a hernia. Hydroceles in infants may communicate with the peritoneal cavity, or they may be noncommunicating. Hydroceles are often associated with inguinal hernias or they may be an isolated finding. Most infants with isolated hydrocele undergo spontaneous closure of the processus vaginalis with resolution of the hydrocele, so reassurance is most appropriate. Referral to a surgeon is indicated for patients with hydroceles that persist beyond the age of 6 months to 1 year (surgeons have different preferences for timing of surgery) or that wax and wane in size, indicating communication with the peritoneal cavity and the associated risk of hernia.

Girls

Vaginal Discharge and Bleeding

Normal newborn girls have well-estrogenized vaginal mucosa because of the transplacental passage of maternal hormones; therefore, a thick white vaginal discharge is a normal finding in a newborn girl. Many newborns also have a scant amount of vaginal bleeding in the first week of life owing to the withdrawal of maternal estrogen. Parents should be reassured that both findings are normal.

HIP EXAMINATION

Infants are examined in the newborn period and at all subsequent visits for the presence of developmental dysplasia of the hip (DDH), which includes unstable, subluxed, or dislocated hips. These conditions have an incidence of 1 in 1,000 newborns with instability and 1 to 1.5 in 1,000 infants with dislocation. The incidence is higher in girls, infants with a family history of DDH, infants with breech presentation, and infants with other risk factors such as neuromuscular conditions and oligohydramnios. The Ortolani and Barlow maneuvers are used to assess hip stability in the newborn (see Chapter 2, "The Physical Examination"). The Ortolani maneuver detects a dislocated femoral head that is reduced into the acetabulum, and the Barlow maneuver detects a hip that can be dislocated posteriorly by gentle adduction and posterior pressure. They are only present for the first 2 to 3 months of age. Other signs that are suggestive of hip dislocation are asymmetry of thigh folds or buttock creases, a positive Galeazzi sign (relative shortness of the femur with the hips and knees flexed), discrepancy of leg lengths, and limited hip abduction.

If a true positive Ortolani or Barlow sign is found, the infant should be referred to an orthopedist. Infants with other equivocally positive signs such as a soft click should have a follow-up examination in 2 weeks. If findings persist, infants may be referred to an orthopedist or have ultrasonography of their hips by 3 weeks of age. For infants detected with concerns who are >4 months of age, plain radiography of the hips is the preferred imaging modality. Because of the high risk of DDH in girls who are born breech (absolute risk of DDH is 12 of 1,000) and girls with a positive family history of DDH (absolute risk of 44 of 1,000), imaging with ultrasonography at 6 weeks of age or plain radiography of the pelvis and hips at 4 months of age is recommended in these select groups.

URINATION AND DEFECATION

Urate Crystals ("Pink Diaper Syndrome")

Parents may notice a **pink crystalline substance** in the diaper or a **salmon-pink residue** on the surface of the diaper, resulting from the deposition of urate crystals. Urate crystals are usually easily distinguished from blood on the basis of appearance, but occult blood testing can also be performed. Urate crystals are typically found in the setting of concentrated urine and **may indicate dehydration,** so a careful assessment for hydration status is warranted (including frequency of wet diapers, vital signs, and presence of a sunken fontanelle or dry mucous membranes). Parents should be counseled to increase the frequency and amount of feedings if there are concerns about an infant's hydration.

Meconium, Transitional Stool, and Typical Stool

Passage of some amount of **meconium** usually occurs within the first 12 hours of life, with 99% of all term infants and 95% of preterm infants passing meconium within the first 48 hours of life. **Transitional stools** follow the passage of meconium until the passage of the typical stool of the newborn is established. Typically, the stool is described as yellow and seedy in breast-fed infants and yellow or brown in formula-fed infants.

Failure to pass meconium can occur as a result of imperforate anus, functional intestinal obstruction (i.e., Hirschsprung disease), illness, or hypotonia. Failure to pass transitional stools following the passage of meconium may be indicative of a volvulus or malrotation. Any newborn who fails to pass meconium or fails to progress to passing **typical stools** should be evaluated in a timely fashion to rule out the presence of intestinal obstruction.

Establishment of a Bowel Pattern and Constipation

In each newborn, the establishment of a **normal bowel pattern** occurs over time and varies as the newborn grows. The typical breast-fed baby passes a bowel movement after each feeding initially, but by the age of 1 month, normal patterns vary from a bowel movement after each feeding to one every 1 to 7 days. The typical formula-fed baby has a bowel movement every 1 to 3 days.

Constipation is the infrequent passage of hard or painful bowel movements or a decrease in the frequency of bowel movements from an established pattern. Constipation can occur at any age. It is important to discuss with the parents of a newborn the fact that the consistency and regularity of the passing of stool varies over time. Parents should be advised to contact the physician if the infant develops abdominal distention, vomiting, refusal to eat, bloody stools, or extremely hard stools. These clinical signs and symptoms may indicate pathology, including many of the entities discussed in Chapter 22, "Constipation."

COMMON CONCERNS

Recommended Sleeping Position

The American Academy of Pediatrics (AAP) recommends placing healthy term infants to sleep in a nonprone position. **Sleeping supine confers the lowest risk of sudden infant death syndrome (SIDS)** and is preferred. This recommendation is based on analysis of a number of studies from around the world that demonstrate an association between the prone sleeping position and an increased risk of SIDS. In the United States, there has been a reduction in prone sleeping from 70% to 20% of infants since 1992, with a concomitant 40% reduction in the rate of SIDS.

In addition, parents should be instructed not to put infants to sleep on waterbeds, sofas, or soft mattresses. They should not place any soft objects (such as pillows, quilts, sheepskins, or stuffed toys) in an infant's sleeping environment, and they should recognize that loose bedding may also present a hazard to a small infant. Overheating and overbundling should be avoided.

Hiccups

Many babies hiccup. The precise cause is unknown, although many feel it is a reflection of an immature nervous system. If hiccups persist for 5 to 10 minutes and are distressing to those caring for the baby, nursing or a few sucks on a bottle of sugar water may relieve the hiccups.

Sneezing and Coughing

In babies, sneezing and coughing can be a protective mechanism to clear material from the respiratory passages. Therefore, intermittent sneezing or coughing should not be of concern. Persistent coughing or sneezing may be a sign of a problem and requires evaluation by a physician.

Chin Quivering

A baby's chin may intermittently quiver. This motion is a reflection of an immature nervous system, and the quivering stops as the nervous system matures.

Suggested Readings

American Academy of Pediatrics, Task Force on Infant Sleep Position and Sudden Infant Death Syndrome: Changing concepts of sudden infant death syndrome: implications on infant sleep environment and sleep position. *Pediatrics* 105(3):650–655, 2000.

American Academy of Pediatrics, Committee on Quality Improvement, Subcommittee on Developmental Dysplasia of the Hip. Clinical Practice Guideline: Early detection of developmental dysplasia of the hip. *Pediatrics* 105:896–905, 2000.

Brook I. Cutaneous and subcutaneous infection in newborns due to anaerobic bacteria. *J Perinatol Med* 30:197, 2002.

Gill B, Kogan S: Cryptorchidism. Current concepts. *Pediatr Clin North Am* 44(5):1211–1227, 1997.

Joint Committee on Infant Hearing, Year 2000 Position Statement: Principles and guidelines for early hearing detection and intervention programs. *Pediatrics* 106:798–817, 2000.

Kaye, CI and the Committee on Genetics: Introduction to the Newborn Screening Fact Sheets. *Pediatrics* 118:1304–1312, 2006.

Kendig JW: Care of the normal newborn. *Pediatr Rev* 13:262–268, 1992.

Komotar RJ, Zacharia BE, Ellis JA, et al.: Pitfalls for the pediatrician: positional molding or craniosynostosis? *Pediatr Ann* 35(5):365–375, 2006.

MacDonald MG, Mullett MD, Seishia MM: *Avery's Neonatology: Pathophysiology and Management of the Newborn.* Philadelphia, Lippincott, Williams & Wilkins, 2005.

Mullany LD, Darmstadt GL, Tielsch JM: Role of antimicrobial applications to the umbilical cord of neonates to prevent bacterial colonization and infection: a review of the evidence. *Pediatr Infect Dis* 22:996–1002, 2003.

Paller AS, Mancini AJ: *Hurwitz Clinical Pediatric Dermatology: A Textbook of Skin Disorders of Childhood and Adolescence.* Philadelphia, Elsevier Saunders, 2006.

Scheinfeld N: Diaper dermatitis: a review and brief survey of eruptions of the diaper area. *Am J Clin Dermatol* 6(5):273–281, 2005.

Scheree LR, Grosfels JL: Inguinal hernia and umbilical anomalies. *Pediatr Clin North Am* 40(6):1121–1131, 1993.

Seth R, Heyman MB: Management of constipation and encopresis in infants and children. *Gastroenterol Clin North Am* 23(4):621–636, 1994.

Shusterman S: Pediatric dental update. *Pediatr Rev* 15:311–319, 1994.

PART two

Problems

chapter 8

Abdominal Mass

Sabreen Akhter and Marc H. Gorelick

INTRODUCTION

In children, abdominal masses present in variable ways. **Some produce symptoms or signs; others remain silent** even when large. An abdominal mass may be discovered by a parent or caregiver, or it may be an incidental finding during physical examination. The **age of the child is an important factor** in the differential diagnosis: Most masses discovered in neonates are benign, whereas up to 50% of masses in older children are malignant (Table 8-1). Table 8-2 lists the most common sites of origin of abdominal masses according to the age of the patient

> **HINT:** In newborns, the bladder is an abdominal organ.

> **HINT:** An abdominal mass in a neonate is usually renal in origin—hydronephrosis and multicystic kidney are the most common causes of abdominal mass in neonates.

DIFFERENTIAL DIAGNOSIS LIST

Infectious Causes
Appendiceal abscess
Tubo-ovarian abscess
Hepatic abscess
Perinephric abscess

Neoplastic Causes

Malignant
Wilms tumor (nephroblastoma)
Neuroblastoma
Lymphoma

Rhabdomyosarcoma
Rhabdoid tumor
Hepatoblastoma
Sarcomas (retroperitoneal, embryonal)
Ovarian tumor
Metastatic disease

Benign
Ovarian teratoma
Sacrococcygeal teratoma
Mesonephric blastoma

TABLE 8-1 Common Abdominal Masses

Neonates	Infants	Older Children
Hydronephrosis	Hydronephrosis	Constipation
Ureteropelvic obstruction	Wilms tumor	Wilms tumor
Multicystic kidney	Neuroblastoma	Neuroblastoma
Distended bladder	Distended bladder	Hydronephrosis
Ectopic kidney	Multicystic kidney	Appendiceal abscess
Hydrometrocolpos	Pyloric stenosis	Ovarian cyst
Gastrointestinal duplication	Intussusception	
Posterior urethral valves	Hydrometrocolpos	
Mesonephric blastoma		

Traumatic Causes

Perinephric hematoma
Pancreatic pseudocyst
Adrenal hematoma
Duodenal hematoma

Congenital or Vascular Causes

Cysts—ovarian, choledochal, hepatic, mesenteric, urachal
Hydrometrocolpos or hematocolpos
Anterior myelomeningocele
Renal vein thrombosis
Hepatic hemangioma

Gastrointestinal System Causes

Gastrointestinal (bowel) duplication
Constipation
Pyloric stenosis
Hepatitis
Intestinal distention—intussusception, imperforate anus, Hirschsprung disease, volvulus, meconium ileus
Gallbladder hydrops

Genitourinary System Causes

Hydronephrosis
Polycystic or multicystic kidney
Ectopic or horseshoe kidney
Posterior urethral valves
Distended bladder
Pregnancy (intrauterine or ectopic)

> HINT: The patient's age is an important key in helping narrow down the possible differential diagnosis of an abdominal mass because its causes differ among neonates, infants, and children.

TABLE 8-2 Sites of Origin of Abdominal Masses

	Renal	Retroperitoneal	Gastrointestinal	Genital
Neonates	20%	15%	55%	10%
Infants and older children	55%	23%	18%	4%

DIFFERENTIAL DIAGNOSIS DISCUSSION

Constipation

Constipation is discussed in Chapter 22, "Constipation."

Intussusception

Intussusception is discussed in Chapter 9, "Abdominal Pain, Acute."

Appendiceal Abscess

Etiology

Untreated acute appendicitis leads to perforation with abscess formation.

Clinical Features

A child with an appendiceal abscess appears generally ill. **Fever and abdominal pain** are common symptoms. Although many children have a history highly suggestive of appendicitis (see Chapter 9, "Abdominal Pain, Acute"), others have an atypical history characterized by a subacute course, with symptoms present for days to weeks.

> **HINT:** Patients (especially young children) with appendiceal abscess may not show typical abnormalities associated with appendicitis, such as anorexia and peritoneal signs.

Evaluation

A **tender mass** is located in the **right lower quadrant,** and signs of peritoneal irritation are often, but not invariably, present. The mass may be palpable on rectal examination. In **postpubertal females, a pelvic examination** is important to exclude pelvic inflammatory disease.

Leukocytosis with a left shift is a helpful supportive finding. If the diagnosis of appendicitis is clear, additional studies are unnecessary. In difficult cases, an abdominal radiograph may provide confirmatory evidence (e.g., a fecalith, present in <10% of cases, free intraperitoneal air, or a right lower quadrant mass effect with ileus); however, **ultrasound** is the diagnostic study of choice.

Treatment

Urgent surgical consultation is necessary. Preoperatively, patients should receive broad-spectrum parenteral **antibiotics** to cover Gram-negative and anaerobic organisms.

Distended Bladder

Etiology

A palpably distended bladder results from **obstruction** (e.g., posterior urethral valves in boys, extrinsic mass, stricture), **neurologic dysfunction** (e.g., spinal cord injury, myelomeningocele, anticholinergic medication), or **voluntary retention** (as a result of dysuria).

Evaluation

The history should include questions about urinary frequency, dysuria, and the quality of the stream, as well as bowel function, which may also be affected in cases of neurogenic bladder.

Palpation of the abdomen reveals a **smooth suprapubic mass,** which may be somewhat tender if the abdomen is grossly distended. The mass is cystic to percussion. Look for evidence of urethral or vaginal irritation and evaluate **neurologic function.** The innervation of the bladder is S2-S4, the same area as the sacrum, so **testing the anal wink** identifies those patients with disruption of bladder innervation.

An **ultrasound** confirms that the mass is the bladder, and a **voiding cystourethrogram** may help identify the cause of the distention. **Urinalysis** should be performed if dysuria suggests cystitis.

Treatment

Urethral catheterization relieves the distention. Definitive treatment depends on the underlying cause of the obstruction, but usually referral to a urologist is required.

Hydronephrosis

Etiology

Hydronephrosis **(dilation of the renal collecting system)** results from **partial or complete obstruction of urine flow.** Causes include ureteropelvic junction obstruction, posterior urethral valves, vesicoureteral reflux, ureterocele, and duplication of the collecting system. Hydronephrosis can be unilateral or bilateral.

Clinical Features

Many children with hydronephrosis are **asymptomatic;** others present with **abdominal pain** (often chronic or recurrent) or, in rare cases, evidence of **renal failure.** Hydronephrosis tends to be more common in males and more commonly involves the left kidney.

Evaluation

Abdominal examination reveals a **palpable unilateral or bilateral smooth flank mass,** especially in infants. **Any palpable kidney in a child >3 years** of age is suspicious, as is **asymmetry in younger children.**

Ultrasound is diagnostic. It shows a dilated renal pelvis surrounded by several cystic structures (calyces).

Treatment

Most causes of hydronephrosis are treated with **surgical repair.**

Wilms Tumor (Nephroblastoma)

Etiology

Wilms tumor, the **second most common intra-abdominal malignancy in children,** accounts for virtually all pediatric renal neoplasms. Wilms tumor is associated with certain **congenital anomalies:** genitourinary malformations, hemihypertrophy, sporadic aniridia, cryptorchidism, Beckwith-Wiedemann syndrome, Denys-Drash syndrome, and the Wilms (tumor), aniridia, genitourinary (abnormalities), and (mental) retardation (WAGR complex). There is also a **familial form** of Wilms tumor.

Clinical Features

Peak incidence is at **3 years** of age. Most patients present with an **asymptomatic abdominal mass** or **abdominal distention.** It can go unnoticed owing to the tumor's retroperitoneal location and painless quality. This diagnosis should be considered in any young child with a large abdomen. Occasional symptoms include abdominal pain, vomiting, hematuria, and hypertension.

Evaluation

The mass is **smooth and firm,** rarely crossing the midline; in 5% to 10% of patients, masses are **bilateral.** In some cases, the mass is so large (mean diameter of 11 cm at the time of diagnosis in one study) that **diffuse distention,** rather than a discrete mass, is felt.

Although it may show microscopic hematuria, urinalysis is too nonspecific to be helpful. An **abdominal sonogram** or **computed tomography (CT) scan** shows a solid intrarenal mass.

Treatment

Wilms tumor is treated with a combination of **surgical resection (nephrectomy)** and **chemotherapy.** Success rates depend on the extent of disease and the clinical stage at the time of diagnosis. Approximately 15% are metastatic at diagnosis, most commonly to the lungs.

> **HINT:** The most common solid renal tumor in a neonate is congenital mesoblastic nephroma. This is different from Wilms tumor in that it is benign and usually occurs in the first 3 months of life, whereas Wilms tumor usually presents after 6 months of life.

Neuroblastoma

Etiology

A malignancy arising from neural crest cells, neuroblastoma is the **second most common solid tumor of childhood and the most common extracranial**

solid tumor in childhood. In approximately two thirds of patients, the primary site is in the **abdomen** (usually adrenal); the **thoracic region** is the next most common site.

Clinical Features

Like Wilms tumor, neuroblastoma may present as an **asymptomatic mass.** However, patients tend to be somewhat **younger** (median age, 2 years) and they appear **more ill**—an indication of the high incidence of metastatic disease at diagnosis (approximately 60%).

Associated symptoms may include **abdominal pain, urinary obstruction, flushing, sweating, diarrhea** (caused by tumor secretion of vasoactive intestinal peptide), **anorexia, malaise,** and **site-specific symptoms** from metastases to the bone, skin, liver, or central nervous system. Although most tumors produce catecholamines, rapid metabolism makes symptoms of hypertension and irritability rare.

> **HINT: Opsomyoclonus, consisting of myoclonic jerks, ataxia, and jerky eye movements ("dancing eyes, dancing feet"), is a unique paraneoplastic syndrome associated with neuroblastoma. Findings suggestive of opsomyoclonus should prompt a search for an occult neuroblastoma, even in the absence of an abdominal mass.**

Evaluation

A **firm, irregular, nontender mass** is palpable in the **abdominal region.** Other physical examination findings include **pallor, subcutaneous nodules,** and **hepatomegaly.**

> **HINT: Neuroblastoma is one of the few causes of massive hepatomegaly.**

Urinary levels of catecholamine metabolites, which are elevated in 90% to 95% of patients (i.e., vanillylmandelic acid, homovanillic acid, and metanephrine), were used for screening in the past, but abdominal ultrasound or CT is the current diagnostic procedure of choice. Identification of a solid adrenal or paraspinal mass, which is calcified in 80% of patients, strongly suggests neuroblastoma. Findings usually produce biliary tract obstruction with jaundice and acholic stools. Bone scan and skeletal radiographs are helpful to delineate bony involvement.

Treatment

Treatment may include **bone marrow transplantation, chemotherapy, radiation therapy,** and **surgical debulking or resection.** The prognosis depends on the stage of the disease, the age of the patient, the site of the primary tumor, and the findings on histologic evaluation. N-*myc* onco-gene amplification is associated with a poorer prognosis and occurs in about 20% of patients. Patients with stage IV-S disease, which often presents in the first few months of life, may experience spontaneous regression of the primary tumor.

Cysts

Etiology

Cysts may arise as **developmental variants** from any number of structures.

Clinical Features

Symptoms are **variable** and depend on the site of the cyst; **nonspecific abdominal pain** is most common. An ovarian cyst may cause cyclic pain in menarchal girls; a choledochal cyst usually produces biliary tract obstruction with jaundice and acholic stools.

Evaluation

Many cysts are palpable on abdominal or pelvic examination as a **smooth, soft, or firm mass** at the site of the organ of origin.

A **sonogram** is the optimal diagnostic tool.

Treatment

Ovarian or mesenteric cysts discovered as an incidental finding may be followed because they spontaneously regress much of the time; cysts causing **significant symptoms** require **excision.**

Renal Cystic Disease

Types of Renal Cystic Disease

- **Multicystic dysplastic renal disease.** This is one of the most common causes of abdominal masses in neonates. The affected kidney consists of a mass of cysts with little or no identifiable renal tissue ("grape cluster" appearance on ultrasound). These are usually unilateral and sporadic with symptoms that may include abdominal pain, hematuria, and urinary tract infections; bilateral cases are associated with renal failure.

- **Polycystic renal disease.** In polycystic renal disease, one or both kidneys contain multiple cortical and medullary cysts consisting of dilated tubules. The more common autosomal dominant form usually presents in adulthood but is sometimes diagnosed in children. The autosomal recessive form, which is more severe and more likely bilateral, usually manifests itself in infancy. Both forms are uncommon in children. Ultrasound findings show many small cysts in the collecting ducts with no intrinsic renal dysplasia.

> **HINT:** The majority of infants with autosomal recessive polycystic kidney disease also have hepatic cysts, sometimes leading to severe liver disease.

Clinical Features

Except for those with bilateral involvement, infants with multicystic dysplastic kidney present with an **asymptomatic flank mass** that is irregular and nontender. Infants with bilateral cystic kidneys may have a history of **oligohydramnios** and, in severe cases, findings of **Potter syndrome.** Children with multicystic dysplastic kidney have a high incidence of **associated urinary tract anomalies** and require **complete urologic evaluation.**

Patients with polycystic kidney disease often have concomitant **hematuria** (gross or microscopic) or **hypertension,** but renal failure is rare. Again, a **unilateral or bilateral flank mass** is palpated.

Evaluation

In all cases, **ultrasound** confirms the diagnosis.

Treatment

Patients with renal cystic disease require close follow-up to monitor for signs of **renal insufficiency** or **hypertension.** These patients are usually on dialysis until transplantation can occur.

Gastrointestinal (Bowel) Duplication

Etiology

Occurring in any part of the gastrointestinal tract, but most commonly in the **region of the ileocecal valve,** duplication cysts result from a **morphogenetic defect.** The cyst varies in size, has a tubular or spherical shape, and may or may not communicate with the true intestinal lumen, producing a closed cystic mass. These can present as asymptomatic abdominal distension or with signs of obstruction, bleeding, or perforation. Gastrointestinal (bowel) duplication is the **most common cause of neonatal gastrointestinal masses.**

Evaluation

Bowel duplications may be **asymptomatic** or they may cause **intestinal obstruction.** They are typically compressible and mobile and either round or tubular. The diagnosis is made by **ultrasound** or a **gastrointestinal contrast study.**

> **HINT:** The mucosa of the cyst may arise from any part of the gastrointestinal tract, regardless of location; when gastric mucosa is included, ulceration or perforation may result. A Meckel's scan may be useful in cases where gastric mucosa may be present.

Treatment

Surgical resection is generally curative.

Hydrometrocolpos and Hematocolpos

Etiology

Imperforate hymen leads to accumulation of secretions in the vagina; if undetected until puberty, accumulated menstrual blood causes hematocolpos.

Clinical Features

The distended vagina may **interfere with voiding or defecation**, but infants are otherwise **asymptomatic**.

Evaluation

The **mass is smooth, suprapubic,** and **frequently palpable** on rectal examination. The imperforate hymen may also be seen bulging externally.

An **ultrasound** shows the dilated, fluid-filled vagina.

Treatment

Resection of the imperforate hymen is required.

EVALUATION OF ABDOMINAL MASS

Patient History

The following items should be noted:

- In neonates: maternal pregnancy complicated by oligohydramnios/polyhydramnios, or any interventions (such as amniocentesis)
- Symptoms (e.g., fever, abdominal pain, vomiting, jaundice)
- Stooling pattern (frequency, consistency)
- Voiding pattern (frequency, hematuria)
- History of trauma
- Menstrual history
- History of abdominal surgery or umbilical catheterization

Physical Examination

The following should be noted or sought on physical examination:

- Size and location of mass (asymmetry, position of the umbilicus)
- Presence of tenderness
- Findings on percussion
- Texture (solid or cystic)
- Blood pressure
- Presence of scleral icterus
- Evidence of dehydration

Laboratory Studies

The choice of laboratory studies is guided by the type of symptoms and signs that are involved. Studies to be considered include:

- Urinalysis
- Complete blood cell count
- Blood urea nitrogen and creatinine
- Electrolytes
- Hepatic transaminases and bilirubin

Diagnostic Modalities

- **Ultrasound.** The diagnostic study of choice in most cases of abdominal mass is ultrasound. Exceptions include clinically diagnosed constipation, intrauterine pregnancy, and appendicitis, where further studies are generally unnecessary, or intussusception, where a contrast enema is both diagnostic and therapeutic. Ultrasound examination provides information regarding the location and character (cystic versus solid, homogeneous versus heterogeneous, calcified) of the abdominal mass and should be the initial study in most cases.
- **Abdominal radiographs.** Although these are frequently obtained, provide little information in a relatively asymptomatic child. Some exceptions are the use of radiographs to detect calcifications in a mass, organomegaly, or displacement of the intestines, all of which may help narrow the differential diagnosis (Table 8-3).
- **Abdominal CT.** It which provides more detailed anatomic information than ultrasound, should be reserved for further delineation of certain masses but may be a substitute when ultrasound is unavailable.

TABLE 8-3 Abdominal Masses Commonly Associated with Calcification

Neuroblastoma
Teratoma
  Ovarian
  Sacrococcygeal
Adrenal hematoma
Hepatic hemangioma
Meconium peritonitis

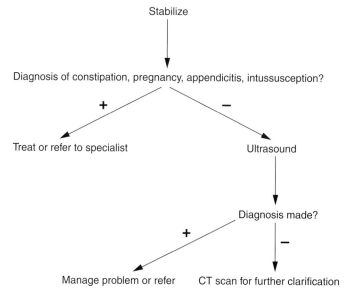

Figure 8-1 ▪ Evaluation of a patient with an abdominal mass
CT = computed tomography.

▪ **Intravenous urography.** Once the initial study of choice, has now been supplanted by the preceding methods.

APPROACH TO THE PATIENT (FIGURE 8-1)

The workup of an abdominal mass should be accompanied by **supportive care** and **resuscitation** in an ill-appearing child, including **fluid therapy** in the presence of dehydration, **supplemental oxygen** and **assisted respiration** in patients with respiratory compromise, and **control of blood pressure** in patients with symptomatic hypertension. The initial study in these patients is an **abdominal series** (flat and upright) to evaluate for obstruction or perforation. Once the child is stabilized, additional studies may be undertaken.

Suggested Readings

Cass DL, Hawkins E, Brandt ML, et al.: Surgery for ovarian masses in infants, children, and adolescents: 102 consecutive patients treated in a 15-year period. *J Pediatr Surg* 36(5):693–699, 2001.
Caty MG, Shamberger RC: Abdominal tumors in infancy and childhood. *Pediatr Clin North Am* 40:1253–1271, 1993.

Chandler JC, Gauderer MW: The neonate with an abdominal mass. *Pediatric Clin North Am* 51: 979–997, 2004.

Kim S, Chung DH: Pediatric solid malignancies: neuroblastoma and Wilms tumor. *Surgical Clin North Am* 86: 469–487, 2006.

Kuppermann N, O'Dea T, Pinckney L, et al.: Predictors of intussusception in young children. *Arch Pediatr Adolesc Med* 154(3):250–255, 2000.

Merten DF, Kirks DR: Diagnostic imaging of pediatric abdominal masses. *Pediatr Clin North Am* 32:1397–1425, 1985.

Morrison SC: Controversies in abdominal imaging. *Pediatr Clin North Am* 44(3):555–574, 1997.

Neville HL, Ritchey ML: Wilms' tumor. Overview of National Wilms' Tumor Study Group results. *Urol Clin North Am* 27(3):435–442, 2000.

Ota FS, Maxson RT, Abramo TJ: Ominous findings in toddlers with increasing abdominal girth: two unusual cases and a review of the clinical evaluation. *Ann Emerg Med* 45(5): 517–523, 2005.

chapter 9

Abdominal Pain, Acute

Paul Ishimine

INTRODUCTION

The evaluation of acute abdominal pain in a child presents a challenge to any clinician. A common chief complaint, the causes of abdominal pain range from benign to life-threatening processes. Furthermore, abdominal pain can originate from both intraabdominal organs and from sources outside the abdomen (see Chapter 59, "Pelvic Pain" and Chapter 70, "Sexually Transmitted Diseases"). An ordered approach to evaluation is required and is guided by the age of the patient, the history and physical examination, and selected laboratory and imaging studies. In many cases, a definitive diagnosis may not be made on a single patient encounter, and repeated evaluation is required.

DIFFERENTIAL DIAGNOSIS LIST

Gastrointestinal

Constipation
Appendicitis/appendiceal
  abscess
Peptic ulcer disease/gastritis
Gastroenteritis
Esophagitis/gastro-
  esophageal reflux
Foreign body ingestion
Cholecystitis
Pancreatitis/pancreatic
  pseudocyst
Hepatitis
Bowel obstruction
Incarcerated hernia
Intussusception
Abdominal trauma
Hirschsprung disease
Inflammatory bowel disease
Peritonitis
Necrotizing enterocolitis
Mesenteric adenitis
Malrotation with volvulus
Infectious colitis
Antibiotic-associated
  (pseudomembranous) colitis
Food allergy (e.g., milk or soy
  protein)

Genitourinary

Urinary tract infection (e.g.,
  cystitis, pyelonephritis)
Renal calculus
Pregnancy (e.g., intrauterine,
  ectopic)
Pelvic inflammatory
  disease
Ovarian cyst
Adnexal torsion
Mittelschmerz
Dysmenorrhea
Endometriosis
Hematocolpos/
  hydrometrocolpos
Testicular torsion/torsion of
  the appendix testis
Orchitis
Epididymitis

Respiratory
Pneumonia
Streptococcal pharyngitis
Asthma

Malignancy
Wilms tumor
Neuroblastoma
Leukemia
Lymphoma
Hepatoblastoma
Ovarian tumor
Teratoma
Typhlitis
Rhabdomyosarcoma

Systemic disorders
Diabetic ketoacidosis
Vasculitis (e.g.,
  Henoch-Schönlein
  purpura)

Collagen vascular disease
  (e.g., lupus, polyarteritis
  nodosa, juvenile dermato-
  myositis, scleroderma)
Kawasaki disease
Hemolytic uremic syndrome
Infectious mononucleosis
Sickle cell disease
Cystic fibrosis
Porphyria

Miscellaneous
Functional
Colic
Toxins (e.g., caustic ingestion,
  black widow spider bite)
Orthopedic (e.g., septic
  arthritis/osteomyelitis/diskitis)
Abdominal migraine
Herpes zoster
Heat cramps

Any of the causes of chronic abdominal pain can present with acute exacerbations of pain (see Chapter 10, "Abdominal Pain, Chronic")

DIFFERENTIAL DIAGNOSIS DISCUSSION

Acute Gastroenteritis
Acute gastroenteritis is discussed in Chapter 27, "Diarrhea, Acute."

Adnexal Torsion
Adnexal torsion is discussed in Chapter 59, "Pelvic Pain."

Appendicitis

Etiology
Appendicitis is a common cause of abdominal pain, occurring in children of all ages. Appendicitis is typically caused by obstruction of the appendiceal lumen, resulting in appendiceal distention, inhibition of lymphatic and vascular drainage, edema, and perforation.

Clinical Features
The classic symptoms of appendicitis are periumbilical abdominal pain, followed by fever, anorexia, and vomiting. As the disease progresses,

pain localizes to the right lower quadrant (i.e., McBurney point). However, patients with appendicitis often present atypically and with nonspecific symptoms. An appendix situated in the lateral colonic gutter may cause flank pain; an appendix positioned more medially may irritate the bladder and cause dysuria and suprapubic pain. Alternatively, an appendix positioned in the pelvis may cause diarrhea if the inflamed appendix irritates the sigmoid colon. Patients may prefer to lie still because of the peritoneal irritation caused by an inflamed appendix, and children may report increasing pain with coughing.

> **HINT:** Patients with appendicitis are frequently misdiagnosed because of misleading symptoms, such as diarrhea, constipation, dysuria, or lethargy, that suggest other diagnoses.

Unfortunately, making the diagnosis of appendicitis can be challenging, especially in preverbal children in the early stages of the disease process. As a result, young patients frequently present after the appendix has perforated. These patients may report transient improvement of their pain immediately after perforation but soon complain of diffuse abdominal pain from peritonitis. Patients with appendiceal perforation may go on to develop intra-abdominal abscesses (see Chapter 8, "Abdominal Mass").

Evaluation

The physical examination frequently reveals a fever and tenderness in the right lower quadrant, although tenderness may be found in the flank or elsewhere in the abdomen, depending on the location of the appendix. The Rovsing sign (pain in the right lower quadrant with palpation of the left lower quadrant), the psoas sign (pain in the right lower quadrant with extension of the right thigh while the patient is lying on his or her left side), and the obturator sign (pain in the right lower quadrant when the flexed thigh and knee are held and the hip is rotated internally) are all signs that may be seen with appendicitis. A rectal examination may reveal irritation of the rectal wall by an inflamed appendix. If the appendix has perforated and the child has developed peritonitis, he or she may have diffuse abdominal tenderness, rebound tenderness, and abdominal wall rigidity. These children frequently also have signs of systemic toxicity, such as a higher fever, tachycardia, and tachypnea.

Laboratory studies can be helpful in cases where the history and physical examination are equivocal. A complete blood count (CBC) often reveals a mild leukocytosis with an increasing left shift as the appendix becomes more gangrenous or ruptures; however, a normal white blood cell count does not rule out appendicitis. Electrolytes are usually not abnormal unless significant dehydration exists. A few white blood cells in the urine may be found if the appendix lies near the bladder or the ureter. Radiographs of the abdomen may occasionally reveal an appendicolith. More commonly, however, the radiographic findings are nonspecific. Diagnostic accuracy is enhanced in equivocal patients by the use of either abdominal ultrasound and/or abdominal computed tomography (CT) scan. Both of these imaging studies have high sensitivities and specificities for the diagnosis of appendicitis. Ultrasound spares the child from ionizing radiation but is more operator dependent than CT scanning. CT scans are better at identifying other diagnoses that might cause abdominal pain and are generally more easily obtainable than ultrasound studies, but young patients frequently require sedation for CT studies.

> **HINT:** Appendicitis is primarily a clinical diagnosis, and normal lab values and imaging studies do not exclude the diagnosis. If a child has normal studies but a worrisome history or examination, he or she should be undergo a period of close observation with serial abdominal examinations.

Treatment

The treatment for appendicitis is appendectomy, and therefore surgical consultation should be requested promptly once the diagnosis of appendicitis is suspected. Pain management and supportive care should be provided while awaiting operative intervention. Antibiotic therapy should be initiated prior to surgery in patients with suspected perforation.

Constipation

Constipation is discussed in Chapter 22, "Constipation."

Henoch-Schönlein Purpura

Henoch-Schönlein purpura is discussed in Chapter 18, "Bleeding and Purpura."

Intussusception

Etiology

Intussusception occurs when a proximal segment of bowel telescopes into a distal portion of intestine, causing edema, lymphatic obstruction, and vascular compromise. Intussusception is typically ileocolic but can also be ileoileal or colocolic. If a diagnosis is not made in a timely fashion, this ischemic portion of bowel becomes gangrenous and eventually perforates, leading to peritonitis. Most cases are idiopathic; however, intussusception may arise from an intestinal lead point. In infants, hypertrophied Peyer patches may create a lead point, whereas in older children tumors, polyps, Meckel diverticula, duplications, or intestinal lesions associated with Henoch-Schönlein purpura are most often identified as lead points. The first oral rotavirus vaccine (RotaShield) was associated with an increased risk of intussusception and withdrawn from use in 1999; newer rotavirus vaccinations do not seem to be associated with an increased risk of intussusception.

Intussusception is the most common cause of intestinal obstruction in young children and occurs most commonly in patients 4 to 12 months of age. The classic symptoms of intussusception are episodic abdominal pain, vomiting, and stools with the appearance of "currant jelly." Periods of severe pain, often causing the child to pull up his legs, are followed by periods of no obvious discomfort. Occasionally, however, the child appears lethargic between the painful episodes. Eventually, the child begins to vomit and develops more consistent pain as the intestine becomes more edematous and ischemic. This circulatory compromise causes sloughing of the intestinal mucosa, which results in passage of currant jelly stools, and represents a late finding in intussusception.

Evaluation

Patients with intussusception may look well or may be quite ill appearing with unstable vital signs. Abdominal examination may reveal distention because of either partial or complete obstruction. Occasionally, a sausagelike mass can be palpated, most often in the right upper quadrant. Rectal examination may reveal heme-positive stool. Laboratory studies are generally unhelpful in the diagnosis of intussusception. An abdominal radiograph may show varying degrees of small bowel obstruction, a paucity of gas in the right lower quadrant, and an intracolonic mass. Rarely, free air may be noted because of intestinal perforation. These radiographic findings are helpful if present, but frequently, the plain radiographs show nonspecific gas patterns. A contrast enema is the imaging study of choice for patients with suspected intussusception because it is also potentially therapeutic. Intussusception can also be seen with ultrasound (an option when clinical suspicion of intussusception is not high to avoid an invasive procedure) and CT.

Treatment

Intravenous fluids should be provided for presumed dehydration and a nasogastric tube placed to decompress the stomach and intestines. The administration of broad-spectrum antibiotics is recommended just prior to attempted reduction. An air or barium emesis contrast enema can be both a diagnostic and therapeutic maneuver in suspected intussusception. If barium enema or air insufflation is unsuccessful, or if the child appears systemically toxic prior to the enema, intraoperative reduction is necessary. Because of the potential for failure of enema reduction, and because contrast enemas can occasionally cause perforation, early surgical consultation is advised when intussusception is suspected. The recurrence rate after successful nonoperative reduction is reported to be 5% to 10%; recurrence is more common in an older child with a lead point.

Malrotation with Volvulus

Etiology

Intestinal malrotation is a consequence of abnormal embryonic development, resulting in abnormal fixation of the mesentery of the intestines. Although malrotation can be asymptomatic, this predisposes children to volvulus, the twisting of loops of bowel around its mesenteric base, leading to bowel obstruction. Furthermore, because the vascular supply to the intestines is carried within this mesenteric stalk, this twisting leads to ischemia and abdominal pain and can cause intestinal necrosis within hours. Malrotation with volvulus is most commonly seen in young infants, but more indolent forms of malrotation can present later in childhood. Patients who present at an older age more commonly have symptoms such as feeding difficulties with intermittent bilious emesis, or with failure to thrive because of feeding intolerance.

Young infants with volvulus commonly present with the sudden onset of emesis and abdominal pain. The emesis is usually bilious, and the abdominal pain is constant. The patient appears ill and in distress and may present with unstable vital signs if necrosis has already occurred. The abdomen is tender on examination, and there may be varying degrees of abdominal distension, depending on the location of the malrotation. The presence of blood on rectal examination implies that ischemic injury to the intestinal mucosa has already occurred and is a late finding with volvulus.

Evaluation

Patients with clinical findings suggestive of volvulus need to be evaluated immediately. Plain radiographs may reveal air-fluid levels and dilated loops of bowel; there may also be a paucity of air in the lower gastrointestinal (GI) tract. Both the "double-bubble" sign, dilation of the stomach and the proximal duodenum, and the presence of loops of small bowel overlying the liver shadow suggest a volvulus. However, plain radiographs may be normal in a patient with volvulus. An upper GI series with contrast is the diagnostic study of choice and may reveal a corkscrew-like appearance of the contrast within the twisted intestinal loops.

Treatment

Malrotation is a surgical emergency. Both patient survival and intestinal viability are directly related to the timeliness of making this diagnosis. As a consequence, a young infant with bilious emesis and abdominal pain should be presumed to have malrotation with volvulus until this diagnosis is excluded. Immediate surgical consultation is mandatory and should not be delayed for the results of abdominal imaging. A child with suspected malrotation with volvulus should have a nasogastric tube and intravenous access. Patients who are unstable need to undergo fluid resuscitation and should receive antibiotics. Plans should be made for emergent surgery because the only definitive treatment for volvulus is operative intervention.

Respiratory Tract Infections

Group A Streptococcal Pharyngitis

Patients with group A streptococcal pharyngitis sometimes present with abdominal pain in addition to throat pain, fever, and cervical adenopathy (see also Chapter 72, "Sore Throat). Patients with abdominal pain and suspected strep throat should have their posterior pharynx swabbed and evaluated either by a rapid streptococcal antigen detection test or by throat culture. Patients with streptococcal pharyngitis should be treated with antibiotics.

Lower Lobe Pneumonia

Children with lower lobe pneumonia can present with respiratory symptoms and abdominal pain. Evidence for pneumonia can be as subtle as an increased respiratory rate or unexplained high fevers. Lower lobe pneumonias are sometimes discovered incidentally on abdominal radiographs taken for evaluation of abdominal pain. Treatment consists of analgesics and appropriate antibiotics for pneumonia.

Testicular Torsion (See Chapter 67, "Scrotal Pain, Acute")

Toxin Exposures and Foreign Body Ingestions

Although many substances can cause nausea and vomiting when ingested, some toxins are more commonly associated with abdominal pain. Examples include iron, aspirin, caustic ingestions, and lead and other heavy metals. Specific antidotes (e.g., deferoxamine for iron toxicity) can be given in addition to activated charcoal and other GI decontamination measures as indicated. Treatment of the patient who has a toxic ingestion should be coordinated with a poison control center. Many swallowed foreign bodies may not result in symptoms, but some, such as needles or disc batteries, can cause abdominal pain by irritating or perforating the GI mucosa. Most swallowed foreign bodies travel through the GI tract without difficulty, but foreign bodies that cause symptoms or are at high risk of causing perforation or other complications should be removed by a gastroenterologist, otolaryngologist, or surgeon, depending on the location of the foreign body. A unique toxic exposure causing abdominal pain is a black widow spider bite. Venom from the black widow spider (*Latrodectus mactans*) can cause severe abdominal cramping as well as cardiovascular collapse in young children. Black widow spider antivenin may be indicated in the presence of systemic symptoms.

Trauma

Etiology

The history is an important consideration in evaluating a child with abdominal trauma. Abdominal trauma is categorized as either blunt or penetrating, and most children with abdominal trauma have blunt trauma. Common mechanisms of injury include falls, motor vehicle–related injuries, and child abuse. Although the history is crucial in evaluating children with abdominal trauma, children injured because of child abuse may have inaccurate or deceptive histories.

> **HINT:** Consider child abuse in patients with more severe or multiple injuries if the reported mechanism of injury does not seem to correlate with physical findings, or if the caretakers provide inconsistent histories.

Clinical Features and Evaluation

Abdominal symptoms may be subtle immediately after an injury and may be further limited by distracting injuries and alterations in mental status. A high index of suspicion for abdominal injury is appropriate in the evaluation of the patient with trauma. Patients with abdominal trauma must be thoroughly examined. Children with blood loss present initially with tachycardia; hypotension is a late sign, developing only after significant bleeding. Children may present with tachypnea and shallow respirations in an attempt to minimize abdominal pain associated with breathing. Pain and tenderness may be focal because of a solid organ injury or diffuse because of peritoneal irritation from a perforated viscus or intraperitoneal blood. Bruising on the abdominal wall from a seat belt increases the risk of intra-abdominal injury in children who have been involved in motor vehicle crashes. The presence of gross blood on rectal examination suggests a hollow viscus injury.

Further evaluation of the patient's abdominal pain depends on the results of the history and physical examination. In a child in whom the suspicion of injury is low, observation and repeated physical examinations are appropriate. However, in patients with worrisome findings, additional evaluation is warranted. Laboratory studies commonly include CBCs, liver function tests, pancreatic function tests, urinalyses, and blood type and screen. These tests may suggest intra-abdominal injury if abnormal; however, normal values do not rule out intra-abdominal injury and thus should not supplant imaging studies if the clinical suspicion is high. With the exception of pelvis radiograph to look for fracture, radiographs are of limited value in the evaluation of abdominal trauma. The imaging study of choice is an abdominal CT scan, frequently with intravenous and oral contrast. The sensitivity for detecting solid organ injury is excellent. The CT scan is less sensitive in detecting hollow viscus and pancreatic injury.

Diagnostic peritoneal lavage (DPL) is performed in rare circumstances (e.g., when a patient is too unstable to go to the CT scanner). Although DPL is even more sensitive than CT scan in detecting intra-abdominal blood, the DPL is less specific for injuries that need surgical repair because many solid injuries that cause a positive DPL are managed nonoperatively. Abdominal ultrasound is being used more extensively in adult trauma patients, but its role in the evaluation of the pediatric trauma patient is less clear. Immediate surgical consultation is indicated for patients with significant abdominal trauma.

Treatment

Patients with abdominal trauma should have their life-threatening conditions addressed first. After the patient's airway, breathing, circulation, and cervical spine have been stabilized, the patient's abdominal injuries can then be addressed. Penetrating trauma of the abdomen is a surgical emergency, and wounds that violate the peritoneal cavity are generally explored in the operating room. Patients with solid organ injury are frequently managed nonoperatively, but these management decisions should be directed in conjunction with a trauma surgeon. For those patients who do not have any obvious injuries after initial evaluation with persistent posttraumatic abdominal pain, close observation is indicated.

Evaluation of *Acute* Abdominal Pain

The differential diagnosis of acute abdominal pain in a child is extensive, and determining the etiology of a patient's abdominal pain often taxes a physician's diagnostic abilities.

History

Type and Location of Pain

- Visceral pain is caused by stretching of the nerve fibers surrounding an abdominal organ and is a poorly localized, aching pain.
  - Epigastric pain originates from structures derived from the foregut (e.g., the stomach, duodenum, pancreas, liver, and biliary tree).
  - Periumbilical pain arises from involvement of the midgut structures (e.g., the jejunum, ileum, and large intestine up to the splenic flexure).
  - Suprapubic pain is produced by hindgut structures (e.g., the distal colon and rectum).
- Somatic pain occurs when pain fibers in the parietal peritoneum are irritated either by inflammation of the peritoneum itself or by an adjacent inflamed organ. Somatic pain is better localized than visceral pain and typically worsened by movement.
- Referred pain to the lower neck and shoulders is associated with phrenic nerve irritation from pancreatitis, splenic pathology, or hepatobiliary disease.

Characteristics of Pain

- Sudden onset suggests perforation of a visceral organ or ischemia.
- Gradual onset suggests inflammation, such as pain associated with appendicitis.
- Colicky pain suggests pain from a hollow viscus, such as kidney stones or gallstones.

Associated Symptoms

- Fever or chills.
- Nausea or vomiting (specifically if there is bile or blood in the emesis).
- Abdominal distention.
- Stool irregularities (e.g., constipation, diarrhea, hematochezia, melena, or mucus in the stools).
- Other complaints, such as sore throat, dyspnea, cough, dysuria or urinary frequency, and extra-abdominal pain.
- Adolescents should be asked about their sexual history. Ask adolescent girls about menstrual history, vaginal bleeding, or discharge.
- Previous episodes of similar pain.
- Previous surgeries.
- Past medical history and medications.

Physical Examination

A complete physical examination of should be performed on patients with abdominal pain prior to examining the abdomen itself, with emphasis on:

- Vital signs and general appearance.
- Head, ears, eyes, nose, throat (HEENT): Eyes and mucous membranes should be checked for icterus, and the pharynx should be inspected.
- Lungs and heart.
- Lower extremities: Inspection of the legs may reveal purpura seen with Henoch-Schönlein purpura.

The abdomen should be examined in the following order:

- Inspection: look for scars, bruising, masses, distension, and peristalsis.
- Auscultation: may reveal high-pitched bowel sounds typical of bowel obstruction or the absence of bowel sounds as seen in a patient with an ileus.
- Palpation: In a verbal child, ask the patient which part of his or her abdomen hurts the most; this should be the last area palpated. Palpation may reveal masses or guarding.
- A rectal examination including testing for occult blood should be considered in patients with unexplained abdominal pain. A genital examination is important for both males and females. A pelvic

examination should be considered in all postpubertal females. In prepubertal females, the external genitalia should be inspected.

> **HINT:** Patients often have pain radiating to the abdomen because of genitourinary pathology and are reluctant to volunteer this information.

Laboratory Studies

The following laboratory tests may be helpful:

- CBC and erythrocyte sedimentation rate may be abnormal in the setting of infection but are neither sensitive nor specific.
- Electrolytes, blood urea nitrogen, and creatinine are of limited diagnostic utility but may help in the management of fluid repletion.
- A glucose level is helpful in patients suspected of having diabetic ketoacidosis.
- Liver function tests and amylase and lipase levels should be sent when hepatic or pancreatic disease is suspected.
- Blood type and crossmatch should be sent if transfusion is a possibility.
- Urinalysis may reveal infection or hematuria.
- Urine pregnancy test should be performed in all pubertal females with abdominal pain.
- Throat, stool, cervix, and urine cultures should be ordered if infection is suspected.

Imaging Modalities

Various imaging studies can be used in evaluation of the patient:

- Plain abdominal radiographs: a two-view abdominal obstruction series is more helpful than a single film of the abdomen and may reveal a bowel obstruction, ileus, fecalith, free air, or abdominal masses. A chest radiograph may reveal thoracic pathology causing abdominal pain.
- Radiographic studies with contrast can be helpful when looking for malrotation (upper GI series) or intussusception (air or contrast enema).
- Ultrasound can help evaluate right upper quadrant pain, the kidneys, gynecologic causes of abdominal pain, and suspected appendicitis.
- Abdominal CT is helpful in the evaluation of abdominal masses and solid organ injury. CT is also being used more frequently in the evaluation of appendicitis.

Approach to the Patient (See Table 9-1)

TABLE 9-1 Differential Diagnosis of Acute Abdominal Pain by Age and Location

	<2 years	2–5 years	5–12 years	Adolescence
Localized pain	Appendicitis (late) Incarcerated hernia Urinary tract infection	Appendicitis (late) Urinary tract infection Sickle cell disease	Appendicitis (late) Urinary tract infection Infectious mononucleosis Peptic ulcer disease	Appendicitis (late) Urinary tract infection Infectious mononucleosis Peptic ulcer disease Cholecystitis Pelvic inflammatory disease Ovarian cyst/torsion Pregnancy/ectopic
Diffuse pain	Appendicitis (early or perforated) Intussusception Volvulus/malrotation Colic Food allergy Constipation Hemolytic uremic syndrome Necrotizing enterocolitis Gastroenteritis Henoch-Schönlein purpura Hirschsprung disease	Appendicitis (early or perforated) Constipation Gastroenteritis Ingestion Pharyngitis Pneumonia Henoch-Schönlein purpura Diabetic ketoacidosis Asthma Sickle cell disease Inflammatory bowel disease	Appendicitis (early or perforated) Diabetic ketoacidosis Pharyngitis Pneumonia Gastroenteritis Constipation Functional Inflammatory bowel disease Testicular torsion Asthma Sickle cell disease	Appendicitis (early or perforated) Dysmenorrhea Mittelschmerz Functional Inflammatory bowel disease Diabetic ketoacidosis Testicular torsion Gastroenteritis

Suggested Readings

Bundy DG, Byerley JS, Liles EA, et al.: Does this child have appendicitis? *JAMA* 298(4):438–451, 2007.

Doria AS, Moineddin R, Kellenberger CJ, et al.: US or CT for diagnosis of appendicitis in children and adults? A meta-analysis. *Radiology* 241(1): 83–94, 2006.

Justice FA, Auldist AW, Bines JE: Intussusception: trends in clinical presentation and management. *J Gastroenterol Hepatol* 21:842–846, 2006.

McCollough M, Sharieff GQ: Abdominal pain in children. *Pediatr Clin North Am* 53:107–137, 2006.

Milar AJW, Rode H, Cywes S: Malrotation and volvulus in infancy and childhood. *Semin Pediatr Surg* 12(4):229–336, 2003.

Ruddy RM: Pain—abdomen. In *Textbook of Pediatric Emergency Medicine,* 5th ed. Edited by Fleisher GR, Ludwig S, Henretig FM. Philadelphia, Lippincott Williams & Wilkins, 2006, 469–476.

Wegner S, Colletti JE, VanWie D: Pediatric blunt abdominal trauma. *Pediatr Clin North Am* 53:243–256, 2006.

DIFFERENTIAL DIAGNOSIS LIST

Neonate/Toddler

Functional
  Infant colic
  Infant dyschezia
  Infant regurgitation
  Milk-protein allergy and/or
    eosinophilic gastroenteritis
  Gastroesophageal reflux disease

Child/Adolescent

Functional
  Appendiceal colic
  Childhood functional
    abdominal pain
  Childhood functional
    abdominal pain syndrome
  Functional dyspepsia
  Irritable bowel syndrome
  Abdominal migraine
  Functional constipation
  Intestinal pseudo-obstruction
Inflammatory Causes
  Chronic cholecystitis
  Chronic pancreatitis, with
    or without pseudocyst
  Inflammatory bowel disease
  Non-*Helicobacter pylori*-
    mediated esophagitis, gas-
    tritis, and peptic ulcer dis-
    ease (reflux, nonsteroidal
    anti-inflammatory drugs,
    corticosteroids, etc.)
Infectious Causes
  Giardia lamblia enteritis and
    other parasitic infections
  H. pylori–mediated
    esophagitis, gastritis, and
    peptic ulcer disease

Vertebral infection—diskitis,
  osteomyelitis
Anatomic/Mechanical Causes
  Abdominal muscle strain
  Choledochal cyst
  Cholelithiasis
  Chronic nephrolithiasis
  Hematoma, intra-abdominal
  Hernia, internal
  Intestinal duplication
  Malrotation with or without
    volvulus
  Musculoskeletal
  Slipping-rib syndrome
  Ureteropelvic junction
    obstruction
Gynecologic Causes
  Dysmenorrhea
  Endometriosis
  Hematometrocolpos
  Mittelschmerz
  Cystic teratoma
Toxic Causes
  Lead poisoning
Systemic Causes
  Abdominal tumor—Wilms
    tumor, neuroblastoma
  Acute intermittent
    porphyria
  Carbohydrate intolerance/
    malabsorption
  Celiac disease
  Chronic Henoch-Schönlein
    purpura
  Collagen vascular disease
  Hepatitis
  Hereditary angioedema

Leukemia
Lymphoma, including
  gastrointestinal (GI)
  tract lymphomas
Sickle cell disease
Spinal column tumor (e.g.,
  leukemia, osteosarcoma)

Neurologic/Psychiatric
  Conversion reaction
  Depression
  Factitious

DIFFERENTIAL DIAGNOSIS DISCUSSION

Chronic abdominal pain is one of the **most commonly encountered symptoms** in pediatrics. The definition has evolved since first introduced in the 1950s by Apley as intermittent abdominal pain in children between the ages of 4 to 16 that is present for >3 months and affects daily activity. In clinical practice, pain lasting >**2 months** is considered to be chronic. Prevalence studies indicate that as many as 20% of middle and high school students experience frequent abdominal pain. Approximately 90% of these children have **functional or nonorganic abdominal pain,** pain without demonstrable evidence of a pathologic condition, such as an infectious, inflammatory, anatomic, or biochemical mechanism. The remainder of patients have **organic abdominal pain,** whose most common causes are described in detail here.

Abdominal Pain in Infants/Toddlers

Infant Colic

Infant colic is a **functional GI** disorder in an infant <4 to 5 months without a clear organic basis. Whereas the term "colic" implies abdominal pain secondary to obstruction of blood flow from an organ such as the kidney, gallbladder, or intestine, **"infant colic"** is a behavioral syndrome incorporating bouts of **crying and difficult-to-soothe behavior** that is usually influenced by psychosocial issues in a family. No clear evidence indicates that colic pain is from GI organs or from any other body part. Nonetheless, it is often assumed that the cause of the excessive colic is GI in origin.

Etiology

Colic, when referring to the prolonged crying seen in infancy, is technically defined as colic syndrome. The definition of infantile colic has evolved from the seminal definition by Wessel in the 1950s to include paroxysms of crying, irritability or fussiness **lasting >3 hours per day and occurring at least 3 days per week for >1 week.** Organic etiologies such as failure to thrive need to be excluded. The **etiology of colic is not**

well understood, and the mechanisms proposed to cause it are at best vague. The **immaturity of the infant nervous system** may play a role, particularly the transitioning to a more awake state. The gradual decrease in colic symptoms coincides with the acquisition of skills that enable the infant to more adequately maintain a calm awake state. Behavioral factors such as burping abnormalities or crying while feeding leading to ingested air (**aerophagia**) are suggested; however, it is argued that intestinal gas is a result of colic rather than a cause. Baseline **motilin** levels are raised, suggesting that increased gastric emptying increases small bowel peristalsis leading to perceived intestinal pain. Other proposed etiologies include **intolerance to cow's milk,** although little evidence indicates that children with colic have true milk protein intolerance, and the symptoms of that disorder do not include colic-like symptoms.

Evaluation

The **crying** noted in colic typically **peaks in the evening** at the **age of 6 weeks,** generally tapering off by 3 to 4 months of age. Other features include movements and facial features interpreted as being consistent with pain, as well as **GI symptoms** such as gas and abdominal distention. Clearly, these criteria are loose and may fall within the realm of normal infant behavior, albeit at one end of the curve. Physical and laboratory examinations of children with colic are uniformly normal.

Treatment

Treatment of colic is designed to **relieve the parents' stress.** Infants in this age range are targets of abuse, and preventing overstressed parents from harming these children is an important goal. Advice to parents of an infant with colic should always include suggestions on how to manage the stress, such as taking a brief break from caregiving. **Reassurance** that the crying will eventually stop is helpful. **Environmental changes** that facilitate the awake state and reduce crying, such as increasing rhythmic rocking, using a pacifier, increasing background white noise with a vacuum cleaner or washing machine, or taking a ride in the car or stroller, may be helpful. Antispasmodics and anticholinergics are not indicated for use in infants because they are associated with **respiratory distress** and **apnea.** Changing from breast- to formula-feeding is not indicated, and switching formulas should only be done if there is a suggestion of true milk-protein intolerance.

Infant Dyschezia

Etiology

Infant dyschezia is defined as a **functional** GI disorder. It is characterized by otherwise healthy infants <6 months of age experiencing at least **10 minutes of straining and crying** before successful passage of soft stools. Infant dyschezia is secondary to failure to coordinate increased intra-abdominal pressure with pelvic floor relaxation. Crying is analogous to creating increased abdominal pressure (Valsalva maneuver) prior to learning how to coordinate and bear down more effectively.

Evaluation and Treatment

Parents describe screaming, crying, and turning red or purple in the face with effort prior to defecation. **Physical examination**, which should be performed in the presence of the parents to help promote effective reassurance, is **normal**, inclusive of rectal examination. Diagnostic tests are not required. **Avoidance of rectal stimulation** is advised to negate artificial sensory experiences. Infant dyschezia rarely lasts >1 to 2 weeks and responds spontaneously.

Infant Regurgitation

Etiology

Uncomplicated regurgitation of food in otherwise healthy infants ages 3 weeks to 12 months is a **functional** GI disorder. It is defined as regurgitation **two or more times per day for >3 weeks** without evidence of pathologic symptoms such as apnea, failure to thrive, aspiration, feeding difficulties, retching, or hematemesis. When regurgitation contributes to tissue damage or inflammation of the esophagus, it is known as **gastroesophageal reflux disease.**

Evaluation and Treatment

Parents usually describe **irritability or arching of the back** after feeds. Regurgitation occurs in more than two thirds of healthy 4-month-old infants. Daily regurgitation decreases with age to 5% of infants 10 to 12 months of age. Risk factors include abnormalities of the chest, lungs, central nervous system, oropharynx, heart, or GI tract. Milk allergy may be present, especially if associated with eczema or wheezing and may require switching of infant formula. The natural history of infant regurgitation suggests **spontaneous improvement**. Left-sided positioning and thickening of feeds may help reduce symptoms. Improving the parent–child relationship and decreasing familial stress are ways to help provide effective reassurance. Gastroesophageal reflux in infants is treated with **acid blockade**, most commonly a **histamine$_2$-receptor antagonist.**

ABDOMINAL PAIN IN CHILD/ADOLESCENT

Children with functional GI disorders typically exhibit one of three clinical presentations, including isolated paroxysmal abdominal pain, abdominal pain associated with dyspepsia, and abdominal pain associated with irritable bowel syndrome as specified by the **Rome III criteria** and described here and in Table 10-1. Also included in functional

TABLE 10-1 Rome Criteria for the Diagnosis of Functional Abdominal Pain in Children with Pain at Least Once per Week for at Least 2 Months Prior to Diagnosis

Childhood Functional Abdominal Pain	Childhood Functional Abdominal Pain Syndrome	Functional Dyspepsia	Irritable Bowel Syndrome
Episodic or continuous abdominal pain *and*	Episodic or continuous abdominal pain 25% of the time *and*	Persistent or recurrent pain or discomfort in the upper abdomen (above the umbilicus) *and*	Abdominal pain or discomfort at least 25% of the time with two or more of the following: relief with defecation, onset associated with a change in frequency, or onset associated with a change in stool consistency *and*
No structural or biochemical abnormalities to explain the symptoms *and*	Some loss of daily functioning *or*	Symptoms not relieved by defecation or associated with the onset of a change in stool frequency or stool form *and*	Associated with abnormal stool frequency (≤2 times/week or ≥4 times/day), alternating stool character, straining, urgency, passing mucus, bloating, and distension *and*
The child does not satisfy criteria for another type of functional abdominal pain.	Somatic systems such as headache, limb pain, or difficulty sleeping *and* No structural or biochemical abnormalities to explain the symptoms.	No structural or biochemical abnormalities to explain symptoms.	No structural or biochemical abnormalities to explain the symptoms.

disorders are abdominal migraine, appendiceal colic, and functional constipation. Chronic intestinal pseudo-obstruction is a defect in small bowel intestinal motility. Approximately 20% of school-age children, most commonly **4 to 16 years of age,** are believed to have some variety of functional abdominal pain. The mean age of onset is **between 4 and 8 years of age,** with boys and girls affected equally until 9 years of age, at which point more girls are affected. Onset **>14 years** is usually associated with symptoms more consistent with **irritable bowel syndrome,** whereas onset **<4 years** has a greater chance of an **organic etiology.** Although psychological factors are important, there is no correlation of functional abdominal pain with personality traits such as perfectionism or chronic worrying.

Etiology

The factors that produce functional abdominal pain are not entirely clear. Pathophysiologic studies have focused on the autonomic nervous system and GI motility, suggesting a role for **altered gastric motility** and **heightened visceral sensitivity** to intestinal contractions in individuals with functional abdominal pain. Although psychological factors do not distinguish organic from nonorganic etiology, correlation with various psychosocial factors, such as **family stress,** are described. Often there is a family history of alcoholism, behavioral problems, abdominal pain, or migraine headaches. The **family dynamic in response to the pain** is important as well, as often there is positive reinforcement for having abdominal pain, ranging from emotional support to excusing from school or household chores.

Childhood Functional Abdominal Pain

Childhood functional abdominal pain is defined as episodic or continuous pain that occurs **at least once per week for at least 2 months prior to diagnosis** without a clear organic etiology. Childhood functional abdominal pain syndrome includes functional abdominal pain **at least 25% of the time and either some loss of daily functioning or somatic symptoms** such as headaches, limb pain, or difficulty sleeping. Pain is usually generalized or periumbilical, lasts <1 hour, and does not have a temporal relation to meals.

Functional Dyspepsia

Functional dyspepsia is defined as persistent or recurrent abdominal pain or discomfort centered **above the umbilicus and not relieved by defecation or associated with changes in stool frequency or consistency.** There is no evidence of an underlying etiology including an inflammatory, anatomic, metabolic, or neoplastic process that can explain the symptoms that need to be present at least once per week for at least

2 months prior to diagnosis. Often there is a temporal relation between meal ingestion and symptoms. Commonly associated symptoms include nausea, early satiety, postprandial abdominal distention, and excess gas.

Irritable Bowel Syndrome

Irritable bowel syndrome is characterized by abdominal discomfort or pain occurring at least 25% of the time without an underlying etiology and two of the following: **improvement with defecation, a change in stool frequency, or a change in stool consistency.** The symptoms are present at least once per week for at least **2 months** prior to diagnosis. Irritable bowel is usually associated with autonomic-type symptoms and environmental stress, as is isolated functional abdominal pain.

Evaluation

Functional abdominal pain is categorized by the different constellation of symptoms. The pain of functional abdominal pain is **recurrent and paroxysmal.** There is typically **a clustering of the pain episodes** within days or weeks that waxes and wanes over the course of months. The pain is often difficult for the child to describe and often not associated with eating or other activities but frequently occurs at the **same time of day** and usually lasts **<1 hour.** The presence of alarming symptoms such as weight loss, melena, and other red flags listed in Table 10-2 suggests the presence of an organic etiology to the pain.

As with all diagnoses in medicine, a **thorough and careful history** is the most helpful tool in the diagnosis of functional abdominal pain because it reveals the absence of alarming signals. The **physical examination** of the child with functional abdominal pain is **normal,** including rectal exam and stool guaiac. Although indiscriminate testing of these children is

---

TABLE 10-2 **Clinical Features of Abdominal Pain of Organic Etiology**

Age <4 years
Pain localized to the right upper quadrant
Pain referred to the back, chest, shoulder, or lower extremities
Associated joint pain or swelling
Dysuria, flank pain, hematuria, or dark-colored urine
Dyspareunia or vaginal discharge
Constitutional symptoms such as fever, weight loss, growth deceleration, rash, or night sweats
Significant vomiting
Significant diarrhea
Gross or occult blood in the stool
Intermittent fecal incontinence
Perianal disease (tags, fissures, fistulae)
Decreased energy or sleepiness after pain attacks
Abnormal physical examination (i.e., hypotonia)
Abnormal screening laboratory studies, including elevated white blood count or erythrocyte sedimentation rate, hypoalbuminemia, anemia

unwarranted, **normal screening laboratory tests** will reassure the clinician and family there is no organic cause of the abdominal pain. **Laboratory testing** suggested includes complete blood cell count, erythrocyte sedimentation rate, liver function tests including aminotransferases and albumin, urinalysis, and examination of the feces for ova and parasites. **Upper endoscopy** is indicated in patients with **dyspepsia pain** if response to treatment is poor or if symptoms recur after a 4- to 6-week course of medication. **Lactose breath test** is helpful if lactose intolerance is a concern, and **abdominal ultrasound** may be helpful if the child is difficult to examine or if there is concern for an anatomic problem.

In addition to screening for organic causes, the clinician should work with the family to track the course of the pain and to attempt to gain a psychosocial understanding of the child and the family. A **pain diary** kept by the family is often a useful diagnostic and even occasionally therapeutic tool. Despite the clear influence of stress and other psychosocial factors in this disease, it is important that this diagnosis not be arrived at as a last resort, after "more serious" causes of abdominal pain have been "ruled out." As an adjunct in managing the situation, a **psychologist or psychiatrist** may be helpful because abdominal pain of any nature causes stress on the child and the family. Clearly, the clinician should use the tools available to identify the cause of abdominal pain while attempting to avoid overreliance on elaborate tests and unnecessary referrals to specialists.

Treatment

The treatment of functional GI disorders begins with making the diagnosis and letting the family understand this is a **genuine entity.** The goal of therapy is to restore **normality** to the patient's lifestyle and reduce or eliminate the pain. Generally, this involves **explaining that the pain is real**, most likely caused by altered intestinal motility or visceral hypersensitivity. In addition, **addressing the stressors** that seem to be contributing to the pain and **reversing the positive reinforcement** the child may be receiving are important. **School attendance is critical** to breaking the cycle, and school health officials must be instructed of the need for negative reinforcement. Involvement of **mental health professionals** may be helpful for many families in particularly stressful situations. Drug therapy for functional paroxysmal abdominal pain is generally not indicated, and hospitalization should be avoided. For functional dyspepsia, **avoidance** of nonsteroidal anti-inflammatory agents and foods that aggravate symptoms is recommended. The mainstay of treatment for irritable bowel syndrome in adults is a high-fiber diet; results in children, however, are less convincing. Peppermint oil and antispasmodics such as hyoscyamine may be helpful. Calcium channel antagonists and antimuscarinic agents' as well as biofeedback and psychotherapy have also been used. Much of the therapy for irritable bowel syndrome in children relies on **reassurance and education,** with psychological or behavioral support added if necessary.

Chronic Intestinal Pseudo-Obstruction

Etiology

Chronic intestinal pseudo-obstruction refers to a heterogeneous set of **functional GI motility disorders** resulting in **symptoms consistent with obstruction** but **without an actual mechanical blockage.** These diseases appear to result from **decreased contractility of the intestinal smooth muscle** and are generally caused by a multitude of conditions that result in **myopathy or neuropathy,** either localized to the viscera or in systemic diseases such as muscular dystrophy.

Evaluation and Treatment

Symptoms include pain similar to the pain of true obstruction: **vomiting, abdominal distention, constipation,** and **early satiety.** Diagnosis is difficult and requires exclusion of the causes of obstruction but may be suggested by **plain radiographs** or **scintigraphic studies of motility. Intestinal manometry** is helpful, although these tests are not done frequently in children. Treatment is often **supportive** and may include supplemental **enteral feeding** or **intravenous nutrition.** Pharmacological treatment is not consistently advantageous.

Peptic Disease

Etiology

"Chronic peptic disease" is a term that encompasses **ulcers in the small bowel and duodenum** as well as **esophagitis, gastritis,** and **duodenitis.** In children, gastroesophageal reflux, nonsteroidal anti-inflammatory drugs, COX-2 inhibitor or corticosteroid exposure, extensive burns, or head trauma are common etiologies for peptic disease. In older children and adolescents, *H. pylori* infection becomes relatively more common and duodenitis becomes more prevalent, although the other conditions still persist but at a much lower incidence. Often this group has a positive family history of ulcer disease.

Evaluation

The **symptoms** of chronic peptic disease **vary with age. In younger children, pain** is generally present in the **mid to upper abdomen** and has no temporal relation to eating. In contrast, peptic disease in the **older child** is characterized by **epigastric pain,** occasionally associated with vomiting, occurring after meals and in the early morning. Relief of pain during eating is not a characteristic sign of peptic disease in children. In any age child, **blood loss** from inflammation may lead to melena or occult blood in the stool. Diagnosis is established by **endoscopy and biopsy,** although milder cases may be inferred as positive by a successful therapeutic trial of medication. A **pH probe** may be helpful to document reflux-associated pain. **Urea breath tests,** *H. pylori* **serology,** and **stool polyclonal antigen** testing are various methods to detect *H. pylori.*

Treatment

Peptic disease is treated with **acid blockade,** by either a **histamine$_2$-receptor antagonist or a proton pump inhibitor.** If reflux is a concern, a prokinetic agent such as **metoclopramide or erythromycin ethylsuccinate** may be tried after an upper GI series has been obtained to rule out an anatomic cause of reflux such as malrotation. Treatment for *H. pylori* infection involves **acid blockade** using a proton pump inhibitor as well as **double antibiotic therapy** with amoxicillin plus clarithromycin or metronidazole.

Carbohydrate Intolerance

Etiology

Dietary carbohydrates serve as the substrates for bacterial fermentation, resulting in nausea, abdominal distention, and excessive flatulence with resultant abdominal pain and cramps. **Malabsorption of lactose** is by far the **most common type of carbohydrate intolerance.** Intolerance of lactose is caused by deficiency of the enzyme lactase, an inhabitant of the small intestinal brush border. Congenital lactase deficiency is extraordinarily rare, and the **most common causes of true lactase deficiency** are a **genetic late-onset lactase deficiency** or **mucosal injury.** The genetic form of late-onset lactase deficiency is least common in those of Scandinavian and Northwest European descent and most common in those of Native American, Southeast Asian, Turkish, Italian, and African descent. Mucosal injury may occur after gastroenteritis, particularly that caused by rotavirus, parasitic infections such as *Giardia,* celiac disease, Crohn disease, and radiation or drug exposure. **Sorbitol** and **fructose** are two carbohydrates that are frequent offenders. **Sorbitol** is found in **many sugar-free items,** and **fructose** is the primary sweetener in **most foods,** including soda and juices.

Evaluation

Ingestion of lactose-containing food usually results in abdominal distention, **excessive flatulence,** and nausea progressing to **periumbilical abdominal pain, cramps,** and finally **watery diarrhea.** Occasionally in adolescents there may be vomiting. Diagnosis may be made by history alone, although the gold standard of diagnosis is a **lactose breath test.** In this test, patients are fed lactose and breath is collected for hydrogen gas produced by fermentation of undigested lactose by colonic bacteria.

Treatment

Treatment involves **avoidance** of the offending sugar. Multiple dairy products, including formula, do not contain lactose. In addition, **dietary supplements of lactase** can predigest the lactose before consumption. Avoidance of other carbohydrates is more difficult, although there are special formulas and nutritional supplements for many types of carbohydrate intolerance. Complete resolution of symptoms with removal of the offending agent confirms the diagnosis.

Celiac Disease

Etiology

Celiac disease is an inheritable disorder of the small intestine. It is characterized by an inflammatory T-cell response to proteins in **wheat, rye,** and **barley** (collectively known as **gluten**). Although it has been demonstrated that the use of oats as part of a gluten-free diet in adults does not have unfavorable results, a few celiac patients show intolerance to oats. If untreated, celiac disease can lead to **anemia, infertility, osteoporosis** and **intestinal lymphoma.** Celiac disease is most common in **whites,** frequent in Asians from India, Pakistan, and Iran, and rare in Native Americans, Japanese, and Chinese.

Evaluation

The most common presenting symptoms include chronic diarrhea, steatorrhea, **iron deficiency anemia,** abdominal distention, muscle wasting, **short stature, and failure to thrive.** Abdominal pain usually accompanies other symptoms and is frequently associated with irritable bowel syndrome. Diagnosis is based on history, laboratory, and endoscopy findings. Serological markers include the **IgA antibodies to tissue transglutaminase (tTG) and endomysium (EMA) IgA antibodies and IgA levels.** Selective IgA deficiency occurs more frequently in children with celiac disease. Antigliadin antibodies have a poor positive predictive value. **Upper endoscopy** is the gold standard of diagnosis with biopsies taken from the distal duodenum or proximal jejunum while the patient is on a diet containing gluten, with resolution when gluten is removed from the diet. Endoscopic findings include total or subtotal villous atrophy, crypt elongation, surface cell damage, an increase in intraepithelial lymphocytes, and infiltration with inflammatory cells. Celiac disease is also associated with genetic factors encoded by the HLA complex, specifically **HLA-DQ2** and **HLA-DQ8.**

Treatment

Treatment involves **removing gluten from the diet. Wheat, rye,** and **barley** are the predominant grains containing the peptides. A gluten-free diet should result in a rapid clinical response, with histological recovery over 2 years. Strict adherence to the diet is difficult for many patients, especially among adolescents. Minute amounts of gluten in the diet induce change in the small bowel.

Inflammatory Bowel Disease

Etiology

Inflammatory bowel disease (IBD) commonly refers to **Crohn disease (CD) and ulcerative colitis (UC),** inflammatory conditions of the GI tract that cause chronic abdominal pain in children and adolescents. The etiology is unclear but thought to be multifactorial. A multitude of environmental, genetic, and immune factors lead to the development of IBD. Both CD and UC are more prevalent in the Northern Hemisphere and in industrialized nations.

Evaluation

History and physical examination are imperative in evaluating patients with IBD because the symptoms depend on the site and extent of mucosal inflammation and include extraintestinal manifestations in a subset of patients. Family history and growth charts are necessary. The most common presentations include abdominal pain, weight loss, bloody or nonbloody diarrhea, skin lesions, fevers, arthralgias, and growth failure. In CD, **abdominal pain** is most commonly in the **right lower quadrant** because most patients have disease in the terminal ileum and ascending colon, whereas in UC the **abdominal pain** is usually limited to **times of defecation** because most have rectosigmoid disease. Perirectal disease is most commonly associated with CD. **Laboratory testing** suggested includes evaluation of iron deficiency anemia, inflammatory markers, and nutritional status with albumin and prealbumin. *Anti-Saccharomyces cerevisiae* antibody (ASCA) and perinuclear antineutrophil cytoplasmic antibody (pANCA) assays are associated with CD and UC, respectively. **Upper GI series with small bowel** followthrough is essential for evaluating the small bowel, which may be affected in CD. Diagnosis is by **endoscopy with biopsies.** UC usually involves the rectum and extends proximally, whereas CD may involve any portion of the GI tract and may have skip lesions. The presence of granulomas on histology is diagnostic of CD.

Treatment

The goals of therapy are aimed at **decreasing bowel inflammation and preventing recurrent or worsening disease.** Initial therapy for mild symptoms is 5-aminosalicylates (5-ASA) and, if the symptoms are severe, corticosteroids. Patients with severe disease may need immunomodulatory therapy. Nutritional support with oral supplements or nasogastric or gastrostomy feedings may be critically important in addressing growth failure. Patients who fail to respond to medical therapy may require surgery. Colonic cancer and sclerosing cholangitis are associated risk factors.

Chronic Pancreatitis

Etiology

Chronic pancreatitis, more correctly termed **recurrent acute pancreatitis,** is typified by **recurrent bouts of abdominal pain with periods of intervening wellness** that **may progress to pancreatic insufficiency.** The etiology of chronic pancreatitis in children is often unclear. The differential includes hereditary pancreatitis, congenital or acquired pancreatic duct anomalies, cystic fibrosis, trauma, hypercalcemia, organic acidemias, and various hyperlipidemia syndromes. Occasionally, chronic pancreatitis is associated with pseudocyst formation.

Evaluation

Symptoms of chronic pancreatitis include **midepigastric pain** that may be **associated with stress or a large fatty meal.** Pain may radiate to the back, and **nausea and vomiting** are frequently associated. The episode usually **resolves within 1 week.** Occasionally, symptoms are associated with pancreatic insufficiency or diabetes mellitus. Diagnosis is based on history and laboratory findings of **elevated amylase and lipase,** although the levels may not correlate with the intensity of the pain. Amylase typically peaks 3 days after the onset of pancreatitis; the timing of the elevation of lipase is variable. With pancreatic insufficiency, serum amylase and lipase can be normalized. Late in the disease, fat-soluble vitamin deficiency, hypoalbuminemia, glucose intolerance, and abnormalities in liver enzymes can be seen. **Abdominal ultrasound or computerized tomography (CT) scan** may show enlargement or inflammation of the pancreas. Endoscopic retrograde cholangiopancreatography (**ERCP**) and noninvasive magnetic resonance cholangiopancreatography (**MRCP**) are useful in patients in whom gallstones are suspected (unusual in children) or in whom there is a concern for anatomic abnormalities.

Treatment

Treatment of acute pancreatitis involves **bowel rest and pain control.** Chronic pancreatitis may require **parenteral nutrition.** For those children in whom pancreatic insufficiency is suspected, **pancreatic enzyme supplementation** may be helpful. **Drainage or removal of a pseudocyst** is indicated if present to prevent possible infection or rupture.

Ureteropelvic Junction Obstruction and Other Genitourinary Disorders

Ureteropelvic junction obstruction refers to a **kink in the ureter at the outlet from the renal pelvis.** Ureteral obstruction leads to abdominal pain and occasional renal damage in children. The condition is **more common in males,** more often **left sided,** and frequently associated with **vomiting.** Symptoms vary with age. **Infants** often present with a **palpable abdominal mass or pyelonephritis,** whereas in **children** the presentation is more frequently **abdominal pain.** The pain is crampy and intermittent, occasionally as infrequent as twice per week, and may radiate to the groin or flank. **Older children** may have a **palpable abdominal mass or abnormalities on urinalysis** such as hematuria, but the absence of these findings does not rule out an obstruction. Diagnosis is made by **renal ultrasound or CT scan** of the abdomen. Treatment involves **surgical relief** of the obstruction.

Other genitourinary disorders may cause abdominal pain as well. **Chronic nephrolithiasis** may present as recurrent bouts of abdominal and/or groin pain, usually associated with hematuria. **Cystic teratoma of the ovary** may lead to chronic or recurrent abdominal pain, generally in the lower quadrants or pelvic region. As with ureteropelvic junction obstruction, **ultrasound** is the diagnostic method of choice for both of these entities. Treatment of nephrolithiasis in children is **supportive,** although further diagnostic evaluation for a cause may be indicated, especially in young children.

Parasitic Infections

Etiology

The most common parasitic infection associated with chronic abdominal pain is **giardiasis,** caused by the protozoan *Giardia lamblia.* This infection is most frequently associated with **drinking contaminated fresh water,** although **day care** may be a source in children.

Evaluation and Treatment

Symptoms usually **resolve over weeks,** but **occasionally children develop chronic symptoms** of diffuse, crampy abdominal pain, nausea, abdominal distention, increased flatulence, watery diarrhea, and weight loss from malabsorption. Diagnosis may be made by **collecting the stool** specifically to **look for the cysts or trophozoites,** or if these are negative and the suspicion is high, examination of **duodenal aspirates or biopsy specimens** may be revealing. Treatment is with **metronidazole.**

Infection with other parasites such as *Ascaris lumbricoides, Trichuris trichiura,* which is more common in the tropics, *Blastocystis hominis,* or *Dientamoeba fragilis* may lead to abdominal pain. Associated symptoms include anorexia, diarrhea, rectal prolapse, and occasionally small bowel obstruction. Diagnosis is made by screening the **stool for ova and parasites.** Peripheral eosinophilia may be observed in *D. fragilis.* **Treatment** of these helminths is mebendazole or albendazole for *Ascariasis* or *Trichuriasis.* Iodoquinol is the drug of choice for *D. fragilis;* metronidazole, iodoquinol and trimethoprim-sulfamethoxazole are effective to eradicate *B. hominis.* Improvement of sanitation is necessary for population-wide eradication.

History: Important Questions
- Duration and location of the pain?
- Association of the pain with menses?
- Any ingestion of toxins such as lead?
- Any medications: prescribed, herbal, or over the counter?

History: Alarming Points
- Associated fever, weight loss, joint pain, or rash
- Associated vomiting, especially bilious or bloody emesis
- Associated change in stool pattern, especially diarrhea, bloody stool, or melena

History: Does not Distinguish Between Functional and Organic
- Pain quality is altered by eating or stooling.
- Pain wakes patient up at night.
- Family history of inflammatory bowel disease, peptic ulcer disease, functional abdominal pain, migraines.

Physical Examination: Important Clues
- Vital signs, general appearance, interactions with others
- Weight and height percentile patterns
- Mouth: Ulcers? Destruction of tooth enamel?
- Abdominal exam: Distended? Tender? If so, location? Rebound? Mass or stool palpable? Hepatosplenomegaly?
- Rectal examination: Tone of rectum? Size of rectal vault? Perianal disease? Hard stool? Grossly bloody or occult blood?
- Skin: Jaundice? Rash?
- Musculoskeletal: Joint swelling, redness, or tenderness?

Supportive Laboratory Studies
- Complete blood cell count
- Erythrocyte sedimentation rate
- Liver function tests: aminotransferases, albumin, bilirubin
- Amylase and lipase
- Urinalysis and culture
- Electrolytes, blood urea nitrogen, creatinine
- Stool ova and parasites

TABLE 10-3 Distinguishing Characteristics of Various Causes of Chronic Abdominal Pain

Diagnosis	Historical Clues	Physical Examination Clues	Lab/Diagnostic Study Clues
Infant colic	■ Irritability or fussiness for ≥3 hours per day, at least 3 days per week, for at least 1 week ■ Occurs sporadically and usually in the evening	Normal examination	Normal lab findings.
Childhood functional abdominal pain	■ Episodic or continuous ■ Duration >2 months ■ Pain not associated with eating or stooling ■ Functional abdominal pain syndrome includes some loss of daily functioning or somatic symptoms	Normal examination	Normal lab findings.
Functional dyspepsia	■ Abdominal pain above the umbilicus ■ Duration >2 months ■ Pain not associated with stooling	Normal examination	Normal labs and studies, including endoscopy.
Irritable bowel syndrome	■ Duration >2 months ■ Associated with straining, urgency, passing mucus, bloating, and distension ■ Pain relieved by defecation or associated with a change in bowel pattern	Normal examination	Normal lab findings.
Abdominal migraine	■ Intense paroxysmal periumbilical pain that interferes with normal activity ■ Intervening periods of usual health ■ May be associated with headache, vomiting, photophobia, pallor, anorexia, or nausea ■ Family history of migraine	Normal examination	■ May respond to antimigraine medications. ■ Trigger avoidance.

(Continued)

TABLE 10-3 Distinguishing Characteristics of Various Causes of Chronic Abdominal Pain *(continued)*

Diagnosis	Historical Clues	Physical Examination Clues	Lab/Diagnostic Study Clues
Chronic intestinal pseudo-obstruction	■ Intermittent crampy pain, vomiting, and decreased flatus ■ Vomiting may be bilious ■ May have history of previous abdominal surgery	■ Abdominal distension and tenderness ■ May have scars from previous surgery on abdomen	■ Abdominal radiograph frequently shows fixed air-fluid levels with decreased air distally.
Functional constipation	■ Diffuse, vague pain ■ Decreased stool frequency; hard or voluminous stool ■ Large-diameter stools that may obstruct toilet ■ May have withholding or encopresis	■ Often large fecal mass on rectal exam ■ Often dilated rectal vault	■ Normal lab findings. ■ Abdominal radiograph may show abundant stool, dilated colon.
Peptic disease	■ Epigastric pain ■ Pain often, but not always, after meals ■ Family history of ulcers possible	■ May have epigastric tenderness ■ Heme-positive stools possibly present	■ Anemia possible. ■ A pH probe may be helpful. ■ Endoscopy shows esophagitis, gastritis, duodenitis, or ulcers. *Helicobacter pylori* studies may be positive.
Carbohydrate intolerance	■ Diffuse, crampy pain after meals ■ Watery diarrhea typical ■ May have poor weight gain ■ May be postinfectious ■ More common in certain ethnic groups	■ Usually normal	■ Breath tests for the offending sugar are the tests of choice.
Celiac disease	■ May have chronic diarrhea ■ May have failure to thrive ■ May have abdominal distention	■ Tooth discoloration/loss of enamel possible ■ Rash possible	■ Iron-deficiency anemia. ■ Abnormal anti-tissue transglutaminase and anti-endomysial antibodies. ■ Endoscopy and histology show flattened villi in duodenum/jejunum.

Condition	History/Symptoms	Physical Examination	Diagnostic Evaluation
Inflammatory bowel disease	■ Pain diffuse or localized ■ Constitutional symptoms such as fever, weight loss, rash, joint pain common ■ Diarrhea or bloody stool possibly present ■ Vomiting possible ■ Mouth ulcers or perianal disease possibly present	■ Fever, tachycardia ■ Abdominal tenderness ■ Heme-positive stools frequent ■ Rash or joint findings possible	■ Elevated erythrocyte sedimentation rate, anemia, hypoalbuminemia are common. ■ Upper GI-small bowel series may show strictures in Crohn disease. ■ Endoscopy and biopsy needed for diagnosis.
Chronic pancreatitis	■ Midepigastric pain ■ May radiate to back ■ May have vomiting or loss of appetite ■ May have malabsorptive symptoms	■ May be ill appearing or cachectic ■ Midepigastric tenderness common	■ Elevated amylase and lipase. ■ May have enlargement of pancreas or pseudocyst by ultrasound or CT.
Ureteropelvic junction obstruction	■ Diffuse intermittent pain that may radiate to groin or flank ■ May have hematuria ■ Frequently associated with vomiting	■ May have palpable abdominal mass ■ May have costovertebral angle tenderness	■ Ultrasound or CT scan shows anomaly.
Nephrolithiasis	■ Severe intermittent crampy pain in abdomen and/or flank, occasionally radiating to groin ■ Often associated with hematuria ■ Often associated with nausea and vomiting	■ May have abdominal or costovertebral angle tenderness	■ Ultrasound or CT scan may show presence of stone.
Giardiasis	■ Diffuse, crampy pain ■ Weight loss or poor weight gain ■ Nausea, watery diarrhea, bloating, increased flatulence common ■ Exposure through day care or contaminated fresh water	■ Abdominal distention common	■ Stool examination may show cysts or trophozoites. ■ May need to perform duodenal aspirates or endoscopy.

(Continued)

147

TABLE 10-3 Distinguishing Characteristics of Various Causes of Chronic Abdominal Pain *(continued)*

Diagnosis	Historical Clues	Physical Examination Clues	Lab/Diagnostic Study Clues
Biliary colic	■ RUQ or midepigastric crampy pain after meals, especially fatty foods ■ May have vomiting ■ May be obese or have concurrent illness	■ RUQ or midepigastric tenderness possible	■ May have elevated bilirubin or transaminases. ■ Ultrasound shows gallstones or thickened gallbladder wall.
Ovarian teratoma	■ Intermittent lower quadrant pain, often one sided ■ Vomiting possible	■ Lower-quadrant fullness, tenderness	■ Ultrasound or CT scan will show anomaly. ■ Ultrasound can also determine blood flow.
Dysmenorrhea	■ Crampy lower abdominal pain, occurring during menses ■ Often a family history of dysmenorrhea	■ Normal examination	■ Normal studies, although some may have endometriosis.
Lead poisoning	■ Diffuse pain ■ Often a history of pica ■ In high-risk exposure area	■ Usually normal	■ Elevated serum lead level. ■ Microcytic anemia. ■ May see basophilic stippling.

CT = computed tomography; EEG = electroencephalogram; GI = gastrointestinal; RUQ = right upper quadrant; WBC = white blood cell.

Diagnostic Tests: Based on Clinical Suspicion

- Abdominal two-view radiograph
- Abdominal ultrasound
- Lactose or other breath tests
- Endoscopy and biopsy

Table 10-3 displays distinguishing characteristics of the different causes of chronic abdominal pain. The determination of the exact cause of a child's abdominal pain may require multiple visits. Occasionally, referral to a specialist is indicated. It is critical that all involved work as a team and address all of the factors that have produced chronic abdominal pain in the child.

Suggested Readings

Altschuler SM, Liacouras CA (eds): *Clinical Pediatric Gastroenterology.* Philadelphia, Churchill Livingstone, 1998.

Boyle JT: Recurrent abdominal pain: an update. *Pediatr Rev* 18:310–320, 1997.

Diefenbach KA, Breuer CK: Pediatric inflammatory bowel disease. *World J Gastroenterol* 12(20):3204–3212, 2006.

DiLorenzo C, Colletti RB, Lechmann HP, et al.: Chronic abdominal pain in children: a clinical report of the American Academy of Pediatric and the North American Society for Pediatric Gastroenterology, Hepatology and Nutrition. *J Pediatr Gastroenterol Nutr* 40:245–248, 2005.

Drossman DA: The functional gastrointestinal disorders and the Rome III process. *Gastroenterology* 130:1377–1390, 2006.

Gold BD, Colletti RB, Abbott M, et al.: *Helicobacter pylori* infection in children: recommendations for diagnosis and treatment. *J Pediatr Gastroenterol Nutr* 31:490–497, 2000.

Hyman PE, Milla PJ, Benninga MA, et al.: Childhood functional gastrointestinal disorders: neonate/toddler. *Gastroenterology* 130:1519–1526, 2006.

Mearin ML: Celiac disease among children and adolescents. *Curr Probl Pediatr Adolesc Heath Care* 7(3):86–105, 2007.

Megraud F: Comparison of non-invasive tests to detect *Helicobacter pylori* infection in children and adolescents: results of a multicenter European study. *J Pediatr* 146:198–203, 2005.

Rasqion A, DiLorenzo C, Forbes D, et al.: Childhood functional gastrointestinal disorders: child/adolescent. *Gastroenterology* 130:1527–1537, 2006.

Red Book 2006: Report of the Committee on Infectious Disease, 27th ed. Edited by Pickering LK. Elk Grove Village, Il, American Academy of Pediatrics, 2006.

Walker WA, Durie PR, Hamilton JR, et al. (eds): *Pediatric Gastrointestinal Disease: Pathophysiology, Diagnosis, Management,* 4th ed. Hamilton, Ontario, BC Decker, 2004.

Wyllie R, Hyams JS (eds): *Pediatric Gastrointestinal and Liver Disease,* 3rd ed. Philadelphia, WB Saunders, 2006.

11 *Alopecia*

Janet H. Friday

INTRODUCTION

Tinea capitis, trichotillomania, alopecia areata, and telogen effluvium account for >95% of cases of alopecia in children. The growth cycle of hair consists of an active growth phase (anagen), a transition phase (catagen), and a resting phase (telogen). After the telogen phase, the hair is shed and replaced by a new anagen bulb. On a normal scalp, approximately 85% to 90% of the hair is in the anagen phase. There are 100,000 hairs on the normal scalp. Hair loss is only clinically apparent when a person has lost 25% to 50% of his hair.

DIFFERENTIAL DIAGNOSIS LIST

Infectious Causes
Tinea capitis
Secondary syphilis

Toxic Causes
Cytotoxic agents
Anticonvulsants
Radiation
Hypervitaminosis A
Anticoagulants

Neoplastic Causes
Histiocytosis

Traumatic Causes
Trichotillomania
Traction alopecia
Friction alopecia

Congenital Causes
Aplasia cutis congenita
Nevus sebaceous
Epidermal nevus
Hemangioma
Loose anagen syndrome

Ectodermal dysplasia
Hair shaft defects

Metabolic or Genetic Causes
Androgenic alopecia
Acrodermatitis enteropathica
Anorexia nervosa
Malnutrition
Hypo- or hyperthyroidism
Hypopituitarism
Diabetes mellitus

Inflammatory Causes
Alopecia areata
Systemic lupus
  erythematosus
Scleroderma

Miscellaneous Causes
Atopic dermatitis
Seborrheic dermatitis
Psoriasis
Telogen effluvium
Anagen effluvium

DIFFERENTIAL DIAGNOSIS DISCUSSION

Tinea Capitis

Etiology

Caused by **dermatophyte** infection of the scalp hairs, tinea capitis is responsible for **<50% of cases of hair loss** in children. Currently, the most prevalent fungus causing tinea capitis is *Trichophyton tonsurans*.

Clinical Features

Tinea capitis is seen most commonly in school-age children. The infection causes **patchy hair loss** that may or may not be accompanied by **scale**. Some areas may seem completely bald and indistinguishable from alopecia areata, but on closer examination the scalp contains **very short hairs**, called "black-dot" tinea capitis.

Evaluation

Unlike *Microsporum canis*, which caused epidemic outbreaks of tinea capitis during the 1940s, *T. tonsurans* does not show immunofluorescence under Wood lamp examination. Diagnosis can be confirmed using a **potassium hydroxide (KOH) preparation** and by **fungal culture** of the hair and scale. A KOH preparation reveals organisms inside the hair shaft.

Treatment

Oral griseofulvin dosed at 15 to 20 mg/kg once daily for 6 to 8 weeks is the standard therapy for tinea capitis in children. It is best absorbed when taken with **fatty foods**. The medication is **safe in children;** it is not necessary for the patient to undergo laboratory testing before initiating drug therapy. Newer antifungal medications such as **fluconazole, itraconazole,** and **terbinafine** may also be effective and require a shorter course of therapy. An **antifungal or selenium shampoo** may hasten resolution in combination with systemic antifungal medication. An effort should be made to identify and treat infected household contacts to avoid reinfection.

> **HINT:** The infection may be accompanied by a hypersensitivity reaction called a kerion, which is a boggy, inflammatory mass. The surface may contain pustules, and cervical lymphadenopathy is usually present. Although it may appear to be superinfected, the lesion can usually be treated successfully with griseofulvin and oral prednisone.

> **HINT:** Tinea capitis mimics many other conditions and should be considered the diagnosis of exclusion in all cases of acquired localized alopecia.

Alopecia Areata

Etiology

Alopecia areata is the **second most common cause** of alopecia in children and may appear insidiously in an otherwise healthy school-age patient. Multiple factors are implicated in the pathophysiology, including genetic, organ-specific autoimmune, and nonspecific immune components.

Clinical Features

The hair loss occurs in **variably sized patches** completely **devoid of hair.** Hairs surrounding the area of alopecia may demonstrate a narrow waist on microscopic examination ("exclamation point" hairs). The **entire scalp** is **involved in alopecia totalis,** and the **entire body** is **involved in alopecia universalis.** Accompanying features may include **pitting** or a **scotch-plaid pattern** on the **nails.** Other autoimmune disorders may occur in these patients, such as Hashimoto thyroiditis, diabetes mellitus, vitiligo, Addison disease, and inflammatory bowel disease.

Evaluation

Hair pluck with microscopy should be performed to look for classic **"exclamation point" hairs,** which confirm the diagnosis of alopecia areata.

Treatment

Treatment for this disorder is less than straightforward. Modalities such as topical and systemic steroids, minoxidil, and anthralin have been used; unfortunately, none have proved effective in reversing the course of disease. In **a third of patients,** the **condition regresses spontaneously** within 6 months. More extensive cases are less likely to resolve. A frank discussion with the patient and family and **close follow-up** are mandatory. A **wig or hairpiece** may be necessary to counteract the psychological trauma of this disease. **Referral to a pediatric dermatologist** should be considered in all cases in which aggressive therapy seems warranted.

Trichotillomania

Etiology

Seen more commonly in children than in adults, trichotillomania is an **uncontrollable urge to pull out one's own hair.** Adolescent girls are most commonly afflicted; however, in children <6 years, it is more common in boys.

Clinical Features

The hair-pulling results in **ill-defined areas of baldness** in **unusual distributions.** The diagnosis is usually made clear by the presence of **many** broken hairs of various lengths. The sites involved are varied, although a predilection for the side of handedness may be seen. The periphery of the scalp is usually spared. Other body hair may also be involved in severe cases. Often nail biting, thumb sucking, and **other compulsive behaviors** are also present.

Evaluation

Hair pluck should be performed to rule out alopecia areata. A **scalp biopsy** may be necessary to confirm the diagnosis.

Treatment

This diagnosis may be difficult for the family to accept. Treatment strategies include **cognitive behavior therapy.** Severe cases should be **referred to a psychiatrist** for adjuvant pharmacotherapy.

Telogen Effluvium

Telogen effluvium occurs when a **large percentage of scalp hairs enter the resting phase** after a **stressful event** and are shed 2 to 4 months later. The precipitant may be childbirth, major surgery, anesthesia, febrile illness, crash dieting, or psychological trauma. The hallmark of telogen effluvium is **diffuse acute hair loss** that **spontaneously resolves** over several months. Hair pluck reveals a disproportionate number of hair follicles in the telogen phase. Eventually, **full recovery** of hair growth ensues and no treatment is necessary.

Traction Alopecia and Friction Alopecia

Tension on the hair shaft can cause hair loss in areas most affected (traction alopecia). Tight braiding of the hair, ponytails, cornrows, and hot combs are the worst culprits. In a similar fashion, hair in **areas of pressure,** such as the occiput in a supine infant, may exhibit hair loss, although the scalp is functionally normal (friction alopecia). Hair loss occurs in a **classic distribution.** Diagnosis is made on a clinical basis. If the alopecia fails to respond to conservative management, the diagnosis should be reevaluated. The hairstyle or positioning should be altered. Normal hair growth should follow.

Anagen Effluvium

Like telogen effluvium, anagen effluvium is characterized by **diffuse acute hair loss.** In anagen effluvium, hair loss results from **disruption of the normal hair growth cycle** following a toxic insult to the hair follicle. The causes are usually cytotoxic agents such as vincristine and cyclophosphamide. Heavy metal toxicity, hypothyroidism, and severe malnutrition are also implicated. If the cause is not apparent, hair pluck differentiates anagen effluvium from telogen effluvium. The **hair regrows following**

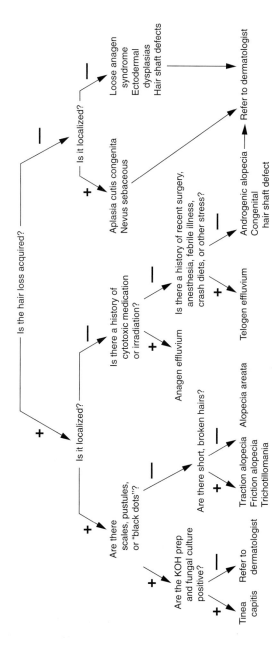

Figure 11-1 ■ Evaluation of a patient with alopecia.
KOH prep = potassium hydroxide preparation.

removal of the offending agent, although the color and texture of the new hair may be different.

EVALUATION OF ALOPECIA

Patient History

The elements of the history most crucial to the diagnosis of alopecia disorders are as follows:

- Time of onset—congenital versus acquired
- Associated stressors—childbirth, recent surgery, toxic exposures, seizures, and febrile illnesses
- Any abnormal behaviors—for example, thumb sucking, nail biting

Physical Examination

Physical examination should focus on **distribution of hair loss, presence of scale, presence of broken hairs,** and **nail findings.** A magnifying glass and good lighting aid in detection of subtle scalp findings.

Laboratory Studies

A **KOH preparation** is important when the diagnosis of tinea capitis is suspected, and **fungal culture** should be obtained. A **hair pluck** is used to diagnose telogen effluvium or alopecia areata. **Morphologic examination of the hair shaft** allows detection of structural defects.

> **HINT:** If a diagnosis is still unclear after an initial evaluation, referral to a dermatologist may be warranted.

APPROACH TO THE PATIENT (FIGURE 11-1)

Suggested Readings

Atton AV, Tunnessen WW: Alopecia in children: the most common causes. *Pediatr Rev* 12(25):25–30, 1990.

Verbov J: Hair loss in children. *Arch Dis Child* 68:702–706, 1993.

Additional References

Levy ML: Disorders of the hair and scalp in children. *Pediatr Clin North Am* 38(4):905–919, 1991.

Madani S, Shapiro J: Alopecia areata update. *J Am Acad Dermatol* 42(4):549–566, 2000.

Raimer SS: New and emerging therapies in pediatric dermatology. *Dermatol Clin* 18:1, 2000.

Woods DW: Understanding and treating trichotillomania: what we know and what we don't know. Psychiatr Clin North Am 29:2, 2006.

Zhang AY, Camp WL, Elewski BE: Advances in topical and systemic antifungals. *Dermatol Clin* 25:165–183, 2007.

Ambiguous Genitalia

Lorraine E. Levitt Katz

INTRODUCTION

Genitalia are defined as ambiguous when it is not possible to categorize the gender of the child based on outward appearances. Ambiguous genitalia may be associated with genotypic **females who are virilized,** genotypic **males who are undermasculinized,** and problems of **gonadal differentiation.**

Sexual Differentiation

Management of patients with sexual ambiguity requires an understanding of normal sexual differentiation. The primitive gonad is bipotential, containing both ovarian (cortical) and testicular (medullary) components. Sexual differentiation is determined by the genetic information contained in the sex chromosomes, as well as by hormonal factors.

Male Sexual Differentiation

The SRY gene (i.e., the sex-determining region) on the short arm of the Y chromosome is the **primary testis-determining factor (TDF).** Additional genetic factors that are important to sexual differentiation include DAX-1, SOX-9, and Wnt 4. The transcription factors WT1 and SF 1 are necessary for gonadal development. TDF induces the bipotential gonads to develop as testes by 6 to 7 weeks of gestation. At 7 to 8 weeks of gestation, Sertoli cells in the testes secrete anti-müllerian hormone (AMH), also called müllerian-inhibiting substance (MIS), which causes regression of the müllerian ducts in the male fetus.

Human chorionic gonadotropin (HCG) and fetal pituitary gonadotropin stimulate the Leydig cells in the fetal testes to secrete **testosterone,** which causes the wolffian structures to develop into the vas deferens, epididymis, and seminal vesicles. Testosterone is converted locally to dihydrotestosterone (DHT) by 5α-reductase. DHT is necessary for the development of the scrotum and phallus from the labial scrotal folds and the genital tubercle.

Although the formation of the male genitals is complete by 12 weeks of gestation, MIS stimulates abdominal descent of the testes in the second trimester. During the second and third trimesters, further testicular descent and penile growth are stimulated by testosterone.

Female Sexual Differentiation

The differentiation of the bipotential gonad into an ovary by 10 weeks of gestation requires that two X chromosomes be present and that the

Y chromosome (i.e., the SRY gene) be absent. Because MIS is not produced, the müllerian ducts develop into the uterus, the fallopian tubes, and the upper two thirds of the vagina. In the **absence of androgens**, the wolffian ducts degenerate, the external genitalia differentiates as the clitoris and labia, and the urogenital sinus becomes the lower third of the vagina and urethra.

DIFFERENTIAL DIAGNOSIS LIST 🔓

Virilized Female
Pseudohermaphroditism
Congenital adrenal hyperplasia (CAH)—21-hydroxylase deficiency, 3β-hydroxysteroid dehydrogenase deficiency, 11-hydroxylase-deficiency
Maternal androgen exposure—exogenous, excess androgen production
Associated anatomic anomalies
Chromosomal Aberrations
XO/XY
XX/XY
True hermaphroditism
Idiopathic

Undervirilized Male
Pseudohermaphroditism
CAH—StAR deficiency, 17,20-desmolase deficiency, 3β-hydroxysteroid dehydrogenase deficiency, 17α-hydroxylase deficiency
Other androgen synthesis defects—17-lyase deficiency, 17-ketosteroid reductase deficiency, 5α-reductase deficiency, Smith Lemli-Opitz syndrome
Partial androgen receptor defects
Associated anatomic abnormalities
Deficient AMH
Gonadal (testicular) dysgenesis
Leydig cell hypoplasia
True hermaphroditism
Idiopathic

DIFFERENTIAL DIAGNOSIS DISCUSSION

Gonadal (Testicular) Dysgenesis
Etiology
- In **pure gonadal dysgenesis,** dysgenesis of the genital ridges results in gonads that are hypoplastic. The condition may be inherited or caused by teratogenic agents.
- In **partial gonadal dysgenesis,** teratogenic factors or vascular accidents may damage the gonads following differentiation into testes (in genetic males).
- In **mixed gonadal dysgenesis,** individuals with the mosaic genotypes XO/XY and XX/XY have gonads that contain both medullary and cortical elements.

Clinical Features

- In **pure gonadal dysgenesis**, the phenotype is that of a normal female.
- In **partial gonadal dysgenesis**, AMH has been secreted and the müllerian structures have degenerated, but the development of male external genitalia (which depends on the conversion of testosterone to DHT) does not occur. External genitalia are phenotypically female or ambiguous, but there are no gonads or müllerian structures. Testicular damage that occurs during the second and third trimesters may be less severe and may result in micropenis (i.e., a normally formed, appropriately positioned phallus with a length <2.5 standard deviations below the appropriate mean for the patient's age) or cryptorchidism.
- In **mixed gonadal dysgenesis**, external genitalia may be normal female, intersex, or normal male. Patients with XO/XY mosaicism often have many of the classic features of Turner syndrome. The presence of testicular tissue in patients with mixed gonadal dysgenesis increases the likelihood of androgenic hormonal function and the presence of wolffian duct structures.

Evaluation

The diagnosis is made by chromosomal analysis. In some cases, gonadal biopsy is indicated.

Treatment

Individuals with mixed gonadal dysgenesis have an increased risk of malignant degeneration of gonadal tissues, and gonadectomy is recommended.

True Hermaphroditism

True hermaphrodites possess both ovarian and testicular elements. They may have a separate ovary and a testis on the contralateral side or a combination of the two gonads ("ovotestes").

Etiology

True hermaphrodites include patients with mixed gonadal dysgenesis, as well as those with the karyotype 46,XX and (less commonly) 46,XY. The differentiation of the internal duct structures corresponds to the amount of testicular tissue present in the gonad on the same side. Müllerian duct structures may develop on the side of an ovary with contralateral wolffian duct structures, thus indicating that MIS acts locally.

Clinical Features

The degree of functioning testicular tissue determines the appearance of the external structures.

Evaluation

After ruling out hormonal causes of ambiguous genitalia, the definitive diagnosis can be made by gonadal biopsy demonstrating both ovarian and testicular tissue.

Treatment

Ovotestes and dysgenetic testes should be removed because of the risk for malignant degeneration.

Female Pseudohermaphroditism

Pseudohermaphroditism occurs when the external genitalia do not correspond to the chromosomal or gonadal sex (i.e., an XX female who is masculinized or an XY male who is inadequately masculinized). The internal genitalia develop normally.

Etiology

Virilization of the genotypic female fetus is usually caused by **androgens** produced by the fetus or transferred across the placenta. Androgen exposure before 12 weeks of gestation results in interference of septation of the urogenital sinus and some degree of labial scrotal fusion. After 12 weeks of gestation, androgen exposure can cause clitoral enlargement but not labial scrotal fusion. The following are sources of androgen exposure:

- **CAH.** Can 21-Hydroxylase, 11-hydroxylase, and 3β-hydroxysteroid dehydrogenase deficiencies are associated with the production of excessive amounts of adrenal androgens and are the most common causes of virilization in newborn females; 21-hydroxylase deficiency represents 90% of cases of CAH.
- **Exogenous androgens.** The use of progestational agents in the first trimester of pregnancy for prevention of spontaneous abortion is associated with female virilization; as a result, the use of these agents has decreased.
- **Exposure to maternal androgens.** The production of androgens by the mother, either as a result of poorly controlled CAH or as a result of an ovarian or adrenal tumor, may also cause masculinization of the female fetus.
- **Idiopathic.** Anomalies of the gastrointestinal and urinary tract may be associated with virilization of the female external genitalia without exposure to androgens. Rarely, female pseudohermaphroditism may occur independently of anatomic abnormalities or androgen exposure.

Clinical Features

The external genitalia are virilized. Patients with 21-hydroxylase or 3-hydroxylase deficiencies may present with salt-losing crises within a few weeks of birth.

Evaluation

In patients with pseudohermaphroditism caused by CAH (i.e., 21-hydroxylase deficiency, 3β-hydroxysteroid dehydrogenase deficiency, or 11-hydroxylase deficiency), the diagnosis can be made by obtaining baseline steroid measurements and steroid measurements following adrenocorticotropic hormone (ACTH) administration (Tables 12-1 through 12-3). Baseline and stimulated steroid levels are elevated.

In patients with other causes of pseudohermaphroditism, the androgen levels are not elevated and the diagnosis can usually be made on the basis of the patient's history and physical examination.

Treatment

Patients with pseudohermaphroditism caused by CAH should receive cortisol and mineralocorticoid replacement as needed. Cosmetic surgical repair may be appropriate for all patients.

Male Pseudohermaphroditism

Etiology

Inadequate masculinization of the genotypic male fetus can be caused by enzyme disorders of testosterone synthesis or a lack of responsiveness to testosterone action (androgen resistance syndromes).

- **CAH.** Can result in undervirilization of the male fetus when the adrenal enzymes necessary for testosterone synthesis (i.e., 3β-hydroxysteroid, 17α-hydroxylase, cholesterol desmolase) are also deficient in the testes. 3β-Hydroxysteroid dehydrogenase plays an important role in the early biosynthetic pathway of glucocorticoids, mineralocorticoids, and sex steroids. 17α-Hydroxylase deficiency is a rare disorder that results in the inability to produce sex steroids. Congenital lipid

TABLE 12-1 Clinical and Biochemical Features of Congenital Adrenal Hyperplasia (CAH)

| Enzyme Defect | Sexual Ambiguity | | Additional Clinical Manifestations | Predominant Steroids |
	Female	Male		
StAR, Desmolase	—	+	Salt wasting	. . .
3β-Hydroxysteroid dehydrogenase	+	+	Salt wasting	17-OH-Pregnenolone, DHEA
21-Hydroxylase	+	—	Salt wasting	17-OH-Progesterone, androstenedione
11-Hydroxylase	+	—	Hypertension	11-Deoxycortisol
17-Hydroxylase	—	+	Hypertension	DOC, corticosterone

DHEA = dehydroepiandrosterone; DOC = deoxycorticosterone.

TABLE 12-2 Normal Serum Adrenal Steroid Levels in Newborn Infants

Steroid	Preterm Sick		Preterm Well	Full Term
	24–28 weeks	31–35 weeks	31–35 weeks	
Cortisol (μg/dL)	7.5 ± 4	6 ± 2.7	6.9 ± 3.8	6.2 ± 3.9
17-OH-Preg (ng/dL)	1794 ± 1818	1395 ± 694	942 ± 739	245 ± 291
17-OH-Pro (ng/dL)	651 ± 661	373 ± 317	169 ± 95	36 ± 13*
11-deoxycortisol (ng/dL)	662 ± 548	294 ± 239	111 ± 62	87 ± 42
DHEA (ng/dL)	1872 ± 4038	675 ± 502	920 ± 1227	286 ± 238
DHEAS (μg/dL)	467 ± 312	459 ± 209	341 ± 93	162 ± 88
Androstenedione (ng/dL)	479 ± 1032	206 ± 86	215 ± 134	149 ± 67

Data based on information in Lee MM, Rajabopalan L, Berg G, et al.: Serum adrenal steroid concentrations in premature infants. *J Clin Endocrinol Metab* 69:1133–1136, 1989, and in Wiener D, Smith J, Dahlem S, et al.: Serum adrenal steroid levels in healthy term 3-day-old infants. *J Pediatr* 110(1):122–124, 1987.
17-OH-Preg = 17-OH-pregnenolone; 17-OH-Pro = 17-OH-progesterone; DHEA = dehydroepiandrosterone; DHEAS = dehydroepiandrosterone sulfate.
*17-OH-Pro values in full-term sick newborns may be double or triple the baseline values. No data are available for other steroid hormones in sick full-term infants.

adrenal hyperplasia associated with defects in steroidogenic acute regulatory protein StAR, as well as cholesterol desmolase deficiency, results in insufficient mineralocorticoid, glucocorticoid, and androgen synthesis.

■ **Other androgen synthesis defects.** 17-Ketosteroid reductase deficiency in the testes prevents the conversion of androstenedione to testosterone. 17-Lyase is necessary for the conversion of C21 steroids

TABLE 12-3 Serum Adrenal Steroid Levels in Infants 1-Hour Post-ACTH Administration

Steroid	Preterm Sick (24–28 weeks)	Well Infants (2–12 months)*	
		Female	Male
Cortisol (μg/dL)	18.3 ± 6.8	40 ± 8.1	38.2 ± 4.4
17-OH-Preg (ng/dL)	5730 ± 4461	1610 ± 800	1242 ± 753
17-OH-Pro (ng/dL)	968 ± 876	142 ± 50	196 ± 85

Data based on information in Hingre RV, Gross SJ, Hingre KS, et al.: Adrenal steroidogenesis in very low birth weight preterm infants. *J Clin Endocrinol Metab* 78(2):266–270, 1994, and in Lashansky G, Saenger P, Fishman K, et al.: Normative data for adrenal steroidogenesis in a healthy pediatric population: age- and sex-related changes after adrenocorticotropin stimulation. *J Clin Endocrinol Metab* 73:674–686, 1991.
ACTH = adrenocorticotropic hormone; 17-OH-Preg = 17-OH-pregnenolone; 17-OH-Pro = 17-OH-progesterone.
*No post-ACTH steroid data are available for full-term newborns.

to C19 androgenic steroids in the testes. 5α-Reductase deficiency prevents conversion of testosterone to DHT, which is necessary for the development of the male external genitalia.

- **Syndromes of androgen resistance.** Result from abnormalities in the androgen receptors or postreceptor defects. Testicular feminization is the classic X-linked androgen resistance syndrome. Affected patients have normal female external genitalia with absent wolffian and müllerian structures.

Clinical Features

Patients with male pseudohermaphroditism may show micropenis, hypospadias, a poorly developed scrotum, or undescended testes. Alternatively, a normal female phenotype may be present.

- **CAH.** Patients with 3β-hydroxysteroid dehydrogenase deficiency or StAR protein deficiency exhibit severe salt wasting in addition to ambiguity of the external genitalia. 17α-Hydroxylase–deficient individuals may be hypertensive because this disorder also results in increased mineralocorticoid production.
- **Other androgen synthesis defects.** Individuals with 17-ketosteroid reductase deficiency and 17-lyase deficiency have variable degrees of undervirilization. Patients with 5α-reductase deficiency have a blind vaginal pouch, small phallic structure, and severe hypospadias; some infants are assigned a female sex at birth. Because the testis produces both MIS and testosterone, regression of the müllerian ducts and normal development of wolffian structures occur. With increasing testosterone concentrations at puberty, individuals develop penile enlargement, testicular descent of inguinal testes into the labial scrotal folds, and secondary sexual characteristics (e.g., pubic hair, increased muscle mass).
- **Syndromes of androgen resistance.** Patients with incomplete forms of androgen resistance often present with sexual ambiguity, whereas individuals with complete androgen resistance appear phenotypically female. A blind vaginal pouch (caused by MIS secretion by the testes) is present. Testes may be located in the abdomen, inguinal canal, or in an inguinal hernia. There is no virilization at puberty, and breasts develop as the result of peripheral conversion of high levels of testosterone to estradiol. Most affected patients develop little or no pubic hair.

Evaluation

- **CAH.** The diagnosis can be made by measuring elevated steroids in the serum at baseline and after ACTH stimulation (see Tables 12-1 through 12-3).
- **17-Ketosteroid reductase deficiency.** Can be diagnosed by an abnormal ratio of androstenedione to testosterone, either at baseline or after stimulation with HCG.

- **17-Lyase deficiency.** Suggested by low androgen levels and increased gonadotropin levels.
- **5α-Reductase deficiency.** The testosterone-to-DHT ratio is normally <16 basally and following HCG stimulation; a ratio >30 suggests the diagnosis of 5α-reductase deficiency. The diagnosis is confirmed by finding reduced 5α-reductase activity in fibroblasts in genital skin samples.
- **Syndromes of androgen resistance.** Patients have an XY karyotype, no müllerian structures, and elevated testosterone and LH levels in the newborn period.

Treatment

Patients with CAH should receive cortisol and mineralocorticoid replacement as needed. Cosmetic surgical repair may be necessary.

Other Defects in Male External Genital Development

Hypospadias may be a finding in various intersex disorders. Although isolated first-degree hypospadias is usually not associated with endocrine abnormalities, the incidence of associated intersex disorders increases as the severity of the hypospadias increases and with the presence of bilateral undescended testes. **Micropenis** may occur with congenital hypopituitarism, isolated gonadotropin deficiency (Kallmann syndrome), testicular dysfunction, or partial androgen resistance.

EVALUATION OF AMBIGUOUS GENITALIA

Patient History

The following information should be sought:

- A careful maternal obstetric history that focuses on drug ingestion and exposure to teratogens or infections during the pregnancy, particularly during the first trimester
- A careful family history, focusing on any androgenic changes in the mother or anything suggestive of CAH in other family members (e.g., neonatal death, virilization, or precocious adrenarche)

Physical Examination

The following information needs to be noted:

- Palpable gonads, which imply the presence of Y chromosome material
- The length and diameter of the penis (**Table 12-4**) **and the position of the urethra**
- The existence of a vagina, the degree of fusion of the labia, and the length of the clitoris (Table 12-4)
- Other dysmorphic features, especially those involving the urinary tract and anus

TABLE 12-4 Penile and Clitoral Length in the Newborn Infant

Gestational Age	Length
Males[*]	
30 weeks	2.5 ± 0.4 cm
34 weeks	3.0 ± 0.4 cm
Term	3.5 ± 0.4 cm
Females[†]	
Term[‡]	4.0 ± 1.24 mm

Data based on information in Feldman KW, Smith DW: Fetal phallic growth and penile standards for newborn male infants. *J Pediatr* 86:395, 1975, and in Oberfield S, Mondok A, Shanrivar F, et al.: Clitoral size in full-term infants. *Am J Perinatol* 6(4): 453, 1989.

[*]Measure from the pubic ramus to the tip of the glans with gentle pressure applied.
[†]Measure with the labia majora separated and the prepuce skin retracted.
[‡]The clitoris achieves full size by 27 weeks of gestation and may appear more prominent in premature infants relative to the labia.

Laboratory Studies

- **Karyotyping.** Blood and bone marrow samples should be submitted for karyotyping. Some laboratories can have a karyotype result from a bone marrow specimen available within 6 hours. A standard chromosome analysis should be performed as well because bone marrow karyotyping can miss mosaicism.
- **Serum levels** of **17-hydroxyprogesterone, 17-hydroxypregnenolone, dehydroepiandrosterone, testosterone, DHT, 11-deoxycortisol,** and **androstenedione** should be obtained. Table 12-5 lists the normal values for serum testosterone and DHT. Recall that adrenal steroid levels are elevated in premature infants, particularly when the child is ill and under stress (see Tables 12-2 and 12-3).
- **Serum levels** of **luteinizing hormone (LH)** and **maternal androgens** may be appropriate to obtain.
- **AMH** levels are a marker for testicular tissue.
- **Biopsy samples.** A gonadal biopsy or skin biopsy to evaluate testosterone metabolism may be indicated.
- **DNA** analysis for specific disorders following the initial evaluation.

Diagnostic Imaging Studies

- **Pelvic ultrasound** can demonstrate a uterus and gonads.
- **Vaginogram.** The injection of contrast dye into urethral or vaginal openings demonstrates müllerian ducts (if any are present). The absence of a müllerian system implies functioning testicular tissue early in gestation and the secretion of MIS.

TABLE 12-5 Normal Laboratory Values for Serum Testosterone and Dihydrotestosterone (DHT)

	Testosterone (ng/dL)		DHT (ng/dL)	
	Male	Female	Male	Female
Cord blood	13–55	5–45	<2–8	<2–8
26–28 weeks of gestation	59–125	5–16	. . .	. . .
31–35 weeks of gestation	37–198	5–22	10–53	2–13
Full term	75–400*	20–64†	5–60‡	<2–15§

Data provided by the Esoterix Endocrinology Laboratory, Los Calabasas Hills, California.
*Levels decrease to 20 to 50 ng/dL during week 1 and then increase to 60 to 400 ng/dL at 20 to 60 days. Levels decrease to prepubertal values by 7 months.
†Levels decrease to <10 ng/dL during the first month and remain at that level untilpuberty.
‡Levels decrease during week 1 and then increase to 12 to 85 ng/dL by 30 to 60 days. Levels decrease to prepubertal values by 7 months.
§Levels decrease to 3 ng/dL during the first month and remain at that level until puberty.

- **Radiologic studies,** such as intravenous pyelography (IVP), bone age, or a barium enema, may be indicated.

APPROACH TO THE PATIENT (FIGURE 12-1)

Ambiguous genitalia in the neonate should be treated as a **medical emergency** and the diagnostic evaluation undertaken as soon as possible. A team approach with consultations from endocrinology, genetics, urology, and psychiatry is useful.

Often, it is advisable for parents to delay naming or announcing the birth of their child until the definitive gender is assigned. The parents should be informed that the definitive gender will be determined within 48 to 72 hours. **Gender assignment** usually can be made on the basis of the physical examination, karyotype, and internal pelvic structures while awaiting the results of serum studies; however, karyotype should not be the only factor in gender determination because gonadal function and future sexual function are also important. In addition, the size of the phallus and the degree of hypospadias need to be considered. For families known to carry CAH mutations, prenatal diagnosis and treatment may help reduce virilization of the female fetus.

> **HINT:** Females with CAH, even when severely virilized, should be raised as females because cosmetic repair can be managed surgically, and patients have good future potential for sexual function and reproduction.

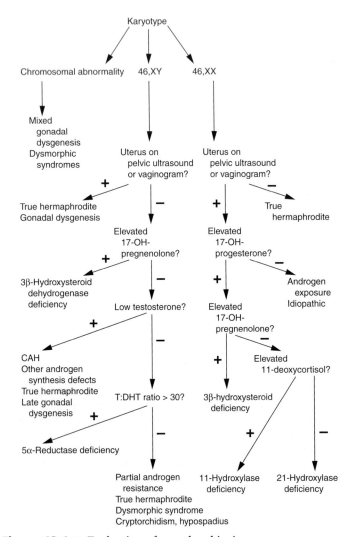

Figure 12-1 ■ Evaluation of sexual ambiguity

T:DHT ratio = testosterone-to-dihydrotestosterone ratio.

Suggested Readings

Hughes IA, Hook C, Ahmed SF, et al.: Consensus statement on management of intersex disorders. *Arch Dis Child* 91(7):554–563, 2006.

Seizer PW, White PC: Congenital adrenal hyperplasia. *N Engl J Med* 349:776–788, 2003.

Additional References

McLaughlin DT, Donahoe PC: Sex determination and differentiation. *N Engl J Med* 350:367–378, 2004.

New MI: Inborn errors of adrenal steroidogenesis. *Mol Cell Endocrinol* 211:75–83, 2003.

Ogilvy Al, Brani CE: Early assessment of ambiguous genitalia. *Arch Dis Child* 89:401–407, 2004.

Vaiman D, Pailhoux E: Mammalian sex reversal and intersexuality: deciphering the sex-determination cascade. *Trends Genet* 16(11):488–494, 2000.

Yong EL, Lim J, Qi W, et al.: Molecular basis of androgen receptor diseases. *Ann Med* 32(1):15–2, 2000.

13 *Amenorrhea*

Valerie Lewis
Marina Catallozzi and Jonathan Plechter (Third Edition)

INTRODUCTION

Amenorrhea, defined as the **absence of menses,** is common during adolescence. Determining the underlying cause of amenorrhea necessitates an understanding of the normal menstrual cycle. Although the broad differential diagnosis includes genetic, endocrine, structural, environmental, and psychological disorders, **pregnancy should always be considered.** Evaluation should begin soon after amenorrhea is noted because underlying pathologic conditions can cause physical and emotional sequelae.

Menarche, a pivotal event of puberty, requires intact and functioning interactions between the hypothalamus, pituitary, ovaries, and uterine endometrial lining. Successful menstrual cycles also require the presence of an unobstructed uterus, cervix, and vagina. The body must have an adequate amount of fat and not be under any extremes of stress (e.g., extreme exercise, emotional stress). Normal cycles indicate the presence of ovulation. **Menarche is one of the latest signs of puberty in females,** occurring at Tanner stage (or sexual maturity rating) IV in the majority of adolescents. Menarche generally occurs 2 to 2.5 years after thelarche and 1 year after the growth spurt. In the United States, 12.8 years is the average age of menarche for white females (the range is 9 to 16 years, and the average age is slightly lower for black females). Race, nutritional status, body fat, and maternal age at menarche all influence an individual's age of menarche. The majority of cycles are anovulatory for the first year and remain so for an average of ≥ 2 years. Normal menstrual cycles have 21- to 45-day cycles (depending on the individual), have flow lasting 2 to 7 days, and have an average blood loss of between 30 and 40 mL.

> **HINT:** Although the arbitrary age of primary amenorrhea is 16.5 years, if a girl ≥ 14 years presents with absence of breast budding, diagnostic evaluation should be performed immediately because it is unlikely that she will menstruate within the next 2 years.

The menstrual cycle begins with pulsatile release of gonadotropin-releasing hormone from the hypothalamus, causing secretion of follicle-stimulating hormone (FSH) and luteinizing hormone (LH) from the pituitary. Ovarian follicles grow and develop under the influence of FSH. Theca cells produce androgens that are converted to estrogen by granulosa cells. This increased estrogen not only inhibits the pituitary release of FSH, causing follicles to involute, but it also stimulates uterine development and endometrial growth. In the first part of the cycle, increased estrogen leads to decreased FSH release. Midcycle, FSH results in LH surge and ovulation. In **early adolescence,** although estrogen levels are high, the feedback patterns are not mature, and **menses are anovulatory,** representing sloughing of a proliferative endometrium rather than shedding secondary to the luteal phase of an ovulatory cycle. Clinically, this may be characterized by irregular or heavy bleeding (dysfunctional uterine bleeding) and lack of dysmenorrhea.

Primary amenorrhea is the **absence of menarche (with normal pubertal development) by 16 years of age, 14 years of age (without normal pubertal development), or 2 years after completion of sexual maturation.** Secondary amenorrhea is the **absence of menstruation for three cycle lengths** (usually between 6 and 12 months, depending on whether the patient was oligomenorrheic). Although primary and secondary amenorrhea are helpful in describing menstrual cycle interruption in regard to timing, the terms do not indicate an underlying cause or offer information about treatment or prognosis. Although the differential diagnosis of amenorrhea can be presented on the basis of timing, because several of the processes that cause amenorrhea can present as primary or secondary, the evaluation and diagnostic strategy is based on pubertal physiology and sexual development.

DIFFERENTIAL DIAGNOSIS LIST

Amenorrhea with Delayed Puberty

Hypergonadotrophic Hypogonadism
   Gonadal Failure
   Congenital causes:
   Genetic: Turner syndrome (45, XO)
   Ovarian: Pure or mosaic karyotype gonadal dysgenesis
   Acquired causes (affecting ovaries):

Medications, chemotherapy/ radiation
Gonadotropin-resistant ovary syndrome
Autoimmune oophoritis
Infiltrative, ischemic, or destructive disorders
   Receptor Defect
   Congenital causes:
   Androgen insensitivity or testicular feminization
Hypogonadotrophic hypogonadism

Disorders Of The
Hypothalamus
And/Or Pituitary

Congenital causes:
Abnormal hypothalamic
development (e.g.,
Kallmann syndrome)

Acquired causes: central
nervous system (CNS)
tumors (pituitary
adenoma); head trauma;
medications, chemotherapy/
radiation; infiltrative,
ischemic, or destructive
disorders; chronic illness;
weight loss (anorexia
nervosa); exercise, stress;
marijuana

Endocrine
Chronic disease: Thyroid
disease, diabetes, Addison
disease
Hyperprolactinemia:
Pituitary adenoma, renal
failure, psychoactive drugs
(e.g., Haldol, a dopamine
antagonist)

Others
Constitutional delay
Structural genital tract
defects: *Uterus/vagina:*
Congenital absence of
the uterus, outflow tract
obstruction

Amenorrhea with Normal Puberty

Hypergonadotrophic
hypogonadism
Gonadal Failure
Acquired causes (affecting
ovaries): Medications,
chemotherapy/radiation;
premature menopause;
autoimmune oophoritis;
infiltrative, ischemic, or
destructive disorders

Hypogonadotrophic
hypogonadism
Acquired causes: CNS
tumors (pituitary
adenoma); head trauma;
medications, chemotherapy/
radiation; infiltrative,
ischemic, or destructive
disorders; chronic illness;
weight loss (anorexia
nervosa); exercise, stress;
marijuana

Endocrine
Chronic disease: Thyroid
disease, diabetes, Addison
disease
Hyperprolactinemia:
Pituitary adenoma, renal
failure, psychoactive
drugs (e.g., Haldol,
a dopamine antagonist)
Hyperandrogenism:
Polycystic ovary
syndrome, late-onset
congenital adrenal
hyperplasia, Cushing
disease, ovarian or
adrenal tumors,
hyperthecosis (hypertro-
phy of ovarian stroma)
Anovulatory cycles:
Owing to immaturity
of hypothalamic-pituitary-
ovarian axis

Others
Pregnancy
Lactation

DIFFERENTIAL DIAGNOSIS DISCUSSION

> **HINT:** Pregnancy is the most common cause of secondary amenorrhea in women of reproductive age, and this possibility should always be ruled out first.

Gonadal Failure

Etiology

Gonadal failure (i.e., lack of ovarian estrogen production) is the **most common cause of primary amenorrhea,** accounting for almost 50% of cases. Sometimes it is a consequence of therapies (chemo or radiation) or disease processes, but it is usually caused by a **chromosomal disorder or deletion of all or part** of an X chromosome. The chromosomal disorders that cause gonadal failure are usually the result of a **random** meiotic or mitotic **abnormality** (i.e., they are not inherited). If the chromosomes are normal (46,XX or 46,XY [pure gonadal dysgenesis]), a gene disorder may be the cause of the primary amenorrhea. Because two X chromosomes are necessary for normal ovarian development, patients with **Turner syndrome (45,X), mosaicism** involving an X chromosome, **or an abnormal X chromosome** may develop **streak ovaries,** which are masses of fibrous tissue located in the normal anatomic position of the ovary. These streak ovaries **do not produce estrogen;** therefore, estrogen-induced negative feedback inhibition of the hypothalamic–pituitary axis fails to occur, and gonadotropins remain elevated.

Evaluation

An **FSH level >40 mIU/mL** suggests a lack of functioning ovarian follicles, confirming the diagnosis of gonadal failure.

Androgen Insensitivity (Testicular Feminization)

Etiology

Androgen insensitivity is a syndrome caused by the **absence of a gene on the X chromosome** for the testosterone receptor. It is inherited in an **X-linked recessive** or sex-limited autosomal dominant fashion with transmission **through the mother.** Patients are **genetically normal males** with a 46,XY karyotype and normally functioning testes that produce normal male levels of testosterone and dihydrotestosterone. Because there are no testosterone receptors, there is **no development of external or internal male genitalia.** In the absence of sex steroids, **female development** occurs. The fetal testes produce müllerian-inhibiting substance, which causes müllerian-duct regression (explaining the absence of the uterus).

Clinical Features

Patients have **normal female external genitalia** and a **short or absent vagina.** **Pubic and axillary hair is absent or scanty** because of the lack of androgen receptors, but **breast development is normal or excessive** because there is no androgenic opposition to the small amounts of estrogen produced by the testes and adrenals. The **gonads** in these patients are **abnormal,** and 20% develop a **malignancy** (gonadoblastoma or dysgerminoma).

> **HINT:** Patients with testicular feminization can be differentiated from patients with uterine agenesis by the absence of normal pubic hair.

Treatment

Patients with testicular feminization are **phenotypically female** and have been raised as such. They should be told they are **sterile** because of a missing piece of the X chromosome and that the **gonads must be removed** because they are at risk of developing a malignancy. These malignancies rarely occur <20 years of age; therefore, it is recommended that the gonads be left in place until after puberty to allow normal sexual maturity.

Hypothalamus and Pituitary Disorders

Etiology

Patients with **normal female internal genitalia** but **absent secondary sex characteristics** as a result of a central nervous system (CNS)–hypothalamus–pituitary disorder have **low levels of gonadotropin and estrogen.** In addition, any **anatomic lesion** of the hypothalamus or pituitary gland can cause low gonadotropin production. These lesions can be **congenital** (e.g., aqueductal stenosis or absence of the sellar floor) or **acquired** (e.g., tumors). The most common tumors are **pituitary adenomas,** which result in **elevated levels of prolactin.** (Most, but not all, pituitary tumors secrete prolactin; chromophobe adenomas are the most common non-prolactin-secreting pituitary tumors.)

Evaluation

Patients with suspected CNS–hypothalamic–pituitary disorders should undergo **magnetic resonance imaging** (best modality) or **computed tomography** of the hypothalamic–pituitary region to rule out the presence of a lesion. Pituitary adenoma can be detected by finding an elevated **serum prolactin level.**

Structural Genital Tract Defects

Etiology

Congenital absence of the uterus (uterine agenesis, uterovaginal agenesis, Rokitansky-Kuster-Hauser syndrome) is the **second most common** cause of primary amenorrhea, after gonadal failure. **Congenital** absence of the uterus accounts for approximately 15% of cases of primary amenorrhea, and occurs in 1 of every 4,000 to 5,000 female births. Congenital absence of the uterus is typically a sporadic event and only rarely genetically inherited. Patients have no underlying endocrine abnormality, but they are amenorrheic because of absence of the end organ.

Clinical Features

Patients have normal breasts and pubic and axillary hair, but the **vagina is shortened or absent** and the **uterus is absent.** The ovaries are present and function normally, with ovulation occurring cyclically. Approximately 33% of patients with congenital absence of the uterus have **congenital renal abnormalities,** and 12% have **skeletal abnormalities. Cardiac and other congenital abnormalities** occur with increased frequency.

EVALUATION OF AMENORRHEA

Patient History

Delayed or absent menstruation can be very anxiety provoking. Be sensitive to the parent and adolescent's level of concern during the history. Review of growth and development, detailed menstrual history (e.g., menarche, dysmenorrhea, duration, and flow), history of illnesses, and medications can all be discussed with the patient and parent. To obtain accurate information, the **sexual history, psychosocial assessment,** and **substance use** history should be **obtained privately with the patient.** Questions regarding diet, physical activity (duration and intensity), weight change, and body image can give an indication if there is an eating disorder. Review of symptoms should focus on:

- New-onset virilizing symptoms: acne, hirsutism, clitoromegaly
- Vasomotor symptoms (e.g., hot flashes, associated with low circulating estrogens)
- Galactorrhea (hyperprolactinemia)
- Cyclic abdominal pain, bloating, or breast changes (vaginal outlet obstruction)
- Palpitations, fatigue, or nervousness (hyperthyroidism)

Physical Examination

Height (**short stature**), weight, body habitus, and vital signs (**hypertension** may indicate some of the causes of hyperandrogenicity such as Cushing disease) should be measured. Signs of **anorexia nervosa** include bradycardia, hypotension, and hypothermia. A thorough funduscopic and neurologic examination can help rule out **pituitary or other CNS lesions.** Other areas of focus should include the **thyroid,** the **breasts** (for Tanner staging

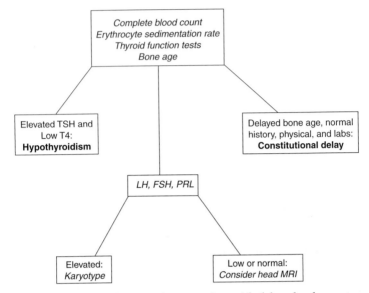

Figure 13-1 ▪ Evaluation of amenorrhea with delayed puberty
(Modified from Pletcher JB, Slap GB: Menstrual disorders. Amenorrhea. Pediatr Clin North Am 46(3):505–518, 1999.)

and galactorrhea), and the **genital area** (Tanner stage and hyperandro-genism, virilization, imperforate hymen; consider a pelvic examination to rule out ovarian mass). **Pelvic examination** is not necessary if the patient has never been sexually active and genital anomalies are not suspected. Otherwise, pelvic examination can help evaluate for the presence of uterus and ovaries. Laboratory workup depends on the pubertal development. See **Figures 13-1 through 13-3 for stepwise workup.**

TREATMENT OF AMENORRHEA

Apart from specific therapies with regard to the diagnoses listed in the differential diagnosis list, the principles behind management of amenorrhea are the same regardless of the etiology:

- Restore ovulatory cycles to ensure good long-term prognosis.
- If ovulatory cycles do not occur spontaneously, estrogen–progestin therapy is indicated (for bone protection and to counteract the effects of unopposed estrogen on the endometrial lining).
- Reassure the patient and parent.
- Reevaluate frequently.

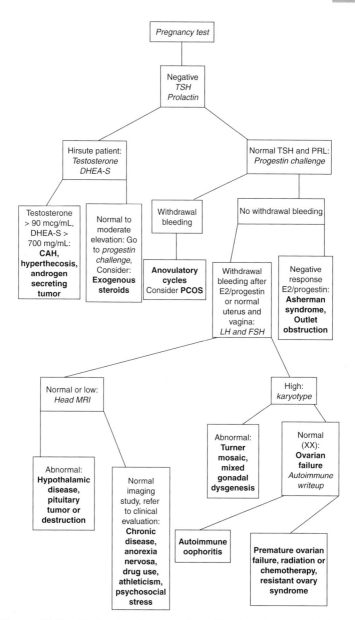

Figure 13-2 ■ Evaluation of amenorrhea with otherwise normal puberty
(Modified from Pletcher JB, Slap GB: Menstrual disorders. Amenorrhea. Pediatr Clin North Am 46(3):505–518, 1999.)

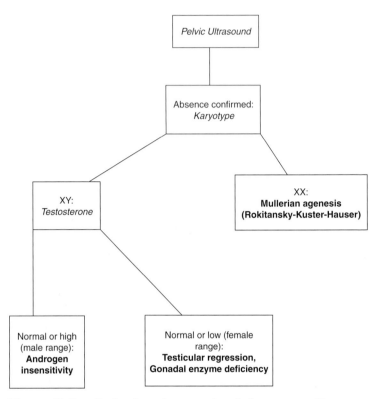

Figure 13-3 ■ Evaluation of suspected genital tract anomalies
(Modified from Pletcher JB, Slap GB: Menstrual disorders. Amenorrhea. Pediatr Clin North Am 46(3):505–518, 1999.)

Suggested Readings

Emans SJ: Amenorrhea in the adolescent. In *Pediatric and Adolescent Gynecology*, 5th ed. Edited by Emans SJ, Laufer MR, Goldstein, DP. Philadelphia, Lippincott, Williams & Wilkins, 2005.

Folch M, Pigem I, Konje JC: Müllerian agenesis: etiology, diagnosis, and management. *Obstet Gynecol Surv* 55(10):644–649, 2000.

Golden NH, Jacobson MS, Schebendach J, et al.: Resumption of menses in anorexia nervosa. *Arch Pediatr Adolesc Med* 151(1):16–21,1997.

McIver B, Romanski SA, Nipploldt TB: Evaluation and management of amenorrhea. *Mayo Clin Proc* 72(12):1161–1169, 1997.

Mishell DR: Primary and secondary amenorrhea: etiology, diagnostic evaluation and management. In *Comprehensive Gynecology*, 3rd ed.

Edited by Mishell DR, Stenchever MA, Droegemueller W, et al. St. Louis, Mosby-Year Book, 1997.

Pletcher JR, Slap GB: Menstrual disorders. Amenorrhea. *Pediatr Clin North Am* 46(3):505–518, 1999.

Speroff L, Glass RH, Kase NG: Amenorrhea. In *Clinical Gynecologic Endocrinology and Infertility*, 5th ed. Edited by Speroff L, Glass RH, Kase NG. Baltimore, Williams & Wilkins, 1994.

INTRODUCTION

Humans have contact with animals in a variety of occupational and recreational settings, and more than half of households in the United States have at least one pet. Animal and human bite wounds are frequent in the pediatric population and are seen in primary care offices and emergency departments. As a result, all pediatric practitioners should become familiar with evaluation and management of the most common animal bite wounds. The complex microbiology of animal bite wounds makes management a challenging clinical problem, and therapy is often empirical.

DIFFERENTIAL DIAGNOSIS LIST

Local bacterial wound infection —mouth flora vary by species (Table 14-1)

Rabies—many animals, especially dogs, cats, bats, foxes, raccoons, skunks

Tularemia—many animals, especially rabbits, cats, squirrels, pigs, sheep, coyotes, ticks

Rat-bite fever

Cat-scratch disease (CSD)

DIFFERENTIAL DIAGNOSIS DISCUSSION

Dog and Cat Bites

Dog and cat bites make up the **majority of bite wounds.** Because of their inquisitive nature, children are bitten by dogs and cats more frequently than adults, with most bites occurring in the 5- to 9-year-old age group. Their size relative to an animal causes children to sustain **more facial bites,** resulting in greater severity of **laceration, infection, disability,** and **death,** especially when large dogs are involved. **Cat bite wounds** are typically **puncture wounds** that involve the hand or extremity. Because of the sharp and slender nature of cat teeth, they are able to **penetrate bones,** which may lead to greater morbidity from complicated wounds.

Dog bites have an infection rate of approximately 5% to 15%, the lowest of all mammalian bites. **Cat bites become infected more frequently** (approximately 50%). Wound characteristics and initial wound care determine the risk of infection. Puncture wounds, wounds on the hands or feet, those involving joints, tendons, or other deep structures,

TABLE 14-1 Organisms Commonly Associated with Bite Wounds

Animal	Organism	Special Considerations
Dog and cat	Pasteurella species Streptococcus species Staphylococcus aureus Neisseria species Anaerobes: Bacteroides, Fusobacterium, Porphyromonas, Prevotella	Rabies prophylaxis based on immunization status, ability to observe animal, local epidemiology
Horse	Similar to dog and cat	Crush injury, osteomyelitis
Pig and sheep	Dog and cat flora + Francisella tularensis and others	
Rat	Dog and cat flora + Streptobacillus moniliformis, Leptospira	Rabies prophylaxis generally not needed
Ferret and gerbil	Rat flora + Acinetobacter anitratus	Antipseudomonal penicillin
Raccoon, bat, fox	High risk for rabies	RIG, HDCV
Squirrel	Francisella tularensis	Gentamicin
Aquatic	Aeromonas hydrophila, Vibrio, Enterobacter, Pseudomonas	
Avian	Staphylococcus, Clostridium, Aspergillus, Bacteroides, Pseudomonas	
Human	Streptococcus species Staphylococcus species Eikenella corrodens Anaerobes: Prevotella, Fusobacterium, Veillonella, Peptostreptococcus	Hand injuries high risk
Monkey	Human flora + Herpes B	Antiviral therapy

Note: This table is not an exhaustive list of organisms.
HDCV = human diploid cell vaccine; RIG = rabies immune globulin.

and those in hosts with comorbid illness or immunosuppression are at higher risk for infection. Wounds treated >12 hours after injury and those not properly irrigated and debrided are more likely to become infected. The microbiology of infected dog and cat bite wounds is well studied (see Table 14-1). Most bite wound infections are **polymicrobial** and include anaerobic organisms.

Human Bites

Following dog and cat bites, **human bites** are the **next most common** types of mammalian bite injuries. Human bites are most commonly seen in **teenage or young adult men** and are often related to **aggressive behavior, sports,** and **sexual activity. Wound infections** occur in about 15% to 50% of human bites. **Delays in care,** which are common as a result of the circumstances of injury, **have a direct effect on infection** rates and prognosis. **Simple bites** that occur from occlusion of the teeth on skin, such as bites occurring in child care, **rarely become infected.** Human bite infections are **polymicrobial** with a mixture of anaerobes and aerobes (see Table 14-1). *Eikenella corrodens* deserves special mention, as it is present in 25% of isolates from clenched fist injuries. It has also exhibited synergistic growth with other aerobic organisms.

> **HINT:** When a bite occurs as the result of a direct blow of the victim's hand into the biter's mouth, there is typically a puncture wound overlying one of the metacarpal-phalangeal joints on the dorsum of the hand (clenched-fist syndrome). Penetration of the joint capsule may occur with tendon, nerve, or bone damage. These wounds may appear mild at first, but they are deceiving and can result in extensive infection that requires surgical exploration, debridement, and intravenous antibiotics.

Other significant infectious diseases like herpes virus, syphilis, tuberculosis, actinomycosis, tetanus, and hepatitis B and C have also been documented as occurring through human bites. Although no definitive cases of HIV transmission from this route have been reported, detection of HIV in saliva makes this an unlikely but possible way to acquire HIV infection.

Complications

Local Wound Infection

Characteristics of infected bite wounds include **erythema, warmth, fluctuance, purulent drainage,** and **tenderness** at the site, with **surrounding edema** and **regional adenitis.** Local wound infections can also be accompanied by **mild systemic symptoms** such as **fever, chills,** and **malaise,** and they may be associated with **serum leukocytosis.**

Various clinical syndromes may help differentiate the type of organism that predominates in a bite-wound infection. Infection caused by *Pasteurella* species may evolve rapidly with intense cellulitis and lymphangitis within 24 hours. Cellulitis caused by *Staphylococcus* or *Streptococcus* species usually evolves more slowly and may be associated with abscess formation. More **serious infections,** such as **osteomyelitis** or **septic arthritis,** may present with increased pain and decreased range of motion of the affected part. Deep infections may occur after direct inoculation into deeper tissues or by localized extension of cellulitis. **Immunocompromised hosts** can present with local or systemic infections and are at **higher risk for invasive disease.**

Rabies

Individuals often seek medical care after an animal bite wound because of the concern for rabies. Rabies is caused by a rhabdovirus and is **transmitted via the saliva of an infected animal through a bite or scratch.** Cases often result from an unrecognized exposure or from failure to administer prophylaxis. In the United States, the Centers for Disease Control and Prevention (CDC) reported 51 cases of human rabies between 1990 and 2006. **Rabies prophylaxis recommendations vary by the geographic area and the type of animal** involved. Bats, skunks, raccoons, foxes, dogs, and coyotes serve as the primary reservoirs of rabies, and bats are responsible for the majority of cases. Individuals who awake to find a bat in the room should be considered exposed. Treatment is discussed later.

> **HINT:** In 2004, a teenage girl became the first known person to survive rabies infection. Timely postexposure prophylaxis remains the only reliable strategy to prevent the development of clinical disease. Once rabies develops, the outcome is almost always fatal.

The clinical syndrome of rabies is characterized by **fever, malaise, headache,** and **anxiety** in the early stages. This is followed by **progressive neurologic symptoms** including muscle spasm, autonomic instability, altered mental status with hallucinations, respiratory muscle paralysis, lacrimation, salivation, perspiration, and coma. Infection can be confirmed with **specific serologic testing.**

Tularemia

Tularemia, caused by infection with *Francisella tularensis,* is primarily a **tick-borne disease** but may be transmitted by **bites from animals** such as rabbits, cats, squirrels, pigs, sheep, and coyotes. The clinical syndrome is characterized by an **abrupt onset of fever, chills, headache, anorexia, malaise,** and **fatigue.** The ulceroglandular syndrome is characterized by a **painful ulcer** associated with **tender regional lymph nodes** that can drain spontaneously. The diagnosis can be confirmed with **serologic testing,** and treatment is usually with **streptomycin, gentamicin, or amikacin.**

Rat-Bite Fever

Rat-bite fever is caused by *Streptobacillus moniliformis.* The organism is found in the oral flora of **wild, pet, and laboratory rats** and is transmitted by **bites, scratches, and handling of dead rats.** There is a 3- to 10-day incubation period after exposure, followed by **acute onset of fever, chills,** arthritis, muscle pain, and maculopapular rash, which often involves the palms and soles. The rash may take on other forms such as petechiae, purpura, vesicles, or desquamation. There also may be associated septic polyarthritis, and more rarely endocarditis, pericarditis, and brain abscess. Fatality occurs in 7% to 10% of untreated patients.

The organism can be cultured from blood, synovial fluid, and vesicle fluid, and the receiving laboratory should be informed that *Streptobacillus moniliformis* is the organism of interest. Cultures should be held up to 3 weeks. *Streptobacillus* is sensitive to penicillin, and therapy should be initiated with this drug. Alternative drugs are ampicillin, cefuroxime, cefotaxime, and doxycycline. Recovery is excellent.

Cat-Scratch Disease

CSD is caused by *Bartonella henselae,* a Gram-negative bacillus. It is transmitted primarily to individuals who have close contact with a cat via bites or scratches.

Patients with uncomplicated CSD develop a nontender papule at the site of inoculation followed by regional lymphadenopathy that persists for weeks to months. The most common involved nodes are axillary, cervical, submandibular, and inguinal. Nodes may suppurate and be accompanied by symptoms such as fever, malaise, anorexia, and headache. Complicated CSD is more common in immunosuppressed patients and may cause neurologic symptoms such as encephalopathy, peripheral neuropathy, or vision loss, as well as pneumonia, endocarditis, and osteomyelitis.

Diagnosis is made by serology. Many cases of CSD resolve spontaneously without specific therapy. Painful suppurative nodes can be treated with needle aspiration. Incision and drainage should be avoided. Antimicrobial therapy with macrolides, ciprofloxacin, trimethoprim-sulfamethoxazole, or rifampin can hasten recovery. Routine antimicrobial treatment is not recommended for otherwise healthy individuals with regional lymphadenitis.

EVALUATION OF ANIMAL BITES

Patient History

Unstable patients should be evaluated immediately for massive blood loss and wounds that interfere with a patent airway (tracheal or laryngeal location) or breathing (pneumothorax). Important facts to elicit when taking a history from a bitten individual include type of animal, provoking factors for the bite, allergies, medications, and comorbid conditions, especially those associated with immune suppression. Obtain a history of tetanus immunization as well as any previous bites or rabies immunizations.

Physical Examination

The following items should be noted during examination of a bite wound:

- Body location
- Depth of the wound
- Range of motion of the affected part
- Type of wound—puncture, crush, laceration, abrasion
- Involvement of deeper structures—tendon, nerve, vessel, bone
- Function of tendons and nerves
- Signs of inflammation or infection—edema, erythema, warmth, induration, fluctuance, exudates, adenopathy, foreign debris

The **physical examination** may need to take place **after local anesthesia** to maximize the ability to explore the wound. **Photographs or diagrammatic drawings** of wounds are helpful.

Imaging

When **fractures** or **foreign bodies** such as tooth fragments are suspected, a radiograph should be obtained.

Laboratory Evaluation

Routine wound cultures are not needed for animal or human bites that do not have any signs of infection. As a general rule, most bite wounds at this point are more likely to reflect the indigenous flora of the animal's mouth and are not predictive of future infection. **Older wounds** or those with **evidence of infection** should be cultured for both **aerobic and anaerobic organisms** after superficial crusts are removed. It is imperative to **notify the laboratory of the source of a bite-wound culture** and of any suspected organisms.

TREATMENT OF ANIMAL BITES

Wound Management

Experts advocate **copious irrigation** of bite wounds as well as **surface cleaning.** The fluid of choice is **normal saline** (1% povidone-iodine may be added) using a volume of at least 250 mL. Irrigation should be performed **under pressure** with an 18- or 19-gauge catheter attached to a syringe, and **devitalized tissue should be debrided. Puncture and other small wounds should never be injected** because this may inoculate bacteria into deeper structures, increasing tissue trauma and the risk of infection.

The decision to suture a bite wound primarily is made on a case-by-case basis and depends on many factors, including the length of time between the bite and presentation, the location of the wound, the appearance of the wound, and the comorbidities of the patient. Studies have suggested that carefully selected bite wounds are safe for primary closure. **Wounds that are candidates for primary closure** are those to the **head and face** and wounds in other **low-risk areas** such as the proximal extremities and the trunk.

It is generally agreed that all **bites older than 24 hours, bites to the hand, and bites with evidence of infection should not be sutured.** Delayed primary closure 72 hours after antimicrobial prophylaxis has begun is a consideration for high-risk wounds. Aftercare should consist of explicit **instructions for wound cleansing, dressing changes, and antibiotic use** (topical or oral as indicated), as well as **signs and symptoms of possible infection. Large wounds or those over joint surfaces** should be **splinted and elevated.** Appropriate **analgesics** should be prescribed for several days. **Close follow-up** should be arranged for all bite wounds.

Antimicrobial Prophylaxis

Prophylactic antimicrobial therapy is generally recommended for the following:

- All bites to the hand
- Wounds with moderate-to-severe tissue destruction (crush)
- Puncture wounds
- Cat bites
- Injuries involving bone or joint
- Wounds to patients with comorbid conditions or immunosuppression

Amoxicillin–clavulanate is the drug of choice for prophylaxis of an animal bite wound, with an appropriate spectrum of activity against common flora in the mouths of dogs, cats, and humans. An alternative regimen for penicillin-allergic patients is **a second- or third-generation cephalosporin or trimethoprim-sulfamethoxazole *plus* clindamycin.** Postpubertal non-pregnant patients may receive **doxycycline** or **tetracycline.**

Antimicrobial Treatment for Infected Wounds

Infected wounds that have **failed outpatient therapy** require **hospitalization.** *Pasteurella multocida* should be considered in any patient with a wound infection **following a dog or cat bite. Ampicillin/sulbactam** is appropriate empirical intravenous therapy. Alternatives for penicillin-allergic patients are **a second- or third-generation cephalosporin or trimethoprim-sulfamethoxazole *plus* clindamycin; or ciprofloxacin or tetracycline** if appropriate for age.

Tetanus Prophylaxis

Tetanus immunization should be given according to standard CDC recommendations when patients are **deficient in immunization status** or in cases of **high-risk wounds.**

Rabies Prophylaxis

Immediate active and passive prophylaxis is indicated for wild animals known to carry rabies and domestic animals with symptoms of rabies; these **animals should be euthanized and the brain examined** in a qualified laboratory. Passive immunization with **rabies immune globulin (RIG)** in a dose of 20 IU/kg should be given as follows: **half of the dose at the site of the bite wound and the other half at a separate intramuscular location.** In **children** the recommended site is the **anterolateral thigh.** Active immunization with the **human diploid cell vaccine (HDCV)** must be initiated and **repeated on days 3, 7, 14, and 28** after the injury. The dose of the vaccine is 1.0 mL intramuscularly given at a site distant from the immune globulin.

Domestic animals with an unknown rabies immune status may be **observed for 10 days.** RIG and HDCV should be initiated at the first sign of rabies symptoms in the animal. Cases in which the animal is unavailable should be treated as recommended by local health officials.

> **HINT:** Animal bites should be reported to the local health department for surveillance as indicated by local jurisdiction. The risk of rabies differs geographically, and appropriate treatment may vary. Reports to law enforcement agencies may also be necessary to facilitate observation of animals for rabies.

HIV Prophylaxis for Human Bites

The risk of HIV transmission from a human bite is controversial but **thought to be rare.** Bites from a person known to be infected with HIV or bites from a person in which there was **visibly blood-tainted saliva** should be **treated prophylactically** with **oral antiviral agents** according to standard CDC recommendations. In all other instances, postexposure prophylaxis should be determined on a case-by-case basis, but **baseline and 6-month HIV testing** of the victim is prudent. All human bite wounds should be **thoroughly cleansed with a virucidal agent** as soon as possible to lessen any risk of HIV transmission.

PREVENTION OF ANIMAL BITES

Because bites frequently lead to infection, efforts to reduce the risk of infection should be aimed primarily at prevention. Adults, especially pet owners, should become familiar with the behavior of cats and dogs and teach children to avoid provoking behaviors. When handling other animals, appropriate precautions should be taken, such as **wearing gloves** and other **protective garments.**

Suggested Readings

American Academy of Pediatrics: *Red Book: 2006 Report of the Committee on Infectious Diseases*, 27th ed. Edited by LK Pickering, CJ Baker, SS Long, et al. Elk Grove Village, Il, American Academy of Pediatrics, 2006, 648–653.

American Academy of Pediatrics: The use of systemic fluoroquinolones. *Pediatrics* 118(3):1287–1292, 2006.

Bunzli WF, Wright DH, Hoang AD, et al.: Current management of human bites. *Pharmacotherapy* 18(2):227–234, 1998.

Chen E, Hornig S, Shepherd SM, et al.: Primary closure of mammalian bites. *Acad Emerg Med* 7:157–161, 2000.

Glaser C, Lewis P, Wong S: Pet-animal, and vector-borne infections. *Pediatr Rev* 21(7):219–232, 2000.

Goldstein EJ: Current concepts on animal bites: bacteriology and therapy. *Curr Clin Top Infect Dis* 19:99–111, 1999.

Goldstein EJC: Bite wounds and infection. *Clin Infect Dis* 14:633–638, 1992.

Griego RD, Rosen T, Orengo IF, et al.: Dog, cat, and human bites: a review. *J Am Acad Dermatol* 33:1019–1029, 1995.

Lion C, Conroy MC, Carpentier AM, et al.: Antimicrobial susceptibilities of *Pasteurella* strains isolated from humans. *Int J Antimicrob Agents* 27:290–293, 2006.

Medeiros I, Saconato H: Antibiotic prophylaxis for mammalian bites. *Cochrane Database Syst Rev* 2:CD001738, 2001.

Moore DA, Sischo WM, Hunter A, et al.: Animal bite epidemiology and surveillance for rabies postexposure prophylaxis. *J Am Vet Med Assoc* 217:190–194, 2000.

Smith PF, Meadowcroft AM, May DB: Treating mammalian bite wounds. *J Clin Pharm Ther* 25:85–89, 2000.

Talan DA, Abrahamian FM, Moran GJ, et al.: Clinical presentation and bacteriologic analysis of infected human bites in patients presenting to emergency departments. *Clin Infect Dis* 37:1481–1489, 2003.

Talan DA, Citron DM, Abrahamian FM, et al.: Bacteriologic analysis of infected dog and cat bites. *N Engl J Med* 340(2):85–92, 1999.

Weber DJ, Hansen AR: Infections resulting from animal bites. *Infect Dis Clin North Am* 5(3):663–679, 1991.

Wiley JF: Mammalian bites: review of evaluation and management. *Clin Pediatr* 29(5):283–287, 1990.

15

Apnea

Thomas Mollen
Michael L. Spear and John L. Stefano (Second Edition)

INTRODUCTION

The *1986 Consensus Statement on Infantile Apnea and Home Monitoring* from the National Institute of Health (NIH) describes an apparent life-threatening event (ALTE) as "an episode that is frightening to the observer and is characterized by some combination of apnea (central or occasionally obstructive), color change (usually cyanotic or pallid but occasionally erythematous or plethoric), marked change in muscle tone (usually marked limpness), choking, or gagging. . . . [I]n some cases, the observer fears that the infant has died. . . . [P]reviously used terminology such as 'aborted crib death' or 'near-miss SIDS' should be abandoned because it implies a possibly misleading close association between this type of spell and SIDS."

DIFFERENTIAL DIAGNOSIS LIST 🔓

Infectious Causes
Sepsis
Pneumonia
Respiratory syncytial virus
(RSV) infection
Meningitis
Pertussis

Gastrointestinal Causes
Gastrointestinal reflux
(gastroesophageal reflux
disease [GRD])

Traumatic Causes
Intracranial hemorrhage
(subdural, subarachnoid)
Munchausen by proxy
syndrome
Child abuse

Cardiovascular Causes
Cardiac arrhythmias
Congenital heart disease
Cardiomyopathy
Vascular ring

Respiratory Causes
Reactive airway disease
Laryngomalacia
Other airway anomalies
Structural lung malformation

Neurologic Causes
Seizure
Intracranial mass
Cerebral dysgenesis
Structural or cerebrovascular
anomalies

Metabolic Causes
Inborn errors of metabolism
Hypoglycemia
Electrolyte imbalance

Miscellaneous Causes
Apnea of prematurity
Idiopathic apnea of infancy
or ALTE
Physiologic periodic breathing
Central hypoventilation
syndromes

Breathholding spells	Tracheoesophageal fistula
Anemia	Choking event
Hypothermia	Upper airway obstruction
Vocal cord paralysis	Drug- or toxin-induced apnea

DIFFERENTIAL DIAGNOSIS DISCUSSION

Infection

Clinical Features

Although apnea can be the only initial symptom of infection, untreated sepsis progresses rapidly, and the infant develops other signs and symptoms that suggest this diagnosis. **Pneumonia** or **bronchiolitis** caused by RSV can be **associated with life-threatening apnea** and is a **significant cause of infant mortality** among **premature infants** after hospital discharge, especially during the **winter months.**

Evaluation

In an infant who presents with acute apnea, a **careful history** and **physical examination** should be performed in an attempt to elucidate the presence of an acute infection. Depending on the history and physical examination findings, appropriate **laboratory tests** can be ordered.

Treatment

Treatment depends on the underlying infection. Effective **antibacterial therapies,** and some **antiviral therapies,** are available. **Prompt diagnosis and treatment are essential.**

Obstructive Apnea

Etiology

Obstructive apnea is the **inability to effectively oxygenate, ventilate, or both,** despite adequate central respiratory drive. Causes include:

- **Gastrointestinal Reflux (GRD).** The most common cause of obstructive apnea is GRD; as many as 20% of premature infants with apnea have an obstructive component.
- **Prematurity.** The incomplete development of cartilaginous structures in a premature infant's airway can lead to kinking of the airway and obstructive apnea.
- **Laryngeal webs** or **laryngomalacia** can also present as obstructive apnea.

Clinical Features

The parents describe the baby as **regurgitating formula or milk,** either during feeding or afterward. Infants may have **"awake apnea,"** which is most commonly caused by GRD. Alternatively, infants may **struggle during feeding,** with **exaggerated respiratory effort.**

Evaluation

If GRD is suspected, a **barium swallow with video** capabilities allows the radiologist and the speech therapist to assess both reflux and swallowing function to determine appropriate therapy. Other causes of obstructive apnea require evaluation by an **otolaryngologist.**

Treatment

Thickened feeds, and **metoclopramide** are used to treat GRD. **Upright positioning** after feeds, with the infant's head elevated to a 45° angle, has also been effective. Home monitoring devices may not detect obstructive apnea because they measure chest wall movement but do not measure airflow.

Trauma

Etiology

Birth trauma (e.g., intracranial or subgaleal hemorrhage, rather than a caput or cephalohematoma) and **child abuse** (including physical abuse and Munchausen by proxy syndrome) can be associated with apnea.

> **HINT:** **Munchausen by proxy syndrome is among the differential diagnoses for recurrent apnea; parents with this psychological disorder can interfere with the proper functioning of home monitoring. In addition, parentally induced suffocation can lead to true apnea; the associated hypoxia can be detected with a monitor capable of storing and downloading the data for physician interpretation.**

Evaluation

A **careful history** and **imaging studies** help in confirming the diagnosis of child abuse or birth trauma. Often the information stored in the **home apnea monitor** can help in determining if events at home are real and when they occurred.

Neurologic Disorders

Seizures, CNS structural abnormalities (e.g., arteriovenous malformation [AVM], Arnold-Chiari deformity), central nervous system (CNS) tumors, and **intracranial hemorrhage** can be associated with an ALTE initially. **Persistent idiopathic apnea** is the **hallmark of central hypoventilation disorders,** the most well known of which is Ondine curse.

Clinical Features

The apnea may be associated with **seizures** or symptoms of **increased intracranial pressure.** If a neurologic diagnosis is suspected, then appropriate **CNS imaging studies,** an **electroencephalogram (EEG),** and **laboratory blood tests** are indicated.

Treatment

Treatment depends on the underlying cause. Either **anticonvulsant therapy** or **surgical intervention** may be necessary. Patients with central hypoventilation syndromes may require **nighttime mechanical ventilation.**

Cardiac Disease

> **HINT:** An infant with an ALTE rarely has cardiac disease.

The most common life-threatening cardiac abnormality is **cardiac arrhythmia.** A prolonged QT interval has been noted in infants who have died of sudden infant death syndrome (SIDS). On rare occasions, **congenital heart disease** presents as an ALTE.

Clinical Features

In addition to apnea, infants with heart disease usually have more obvious signs of heart failure, such as **failure to thrive** or **cyanosis.** A **vascular ring** can be associated with **inspiratory stridor.**

Evaluation

When congenital heart disease is suspected, the initial evaluation usually includes an **electrocardiogram (ECG), chest radiograph,** and an **echocardiogram.**

Treatment

Treatment depends on the underlying pathological condition; **medical therapy** is useful for some arrhythmias, and **surgical therapy** may be required by patients with structural heart disease.

Respiratory Abnormalities

Clinical Features

An infant with apnea caused by a structural lung abnormality is often **tachypneic** and **cyanotic** and may show signs of respiratory distress preceding the apnea. An **abnormal cry** or **inspiratory stridor** is present in patients with vocal cord paralysis. **Choking during feeding** is seen with tracheoesophageal fistula.

Evaluation

A chest radiograph is helpful initially. Flexible laryngoscopy or bronchoscopy often is needed.

Treatment

Some structural lung abnormalities (e.g., cystic adenomatoid malformation, diaphragmatic hernia) are surgically correctable. Vocal cord paralysis may improve spontaneously.

Apnea of Prematurity

Premature infants have a much higher risk for ALTE and SIDS than infants who were born at or near-term gestation (≥37 weeks).

Clinical Features

Apnea of prematurity is characterized by pauses in respiration that last >20 seconds. Accompanying bradycardia may also be present.

Only some of these episodes are detected by hospital personnel or parents. In a study involving tracings of asymptomatic premature infants' respiratory patterns, heart rates, nasal air flow, and oxyhemoglobin saturations, almost 50% of the infants had prolonged apnea and other findings defined as abnormal.

Treatment

Several strategies are proposed to address home monitoring of premature infants. The NIH consensus report to the American Academy of Pediatrics recommends against the routine evaluation of premature infants before discharge with a standard two-channel pneumogram (thoracic impedance and heart rate monitoring) because this test has a high rate of both false-positive and false-negative results and is not a reliable predictor of infants who will suffer an ALTE or succumb to SIDS.

One accepted approach is to monitor all premature infants up to and beyond the postnatal age associated with the highest rate of SIDS (i.e., 2 to 4 months). If the infant is stressed (e.g., by an upper respiratory tract illness), it is speculated that the "normal" pauses in respiration can become pathological and present as an ALTE.

HINT: Periodic breathing (i.e., short intervals of apnea interspersed between short intervals of respirations) can appear pathologic to the parent. However, *isolated periodic breathing* in a premature infant is *not predictive* of ALTE or SIDS.

> **HINT:** Many premature infants have mild GRD and a history of choking dur-
> ing feeding. It can be extremely difficult to determine when these
> episodes are truly ALTEs and when they are merely normal variations.
> If the episode is associated with the factors listed in the NIH's defini-
> tion of ALTE (i.e., apnea, color change, marked change in muscle tone),
> then the infant should be admitted for a more complete evaluation.

EVALUATION OF APNEA

There are several approaches to evaluating an infant who has experienced an ALTE. A thorough **history and physical examination** is the most important component of an apnea evaluation. The event should be described in detail by the witness including **events immediately preceding and subsequent to the event**. A careful history may, in many cases, narrow the focus of your investigation and should include the following:

- Duration of the event
- Relationship to feeding
- Choking, gagging, vomiting
- Muscle tone prior to and after the event
- Level of consciousness prior to and after the event
- Presence of seizure activity or a postictal state
- Recent trauma
- Fever, coryza, or any upper respiratory infection symptoms
- Sleep position
- Resuscitation required
- Household medications
- Prior history of similar events

Once the history and physical examination have narrowed the list of differential diagnoses, the appropriate labs tests will then be decided on but may include:

- EEG
- Electrocardiogram (ECG)
- Chest radiograph
- Complete blood cell count
- Serum electrolyte panel
- Serum calcium level
- Serum glucose level
- Blood urea nitrogen and creatinine level
- Multichannel recordings of the heart rate
- Thermistor nasal air flow
- Respiratory rate

- Pulse oximetry
- Esophageal pH
- Brain scan
- Viral studies

TREATMENT OF APNEA

Treatment of an apneic event or ALTE is immediate **cardiopulmonary resuscitation.** However, most infants present to a clinician for evaluation after the event has resolved when no further resuscitation is required. Treatment thus involves addressing the **underlying cause.** Although **hospitalization is not required for all infants** who present with an ALTE, prolonged cardiovascular monitoring may aid in diagnosis by allowing evaluation of any recurrences. Hospitalization also provides reassurance to caregivers while allowing time for **education in cardiopulmonary resuscitation and SIDS risk factors.**

The **role of home cardiorespiratory monitors remains controversial.** A 2003 policy statement by the Committee on the Fetus and Newborn of the American Academy of Pediatrics suggests that home monitoring may be useful to alert caregivers to a recurrent event when predisposing factors are present but **recommends against routine use.** Caregivers should be counseled that the use of home monitors does not prevent SIDS. If caregivers are involved in the decision and elect to use a home monitor, it is recommended that it be discontinued after 2 months without any apnea alarms.

Suggested Readings

American Academy of Pediatrics Committee on Fetus and Newborn: Apnea, sudden infant death syndrome, and home monitoring. *Pediatrics* 111(4):914–917, 2003.

Claudius I, Keens T: Do all infants with apparent life-threatening events need to be admitted? *Pediatrics* 119(4):679–683, 2007.

DeWolfe CC: Apparent life-threatening event: a review. *Pediatr Clin North Am* 52:1127–1146, 2005.

National Institutes of Health: Consensus development conference on infantile apnea and home monitoring. *Pediatrics* 79:292–299, 1987.

16 *Ascites*

Kathleen Wholey Zsolway and Binita M. Kamath

INTRODUCTION

Ascites is the **pathologic accumulation of fluid** in the **peritoneal cavity.** It can be caused by **decreased plasma oncotic pressure, obstructed lymphatic or venous drainage,** or **irritation of the peritoneum** (e.g., as a result of infection, trauma, or neoplasia).

DIFFERENTIAL DIAGNOSIS LIST

Gastrointestinal / Hepatic Causes

Cirrhosis
Protein-losing enteropathy (PLE) (See Table 16-1 for differential diagnosis)
Pancreatitis

Infectious Causes

Bacterial peritonitis
Chronic tuberculous peritonitis
Congenital toxoplasmosis, other, rubella, cytomegalovirus, and herpes simplex virus (TORCH)infection

Neoplastic Causes

Hodgkin disease
Intraperitoneal tumor

Congenital or Vascular Causes

Hepatic vein occlusion (Budd-Chiari syndrome)
Portal vein obstruction
Renal vein thrombosis
Congestive heart failure
Thoracic duct obstruction (chylous ascites)

Metabolic or Congenital Causes

Lysosomal storage disease

Inflammatory Causes

Chronic adhesive pericarditis
Peritonitis—rheumatic, meconium, bile

Renal Causes

Nephrotic syndrome
Perforation of the urinary tract
Obstructive uropathy
Acute glomerulonephritis
Chronic renal failure

Miscellaneous Causes

Systemic lupus erythematosus
Familial Mediterranean fever
Maternal diabetes
Enlarged lymph node
Pulmonary lymphangiectasia
Malnutrition

TABLE 16-1 Diseases Associated with Enteric Protein Loss

Loss from Intestinal Lymphatics

Intestinal lymphangiectasia
Primary
Secondary (i.e., resulting from cardiac disease)
    Constrictive pericarditis
    Congestive heart failure
    Cardiomyopathy
    Fontan physiology
Obstructive lymphatic disorders
    Malrotation
    Lymphoma
    Tuberculosis
    Sarcoidosis
    Radiation therapy and chemotherapy
    Retroperitoneal fibrosis or tumor
    Arsenic poisoning

Loss from an Abnormal or Inflamed Mucosal Surface

Ménétrier disease
Eosinophilic gastroenteritis
Milk- and soy-induced enterocolitis
Celiac disease
Tropical sprue
Ulcerative jejunitis or colitis
Radiation enteritis
Graft-versus-host disease
Necrotizing enterocolitis
Crohn disease
Hirschsprung disease
Systemic lupus erythematosus
Bacterial overgrowth
Giardiasis
Bacterial and parasitic infections
Common variable immunodeficiency

Modified from Proujansky R: Protein-losing enteropathy. In *Pediatric Gastrointestinal Disease*, 2nd ed. Edited by Walker WA, Durie PR, Hamilton JR, et al. Philadelphia, BC Decker, 1996.

DIFFERENTIAL DIAGNOSIS DISCUSSION

Cirrhosis

In children other than neonates, cirrhosis is the **most common cause** of ascites.

Etiology

Cirrhosis is a process characterized by **increased fibrous tissue** and **nodule formation following necrosis of hepatocytes** within the liver. It represents **irreversible distortion** of the intrahepatic vascular and biliary structures. Cirrhosis may develop in association with chronic viral hepatitis, autoimmune hepatitis, cystic fibrosis, Wilson disease, and structural abnormalities of the biliary system (biliary atresia, sclerosing cholangitis). The differential diagnosis of cirrhosis is extensive and varies with the age at presentation.

The ascites of hepatic cirrhosis is a consequence of **hypoalbuminemia** (secondary to failure of protein synthesis) and **excess salt and water retention (secondary to elevated portal venous pressure and activation of the renin-angiotensin system).** Cirrhosis is commonly associated with **peripheral edema** after the presence of ascites has become evident.

Clinical Features

The physical examination may demonstrate a **firm liver with irregular margins (hepatomegaly)** or a **small liver, spider angiomata, palmar erythema, and splenomegaly,** depending on the degree of cirrhosis.

The two major sequelae of cirrhosis are **portal venous hypertension** and **hepatocellular failure.** The main signs of portal hypertension are **splenomegaly, hematemesis** (as a result of bleeding from esophageal varices), and **bloody stools** as a result of bleeding from hemorrhoids. **Hepatic coma** may also occur.

Evaluation

Serum transaminases, serum albumin levels, prothrombin time, and **blood ammonia levels** are often ordered to assess hepatic inflammation and synthetic function. A **complete blood cell (CBC) count** may reveal anemia, thrombocytopenia, and leukopenia as a result of hypersplenism. Various imaging options are available: **Ultrasound** may reveal increased echogenicity; **radioisotope scanning** may reveal decreased uptake, increased flow to the spleen, and irregular hepatic texture; magnetic resonance cholangiopancreatography (MRCP) is useful to assess the biliary system and hepatic texture. A **liver biopsy** is often needed to identify the cause of the cirrhosis.

Treatment

Dietary and drug regimens should be initiated in a controlled hospital environment. The diet should provide adequate calories for growth and be supplemented with **calcium** and **vitamins D, E, and K. Diuretics** and **decreased sodium** content in the diet may improve the ascites and edema. Albumin infusions are commonly used to reverse ascites.

Additional management of cirrhosis entails the **prevention and treatment of life-threatening complications,** such as variceal bleeding. **Liver transplantation** is considered standard therapy for patients with advanced and decompensated cirrhosis.

Infectious Peritonitis

Etiology

- **Primary peritonitis** is an infection in the peritoneal cavity secondary to microorganism invasion via the blood or lymphatics. Causative organisms include pneumococci, group A streptococci, and, less commonly, Gram-negative bacilli and viruses.

- **Secondary peritonitis** is an infection in the peritoneal cavity that occurs through rupture of an intra-abdominal viscus or extension of an abscess. In children, the most common cause of secondary peritonitis is appendicitis. Other causes include gangrenous bowel, necrotizing enterocolitis, and idiopathic gastric or bowel perforation. The causative organisms are the normal flora of the gastrointestinal tract. Secondary peritonitis may also occur as a complication of a ventriculoperitoneal shunt and in patients receiving peritoneal dialysis. *Staphylococcus epidermidis* can be the causative agent in these patients.

Evaluation

Typically, the history includes the **rapid onset of abdominal pain, fever,** and **vomiting** (e.g., over the course of **48 hours**). Physical examination reveals either diffuse or lower quadrant **severe abdominal tenderness.** **Bowel sounds** are **hypoactive or absent,** and **abdominal rigidity** may be present. The **patient prefers** to lie in a **supine position** and feels severe discomfort with motion or palpation.

Abdominal radiographs of patients with peritonitis often reveal intestinal dilation, edema of the small intestine, peritoneal fluid, and absence of the psoas shadow. Patients with intestinal perforation have radiographic evidence of free air in the peritoneal cavity.

Needle aspiration of the peritoneal fluid should be performed if peritonitis is suspected or if the patient has an unexplained fever and fluid in the abdomen. Analysis of the peritoneal fluid from a patient with infectious peritonitis typically reveals an **elevated protein level** and an **elevated white blood cell count** (i.e., >300 cells/mm^3), of which >25% are polymorphonuclear leukocytes. A **Gram stain** and **culture** of the fluid should be performed to help guide antimicrobial therapy.

Treatment

In patients with peritonitis, careful attention must be paid to **fluid and electrolyte status.** In addition, parenteral **antimicrobial therapy** should be initiated. Combination therapy with ampicillin, gentamicin, and clindamycin provides appropriate initial coverage. Antimicrobial therapy should be modified based on culture and Gram stain results. **Surgical evaluation** should occur early because surgical exploration may be necessary to evaluate for a perforated viscus.

Protein-Losing Enteropathy

Etiology

Protein-losing enteropathy (PLE), the **loss of proteins across the gastrointestinal mucosa,** occurs in a variety of disease states (Table 16-1).

Evaluation

The patient's **history** reflects the underlying disease state. **Edema** may be the presenting physical examination finding, although symptoms of a disturbance in bowel function may be elicited in a careful history.

The primary method of diagnosing enteric protein loss is the **detection of elevated α_1-antitrypsin (α_1-AT) in the stool,** a protein that is not actively secreted, absorbed, or digested by the gastrointestinal tract. Quantification can be performed on a spot stool sample or on stool samples collected over several days. Spot sample results appear to correlate well with those obtained from samples collected over a period of time.

Treatment

Treatment addresses the **underlying cause** of PLE. **Reduction in dietary fat** intake can aid in decreasing the enteric protein loss.

Suggested Readings

Proujansky R: Protein-losing enteropathy. In *Pediatric Gastrointestinal Disease,* 4th ed. Edited by Walker WA, Goulet O, Kleinman RE, et al. Philadelphia, BC Decker, 2004, 194–202.

Hardy S, Kleinman RE: Cirrhosis and chronic liver failure. In *Liver Disease in Children,* 3rd ed. Edited by Suchy FJ, Sokol RJ, Balistreri WF. New York, Cambridge University Press, 2007, 97–137.

Hyams JS: Ascites. In *Nelson Textbook of Pediatrics,* 18th ed. Edited by Kliegman RM, Behrman RE, Jenson HB, et al. Philadelphia, WB Saunders, 2007, 1714.

Nowicki MJ, Bishop PR: Ascites. In *Pediatric Gastrointestinal and Liver Disease,* 3rd ed. Edited by Wyllie R, Hyams JS, Kay M. Philadelphia, Elsevier, 2006, 247–260.

17 | *Ataxia*

Courtney J. Wusthoff
Daniel Licht (Third Edition)
Lawrence D. Morton (Second Edition)

INTRODUCTION

Ataxia is a disturbance of coordination or balance that is not caused by a problem of muscle strength. Ataxia is characterized by errors of motor activity with regard to rate, range, direction, timing, duration, and force. The most obvious and often the initial manifestation is a wide-based and staggering gait, although more subtle findings such as nystagmus, titubation (head bobbing), difficulties in fine control of the limbs (dysmetria and past pointing), and hypotonia may be early signs and equally distressing.

The major causes of acute ataxia differ significantly from those of intermittent or chronic ataxia. However, there can be overlap because slowly progressive ataxia may be unrecognized and appear acutely, sometimes in the context of febrile illness or injury. In addition, one may see chronic disability associated with incomplete recovery from intermittent ataxia. Table 17-1 lists the causes of ataxia.

DIFFERENTIAL DIAGNOSIS LIST

Acute Ataxia

Infectious Causes
Encephalitis
Postinfectious or autoimmune disorders (acute cerebellar ataxia, Guillain-Barré syndrome, acute demyelinating encephalomyelitis, Miller-Fisher syndrome, multiple sclerosis)

Toxic Causes
Ethanol
Anticonvulsants
Antihistamines

Neoplastic Causes
Brainstem tumor
Cerebellar tumor

Paraneoplastic Causes
Opsoclonus-myoclonus-ataxia syndrome
(sometimes called "the syndrome of dancing eyes and dancing feet")

Psychosocial Causes
Conversion disorder

Miscellaneous Causes
Migraine headache (benign paroxysmal vertigo)
Trauma

Intermittent Ataxia

Metabolic or Genetic Causes
Dominant recurrent ataxia
Carnitine acetyltransferase deficiency
Hartnup disease
Maple syrup urine disease
Episodic ataxia type 1 (Paroxysmal ataxia and myokymia)

TABLE 17-1 Causes of Ataxia

Form of Ataxia	Major Causes	Other Causes
Acute ataxia	Ingestion Acute cerebellar ataxia Guillain-Barré syndrome	Migraine Opsoclonus-myoclonus-ataxia
Acute recurrent ataxia	Migraine Metabolic disease	
Chronic Ataxia	Congenital cerebellar malformations	
Chronic progressive ataxia	Posterior fossa mass Opsoclonus-myoclonus-ataxia	Friedreich ataxia Ataxia-telangiectasia

Episodic ataxia type 2 (SCA 6, familial hemiplegic migraine)

Pyruvate decarboxylase deficiency

Miscellaneous Causes

Migraine headache (benign paroxysmal vertigo)

Chronic or Progressive Ataxia

Neoplastic Causes

Neuroectodermal tumor

Posterior fossa tumor

Glioma

Astrocytoma

Ependymoma

Medulloblastoma

Metabolic or Genetic Causes

Ataxia-telangiectasia

Ataxia-oculomotor apraxia

Friedreich ataxia

Refsum disease

Progressive myoclonic epilepsy (formerly known as Ramsay Hunt syndrome)

Miscellaneous Causes

Fixed-deficit ataxia—ataxic cerebral palsy, congenital malformations

Acquired diseases (e.g., systemic lupus erythematosus [SLE], hypothyroidism, vitamin E deficiency)

DIFFERENTIAL DIAGNOSIS DISCUSSION

Acute Ataxia

Brain Tumor

Brainstem or cerebellar tumors that **grow rapidly, acutely hemorrhage, or shift** can cause acute decompensation of the brainstem, leading to acute ataxia.

HINT: Cerebellar hemispheric dysfunction leads to limb ataxia on the same side of the lesion.

Encephalitis

Some agents commonly implicated in brainstem encephalitis include Epstein-Barr virus (EBV), enterocytopathogenic human orphan (ECHO) virus, Coxsackievirus, varicella-zoster virus, *Mycoplasma*, and *Borrelia burgdorferi* (the agent responsible for Lyme disease). Ataxia occurs, often in association with other cranial nerve dysfunctions, in patients who have **diffuse encephalitis with altered awareness and/or seizures**. Many children completely recover, although some are left with significant neurologic impairment.

Postinfectious/Autoimmune Disorders

Acute cerebellar ataxia is characterized by the sudden onset of ataxia 2 to 3 weeks after infection. Varicella and EBV are most commonly identified triggers, but most often no agent is identified. Children between 1 and 5 years of age are most often affected. Diagnosis often relies on clinical signs because confirmatory laboratory studies are not always present. CSF may show a mild pleocytosis (in about half of cases), and magnetic resonance imaging (MRI) may show mildly abnormal signal in the cerebellum (in a minority of patients). Generally, improvement begins within days of presentation, and there is a good outcome within weeks. Corticosteroids are of unproven benefit in the treatment of acute cerebellar ataxia.

Guillain-Barré syndrome is a postinfectious demyelinating disease of the peripheral nerves that can occur in children of all ages. Up to 15% of patients develop a sensory ataxia before other signs of peripheral demyelination are apparent. Intravenous immunoglobulin (IVIG) is the treatment of choice.

Miller-Fisher syndrome is an uncommon variant of Guillain-Barré syndrome, characterized by the acute onset of ataxia, ophthalmoparesis, and hyporeflexia. Complete recovery within several weeks is the rule.

Acute demyelinating encephalomyelitis (ADEM), like Guillain-Barré syndrome, occurs 1 to 3 weeks following an infection. However, ADEM is a central demyelinating process, affecting the spinal cord and/or brain. Brainstem or cerebellar involvement may cause ataxia. Steroids are the preferred first-line therapy.

Opsoclonus-myoclonus-ataxia syndrome is a paraneoplastic/autoimmune phenomena characterized by the triad of myoclonus, opsoclonus, and ataxia, classically seen in patients with neuroblastoma. However, any single symptom or combination of the symptoms may occur in a given patient. When present, the underlying neuroblastoma is often occult. In many cases, there is no underlying tumor, and no trigger for the syndrome is found. The outcome varies widely.

Trauma

Ataxia may persist for weeks in **postconcussion syndrome.** Trauma can also produce basilar or vertebral artery occlusion accompanied by occipital headache and other cranial nerve dysfunction.

Conversion Disorder

Conversion disorder is characterized by **involuntary alteration or limitation of physical function as a result of a psychological conflict.** It is different from malingering, which implies a willful act. Hysterical abnormalities of gait in children are always a diagnosis of exclusion. They are seen most commonly in older children and adolescents and characterized by findings that do not match expected pathophysiology. For example, some patients lurch or stagger when they attempt to stand up but are able to sit down without difficulty, which is incongruent because sitting requires better balance and would therefore be difficult for someone with a true coordination or balance disturbance. When this gait is extreme, it is termed **astasia-abasia.**

Intermittent Ataxia

Postinfectious/ Autoimmune Disorders

Multiple sclerosis (less common in children) is a demyelinating disease characterized by recurrent bouts of neurologic symptoms involving different parts of the central nervous system (CNS). MRI shows numerous white matter "plaques." Acute flares may be treated with high-dose corticosteroids.

Metabolic or Genetic Disorders

Dominant recurrent ataxia is characterized by recurrent bouts of ataxia without an identifiable metabolic cause. Ataxic symptoms, some of which are associated with cerebellar hypoplasia, become apparent in patients before 3 years of age.

Hartnup disease is a rare disorder in which defective amino acid transport in the cells of the proximal renal tubules and the small intestine leads to massive aminoaciduria. Patients are developmentally delayed and have a borderline IQ. They are photosensitive and develop pellagra-like rashes when exposed to sunlight. Episodic ataxia is frequently reported, sometimes with delirium and emotional lability. The ataxia is triggered by intercurrent infections.

Maple syrup urine disease (intermittent form), an amino acidemia caused by deficiency of a branched-chain decarboxylase, leads to bouts of ataxia and encephalopathy. Between attacks of ataxia, the patient's physical examination and IQ are typically normal. During attacks, the blood and urine exhibit elevated levels of branched-chain amino acids.

Episodic ataxia type 1 (paroxysmal ataxia and myokymia) and type 2, an autosomal dominant disorder is characterized by attacks of ataxia that last from minutes to hours. The average age of onset is 5 to 7 years. Patients with this disorder usually respond to acetazolamide therapy.

Most patients with **pyruvate decarboxylase deficiency** have episodic ataxia, dysarthria, and developmental delays (although some develop normally). Triggers for attacks of ataxia include infection and a high carbohydrate load. The disorder becomes apparent once the child reaches preschool age. Patients have elevated lactate and pyruvate levels during attacks and occasionally following an oral glucose load. Treatment includes a ketogenic diet and the administration of acetazolamide. The prognosis varies and is related to the percentage of preserved enzyme activity.

Chronic or Progressive Ataxia

Congenital Disorders (Ataxia with Fixed Deficit)

Several congenital disorders produce chronic ataxia, including Dandy-Walker malformations, Chiari malformations, and cerebellar hypoplasia. Appearance of clinical signs usually occurs in infancy or childhood but can be delayed until the patient reaches adulthood. In one recognized variant of cerebral palsy (CP), ataxia is the prominent feature and patients may be hypotonic and hyporeflexic.

Neoplasia

Brain tumors are an important consideration in a child with progressive ataxia, especially those originating in the posterior fossa. Tumors of neuroectodermal origin are most the common solid lesions of the CNS in children and the second most common childhood malignancy. Posterior fossa tumors are most common in children <8 years; tumors involving the telencephalon are more likely in children <2 years and >8 years. The most common posterior fossa tumors include cerebellar astrocytoma, brainstem glioma, and PNET (primitive neuroectodermal tumor) or medulloblastoma. More than two thirds of childhood primary brain tumors are derived from glial elements. CNS tumors arising from the spinal cord account for a very small percentage. Cerebellar astrocytoma generally presents with cranial nerve findings and ataxia as a late symptom. Ependymoma and medulloblastoma frequently present with symptoms of increased intracranial pressure. Medulloblastoma may progress especially rapidly.

Metabolic or Genetic Disorders

Ataxia-telangiectasia is a multisystemic disease that most prominently affects the nervous and immune systems. Truncal ataxia usually develops before the first birthday. Drooling and dysarthria are common.

Telangiectatic lesions, most commonly affecting the conjunctivae and ears, develop after 2 years of age. Complications include frequent sinopulmonary infections (as a result of deficient IgE and IgA) and an increased incidence of neoplasia. Alpha-fetoprotein (AFP) and carcinoembryonic antigen (CEA) levels are elevated, and immunoglobulin levels are decreased. Treatment usually entails vigorous antibiotic support for infections. There is currently no effective therapy for the neurologic symptoms.

Ataxia-oculomotor apraxia is clinically similar to ataxia-telangiectasia. It is autosomal recessive and has the neurologic features of ataxia-telangiectasia, but symptoms start after 1 year of age, and patients have a normal immunologic status.

Friedreich ataxia is a multisystemic disorder affecting the peripheral nerves, spinal cord, and heart. The ataxia usually begins in childhood. Limb ataxia is worse than truncal ataxia. Kyphoscoliosis is common, and there is early loss of position, light touch sensation, and deep tendon reflexes. Diabetes mellitus occurs in 10% to 40% of patients. Cardiomyopathy occurs in the majority of patients and is the highest source of mortality.

Refsum disease is an inborn error of phytanic acid metabolism characterized by retinitis pigmentosa, recurrent polyneuropathy, and ataxia. Elevated serum levels of phytanic acid are found. Treatment is usually dietary.

Progressive myoclonic epilepsy (Ramsay Hunt disease) is characterized by ataxia, myoclonus, and seizures. Although this disease is usually autosomal recessive, autosomal dominant and mitochondrial cases are also described. Seizures and myoclonus may resolve with antiepileptic therapy.

Other hereditary disorders that may present with ataxia include Wilson disease, biotinidase deficiency, adrenoleukodystrophy (X-linked), hypobetalipoproteinemia, juvenile sulfatide lipidosis, sea-blue histiocytosis, Leigh disease, and Leber optic neuropathy.

EVALUATION OF ATAXIA

There are two major pitfalls in diagnosing ataxia. The first is confusing ataxia with other gait disturbances, such as weakness, dizziness, vertigo, and conversion disorders. Misdiagnosis can be avoided by obtaining a careful history of symptoms, noting evidence of cerebellar dysfunction on neurologic examination and observing other findings related to ataxia (e.g., dysmetria, an intention tremor, dysdiadochokinesia).

The second is misidentifying chronic progressive ataxia as acute ataxia. The etiology and possible treatments for acute and chronic ataxia are very different, so distinguishing between the two is important.

> **HINT:** Mild chronic ataxia may be improperly dismissed as clumsiness.

Patient History

After confirming that the symptoms are consistent with ataxia, it is important to characterize the illness in regard to the timing, pattern, and progression of complaints. Isolated gait disturbance can be caused by problems involving the nervous system at various levels as well as being a nonspecific feature of systemic disease, but coexisting scanning speech or discoordination of other limb movements signals true ataxia. Likewise, the presence of headache or vomiting may suggest migraine or elevated intracranial pressure. Other important questions to ask include the following:

- When were symptoms first noticed? Were there any injuries or accidents immediately preceding?
- Is the ataxia acute, intermittent (recurrent), or chronic?
- Are the symptoms constant, fluctuating, or progressive?
- When are the symptoms most notable? (Difficulty with sitting or head control suggests a truncal ataxia, which usually correlates with lesions of the cerebellar vermis. Limb ataxia correlates with lesions of the cerebellar hemispheres.)
- When was the child's last upper respiratory infection or other viral syndrome?
- Are there any medications in the home the child might have ingested?
- Is there any family history of similar symptoms?

Physical Examination

Obviously, all children should have complete general and neurologic examinations. The following pointers can help clarify the diagnosis of ataxia. In the eye examination, careful observation may reveal abnormal movements such as opsoclonus (in the opsoclonus-myoclonus-ataxia syndrome), nystagmus (suggesting brainstem or cerebellar lesion), or abnormal saccades (as in cerebellar lesions). **Papilledema** suggests increased intracranial pressure, as in intracranial mass lesions or hydrocephalus. The presence of **facial weakness, dysarthria, or dysphagia** during the cranial nerve examination is concerning for brainstem or posterior fossa lesion. Strength testing of isolated muscle groups is essential to clarify the nature of the impairment, particularly when gait abnormality is the presenting complaint. Weakness may also exist in Guillain-Barré syndrome. Impaired joint-position sense or vibration sense suggests a problem in the sensory input that guides our movements

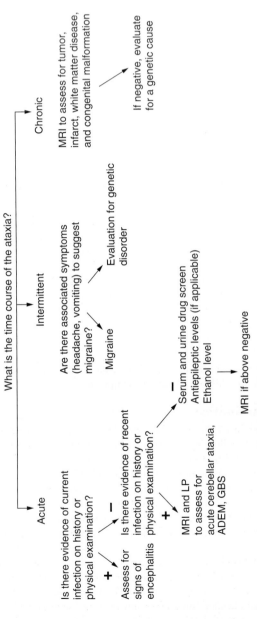

Figure 17-1 ■ **Approach to the patient with acute ataxia.**
ADEM = acute demyelinating encephalomyelitis; GBS = Guillain-Barré syndrome; CSF = cerebrospinal fluid; CT = computed tomography; EEG = electroencephalogram; LP = lumbar puncture; MRI = magnetic resonance imaging.

in space. **Sensory ataxia** is an abnormality of movement caused by impaired sensation of the body's position and movement in space; this leads to the positive **Romberg sign,** in which a patient falls when asked to stand with feet together and eyes closed. Finger-nose-finger testing can clarify asymmetry in ataxia. Rapid alternating hand movements can be useful in demonstrating mild impairments. Problems with fine finger movements are more commonly associated with sensory ataxia than cerebellar ataxia. Gait should be observed for several steps, and it may be helpful to have the patient walk around obstacles or perform tandem gait to demonstrate deficits.

Laboratory Studies

Complete serum and urine drug screen should be performed on all patients presenting with acute ataxia. **Ethanol levels** need to be ordered specifically when ingestion is suspected. If the child takes antiepileptic medication, or such medication is present in the home, **serum levels** may identify toxicity. CBC with differential may identify concomitant infection; **electrolytes** should be checked for metabolic causes of discoordination. **Liver function tests** and **ammonia** may also be considered. If an infectious or postinfectious illness is suspected, **cerebral spinal fluid (CSF)** should be sent for cell count, protein, glucose, and culture. Pleocytosis suggests infection, or postinfectious illness such as acute disseminated encephalomyelitis (ADEM) or acute cerebellar ataxia. Elevated protein may be seen in postinfectious disease, including Guillain-Barré syndrome. Unless insufficient fluid is collected, it should be sent for specific infectious markers (e.g., **mycoplasma titers**) or markers of demyelination (e.g., **oligoclonal bands**).

Diagnostic Modalities

MRI is the imaging modality of choice when evaluating ataxia. Although computed tomography (CT) may be acceptable as an interim screening study while awaiting MRI, it does not adequately assess the posterior fossa, where likely cerebellar and brainstem lesions would be present. Electromyelogram (EMG) and nerve conduction velocity (NCV) may be useful in assessing for peripheral neuropathy causing sensory ataxia, such as Guillain-Barré syndrome. Figure 17-1 illustrates the approach to a patient with acute ataxia.

Suggested Readings

Casselbrant ML, Mandel EM: Balance disorders in children. *Neurol Clin* 23:807–829, 2005.

Fenichel GM: *Clinical Pediatric Neurology: A Signs and Symptoms Approach,* 5th ed. Philadelphia, WB Saunders, 2005, 219–240.

Menkes JH, Sarnat HB, Maria BL (eds): *Child Neurology,* 7th ed. Baltimore, Lippincott, Williams & Wilkins, 2005.

Swaiman KF, Ashwal S, Ferriero DM (eds): *Pediatric Neurology: Principles and Practice,* 4th ed. St. Louis, Mosby, 2006, 1241–1269.

Tunnessen WW: *Signs and Symptoms in Pediatrics,* 3rd ed. Philadelphia, Lippincott-Raven, 1999, 747–758.

INTRODUCTION

Purpura, that is, **petechiae and ecchymoses (bruises)**, and excessive bleeding are caused by disruptions in one or more of the three stages of normal hemostasis:

- **Vascular phase**—vasoconstriction
- **Primary hemostasis**—platelet plug formation
- **Secondary hemostasis**—fibrin thrombus formation

Disruptions in vascular integrity are characterized by **purpuric lesions;** laboratory tests demonstrate **normal platelet number and function** as well as **normal coagulation.** Disorders of **primary hemostasis** are also characterized by **purpuric lesions,** but **laboratory test results are not normal.** Disorders of **secondary hemostasis** are characterized by **hemarthroses** and **deep bleeding and abnormal coagulation studies.** Unexplained excessive bruising and bleeding occurring in children with normal hemostasis requires a thorough investigation for nonaccidental trauma.

DIFFERENTIAL DIAGNOSIS LIST 🔓✂

Thrombocytopenia
Increased Platelet Destruction
  Immune-mediated
    thrombocytopenia
  Idiopathic (immune)
    thrombocytopenic
    purpura (ITP)
  Evans syndrome
  Neonatal, isoimmune, and
    autoimmune
  Posttransfusion purpura
  Drug related
  HIV infection
  Systemic lupus
    erythematosus (SLE)
  Microangiopathic process
  Hemolytic uremic
    syndrome
  Disseminated intravascular
    coagulation

Thrombotic thrombocy-
  topenic purpura
Decreased Platelet Production
  Congenital amegakary-
    ocytic thrombocytopenia
  Thrombocytopenia with
    absent radii (TAR)
  Inherited bone marrow
    failure syndromes
    (Fanconi anemia,
    dyskeratosis congenital,
    cartilage-hair hypoplasia)
  Aplastic anemia
  **Vitamin B_{12} or folate
    deficiency**
  Viral infection—varicella-
    zoster virus, measles virus,
    rubella, cytomegalovirus,
    Epstein-Barr virus
  Drugs

Bone marrow infiltration
Leukemia
Malignancy metastatic to bone marrow
Myelofibrosis
Storage diseases
Osteopetrosis
Platelet Sequestration
Splenomegaly
Large hemangiomas (Kasabach-Merritt syndrome)

Disorders of Platelet Function

Bernard-Soulier disease
Glanzmann thrombasthenia
Wiskott-Aldrich syndrome
May-Hegglin anomaly
Platelet granule defects
Drug-induced abnormalities (e.g., aspirin, ibuprofen)
Uremia

Disruption in Vascular Integrity

Trauma (accidental or nonaccidental)
Henoch-Schönlein purpura

Telangiectasia syndromes
Drug-induced vasculitis
Purpura fulminans
Bacterial (e.g., *Neisseria meningitidis,* streptococcal toxins)
Viral (e.g., measles, influenza)
Rickettsial—Rocky Mountain spotted fever
Parasitic—malaria
Connective tissue disorders
Ehlers-Danlos syndrome
Osteogenesis imperfecta
Vitamin C deficiency

Clotting Factor Deficiencies

von Willebrand disease
Hemophilia—Factor VIII or IX deficiency
Other congenital factor deficiencies
Vitamin K deficiency
Liver disease
Disseminated intravascular hemolysis
Anticoagulants (heparin, warfarin)

DIFFERENTIAL DIAGNOSIS DISCUSSION I: BLEEDING AND PURPURA IN CHILDREN

Idiopathic (Immune) Thrombocytopenic Purpura

ITP, the **most common cause of low platelet counts** in childhood, can be categorized as **acute** (thrombocytopenia resolves within 6 months of diagnosis) or **chronic**. Although ITP can occur at any age, the **peak incidence** in children is **between the ages of 2 and 6 years.**

Etiology

The exact cause of ITP is unknown, but the disorder is thought to be **immune mediated**. A **viral illness** may precede ITP.

Clinical Features

The child with ITP appears otherwise well but has a rapid onset of purpuric lesions. ITP is rarely associated with significant bleeding episodes, but epistaxis occurs in about a third of patients. Clinical findings of lymphadenopathy and hepatosplenomegaly should alert the physician to a diagnosis other than ITP (e.g., malignancy, metabolic disorder).

Evaluation

A complete blood count (CBC) demonstrates thrombocytopenia. Additional laboratory studies (depending on the situation) may include a direct antibody test (DAT), reticulocyte count, and an antinuclear antibody. Other causes of thrombocytopenia (e.g., SLE) should be considered, particularly in adolescent girls.

> **HINT:** Evans syndrome (autoimmune hemolytic anemia with immune mediated thrombocytopenia) should be suspected in patients with thrombocytopenia and anemia. Patients with Evans syndrome have a positive DAT, evidence of hemolysis, and usually require more intensive intervention than those with ITP alone.

Routine bone marrow aspiration to evaluate acute ITP is usually not necessary but should be considered prior to initiating steroid therapy to avoid partially treating an unusual presentation of acute leukemia. Increased platelet precursors (megakaryocytes) are often present on histologic examination of bone marrow aspirate in patients with ITP.

Treatment

Many believe that treating patients with acute ITP is often unnecessary. If a child experiences significant bleeding, treatment is warranted. Treatment options include intravenous immunoglobulin (800 to 1,000 mg/kg), steroids (2 mg/kg per day), and, in Rh-positive children, anti-D immune globulin (50 to 75 µg/kg). Intravenous immunoglobulin administration is associated with a more rapid increase in platelet count than steroid therapy. If a patient with known ITP requires therapy, then it is best to use whatever therapy has been beneficial for that patient in the past.

Intracranial hemorrhage and life-threatening hemorrhage, although rare in patients with ITP, may be fatal. Therefore, treatment is mandatory if the ITP patient has major head trauma, an abnormal neurologic examination, or copious blood loss. High-dose steroid therapy with intravenous immunoglobulin administration should be initiated rapidly before more detailed evaluations. In patients with ongoing life-threatening bleeding, continuous platelet transfusions, emergent splenectomy, or both may be necessary.

TABLE 18-1 Causes of Disseminated Intravascular Coagulation (DIC)

Infection—bacterial, viral, fungal, rickettsial
Cardiovascular disorder—shock
Toxins—snake bites
Tumors—myeloid leukemia
Trauma—massive generalized or head trauma
Hematologic disorder—hemolytic transfusion reactions
Miscellaneous causes—burns, purpura fulminans, severe asphyxia

Disseminated Intravascular Coagulation

Etiology

Disseminated intravascular coagulation (DIC) is a **consumptive coagulopathy** that is characterized by **intravascular coagulation** and **fibrinolysis** resulting in clotting factor deficiencies and thrombocytopenia and associated with an underlying disease (Table 18-1).

> **HINT:** Sepsis should be considered as an etiology for any critically ill child until proven otherwise.

Clinical Features

Children with DIC usually **appear ill** and **bleed from multiple sites**. In neonates, DIC usually manifests as **gastrointestinal bleeding** or **oozing from skin puncture sites**.

Evaluation

In patients with DIC, laboratory values show a normal or **decreased platelet count, increased prothrombin time (PT)** and **partial thromboplastin time (PTT),** decreased fibrinogen, and **increased fibrin split products.** A peripheral blood smear is significant for **schistocytes, fragmented red blood cells (RBCs),** and normal or **decreased platelets.**

Treatment

Treatment is directed toward managing the underlying disorder and replacing coagulation factors and platelets.

Henoch-Schönlein Purpura

Etiology and Incidence

Henoch-Schönlein purpura (HSP) is an **acquired inflammatory vasculitis.** The clinical manifestations of HSP are caused by immunoglobulin A subclass 1 (IgA1) deposition in blood vessel walls and the renal mesangium. **HSP is most common in early childhood.**

Clinical Features

Diffuse inflammation of the small vessels causes abdominal pain, arthritis, and palpable purpura. Renal involvement occurs in 50% of patients. Most patients have a prodromal upper respiratory infection 1 to 3 weeks before the onset of illness. The hallmark of this disorder on physical examination is a symmetric pattern of purpura, primarily involving the buttocks and lower extremities. In some patients, purpura are also found on the extensor surfaces of the arms. The palms, soles, and genitalia are spared.

Evaluation

Hematuria, proteinuria, and cellular casts on urinalysis confirm nephritis in patients with Henoch-Schönlein purpura. The CBC, PT, and PTT are normal unless major gastrointestinal blood loss has occurred, in which case the patient may be anemic.

Treatment

Henoch-Schönlein purpura, a self-limited disorder, usually resolves in 1 to 6 weeks. Treatment primarily involves supportive therapy. Corticosteroids, used to manage renal complications, may be helpful to alleviate persistent or severe gastrointestinal and musculoskeletal symptoms.

von Willebrand Disease

Etiology

von Willebrand disease (vWD), the most common inherited bleeding disorder, is characterized by quantitative or qualitative abnormalities in von Willebrand factor. Patients with vWD can be classified as having type 1, type 2, type 3, or platelet-type vWD, according to the clinical history and laboratory test results. Approximately 65% to 80% of vWD patients have type 1 vWD. The mild form of this inherited disease is primarily autosomal dominant; the severe variant is autosomal recessive.

Clinical Features

Children with vWD present with mucocutaneous bleeding, including epistaxis, gum oozing, menorrhagia, easy bruising, and bleeding after surgery. Patients with type 3 (severe) vWD may develop joint and intramuscular bleeding.

Evaluation

Screening coagulation studies may demonstrate a prolonged PTT, although this may be normal in patients with mild vWD. Specific laboratory studies for vWD include vWF Activity (ristocetin cofactor), factor VIII–related antigen (vWF), and factor VIII:coagulant (factor VIII:C) evaluation. Patients with vWD may have decreased factor VIII:C activity, decreased vWF, decreased ristocetin cofactor, or a combination of the three findings.

Treatment

Multiple treatment options are available for patients with vWD, depending on the type of vWD and the reason for treatment. **Desmopressin acetate,** an analog of vasopressin, is often used to treat or prevent bleeding episodes in patients with **type 1 vWD,** although its use is controversial in patients with type 2B and platelet-type vWD. **Type 2B and type 3 patients** can receive **factor VIII concentrate** with retained vWF activity, and those with the rare **platelet-type vWD** may need **platelet transfusions,** depending on their past experience with blood products.

Hemophilia A and B (Factor VIII and Factor IX Deficiencies)

Etiology and Incidence

Factor VIII deficiency (hemophilia A) occurs in 1 of every 10,000 live male births, and factor IX deficiency (hemophilia B) occurs in 1 of every 40,000 live male births. Most patients have a **family history of bleeding disorders,** but spontaneous mutations are responsible for about 30% of cases of hemophilia.

Clinical Features

Children with factor VIII and factor IX deficiencies develop similar clinical features depending on the severity of the factor deficiency. In **infancy,** there can be **excessive bleeding after circumcision or bruising at injection sites.** Later in **childhood,** patients develop **easy bruisability, large hematomas,** and **hemarthroses or intramuscular hemorrhages** (the hallmarks of hemophilia). Patients with severe factor deficiencies can experience **bleeding episodes spontaneously** or **following trauma.** Patients with moderate or **mild factor deficiencies** rarely have spontaneous hemorrhages, but are at risk for **posttraumatic bleeding** and bleeding after **surgical procedures.** The **most common cause of morbidity is recurrent hemarthroses.**

Evaluation

Laboratory evaluation should include a **platelet count,** a **PT,** and a **PTT.** In patients with factor VIII or IX deficiency, the PTT is prolonged, but the PT is normal. Therefore, in patients with an isolated prolonged PTT, levels of factors VIII and IX should be measured. Severe factor VIII or IX deficiency is classified by factor activity levels of $<1\%$. Patients with moderate disease have levels of 1% to 5%, and those with mild disease have levels of 5% to 20%.

Treatment

The most **serious hemorrhages** in patients with hemophilia are **intracranial, retropharyngeal, retroperitoneal,** and those involving the **airway.** The goal of treatment in these circumstances is to achieve a factor activity level of 100% and to offer appropriate supportive therapy.

- **Intracranial hemorrhage.** In patients with severe factor deficiency, intracranial hemorrhage may be spontaneous; therefore, any patient with severe factor deficiency who has a change in mental status or other neurologic findings should be treated for an intracranial hemorrhage until radiologic studies prove negative. Intravenous access and factor replacement should occur before obtaining a head computed tomography (CT) scan. Factor VIII and IX deficiencies cause poor secondary clot formation, so that bleeding usually occurs hours after the initial trauma. Therefore, a negative head CT scan does not exclude a slowly developing intracranial hemorrhage. Many clinicians admit children following head trauma, particularly those who have severe factor deficiency, to inpatient wards for observation, with frequent neurologic examinations.
- **Intramuscular bleeding** can be massive, leading to shock. The muscles of the thigh and the iliopsoas muscle in particular can accommodate large volumes of blood. Patients with hemophilia should be admitted to the hospital for close monitoring and bed rest if bleeding occurs in these areas. Extensive intramuscular bleeding can compromise vascular blood flow and cause compartment syndromes. Tingling, numbness, or loss of pulses in an extremity requires immediate factor replacement to 100% and an orthopedic evaluation.
- **Joint bleeds (hemarthroses)** require treatment with factor products and immobilization to avoid chronic complications (e.g., decreased mobility, contractures). The goal of factor replacement for hemarthroses depends on the child's individual bleeding history, but in general, factor replacement should be aimed at obtaining an activity level of 30% to 50% for 1 to 2 days. If recurrent hemarthroses have developed in the affected joint (the so-called target joint), then higher factor activity levels should be obtained. Today, many patients receive factor on a regular or "prophylactic" schedule to prevent recurrent joint bleeds. This approach to hemophilia treatment requires the guidance of a hematologist or a hemophilia specialist.
- **Moderate hemorrhages** involving muscles, hematomas, or lacerations usually require treatment to reach a peak factor activity level of 30%. Oral mucosa bleeding may require factor correction and α-aminocaproic acid therapy. α-Aminocaproic acid therapy decreases mouth bleeding by inhibiting clot breakdown and is contraindicated in patients with hematuria or DIC.

- **Hematuria** can occur spontaneously in patients with severe hemophilia, or after trauma in patients with moderate-to-mild disease. Treatment is directed toward cessation of bleeding while avoiding obstruction, which could lead to an obstructive uropathy. Factor replacement, hydration, and bed rest are recommended.
- **Replacement therapy for dental or surgical procedures.** Patients with factors VIII and IX deficiencies must receive replacement therapy before dental, surgical, or other general procedures, including laceration repair, suture removal, or spinal tap. The patient's hematologist should be consulted before initiating any procedures.
- **Factor inhibitors.** Of patients with factor VIII deficiency, about 10% to 25% develop factor inhibitors (i.e., antibodies to factor VIII). Patients who do not improve clinically after receiving the appropriate dosage of factor and who have complied with supportive care measures (e.g., splinting, avoidance of weight bearing with hemarthroses) should be evaluated for the presence of a factor inhibitor. Patients with factor inhibitors require alternative treatment options.

Factor XI Deficiency

Factor XI deficiency is an autosomal disorder primarily affecting persons of **Ashkenazi descent.** This bleeding disorder is **mild,** including **epistaxis, menorrhagia,** and **postoperative bleeding.** The **PTT is prolonged** in these patients and the diagnosis is confirmed by a factor-specific assay.

Factor XII Deficiency

This deficiency is characterized by a **prolonged PTT** with a **normal PT and bleeding time.** Factor XII-deficient patients are **not at risk for increased bleeding.**

Infection-related Purpura

An **acute febrile illness** associated with a **petechial rash** may indicate a **benign, self-limited viral process,** or a **severe, life-threatening bacterial illness** (e.g., meningococcal infection). Therefore, ill-appearing **children with fever and petechiae should be considered septic until proven otherwise.**

Infections can cause purpura by a wide variety of mechanisms. Severe bacterial infections are often associated with DIC. Viral illness can be associated with thrombocytopenia from increased platelet destruction (e.g., ITP) or from decreased production. In addition to causing thrombocytopenia, bacterial, fungal, and viral illnesses can cause **platelet dysfunction** and **vascular abnormalities.**

Drug-Related Purpura

Drug-induced thrombocytopenia in the hospital setting is most often caused by **chemotherapeutic agents** that suppress bone marrow activity.

Heparin, quinidine, digoxin, penicillin, and seizure medications (e.g., valproic acid) can cause immune-mediated thrombocytopenia, which generally **reverses when the drug is discontinued**. Some drugs, such as H_2 blockers, are associated with **idiopathic thrombocytopenia**.

Drug-induced platelet dysfunction as a result of cyclooxygenase enzyme inhibition is seen with **aspirin-containing compounds** and to a lesser degree with **nonsteroidal anti-inflammatory drugs** such as ibuprofen. **Penicillins** and **cephalosporins** can also cause platelet dysfunction, particularly in children with systemic disease. Platelet function should **return to normal** 7 to 10 days after the offending drug is discontinued.

DIFFERENTIAL DIAGNOSIS DISCUSSION II: BLEEDING AND PURPURA IN NEONATES

Bleeding and purpura in the neonate presents a slightly different differential diagnosis than bleeding in the child.

> **HINT:** Patients whose mothers took aspirin, phenytoin, warfarin, or thiazide diuretics are at increased bleeding risk during the neonatal period.

Vitamin K Deficiency (Hemorrhagic Disease of the Newborn)

Etiology

In the past, vitamin K deficiency was **primarily a disease of breast-fed infants** because cow's milk contains four to ten times the amount of vitamin K found in human breast milk. As a result, vitamin K prophylaxis is recommended for all newborns at birth to prevent hemorrhagic disease in the high-risk breast-fed group.

Clinical Features and Evaluation

Presently, vitamin K deficiency is most common in breast-fed infants who did not receive vitamin K prophylaxis. Affected infants may present with **excessive bleeding at 2 to 5 days of age** and have prolongation of the PT and PTT.

> **HINT:** Ill neonates who are transferred from other institutions may not have received vitamin K before transport. Infants of mothers taking phenobarbital are at increased risk for hemorrhagic disease of the newborn.

Treatment

Treatment is the administration of **1 mg vitamin K₁ parenterally.** Fresh-frozen plasma can be given if there is significant bleeding.

Neonatal Alloimmune (Isoimmune) Thrombocytopenia

Etiology

Neonatal alloimmune (isoimmune) thrombocytopenia is characterized by **moderate-to-severe isolated thrombocytopenia.** This **antibody-mediated destruction of platelets** is analogous to hemolytic disease of the newborn and occurs when **maternal antibodies** that are directed against paternal antigens found on the patient's platelets cross the placenta, entering the patient's circulation. These antibodies cause increased platelet destruction in the neonate. The most common offending antigen is PLA-1. Thrombocytopenia will persist as long as the maternal antibodies are found in the patient's circulation, usually within **21 days.**

Clinical Features

The infant with neonatal alloimmune (isoimmune) thrombocytopenia is generally well appearing but may have **petechiae, ecchymoses,** and **mucosal membrane bleeding** within the **first 48 hours of life,** depending on the platelet count. Petechiae and ecchymoses can be found at **injection sites** as well as at pressure points, such as the **extensor surfaces of the knees** and on the **abdomen** where diapering causes pressure. **Intracranial hemorrhage** is reported in 10% to 15% of patients.

Evaluation

Thrombocytopenia **can be severe,** with a platelet count of <20,000/mm³. The mother's platelet count is normal. **Finding maternal antibodies to paternal platelets** strongly suggests this diagnosis. The diagnosis is confirmed by isolating alloantibodies in the mother's serum, but the results are often negative.

Treatment

In the absence of bleeding, many recommend keeping the platelet count >30,000/mm³ for the first few weeks of life. **If bleeding is severe or** signs of **intracranial hemorrhage** are present, **treatment is critical. Transfusing the infant with the mother's washed, irradiated platelets** increases the platelet count because the mother's platelets are missing the antigen against which the antibody is aimed. **Intravenous immune globulin** (IVIG) and corticosteroids can increase the infant's counts, and some clinicians prefer the pharmacological approach to therapy. In **emergent situations, PLA-1(–) platelets or single-donor platelets** can be used if maternal platelets are not available.

Neonatal Autoimmune Thrombocytopenia

Etiology

This type of thrombocytopenia is **secondary to an autoimmune disorder in the mother** (e.g., ITP, SLE, lymphoproliferative disorder, hyperthyroidism). Antibodies are found to maternal and patient platelets in patients with this condition.

Clinical Features and Evaluation

Infants are well appearing and may develop **petechiae within the first 2 days of life.** The diagnosis is made by the clinical presentation of the mother and infant. The infant should have a **low platelet count with a normal PT and PTT.**

Treatment

IVIG should be administered to **patients showing signs of bleeding.** Steroid therapy should be considered in **patients who do not respond to IVIG.** Life-threatening hemorrhage should be treated with **high-dose steroids** and **continuous platelet transfusion.**

Nonimmune Causes of Thrombocytopenia

Consumptive coagulopathies (e.g., DIC) and coagulopathies associated with **sepsis, asphyxia, respiratory distress, or necrotizing enterocolitis** are the most common nonimmune causes of thrombocytopenia in ill neonates. Thrombocytopenia **secondary to thrombus formation from renal vein thrombosis or catheter-related thrombi** is also a frequent occurrence. Thrombocytopenia after exchange transfusion or extracorporeal membrane oxygenation is a normal finding. Nonimmune causes of thrombocytopenia in the sick neonate also include **congenital viral infections** and **hyperbilirubinemia treated with phototherapy.** Kasabach-Merritt syndrome should be considered in neonates with thrombocytopenia and hemangioma.

> **HINT:** Patients of diabetic mothers are at increased risk of polycythemia and renal vein thrombosis.

> **HINT:** If congenital anomalies are present on physical examination of a neonate with purpura or abnormal bleeding, TAR, Wiskott-Aldrich syndrome, Fanconi anemia, Chédiak-Higashi syndrome, and trisomy 21 should be considered.

Treatment is directed toward treating the underlying problem, factor replacement with fresh-frozen plasma and cryoprecipitate, and platelet transfusions (if needed).

EVALUATION OF BLEEDING AND PURPURA

Patient History

When evaluating a child with abnormal bleeding, a careful history and physical examination can direct the approach to patient management (Table 18-2). Important questions to ask pertain to the following:

- **Onset of symptoms.** Acute onset of purpura is consistent with an acquired disorder. Recurrent purpura since infancy suggests an inherited abnormality. The physician should ask questions about bleeding or bruising episodes since birth, such as epistaxis, menses, or excessive bleeding after surgical procedures (e.g., circumcision, tonsillectomy, dental extractions). These questions should be made in reference to family members as well as the patient. A child who presents with repeated hemarthroses and a history of requiring a blood transfusion after an uncomplicated surgical procedure most likely has a congenital bleeding disorder, whereas normal hemostasis after major surgical procedures (e.g., a tonsillectomy) makes the diagnosis of an inherited disorder of hemostasis unlikely. An exception is patients with severe hemophilia—50% of those who are circumcised in the newborn period without factor replacement do not have excessive hemorrhage.

> **HINT:** Remember that children may not have been exposed to situations such as surgery that would reveal a disorder of hemostasis.

- **Location.** The location of the bleeding is important. Unilateral epistaxis in a child who frequently traumatizes his nasal mucosa is usually normal. However, prolonged bilateral epistaxis in a child covered with bruises and petechiae is abnormal.
- **Medication history.** Certain drugs, especially aspirin and ibuprofen, are associated with platelet dysfunction. Some drugs can exacerbate bleeding in a patient with an underlying bleeding disorder. Children with vWD may bruise more easily after taking cough preparations or antihistamines.

Physical Examination

The physical examination should include the **skin, mucous membranes, and fundi.** The type of lesions, pattern of lesions, and the location, size, and stage of resolution of the lesions should be documented.

TABLE 18-2 Clinical Evaluation of Pediatric Patients with Suspected Bleeding Disorders

Question	If the Answer is "Yes," Consider . . .
History	
When the child bleeds from an injury, does the bleeding stop and then resume?	Coagulation disorder
When the child bleeds from a superficial cut, is the bleeding profuse?	Platelet disorder
Does the patient have a history of fever?	Infection
Does the patient have a history of fever and neurologic manifestations?	Meningococcemia, TTP
Is there a history of a viral prodrome?	Hemolytic uremic syndrome, ITP
Has the patient had repeated episodes of bleeding gums, prolonged bleeding from cuts, or massive bleeding from surgical procedures? Has the patient developed large hematomas at vaccination sites? Did the patient experience prolonged bleeding as a result of circumcision?	Congenital disorder
Do other family members have problems with easy bruising or abnormal bleeding?	Congenital disorder
Is the patient currently taking aspirin, ibuprofen, antibiotics, antihistamines, steroids, or oral contraceptives?	Drug-related purpura
Has the patient received multiple blood or platelet transfusions in the past as well as recently?	Posttransfusion purpura and alloimmunization
Could the child have ingested rat poison?	Warfarin toxicity
Does the patient have a history of delayed wound healing, rebleeding episodes, or umbilical stump bleeding?	Factor XIII deficiency
If the patient is a neonate, is there a history of a difficult or traumatic delivery? Did the infant have a low Apgar score?	DIC
If the patient is a neonate, did the mother take phenytoin?	Vitamin K deficiency
Physical Examination	
Are predominant findings on examination large ecchymoses or hemarthroses?	Coagulation disorder, nonaccidental trauma
Are predominant findings on examination petechiae or ecchymoses?	Platelet disorder
Are purpura symmetric and predominantly located on the legs and buttocks?	Henoch-Schönlein purpura
Are ecchymotic lesions extensive and in various stages of resolution?	Physical abuse
Is there lymphadenopathy with hepatosplenomegaly?	Leukemia, lymphoma, infection

(Continued)

TABLE 18-2 Clinical Evaluation of Pediatric Patients with Suspected Bleeding Disorders (*continued*)

Question	If the Answer is "Yes," Consider . . .
Are there palpable purpura with a history of minimal trauma?	Platelet disorder, coagulation disorder
Is there umbilical stump bleeding?	Factor XIII deficiency
Is there jaundice and bruising?	Hepatic disease (factor deficiency)

DIC = disseminated intravascular coagulation; ITP = idiopathic (immune) thrombocytopenic purpura; TTP = thrombotic thrombocytopenic purpura.

Types of Lesions

- **Petechiae** are small (<3 mm in diameter), macular, nonblanching erythematous lesions. They are most common on the face and chest but may involve any skin area.
- **Ecchymotic lesions** are large and can be macular, tender, or raised. Recent injuries are usually purple, fading over time to yellowish brown. Palpable ecchymotic lesions (raised lesions with a central nodule) are rarely a normal finding in children but are found often in boys with hemophilia.
- **Purpura fulminans** (purplish black, well-demarcated, stellate lesions with central necrosis) are usually associated with DIC. They can be extensive and painful.

Findings Suggestive of a Bleeding Disorder

A child who meets any of the following criteria should be screened for a bleeding disorder:

- Excessive purpura involving many sites, particularly areas not normally traumatized (e.g., flexor surfaces of the arms or the axillary and inguinal regions)
- Many purpuric lesions of the same stage
- Palpable ecchymotic lesions
- Observed purpura or bleeding that exceeds what is expected for the child's activity level
- Purpura, excessive bleeding, or both in an ill-appearing child

Laboratory Evaluation

The diagnosis of a bleeding disorder in a child may not be straightforward. Children with abnormal laboratory values may not be at risk for excessive bleeding, whereas those with normal laboratory values may be. Children with **factor XII deficiency or lupus anticoagulants** are **not at risk for increased bleeding,** although their PTT values are prolonged. Conversely, children with **factor XIII deficiency or vasculitic disorders** have normal laboratory values but are at **increased risk for bleeding.**

A laboratory screening evaluation includes the following:

- **CBC with a platelet count.** Thrombocytopenia is a platelet count <150,000/mm^3. Thrombocytopenia determined by automated systems should be confirmed by peripheral blood smear examination.
- **PT and PTT.** Normal values for PT and PTT vary according to the patient's age and the testing system used in the coagulation laboratory. PT measures the activity of factors II, V, VII, and X. PTT measures factors V, VIII, IX, X, XI, and XII. The PT reflects the extrinsic and common pathways of coagulation, whereas the PTT evaluates the intrinsic and common pathways.

HINT: Blood for PT and PTT analysis must be obtained from a blood vessel large enough to provide free-flowing blood. Blood obtained for PT and PTT via "difficult sticks" may falsely decrease the laboratory values.

- **Peripheral blood smear.** Platelet, RBC, and white blood cell morphology can be helpful in narrowing the differential diagnosis. Large platelets are seen in ITP, Bernard-Soulier syndrome, and May-Hegglin anomaly. Small platelets are seen in Wiskott-Aldrich syndrome. Schistocytes accompanying a decreased platelet count suggest a microangiopathic process. WBC blasts on the peripheral blood smear suggest leukemia.
- **Bone marrow aspirate and biopsy.** A bone marrow aspirate and biopsy may be obtained to clarify the cause of the thrombocytopenia (i.e., increased platelet destruction or decreased platelet production). Increased megakaryocytes on a bone marrow aspirate and biopsy suggest increased peripheral destruction of platelets, whereas decreased megakaryocytes suggest decreased production.
- **Bleeding time.** Bleeding times reflect platelet number and function, and vWF activity. Bleeding times vary according to the experience of the laboratory technician and the cooperation of the patient. They are not reliable in children and not performed routinely. Platelet aggregation studies can be performed to assess platelet function, although these must be performed in a special coagulation laboratory.

TREATMENT OF BLEEDING AND PURPURA

Life-threatening bleeding in a patient without a known diagnosis must be treated before a specific diagnosis can be established. **Blood products** should be used to stabilize the patient, particularly if active bleeding cannot be controlled by pressure or other mechanical means. At least

TABLE 18-3 Treatment of Common Childhood Bleeding Disorders

Bleeding Disorder	Treatment	Potential Complications of Therapy
Idiopathic (immune) thrombocytopenic purpura (ITP)*	Intravenous immunoglobulin	Headaches, neutropenia, volume overload, aseptic meningitis, allergic reactions, virus transmission
	Steroids	Partial treatment of leukemia, psychosis, fluid imbalance, hypertension
	Anti-D immune globulin	Hemolysis, virus transmission, allergic reactions
	Continuous platelet transfusion (for life-threatening hemorrhage)	Virus transmission, transfusion reactions
Disseminated intravascular coagulation (DIC)	Fresh-frozen plasma	Virus transmission, allergic reactions
	Platelet and packed red blood cell (RBC) transfusion	Virus transmission, transfusion reactions
	Cryoprecipitate	Virus transmission
Henoch-Schönlein purpura	Steroids†	Fluid imbalance, psychosis, hypertension
Neonatal isoimmune thrombocytopenia	Transfusion of mother's washed, irradiated, or PLA-1 negative platelets, IVIG, or steroids	—
Platelet function abnormalities	Platelet transfusion (for life-threatening hemorrhage)	Virus transmission, transfusion reactions
von Willebrand disease (vWD)	Desmopressin acetate (DDAVP)	Thrombocytopenia in patients with type 2B or platelet-type vWD
Type 2B and platelet-type vWD	Platelet transfusion or cryoprecipitate administration	—

*The necessity of treating acute ITP is controversial.
†Considered for patients with gastrointestinal or joint symptoms.

5 mL of blood should be placed in a sodium citrate tube before blood-product transfusion for coagulation studies, a CBC, a PT, and a PTT.

If the **bleeding is not life threatening,** a **diagnosis should be established before treatment.** Once a diagnosis is made, treatment (using the most specific, safest, and cost-effective product) should be initiated in conjunction with a **hematologist** (Table 18-3).

APPROACH TO THE PATIENT (FIGURE 18-1)

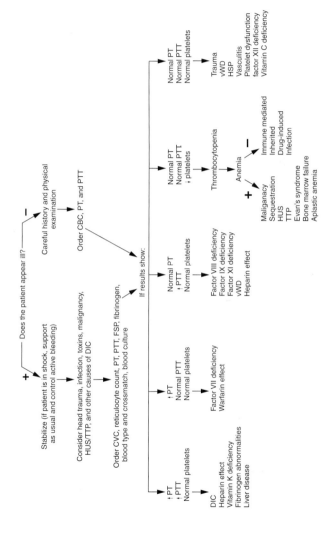

Figure 18-1 ■ Evaluation of a pediatric patient with bleeding or purpura

CBC = complete blood cell count; DC = disseminated intravascular coagulation; FSP = fibrin split products; HSP = Henoch-Schönlein purpura; HUS = hemolytic uremic syndrome; PT = prothrombin time; PTT = partial thromboplastin time; TTP = thrombotic thrombocytopenic purpura; vWD = von Willebrand disease; ↑ = increased; ↓ = decreased.

Suggested Readings

Blanchette VS, Carcao M: Childhood acute immune thrombocytopenic purpura—20 years later. *Semin Thromb Hemost* 29:605–617, 2003.

Geddis AE, Balduini CL: Diagnosis of immune thrombocytopenia purpura in children. *Curr Opin Hematol* 14:520–525, 2007.

Katsanis E, Luike KJ, Hsu Li M, et al.: Prevalence and significance of mild bleeding disorders in children with recurrent epistaxis. *J Pediatr* 113:73–76, 1988.

Khair K, Liesner R: Bruising and bleeding in infants and children—a practical approach. *Br J Haematol* 133:221–231, 2006.

Manno CS: Difficult pediatric diagnoses: bruising and bleeding. *Pediatr Clin North Am* 38:637, 1991.

Medeiros D, Buchanan GR: Idiopathic thrombocytopenic purpura: beyond consensus. *Curr Opin Pediatr* 12(1):4–9, 2000.

Pramanik AK: Bleeding disorders in neonates. *Pediatr Rev* 13:163, 1992.

Saulsbury FT: Henoch-Schönlein purpura. *Curr Opin Rheumatol* 13(1):35–40, 2001.

19 *Chest Pain*

Kan N. Hor and Bradley S. Marino
Bernard J. Clark III (Third Edition)

INTRODUCTION

Chest pain in children and adolescents is **common** and produces a **high level of anxiety** in both patients and families because of its perceived association with fatal heart disease in adults. Chest pain may lead to emergency department visits (accounting for 0.5% of all pediatric visits), school absences, and an unnecessary restriction of activities. Despite the degree of concern it generates, and with the exception of a few uncommon serious conditions, chest pain symptoms in children and adolescents are rarely associated with a cardiac etiology and are usually benign and self-limited. For these reasons, the workup of chest pain is directed toward **ruling out the rare serious causes.** A complete, detailed history and physical examination usually can determine the cause and identify patients who require further evaluation or acute intervention. Cardiac conditions are a rare but potentially serious cause of chest pain and should be considered, particularly when a child presents with chest pain **associated with syncope** or a **family history of syncope or sudden cardiac arrest.**

DIFFERENTIAL DIAGNOSIS LIST

Cardiac Causes

Anatomic Lesions
  Severe aortic stenosis
    (subvalvar, valvar,
    supravalvar)
  Severe pulmonary stenosis
  Aortic root dissection
  Coronary artery anomalies
  Mitral valve prolapse

Acquired Lesions
  Myocarditis
  Pericarditis
  Hypertrophic
    cardiomyopathy
  Coronary vasospasm
    (variant angina) and
    myocardial infarction
  Pulmonary hypertension
  Postpericardiotomy
    syndrome

Arrhythmia
  Sinus arrhythmia
  Supraventricular
    arrhythmia
    Premature atrial
    contractions (PACS)/
    Supraventricular
    tachycardia (SVT)
  Ventricular arrhythmia
  Premature ventricular
    contractions (PVCS)/
    Ventricular tachycardia
    (VT)

Noncardiac Causes
  Idiopathic
  Costochondritis
  Slipping rib
  Precordial catch syndrome
  Overuse pain

Trauma
Pleural effusion
Pneumonia with or
without pleurisy
Pulmonary embolism
Reactive airway disease
Pneumothorax

Upper or lower respiratory
infection resulting in
persistent cough
Gastroesophageal reflux
Hiatal hernia
Gastritis
Peptic ulcer disease

DIFFERENTIAL DIAGNOSIS DISCUSSION

The differential diagnosis for cardiac chest pain in children includes **inflammation** of the myocardium or pericardium, **arrhythmias**, and **structural abnormalities** such as aortic stenosis, subaortic stenosis, coronary artery anomalies, mitral valve prolapse, and rarely, coronary vasospasm and myocardial infarction. A physical examination, **electrocardiogram (ECG)**, and **chest radiograph (CXR)** can rule out many of these possibilities.

Myocarditis and Pericarditis

In patients referred to a pediatric cardiologist for evaluation of chest pain, the most common serious causes of cardiac chest pain are myocarditis and pericarditis.

- **Myocarditis usually follows a febrile viral illness.** Patients typically present with symptoms of **shortness of breath, nonspecific chest pain, anorexia,** or **malaise.** A physical examination may reveal the presence of an **S3 gallop rhythm.** The CXR typically reveals **cardiomegaly,** although early in the illness it may reveal normal heart size. The ECG may reveal **ST segment depression** and **T-wave abnormalities,** especially in the inferior or lateral leads (II, III, AVF, V6, V7). In these patients, the myocardium is inflamed, and ventricular dysfunction and congestive heart failure is common. Myocardial inflammation may also affect the conduction system, and patients with myocarditis may present with **arrhythmias.** These arrhythmias tend to improve when the inflammation resolves. In patients who develop a chronic cardiomyopathy, arrhythmias may persist.
- **Pericarditis** more frequently presents with **acute onset of sharp chest pain,** which is **lessened by leaning forward.** Pericarditis results from inflammation of the pericardium and may result from **infections, uremia, neoplasm, trauma,** or **autoimmune disorders.** In patients with a small pericardial fluid collection, the physical examination may reveal a **friction rub.** In patients with a large pericardial fluid collection around the heart, pericardial tamponade may be present, resulting in distended neck veins, diminished heart sounds, and pulses paradoxus. In the presence of a large pericardial effusion, the ECG may reveal

low-voltage QRS complexes. In patients with pericarditis the CXR usually demonstrates cardiomegaly.

- Myocarditis and pericarditis occur after a viral inflammatory process (e.g., coxsackievirus, adenovirus, echovirus, parvovirus). A viral polymerase chain reaction test on a sample of blood may help determine the specific cause. Because Lyme disease may cause myocarditis, **Lyme titers** should be obtained for a patient who presents with chest pain and a history of a tick bite in an endemic area. Other inflammatory causes of pericarditis include **autoimmune disorders,** such as lupus erythematosus.

Aortic and Subaortic Stenosis

A **history of chest pain** in a child who also has a **significant murmur** may suggest **left ventricular outflow tract obstruction** caused by **aortic stenosis** or subaortic stenosis. In these patients, chest pain may indicate ischemic pain. **Pain occurs during exercise** because the ability to increase cardiac output is limited by the left ventricular outflow obstruction. The limited cardiac output, coupled with a fall in systemic vascular resistance during exercise, results in **coronary hypoperfusion** and subsequent **myocardial ischemia.**

Physical findings in patients with aortic stenosis can include a **systolic ejection click**, a **harsh systolic ejection murmur** over the base of the heart that radiates to the carotid arteries, and frequently a **palpable thrill in the suprasternal notch.** These patients may have a normal ECG or an ECG that suggests left ventricular hypertrophy. A patient with a significant murmur and chest pain should be referred to a cardiologist for an echocardiogram.

Hypertrophic Cardiomyopathy

Another variation of **left ventricular outflow tract obstruction** is **hypertrophic cardiomyopathy.** Because hypertrophic cardiomyopathy may be an autosomal dominant disorder, a **thorough family history** is helpful. These patients have a **systolic murmur** that is **enhanced on standing or subjection to the Valsalva maneuver.** These maneuvers decrease left ventricular volume and thus increase the degree of outflow obstruction.

Coronary Artery Anomalies

Anomalous left coronary artery **is uncommon.** Most patients with anomalous left coronary artery from the pulmonary artery (ALCAPA) present as **infants in a shock-like state.** The pulmonary artery pressure falls as the pulmonary vascular resistance falls during the neonatal period, resulting in a decreased coronary perfusion pressure into the anomalous left coronary artery. This may result in coronary artery hypoperfusion and myocardial ischemia. In children and adolescents with ALCAPA, an anomalous insertion of the left coronary artery into the aorta may result in the coronary artery coursing between the great vessels or having an intramural course; this anatomy is associated with myocardial ischemia and sudden death. The key to diagnosis is a thorough history that reveals symptoms at peak exercise. The pathophysiology is related to inadequate coronary perfusion during exercise, by compression between the great vessels, relative ostial stenosis of the anomalous coronary artery, or coronary steal phenomenon from collateral coronary vessels connecting the right coronary and the anomalous left coronary artery attached to the pulmonary artery. When patients with an anomalous left coronary present, their ECG is often **abnormal** with evidence of **left ventricular hypertrophy** and **abnormal ST segments or inverted T waves** in the left precordial leads.

When a child or adolescent presents with chest pain, it is important to inquire about **previous Kawasaki disease.** Fifteen percent of patients with Kawasaki disease develop **coronary artery aneurysms** in the subacute phase of the illness about 3 to 6 weeks after diagnosis. Studies have reported up a to 2% mortality in patients with Kawasaki disease occurring in the first few months after diagnosis resulting from myocardial infarction or arrhythmia. More than half of all aneurysms resolve spontaneously. Healing of the coronary artery aneurysms following the inflammatory phase may result in areas of stenosis. Similar to any coronary obstruction, myocardial flow reserve and perfusion is decreased during exercise. Therefore, chest pain in children and adolescents with a previous history of Kawasaki disease and coronary artery changes should be considered ischemic until proven otherwise.

Arrhythmia

Patients who present with symptoms of **chest pain** or chest pain and **dizziness** with or without syncope may experience arrhythmias. Younger children may perceive palpitations as chest pain, and the additional symptoms of dizziness or syncope suggest an arrhythmia and require evaluation. All patients suspected of having arrhythmias should have an **ECG** during initial evaluation. In addition to obtaining a rhythm strip to assess for rhythm disturbances, all baseline intervals should be **assessed for heart block** and for **prolonged QTc syndrome.** This interval can be prolonged secondary to electrolyte imbalance (hypocalcemia), medications (class I antiarrhythmics such as quinidine and procainamide, antidepressants, antipsychotics), or because of the long QTc syndrome. Patients with prolonged QTc syndrome are **prone to ventricular arrhythmias** and should be referred to a **cardiologist** for further evaluation and therapy.

Sinus Arrhythmia

Arrhythmias can also present as **isolated chest pain.** In sinus arrhythmia, **normal in children,** the **heart rate slows during inspiration** because of increased venous filling of the heart and thus larger volume for cardiac output. Then the **heart rate increases during expiration** because of the reduced venous return. School-age children, who have increased body awareness, may perceive this arrhythmia as abnormal.

Supraventricular Arrhythmia

The **most frequent pathologic arrhythmia** in infancy and childhood has a supraventricular origin and may be perceived as chest pain in younger children. This includes **premature atrial contractions** and **supraventricular tachycardia (SVT)**. Patients who present to the emergency department with chest pain and tachycardia should first have a **12-lead ECG.** Supraventricular and ventricular arrhythmia can generally be distinguished on the basis of the QRS and P-wave morphology and the rate of tachycardia. SVT is usually a **narrow complex tachycardia** with rates of approximately **200 beats per minute,** depending on the age of the patient. For treatment strategies for SVT see Chapter 75, "Tachycardia."

Ventricular Arrhythmia

Patients with ventricular tachycardia (VT) can also present with **chest pain.** VT generally is noted as a wide QRS tachycardia with a rate of **120 to 240 beats per minute,** generally not as rapid as SVT for the same age range. When present, VT is a **medical emergency** because this rhythm can rapidly **deteriorate into ventricular fibrillation.** For treatment guidelines for VT see Chapter 75, "Tachycardia."

Mitral Valve Prolapse

Mitral valve prolapse (MVP) may also be associated with chest pain and is a common finding in adults. Its prevalence and clinical significance in pediatrics is controversial. In some studies, up to 15% of a normal population have MVP on echocardiography. In children, the incidence of MVP is approximately 6%. Although MVP is usually asymptomatic, a history of nonexertional chest pain, palpitation, and, rarely, syncope may be elicited. However, in the pediatric population, chest pain occurs equally in the normal population and in those with MVP.

The diagnosis of MVP is best made on **physical examination** and confirmed by **echocardiography.** Physical findings include a **mid-to-late systolic click** and possibly a **short systolic murmur** resulting from mild mitral regurgitation. The **click is accentuated** by **standing** or with the **Valsalva maneuver,** which both decrease ventricular filling and move the click from late to midsystole.

Patients suspected of MVP should be referred to a pediatric **cardiologist** for an **echocardiogram** to confirm the diagnosis. There is no longer a requirement for bacterial endocarditis prophylaxis in patients with MVP with mitral regurgitation. Because patients with MVP have a small but finite incidence of arrhythmias, patients with chest pain who are found to have MVP should be considered for **workup for an arrhythmia.**

Aortic Root Dissection

When evaluating chest pain in patients with known or suspected connective tissue disease, the physician must consider aortic root dissection or rupture. The chest pain is unrelenting and becomes quite severe radiating through the back. Patients with aortic dissection may present with significant cardiorespiratory distress with signs of diminished cardiac output. Careful physical examination may reveal stigmata of Marfan syndrome or other connective tissue diseases.

Postpericardiotomy Syndrome

Postpericardiotomy syndrome, a frequent complication of open-heart surgery, is characterized by fever, chest pain, and pericardial and pleural effusions. These signs may develop 1 to 12 weeks after intracardiac surgery in approximately 30% of patients. Although the etiology of the syndrome is unknown, evidence points to a viral and/or autoimmune cause. Postpericardiotomy syndrome is diagnosed after excluding other conditions such as endocarditis and pneumonia. In many cases, the syndrome is self-limiting and occurs only once, but in other cases the symptoms may be recurrent. On physical examination, patients often demonstrate tachycardia and a pericardial friction rub. The pericardial rub disappears either with improvement or with further accumulation of pericardial fluid. Systemic fluid retention and hepatomegaly can also occur. Anti-inflammatory agents, such as salicylates and steroids, represent the drugs most commonly used. Although analgesics with codeine or oxycodone are important for the patient's symptomatic relief, early recognition of the syndrome is the key to limiting the discomfort and possible complications associated with this condition.

EVALUATION OF CHEST PAIN

Patient History

In all patients with a chief complaint of chest pain, it is important to elicit a **thorough history** of events surrounding the onset of chest pain as well as any **aggravating and relieving factors.** Important **general questions** define the type, location, duration, sequence of onset of the pain and association with activity, and syncope. Does the pain awaken the child from sleep? Further questions should be directed to separating out the **specific organ system** most responsible for the symptoms. Pain that **worsens with respiration** or deep breathing may suggest bronchospastic, or pleuritic pain. Patients with an associated **history of cough and fever** are most likely to have pneumonic or bronchospastic chest pain. A **pleural catch** is a sharp sudden pain that limits respiration and can be relieved with a deep breath. **Musculoskeletal chest pain** can be produced with movement, should be well localized, and is reproducible by specific movement or palpation. **Costochondritis** produces pain on palpation of the costochondral joints. **Gastrointestinal pain** can be diffuse, is often pre- or postprandial, and may present as a deep or burning pain.

Physical Examination Findings

The physical examination in the child with chest pain should include complete **cardiac, respiratory,** and **upper body musculoskeletal examination.** **Vital signs** should include blood pressure recordings from the **right arm** and **at least one lower extremity.** The **heart rate and rhythm** should be assessed. Is it regular or irregular? Is the respiratory effort normal? With reference to the cardiac examination, findings of a **murmur,** an **irregular heart rate,** or **additional heart sounds** other than S1 and a split S2 would warrant **further investigation** and may prompt referral to a pediatric **cardiologist.** Respiratory examination should be directed toward the **symmetry of respiratory effort** and the presence of **abnormal sounds.** The musculoskeletal system should be assessed for **palpable abnormalities** or **pain on motion** or palpation.

Laboratory Studies

If one is evaluating a child with a chief complaint of **chest pain,** and a specific diagnosis is not strongly suspected or confirmed by history and physical examination, then a **PA and lateral CXR** and a **12-lead ECG** should be completed. If the history suggests an **arrhythmia,** then, in addition, a **Holter monitor or** a **transtelephonic event monitor** should be used depending on the frequency and duration of the arrhythmia.

APPROACH TO THE PATIENT

Chest pain is a common complaint in the pediatric age group, but the incidence of heart disease in this group is low. The diagnostic approach is to pursue associated signs or symptoms suggestive of cardiac disease (Figure 19-1). These include:

- A history suggestive of myocarditis, such as a recent viral illness, fever, and malaise
- Suspicion of arrhythmia
- Syncope with chest pain
- ECG abnormalities
- Cardiomegaly on CXR
- A significant cardiac murmur

If any of these findings are present with chest pain, further investigation and referral to a pediatric cardiologist are warranted. In patients with

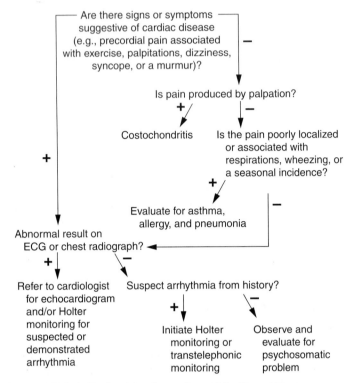

Are there signs or symptoms suggestive of cardiac disease (e.g., precordial pain associated with exercise, palpitations, dizziness, syncope, or a murmur)? **−**

Is pain produced by palpation? **+** / **−**

Costochondritis

Is the pain poorly localized or associated with respirations, wheezing, or a seasonal incidence? **+** / **−**

Evaluate for asthma, allergy, and pneumonia

+

Abnormal result on ECG or chest radiograph? **+** / **−**

Refer to cardiologist for echocardiogram and/or Holter monitoring for suspected or demonstrated arrhythmia

Suspect arrhythmia from history? **+** / **−**

Initiate Holter monitoring or transtelephonic monitoring

Observe and evaluate for psychosomatic problem

Figure 19-1 ■ Evaluation of a patient with chest pain
ECG = electrocardiogram.

respiratory-type chest pain, especially pain brought on by exercise or that limits exercise, referral to a pediatric **pulmonologist** may be useful to establish a diagnosis of **exercise-induced asthma.** In the asymptomatic child with a **normal ECG and CXR, close observation** without referral is appropriate.

Suggested Readings

Kocis KC: Chest pain in pediatrics. *Pediatr Clin North Am* 46(2):189–203, 1999.

Park MK: Special problems. In *The Pediatric Cardiology Handbook Third Edition*. Philadelphia, Mosby, 2003, 201–243.

Selbst SM: Consultation with the specialist: chest pain in children. *Pediatr Rev* 18:169–173, 1997.

Sivarajan VB, Vetter VL, Gleason MM: Pediatric evaluation of the cardiac patient. In *Pediatric Cardiology: The Requisites in Pediatrics*. Edited by Vetter VL. Philadelphia, Mosby Elsevier, 2006, 1–30.

INTRODUCTION

Physicians are responsible for **identifying cases of suspected abuse and reporting them** to the proper authorities for investigation. Diagnosing physical abuse can be challenging. The history provided is often misleading, and the injuries may not be pathognomonic. The presentation varies according to the injury sustained. Possible presentations include single or multiple injuries, unusual or unexplained bruising, a change in mental status, an acute life-threatening event (ALTE), respiratory distress, an inability to use an extremity, nonspecific complaints of gastrointestinal disease, and unexpected cardiorespiratory arrest.

DIFFERENTIAL DIAGNOSIS LIST

Child abuse injuries can result in various physical findings that are also observed in children with physical diseases.

Infectious Diseases

Meningitis
Sepsis
Osteomyelitis
Congenital syphilis
Dermatitis herpetiformis
Impetigo
Staphylococcal scalded skin syndrome
Erysipelas
Purpura fulminans
Disseminated intravascular coagulation (DIC)

Metabolic or Genetic Diseases

Osteogenesis imperfecta
Ehlers-Danlos syndrome
Scurvy
Rickets
Glutaric aciduria type I
Copper deficiency

Congenital or Vascular Diseases

Congenital indifference to pain
Unusual skeletal variants
Arteriovenous malformation (AVM)
Aneurysm
Vasculitis (e.g., Henoch-Schönlein purpura)

Hematologic Diseases

Idiopathic thrombocytopenic purpura (ITP)
Leukemia
Vitamin K deficiency
Hemophilia
von Willebrand disease

Dermatologic Disorders

Mongolian spots
Epidermolysis bullosa
Erythema multiforme
Contact dermatitis, including phytophotodermatitis

Cultural practices—*cao gio* (coining), cupping, moxibustion

Neoplastic Disorders
Brain tumor

Miscellaneous Disorders
Benign external hydrocephalus

COMMON PRESENTATIONS

Bruises

Differential Diagnosis

Abuse should be **suspected in a child** with a given **history of minor trauma** who has **extensive bruises or bruises on multiple body planes.** Bruises that are in **different stages of resolution, centrally located,** or **patterned** (e.g., loop marks, finger marks, belt marks) also suggest abuse. Bruises in **young infants** who are not yet cruising are highly suspicious.

Many conditions can mimic inflicted bruises:

- **Accidental bruises** are usually found over bony prominences and are distally located. They are few to moderate in number.
- **Mongolian spots,** most commonly found in infants with dark complexions, are often located over the buttocks and lower back (but may be found in other locations).
- **Hematologic disorders** (e.g., ITP, leukemia, vitamin K deficiency, coagulopathies, DIC). Children with coagulopathies can have bruising that varies from mild to severe. The distribution of bruises in children with a bleeding diathesis should not be isolated to unusual locations.
- **Dermatologic disorders** (e.g., erythema multiforme, contact dermatitis, including phytophotodermatitis from lime or lemon juice) can be associated with or resemble bruises.
- **Cultural practices** can also be associated with patterned bruises (e.g., coining). It is useful to be familiar with the cultural practices of subpopulations in the community.
- **Genetic diseases** (e.g., Ehlers-Danlos syndrome, osteogenesis imperfecta) are usually associated with other physical stigmata.
- **Henoch-Schönlein purpura** is associated with lesions that are typically located on the buttocks and legs; in addition, joint, abdominal, renal, or central nervous system (CNS) manifestations are usually present.

Evaluation

If child abuse is suspected, the **size, location, shape, and color of the bruises** should be **carefully documented.**

When a bleeding diathesis is suspected, a complete blood cell (CBC) count with platelet count, a prothrombin time (PT), a partial thromboplastin time (PTT), and a von Willebrand panel serve as initial screens. Additional testing will vary depending on the clinical scenario.

Treatment

Most bruises require **no specific treatment** and resolve over days to weeks, depending on their size. Severe beatings, especially over the buttocks or thighs, can result in **myoglobinuria and acute renal failure.** Myoglobinuria is treated with **hydration.**

Burns

Differential Diagnosis

Abusive burns are **most common in infants and toddlers.** Some burn patterns (e.g., immersion burns) are highly specific for inflicted injury. **Immersion burns** are associated with toilet accidents or other behaviors (e.g., vomiting) that require "cleaning" the child. The pattern of burn distribution often identifies the cause—the feet, lower legs, buttocks, and genitals are burned with clear lines of demarcation, but the knees, upper legs, and other parts of the body that were not submerged are spared.

Many conditions can mimic abusive burns:

- **Accidental burns** include burns from hot liquid spills, burns resulting from contact with a clothes iron or curling iron, car-seat buckle burns, chemical burns, and sunburns. Accidental burns are common pediatric injuries, and most pediatric burns are accidental. The history should be compatible with the distribution and severity of the burn.
- **Infection** (e.g., staphylococcal scalded skin syndrome, impetigo, erysipelas) may be associated with fever and an ill appearance. Impetigo can be misidentified as cigarette burns.
- **Cultural rituals** may be associated with burnlike lesions.

Evaluation

Record areas of **partial and full-thickness burns** on an **anatomic chart** and **calculate the percentage of body area burned** using age-appropriate estimates (see Chapter 76, "Thermal Injury"). Additional injuries should be sought. Children <2 years with suspicious burns should have a **skeletal survey** to assess for occult skeletal trauma.

Treatment

Detailed treatment recommendations are provided in Chapter 76, "Thermal Injury."

Fractures

Differential Diagnosis

Although most pediatric fractures are accidental, abuse should be suspected when **unexplained fractures** are identified. Virtually any bone can be injured in cases of child abuse, and no single type of fracture is diagnostic of abuse.

The following are the most commonly seen skeletal injuries:

- **Diaphyseal fractures** are the most common type of fracture in both abusive and accidental trauma cases. This type of fracture should cause more concern for abuse in nonambulatory infants.
- **Spiral fractures** are associated with twisting of the limb. These fractures are often accidental in ambulatory toddlers and children. They should cause more concern for abuse in young infants, especially if the humerus or femur is involved.
- **Metaphyseal fractures** are subtle injuries, most commonly identified by a skeletal survey. These fractures are sometimes associated with abusive head trauma. Although metaphyseal fractures are highly suspicious for abuse, the possibility of healing rickets or congenital syphilis should be considered. These fractures are difficult to date radiographically and usually heal without casting. They are sometimes not visible acutely and may be better identified by a follow-up skeletal survey 2 to 3 weeks after initial presentation.
- **Rib fractures** are common with abusive head trauma and are seen in infants and young children in association with abuse. Only rarely do they result from direct blows to the chest, minor accidental trauma, cardiopulmonary resuscitation, and metabolic bone diseases. Multiple, bilateral, posterior fractures are very specific for child abuse. Rib fractures are difficult to identify acutely, and oblique views of the chest may improve detection of subtle fractures.
- **Skull fractures** may be accidental. In cases of severe abuse, they may be associated with severe CNS injury. Complex, multiple, bilateral fractures are more common in abused children, although none are independently diagnostic of abuse.
- **Other fracture areas** include the clavicle, vertebrae, pelvis, and face (i.e., the mandible, maxilla, or zygoma).

In addition to accidental and inflicted trauma, other causes of fractures must be considered:

- **Birth trauma.** Fractures of the clavicle, humerus, or femur are occasionally seen with difficult or emergency deliveries, large infants, or breech presentations. By 2 weeks of age, birth fractures should show radiographic signs of healing. Rib fractures are rare, but well described in the literature, and they are usually seen in large newborns.
- **Physiologic periosteal changes.** Periosteal new bone formation of the long bones (which is seen with healing fractures) may also represent a physiologic process. Physiologic periosteal changes involve multiple bones, are symmetric, and are typically seen in the first 2 to 3 months of life. They should not be associated with fracture lines.

- **Osteogenesis imperfecta.** Most forms of osteogenesis imperfecta are identifiable on the basis of the patient history, the family history, and the physical examination. Type IV osteogenesis imperfecta is most apt to be confused with abuse. Blue sclerae, hearing impairment, dentinogenesis imperfecta, wormian bones, osteopenia, hypermobility of joints, easy bruising, short stature, a tendency toward bowing and angulation of healed fractures, and progressive scoliosis suggest osteogenesis imperfecta. Definitive diagnosis is made by biochemical analysis of cultured skin fibroblasts or DNA analysis.
- **Congenital syphilis.** The osteochondritis, epiphysitis, and periostitis of congenital syphilis can mimic the metaphyseal fractures and periosteal new bone formation associated with child abuse. Pseudoparalysis of affected limbs and swelling and tenderness of the ends of involved bones suggest the diagnosis of syphilis. In addition, other manifestations are often present. Syphilis can be diagnosed by serologic testing.
- **Rickets.** Vitamin D deficiency, renal and hepatic disease, certain medications (e.g., antacids, anticonvulsants, furosemide), and some rare diseases cause rickets, which predisposes bones to fractures. The diagnosis of rickets depends on clinical suspicion, laboratory data (i.e., calcium, phosphorus, alkaline phosphatase, and vitamin D levels) and radiographic evaluation.
- **Osteomyelitis** is usually diagnosed on the basis of the patient's history, physical examination, C-reactive protein, erythrocyte sedimentation rate, and results of blood or bone aspirate cultures.

Evaluation

The evaluation for suspected fractures usually involves obtaining **skeletal radiographs.** A **skeletal survey** is used to **detect occult or healing fractures** and is recommended for **all children <2 years** who have injuries suspicious for abuse. The skeletal survey is a less sensitive test in children 2 to 5 years of age and is not generally a useful study in children >5 years.

Treatment

Most fractures require **casting.** Some (e.g., **rib fractures, metaphyseal fractures**) usually **do not require specific treatment.**

Abdominal Trauma

Abusive abdominal injuries are uncommon, although they are **under-recognized and underreported.** Severe abdominal trauma is the **second leading cause of death as a result of abuse.** Injuries are usually caused by **blunt trauma** and most often affect the liver and small intestine.

Differential Diagnosis

The **history** is almost always **misleading.** Children who have suffered abdominal trauma as a result of abuse may present with **nonspecific complaints** related to the **gastrointestinal tract** (e.g., bilious vomiting, abdominal pain, anorexia), complaints associated with **peritonitis** (e.g., fever, abdominal pain, lethargy), or **unexplained cardiorespiratory arrest** (as a result of blood loss or sepsis). Approximately 50% of victims have no **external soft tissue evidence** of abdominal injury. Children with minor injuries can be **asymptomatic** yet have laboratory evidence of trauma. The following conditions must be ruled out:

■ **Accidental trauma.** Victims of accidental abdominal trauma tend to be older with injuries to a single solid organ. These accidental injuries occur more often outside the home.
■ **Infection.** Gastroenteritis, peritonitis from a perforated viscus, hepatitis, pancreatitis, and appendicitis must be ruled out.

Evaluation

A simple **hematologic workup** can be used to screen physically abused children for associated abdominal trauma and may reveal abdominal trauma in asymptomatic children. A CBC, liver function tests, amylase and lipase levels, and urinalysis are recommended. **Abdominal imaging** is recommended for children with significantly abnormal laboratory results.

Treatment

Solid organ injuries, unless severe, are **managed conservatively** and usually do not require surgery. **Hollow viscus tears and severe solid organ injuries** require **surgery.** The outcome is generally favorable if the child survives the acute injury.

Head Trauma and Shaking-Impact Syndrome

Head injury, either as a result of blunt trauma, shaking with sudden deceleration forces, or both, is the **leading cause of mortality and morbidity from child physical abuse.** Victims of inflicted head injury are most **often infants and toddlers.** Older children who die of CNS injury more often have signs of blunt impact to the head.

Differential Diagnosis

Children with head trauma as a result of abuse often present with a **change in mental status, respiratory distress, irritability, lethargy, seizures, ALTE,** or an **increasing head circumference.** Variable degrees of **cerebral edema** may be present initially. The following disorders could also account for these findings and need to be ruled out:

■ **Accidental trauma** (e.g., motor vehicle accidents, falls out of windows). Common childhood falls (e.g., falls down the stairs or from the couch or changing table) rarely result in life-threatening head injury.

- **Infection.** Sepsis and meningitis can be differentiated on the basis of the history, physical examination findings, and culture results. Bloody cerebrospinal fluid may be caused by lumbar puncture technique or a subarachnoid hemorrhage. In the latter case, the amount of blood in the fluid does not change significantly from the beginning to the end of the procedure.

- **Gastroesophageal reflux disease (GERD),** central or obstructive apnea, and **inborn errors of metabolism** can be associated with ALTE but are usually distinguished from abuse by a lack of associated traumatic findings. Some physicians advocate a retinal examination as a screen for head trauma in infants who present with ALTEs.

- **Intracranial vascular anomalies** (e.g., AVM, ruptured aneurysm) are usually identified by magnetic resonance imaging (MRI) scan but may not be evident immediately after they hemorrhage.

- **Glutaric aciduria type I,** a rare inborn error of amino acid metabolism, can present with acute encephalopathy and chronic subdural hematomas in infancy. Skeletal or other injuries should not be found. Retinal hemorrhages can be seen. Diagnosis is made by metabolic screening tests.

Evaluation

External physical injuries can be absent and do not rule out the diagnosis of abusive head trauma. **Subtle bruises** may be of significance and should be documented. A **computed tomography (CT) scan** of the brain shows **subdural hemorrhage.** MRI is recommended for all infants with suspected intracranial injuries from abuse. For infants with suspected abusive head trauma, a **complete ophthalmologic examination** and **skeletal survey** are essential.

Treatment

Treatment is aimed at **maintaining cerebral perfusion** and **limiting cerebral edema.** For severely injured children, intubation and intracranial-pressure monitoring may be indicated. Despite aggressive therapy, children with severe injuries often have **poor outcomes.**

Munchausen by Proxy Syndrome

In Munchausen by proxy syndrome, the **parent fabricates or causes a child's illness.** The child is repeatedly presented for medical care, and the parent denies knowing the cause of the "disease." Acute symptoms abate when the parent is separated from the child. Common complaints include apnea, ALTE, gastrointestinal bleeding, hematuria, seizures, recurrent fevers, or recurrent infections.

Diagnosing Munchausen by proxy syndrome requires **eliminating** with reasonable accuracy any **diseases** that may account for the reported symptoms. **Delays are almost universal** because the **perpetrator** (usually the mother) commonly **appears devoted and capable.** The perpetrator is usually alone with the child at the onset of symptoms. The **history** of the acute illness is **often much more severe than the findings** on physical examination.

EVALUATION OF CHILD ABUSE

Patient History

Although many victims of child physical abuse are preverbal, older abused children can often provide a history of abuse, and efforts should be made to **interview an older child alone.** Certain factors in the history given by the caregiver raise the suspicion of abuse:

- A history of trauma that does not correlate with the injuries sustained
- A history that specifically denies trauma to a child with obvious injuries
- A history of injury that does not correlate with the child's development (i.e., the child is developmentally incapable of injuring himself in the manner described)
- A history that changes as more injuries are discovered
- An unexpected or unexplained delay in seeking treatment

Physical Examination

Emphasis should be placed on **detecting subtle signs of injury, neglect, or alternative diagnoses.** Some injury constellations are pathognomonic of abuse. In these cases, the diagnosis can be made even in the absence of a history. The following areas should be covered in the physical examination:

- **Growth.** Plot all growth parameters, and compare with previous points if possible.
- **Skin.** Describe any bruises, burns, scars, or rashes in detail (i.e., size, location, pattern, color). The precise location of burns should be noted, including small splash marks, lines of demarcation, and identifiable patterns. Photographs are often used to document injuries but should not replace careful documentation because they may not accurately reflect the characteristics of the injuries.
- **Head.** Palpate for areas of swelling or bogginess, for stepoffs or depressions overlying fractures, and for cephalohematomas. Inspect the scalp for avulsed hair and bruises. Scalp bruising is often difficult to see because of the overlying hair.

- **Ears.** Look for bruises on the pinna. Battle sign (caused by a basilar skull fracture) may be noted. Examine the middle ear for blood behind the tympanic membrane.
- **Eyes.** Note edema, scleral hemorrhage, hyphema, and bruises. A funduscopic examination is essential for infants or young toddlers with suspected CNS injury.
- **Mouth and oropharynx.** Examine for evidence of trauma. Frenulum lacerations are pathognomonic of child abuse in young infants and are often associated with forced feeding. Examine the teeth for trauma and caries.
- **Chest.** Feel for evidence of healing rib fractures.
- **Heart and lungs.** Assess for tachycardia, which may be a sign of acute blood loss.
- **Abdomen.** Assess for signs of trauma, including bruising, abdominal tenderness, guarding, and rebound tenderness.
- **Back.** Look for bruises and unusual midline masses, which can represent vertebral injuries.
- **Genitalia, anus,** and **rectum.** Assess for signs of trauma (see Chapter 69, "Sexual Abuse").
- **Extremities.** Assess for soft tissue swelling, point tenderness, and function.
- **Neurologic examination,** including rating of the patient according to the Glasgow coma scale, is especially indicated for children with suspected head trauma.

Laboratory Studies

The following laboratory studies may be appropriate:

- **Hematologic evaluation.** A CBC with platelet count, PT, and PTT are indicated for children who present with bleeding or bruising. A von Willebrand panel is sometimes included in the screening process.
- **Toxicology screens** are indicated for infants or children with unexplained neurologic symptoms (e.g., seizures, lethargy, altered mental status, coma). Standard toxicologic screens vary.
- **Aspartate aminotransferase (AST), alanine aminotransferase (ALT), amylase, and/or lipase levels** may be elevated with acute liver or pancreatic injury and are recommended for acutely injured young children in whom the abdominal examination may not be a sensitive indicator of injury.
- **Urinalysis** is used as a screen for renal or bladder trauma, and it can also detect myoglobinuria and hemoglobinuria. Abused children occasionally develop myoglobinuria as a result of severe muscle injury. Urinalysis shows blood by dipstick but no red blood cells

microscopically. An elevated creatine phosphokinase level supports the diagnosis of myoglobinuria and muscle injury in these patients.

Diagnostic Imaging Studies

The following studies are commonly ordered for children with suspected abuse-related injuries:

- A **roentgenographic skeletal survey** is indicated for all infants and children <2 years who are suspected of being physically abused. Repeated surveys done 2 to 3 weeks after initial presentation often yield additional injuries.
- A **radionuclide bone scan** is sensitive for detecting rib fractures that are <7 to 10 days old, subtle diaphyseal fractures, and early periosteal elevation. This test is most often used when the skeletal survey is negative but the physician still suspects abuse.
- A **CT scan** is the method of choice for diagnosing acute intracranial, pulmonary, and solid abdominal organ injuries in a seriously injured child. Significant elevations of AST and ALT should be evaluated with an abdominal CT scan.

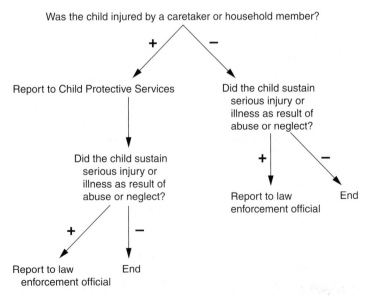

Figure 20-1 ■ Reporting child abuse to officials

TREATMENT OF CHILD ABUSE

Medical treatment is guided by the diagnosed injuries. Hospitalization is required for patients with serious injuries or illnesses from abuse. Occasionally, patients require **hospitalization if a safe environment cannot be guaranteed** at the time of initial diagnosis.

APPROACH TO THE PATIENT

All cases of *suspected* (not proven) **physical abuse** must be **reported to Child Protective Services** (if abuse is committed by a household member or caretaker), **law enforcement officials** (when the injuries are serious or involve a person outside the home), **or both** (**Figure 20-1**).

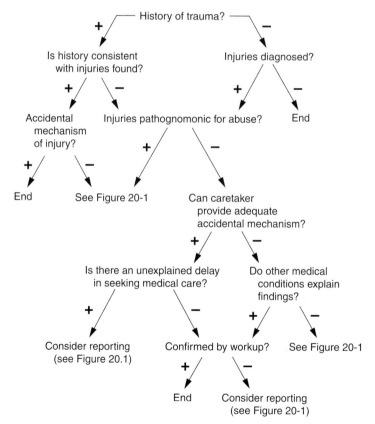

Figure 20-2 ■ Approach to initiating the civil and criminal investigation of suspected abuse

The criteria for reporting suspected child physical abuse depends on the history, examination, and laboratory findings. In some cases, the **injuries alone** are so suggestive of abuse that historical and laboratory data are not needed to reach the threshold for reporting. In other cases, the decision to report is reached only after **considering all factors.** Each state has laws that define child physical abuse, and physicians should be **aware of the laws that apply** in their state of practice.

Figure 20-2 provides a basic approach to initiating the civil and criminal investigation of suspected abuse. Individual state and institutional policies vary and may differ from this general approach. Each case must be weighed individually, with the **safety and well-being of the child** always central to the decision to report.

Suggested Readings

American Academy of Pediatrics Committee on Child Abuse and Neglect: Addendum: distinguishing sudden infant death syndrome from child abuse fatalities. *Pediatrics* 108(3):812, 2001.

American Academy of Pediatrics Committee on Child Abuse and Neglect: Shaken baby syndrome: rotational cranial injuries—technical report. *Pediatrics* 108(1):206–210, 2001.

American Academy of Pediatrics Section on Radiology: Diagnostic imaging of child abuse. *Pediatrics* 105:1345–1348, 2000.

Block RW: Child abuse—controversies and imposters. *Curr Probl Pediatr* 29:249–272, 1999.

Cooper A, Floyd TF, Barlow B, et al.: Major blunt abdominal trauma due to child abuse. *J Trauma* 28:1483–1486, 1988.

Duhaime AC, Christian CW, Rorke LB, et al.: Nonaccidental head injury in infants: the "shaken baby syndrome." *New Engl J Med* 338:1822–1829, 1998.

Jenny C, Hymel K, Ritzen A, et al.: Analysis of missed cases of abusive head trauma. *JAMA* 281:621–626, 1999.

Kellog ND: Committee on child abuse and neglect: evaluation of suspected child physical abuse. *Pediatrics* 119:1232–1241, 2007.

Nimkin K, Kleinman PK: Imaging of child abuse. *Radiol Clin North Am* 39(4):843–864, 2001.

Purdue GF, Hunt JL, Prescott PR: Child abuse by burning—an index of suspicion. *J Trauma* 28:221–224, 1988.

Reece R, Christian CW (eds): *Child Abuse Medical Diagnosis and Management,* 3rd ed. Elk Grove Village, Il, American Academy of Pediatrics, 2008.

21 | *Coma*
Nicholas S. Abend

INTRODUCTION

Consciousness is a state of arousal (wakefulness) with awareness of self and surroundings. Arousal is mediated by the **brainstem** and **subcortical** structures, including the ascending reticular activating system, hypothalamus, and thalamus, as well as the cerebral cortex. Awareness is mediated primarily by the cerebral cortex but also requires subcortical connections. Coma is a state of altered consciousness with loss of both wakefulness and awareness: It is characterized by sustained, pathologic, eyes-closed unarousable unresponsiveness. Between normal consciousness and coma is a spectrum of states of diminished consciousness, subdivided by convention into **lethargy, obtundation,** and **stupor** (Table 21-1). Coma should also be distinguished from delirium, akinetic mutism, locked-in syndrome, minimally conscious state, persistent vegetative state, and brain death (Table 21-2). Coma is a temporary state—there is either return of consciousness, progression to the minimally conscious state or vegetative state, or progression to brain death. Coma is a clinical diagnosis, made by history and physical examination. Diagnostic testing may elucidate an etiology, direct treatment, and clarify prognosis.

> **HINT:** Coma is not a specific disease but a sign of profound nervous system dysfunction. Depression of consciousness requires either dysfunction of both cerebral hemispheres or dysfunction of the reticular activating system of the brainstem.

DIFFERENTIAL DIAGNOSIS LIST

Trauma
Parenchymal Injury
Intracranial Hemorrhage
    Epidural hematoma
    Subdural hematoma
    Subarachnoid hemorrhage
    Intracerebral hematoma
Diffuse axonal injury

Nontraumatic Causes
Toxic/Metabolic
Hypoxic Ischemic
    Encephalopathy

Shock
Cardiopulmonary arrest
Near drowning
Carbon monoxide
    poisoning
Toxins
    Medications (narcotics,
    sedatives, antiepileptics,
    antidepressants, analgesics,
    aspirin)
    Environmental toxins
    (organophosphates, heavy

TABLE 21-1 States of Altered Consciousness	
Lethargy	Reduced wakefulness, deficits in attention
Obtundation	Blunted alertness, diminished interaction with environment
Stupor	Unresponsiveness with little/no spontaneous movement resembling deep sleep; temporary arousal with vigorous stimulation
Coma	Unarousable unresponsiveness

metals, cyanide, mushroom poisoning)
Illicit substances (alcohol, heroine, amphetamines, cocaine)
Systemic Metabolic Disorders
  Substrate deficiencies
    Hypoglycemia
    Cofactors (thiamine, niacin, pyridoxine)
  Electrolyte and acid-base imbalance (sodium, magnesium, calcium)
  Diabetic ketoacidosis
  Thyroid/Adrenal/Other Endocrine Disorders
  Uremic coma
  Hepatic coma
  Reye syndrome
  Inborn Errors of Metabolism
  Urea cycle disorders
  Amino acidopathies
  Organic acidopathies
  Mitochondrial disorders
Infections/Postinfectious/ Inflammatory
  Meningitis and encephalitis (Bacterial, viral, rickettsial, fungal)

Acute demyelinating diseases
  Acute disseminated encephalomyelitis (ADEM)
  Multiple sclerosis
Inflammatory/Autoimmune
  Sarcoidosis
  Sjögren's disease
  Lupus Cerebritis
Mass Lesions
  Neoplasms
  Abscess, granuloma
  Hydrocephalus
Paroxysmal Neurologic Disorders
  Seizures/status epilepticus
  Acute confusional migraine
Vascular
  Intracranial hemorrhage
  Infarcts
  Arterial infarcts
  Venous sinus thromboses
  Vasculitis
Intussusception

EVALUATION OF COMA

History and physical examination are necessary for determining the cause of coma and to mobilize effective therapy. Initial efforts must identify **reversible** causes of coma and normalize vital functions to **prevent secondary brain injury**. Table 21-3 lists an initial approach. Recent guidelines are also published online (see reference list).

TABLE 21-2 **Coma and Other Disease States of Altered Consciousness**

Coma	Arousal and awareness are absent. Sleep/wake cycles are absent. Movements are reflexive and are not purposeful or reproducible. The EEG generally demonstrates diffuse slowing. It is a temporary state that evolves into other states.
Vegetative state	Arousal is present but awareness is absent. Sleep/wake cycles are present. Brainstem and hypothalamic function is sufficiently intact to allow prolonged survival with care. Movements are reflex and are not purposeful or reproducible. The EEG generally demonstrates diffuse slowing. It is considered permanent if it lasts >12 months after traumatic brain injury or 3 months after nontraumatic brain injury.
Minimally conscious state	Arousal is present and there is partial awareness consisting of minimal but definite behavioral evidence of self or environmental awareness such as following simple commands, making verbalizations, making simple nonreflexive gestures, or reacting appropriately to emotional content of stimuli. A sleep/wake cycle is present. The EEG may contain mild slowing or may be normal. Distinguishing from a vegetative state often requires evaluation by a multidisciplinary team trained using a dedicated responsiveness program.
Akinetic mutism	Arousal and awareness are both present, but there is extreme slowing or absence of bodily movement loss and slowed cognition. Sleep/wake cycles are present. The EEG demonstrates diffuse slowing. Caused by damage to bilateral inferior frontal lobes, extensive bihemispheric disease, lesions of the paramedian mesencephalic reticular formation, or posterior diencephalon.
Locked-in syndrome	A state of preserved arousal and awareness, intact sleep/wake cycles, and normal EEG activity with complete paralysis of the voluntary motor systems caused by damage to corticospinal and corticobulbar pathways sparing the midbrain (in which case vertical eye movements may be preserved), or caused by severe neuromuscular disease.
Brain death	Permanent absence of all brain activity, including brainstem function.
Delirium	An acute confusional state characterized by impaired attention, fluctuating level of consciousness, disorganization, perceptual disturbances, and increased or decreased psychomotor activity. It is often associated with acute metabolic, toxic, or endocrine disturbances but may also occur with focal lesions (especially frontal) and seizures.

EEG = electroencephalogram.

History

History taking should include a detailed description of events leading to the onset of coma, with particular attention to **timing, exposures,** and **accompanying symptoms. Rapidly developing somnolence** suggests a metabolic or toxic cause. **Sudden onset of coma without trauma** suggests spontaneous intracranial hemorrhage or seizure. **Slowly progressive loss of**

TABLE 21-3 Initial Evaluation of Coma

- Conduct airway, breathing, and circulation assessment and stabilize.
  - Ensure adequate ventilation and oxygenation.
  - Manage blood pressure depending on underlying coma etiology. If hypertensive encephalopathy or intracranial hemorrhage, then lower blood pressure. If perfusion-dependent state such as some strokes or elevated intracranial pressure, reducing blood pressure may reduce cerebral perfusion.
  - Identify and treat hypoglycemia (thiamine may be given first in adult patients).
- Draw blood for electrolytes, ammonia, arterial blood gas, liver and renal function tests, complete blood count, lactate, pyruvate, and toxicology screen.
- Assess neurologically.
  - Conduct Glasgow Coma Scale.
  - Assess for evidence of raised intracranial pressure and herniation.
  - Assess for abnormalities suggesting focal neurologic disease.
  - Assess for history or signs of seizures.
- If there is concern for infection and lumbar puncture (LP) must be delayed, provide broad-spectrum infection coverage (including bacterial, viral, and possibly fungal).
- Give specific antidotes if toxic exposures are known.
  - For opiate overdose, administer naloxone.
  - For benzodiazepine overdose, consider administering flumazenil.
  - For anticholinergic overdose, consider administering physostigmine.
- Identify and treat critical elevations in intracranial pressure.
  - Neutral head position, elevated head by 20°, sedation.
  - Hyperosmolar therapy with mannitol, 0.5 to 1 g/kg, or hypertonic saline.
  - Hyperventilation as temporary measure.
  - Consider intracranial monitoring.
  - Consider neurosurgical intervention.
- Order head computed tomography (noncontrast).
- Treat seizures with intravenous anticonvulsants. Consider prophylactic anticonvulsants.
- Investigate source of fever and use antipyretics and/or cooling devices to reduce cerebral metabolic demands.
- Conduct detailed history and examination.
- Consider LP, electroencephalogram (EEG) or extended long-term EEG monitoring, magnetic resonance imaging, metabolic testing (amino acids, organic acids, acylcarnitine profile), autoimmune testing (antinuclear antibody panel, antithyroid antibodies), thyroid testing (TSH, T3, T4).

consciousness suggests hydrocephalus, expanding mass lesion, or indolent infection. **Preceding headache** with positional changes or with Valsalva maneuver suggests increased intracranial pressure from hydrocephalus or mass lesion. **Headache with neck pain** or stiffness suggests meningeal irritation from inflammation, infection, or hemorrhage. **Fever** suggests infection, but its absence does not rule it out, particularly in infants <3 months or in immunocompromised children. **Recent fevers or illness** suggests an autoimmune process like ADEM. **Abnormal movements** or a fluctuating mental status may suggest nonconvulsive seizures or a postictal state. Questions about possible toxic ingestions should include a survey of **medications and poisons in the home** and environment, even if not readily accessible to the child. **Travel history** may explain exposure to infections prevalent in certain areas, such as Lyme in the northeastern United States; insect bite history is also helpful but may be misleading. Recent **exposure**

to kittens in a comatose child with axillary or inguinal lymphadenopathy may be a clue to infection with *Bartonella henselae* (cat-scratch
encephalopathy). Discordance between the history of trivial trauma and
findings of extensive injury or delay in seeking treatment should raise suspicion of **child abuse.** A history of recurrent abdominal pain may suggest
intussusception.

Eliciting a **history of trauma,** whether accidental or nonaccidental, is
crucial. Understanding the mechanism of injury can direct further investigation. Delay of hours between trauma and loss of consciousness can
be seen with epidural hematoma. Fractures of the base of the skull may
compromise blood flow or result in dissection of the carotid artery (as it
enters the skull or travels in the petrous canal) resulting in malignant
middle cerebral artery syndromes. Clear fluid leakage from the nose or
ears may suggest skull fractures with an associated cerebrospinal fluid
(CSF) leak.

The child's **past medical history** may provide valuable information.
Prior episodes of unexplained coma suggest intermittent metabolic disease, recurrent toxic ingestions, or **Munchhausen by proxy.** Developmental
delay and preexisting neurologic abnormalities may suggest inborn
errors of metabolism, but they are also independent risk factors for
epilepsy, thus raising suspicion of a prolonged postictal state. Recent
weight changes or other constitutional abnormalities suggest endocrine
dysfunction or an oncologic process. In a child with known cardiac disease, circulatory collapse and hypoxic ischemic encephalopathy from
dysrhythmia should be considered.

Examination

The **Glasgow Coma Scale** (GCS), a reproducible way to rate any patient
with altered consciousness using three areas of response to stimuli, eye
opening, verbal response, and motor response, has been adapted for use
in children (Table 21-4). Intubation and mechanical ventilation often are
indicated in a child with deteriorating mental status whose GCS is ≤8.

> **HINT:** Initial evaluation must focus on the usual ABCs (airway, breathing,
> circulation) of resuscitation because abnormalities may result in
> secondary brain injury.

General examination should be directed toward uncovering clues to
the etiology of coma and to the sequelae of nervous system dysfunction,
starting with vital sign abnormalities. Hypotension, whether from sepsis, cardiac dysfunction (which may be primary or secondary to severe
neurologic injury), or toxic ingestion, may lead to poor cerebral perfusion, resulting in diffuse hypoxic ischemic injury. Hypertension is seen
with increased intracranial pressure as a physiologic response to maintain

TABLE 21-4 Glasgow Coma Scale and Modification for Children

Sign	Glasgow Coma Scale	Modification for Children	Score
Eye opening	Spontaneous	Spontaneous	4
	To command	To sound	3
	To pain	To pain	2
	None	None	1
Verbal response	Oriented	Age-appropriate verbalization, orients to sound, fixes and follows, social smile	5
	Confused	Cries but consolable	4
	Disoriented—inappropriate words	Irritable, uncooperative, aware of environment—irritable, persistent cries, inconsistently consolable	3
	Incomprehensible sounds	Inconsolable crying, unaware of environment or parents, restless, agitated	2
	None	None	1
Motor response	Obeys commands	Obeys commands, spontaneous movement	6
	Localizes pain	Localizes pain	5
	Withdraws	Withdraws	4
	Abnormal flexion to pain	Abnormal flexion to pain	3
	Abnormal extension	Abnormal extension	2

cerebral perfusion pressure. Hypertension with bradycardia and a change in respirations (Cushing triad) is an ominous sign of impending brain herniation (see later). Hypertension in the setting of coma may also be the product of a nonspecific sympathetic response or ingestion of stimulants such as amphetamines. Severe hypertensive encephalopathy can cause seizures with prolonged postictal state or progress to coma. Differentiating reactive or compensatory hypertension from a primary hypertensive encephalopathy may be difficult but is essential in determining how to manage blood pressure.

Abnormalities in respiratory rate and pattern may indicate primary pulmonary pathology, acid-base derangement, or nervous system dysfunction. **Respiratory patterns** may be of some localizing value in patients with primary central nervous system abnormalities, as illustrated **Table 21-5.**

Fever may be an important diagnostic clue for infectious or inflammatory disorders. **Hyperthermia** should be treated aggressively with antipyretic medications or cooling devices to reduce cerebral metabolic demands because outcome in many types of brain injury is worse with hyperthermia. Patients who have coma caused by hypoxic ischemic

TABLE 21-5 Respiratory Patterns in Central Nervous System Disease

Name	Pattern	Description	Localization
Cheyne-Stokes		Alternating hyperpnea and apnea	Extensive bihemispheric dysfunction or diencephalic dysfunction
Central Neurogenic Hyperventilation		Rapid and deep hyperpnea	Midbrain
Apneustic		Prolonged pause at end of inspiration	Lower Pons
Ataxic		Irregular in rate and tidal volume	Medulla

encephalopathy may benefit from hypothermia to further decrease metabolic demand.

A focused general examination should follow vital sign evaluation. Resistance to either flexion of the neck (**Brudzinski sign**) or extension of the knee with the hip flexed (**Kernig sign**) may indicate meningeal inflammation/irritation. Skin examination provides information about trauma (bruises, lacerations), systemic disease, and infection (e.g., superficial lacerations and lymphadenopathy in cat-scratch fever, erythema migrans in Lyme disease, petechiae and purpura in meningococcemia). Organomegaly raises suspicion of metabolic, hematologic, or hepatic disease.

A **detailed neurologic exam** is directed toward localizing brain dysfunction, identifying coma etiology, and determining early indicators of prognosis. In a comatose child, the neurologic examination centers around response to stimuli, brainstem function, and motor function.

> **HINT:** Frequent, standardized, detailed neurologic examinations are critically important in detecting expanding lesions or increasing intracranial pressure, which require immediate treatment.

A comatose child may be flaccid or may display **decorticate** (flexion of the arms and extension of the legs—usually caused by bihemispheric dysfunction with intact brainstem function) or decerebrate posturing (extension and internal rotation of all limbs—usually caused by global metabolic derangements or brainstem pathology. Asymmetries in posture or movement are clues to focal structural cerebral abnormalities.

Cranial nerve examination is important in assessing the brainstem. Pupils are examined first by observing the size of both pupils in dim light and then by assessing reactivity to a bright light shined in each eye. Asymmetric pupil size (**anisocoria**) is caused by unilateral dysfunction of the oculomotor nerve (cranial nerve III) that innervates the pupillary constrictors, or of the sympathetic fibers, originating in the midbrain, which innervate the pupillary dilators. Oculomotor nerve palsy, sometimes caused by **uncal herniation,** causes pupil dilation, ptosis, and ophthalmoparesis in the affected eye. Impairment of sympathetic fibers (**Horner syndrome**) leads to pupil constriction and a small degree of ptosis in the affected eye. In traumatic coma, Horner's syndrome may be an important clue to dissection of the carotid artery. Fixed eye version may suggest an ongoing seizure. Funduscopic examination may reveal **papilledema** associated with increased intracranial pressure (although early in the process papilledema may be absent), **retinal hemorrhages** in shaken baby syndrome, or flame-shaped hemorrhages and **cotton-wool spots** in hypertensive encephalopathy. Abnormalities of eye position and motility may be signs of cortical, midbrain, or pontine

TABLE 21-6 Pupil and Eye Movement Abnormalities in Coma

Etiology/Localization	Pupil Appearance	Eye Movement
Cerebral hemisphere		Fixed conjugate eye deviation (toward side of injury or away from side of ongoing seizure).
Metabolic	Small and reactive	
Hypothalamic	Small and reactive	
Tectal	Large, nonreactive, hippus	
Pontine	Pinpoint	Horizontal gaze palsies.
Midbrain	Midposition and fixed	Vertical and horizontal gaze palsies. Dorsal compression may result in upgaze paresis (so have tonic down gaze), papillary light-near dissociation, lid retraction, and nystagmus.
CN (cranial nerve) III palsy (uncal herniation)	Ipsilateral pupil dilated and fixed	Depression and abduction of eye (down and out).
CN IV palsy (often in traumatic brain injury)		Hypertropic eye.
CN VI palsy (injury or caused by elevated intracranial pressure)		Failure of adduction.
Severe hypoxic ischemic encephalopathy	Bilateral dilated and fixed	
Opiate intoxication	Pinpoint	

dysfunction. Table 21-6 summarizes pupil and ocular movement abnormalities seen in coma.

Oculocephalic reflexes are tested by holding the patient's eyelids open and quickly moving the head to one side. In a comatose patient with an intact brainstem, the eyes move in the direction opposite the head motion (that is, if the head is moved to the right, the eyes move conjugately to the left). After several seconds, the eye may return to a neutral position. Oculocephalic reflexes should not be tested if the patient has sustained cervical spine trauma. The oculovestibular reflex (cold calorics) is also a test of brainstem function. For testing to be accurate, the patient must have an open external auditory canal. With the head of bed at 30°, 120 mL of ice water is introduced into the canal with a small catheter. A conscious patient would experience nystagmus with slow deviation toward to the irrigated ear and fast correction away from the ear (the mnemonic COWS, Cold Opposite, Warm Same, applies to the fast phase). In a comatose patient, the eyes deviate slowly toward the irrigated ear and remain fixed in that position. No movement is seen if the brainstem vestibular nuclei or their connection to eye movement pathways are

TABLE 21-7 Brainstem Reflexes

Reflex	Technique to Examine	Normal Response	Anatomy
Pupils	Response to light	Pupillary constriction	Midbrain Afferent: CN (cranial nerve) II, chiasm Efferent: CN III and sympathetic fibers
Oculocephalic	Turn head side to side	Eyes move conjugately in direction opposite head	Pons Afferent: CN VIII Efferent: CN III and CN VI
Vestibulo-Oculo-Cephalic	Cold caloric	Conjugate deviation toward stimulation with fast nystagmoid movements away	Pons Afferent: CN VIII Efferent: CN III and CN VI
Corneal	Stimulation	Blink	Pons Afferent: CN V Efferent: CN VII
Cough	Stimulation	Cough	Medulla Afferent and Efferent: CN IX and X
Gag	Stimulation	Gag	Medulla Afferent and Efferent: CN IX and X

impaired. Five minutes should be allowed before the second ear is tested to allow rewarming of the first ear. Table 21-7 summarizes other brainstem reflexes.

Further Investigation

All children should have an initial **Dextrostix** upon arrival; laboratory glucose for confirmation should be sent even if normal because hypoglycemia alone may cause coma, and hypoglycemia in association with other etiologies may worsen outcome. Hypoglycemia must be treated urgently with intravenous dextrose infusion. Hyperglycemia may occur in diabetic ketoacidosis and requires specific management. Further laboratory testing should be guided by the suspected etiology. Arterial **blood gases** and **electrolytes** should be considered because abnormalities may cause coma or may occur secondary to intracranial abnormalities. **Liver function tests** should be considered because hepatic encephalopathy may cause coma, and hepatic injury can occur in the setting of systemic hypoxic ischemic injury. A **complete blood count with differential** is indicated to detect infection, anemia, disseminated intravascular coagulopathy, lead encephalopathy, or sickle cell disease. **Blood and urine cultures** should be obtained when an infectious etiology is suspected. **Toxin screens** should be considered in all children and include acetaminophen, salicylate, and ethanol levels. Specific tests for medications found in the home should be carried out as necessary. Ammonia, lactate, and pyruvate levels may be performed to screen for **metabolic disorders.** If abnormal or the history is suggestive of metabolic disease, measurement of organic acids, amino acids, and acylcarnitine profile may be indicated.

Once resuscitation is performed, a **head computed tomography (CT)** (without contrast) should be performed in all children with unknown etiology to look for intracranial bleeds, space-occupying lesions (i.e., tumor or abscess), edema, or focal hypodensities (i.e., acute disseminated encephalomyelitis, herpes simplex encephalitis, infarction, or hydrocephalus).

Lumbar puncture should be performed if the patient is febrile, infection is suspected, or no other etiology can be determined. It should be deferred and treatment initiated for possible infection (bacterial and viral and sometimes fungal) if there is clinical or radiologic evidence for intracranial hypertension. A normal CT does not rule out elevated intracranial pressure, so opening pressure should always be measured. CSF should be tested for cell count (in the case of a traumatic tap, preferably both the first and last tubes to help differentiate true findings), glucose, protein, Gram stain, bacterial culture, viral polymerase chain reaction, additional fungal or tuberculosis cultures when suspected clinically, and lactate (which may be elevated in metabolic/mitochondrial diseases).

An **electroencephalogram** (EEG) can be a helpful adjunctive study. It can detect significant background changes (e.g., triphasic waves suggestive of metabolic encephalopathy or focal slowing with sharp waves associated with herpes simplex encephalitis) and may identify subclinical seizure activity. As described later, a prolonged EEG may be required to detect subclinical seizures.

If the cause of coma remains unknown, additional studies may be directed at uncommon causes of coma in pediatrics such as Hashimoto encephalitis (**thyroid** function tests and thyroid autoantibodies), cerebral **vasculitis** (erythrocyte sedimentation rate, antinuclear antibody panel, and possibly angiography), or paraneoplastic disorders. Once the patient is stabilized, and if the etiology of coma remains unclear, brain magnetic resonance imaging (MRI) may be performed for diagnostic and prognostic purposes.

Treatment

Recent guidelines including evaluation and management flowcharts are published online (see reference list). Evaluation of the ABCs must begin the assessment, and continuous cardiopulmonary monitoring and frequent GCS assessment are crucial. Hypoxia, hypotension, hypoglycemia or hyperglycemia, hyperthermia or hypothermia, and anemia worsen the prognosis of coma and must be treated aggressively and quickly. Frequent examinations are required to detect any change that may require urgent management. Two issues that often arise as the primary problem is treated include elevated intracranial pressure and seizures.

Elevated Intracranial Pressure

Causes of increased intracranial pressure in coma include intracranial hemorrhage, other space-occupying lesions, and cerebral edema. Cerebral edema may be vasogenic (leakage of fluid from blood vessels into the interstitial space with altered blood-brain barriers) or cytotoxic (accumulation of intracellular water after failure of energy-dependent sodium potassium pumps). **Herniation** may result in brainstem compression and may compress arteries resulting in secondary infarction. Thus herniation syndromes often herald impending catastrophic deterioration and death unless intracranial pressure is lowered rapidly by medical or surgical means. Other than the Cushing triad, signs of herniation depend on the location of the herniation syndrome, summarized in Table 21-8. Initial management of critically raised intracranial pressure includes intravenous **hyperosmolar therapy** (mannitol or sodium) and **hyperventilation** to achieve a PCO_2 of 35 mm Hg. Further reduction in PCO_2 may be necessary to achieve rapid but temporary reductions in cerebral blood flow and thus intracranial pressure, but excessive or prolonged hyperventilation may lead to vasoconstriction, further compromised cerebral perfusion, and exacerbation of hypoxic ischemic injury. Barbiturate coma or moderate hypothermia may reduce cellular energy requirements and may thus help protect the brain during periods of hypoxia and ischemia. Similarly, providing adequate sedation and paralysis may further reduce energy demand and prevent spikes in intracranial pressure. Maintaining a neutral neck position and head of bed elevation at 20° to 30° may improve venous drainage. **Surgical decompression** by removal of mass lesions or craniotomy to provide more space may be lifesaving.

> **HINT:** Herniation syndromes suggest impending catastrophic deterioration and must be recognized and treated rapidly.

Seizures

Subclinical seizures in critically ill patients are an underrecognized phenomenon, so the index of suspicion in a comatose child should be high.

TABLE 21-8 Herniation Syndromes

Herniation Syndrome	Location	Signs
Subfalcine herniation	Increased pressure in one cerebral hemisphere leads to herniation of cingulated gyrus underneath falx cerebri.	Anterior cerebral artery compression and infarction leads to paraparesis.
Uncal herniation	Uncus of the temporal lobe is displaced medially over the free edge of the tentorium.	Ipsilateral third nerve palsy (ptosis, pupil fixed and dilated, eye deviated down and out). Ipsilateral hemiparesis from compression of the contralateral cerebral peduncle (Kernohan notch). Other signs of brainstem dysfunction from ischemia secondary to compression of posterior cerebral artery.
Cerebellar tonsillar herniation	Increased pressure in the posterior fossa leads to brainstem compression.	Loss of consciousness from compression of reticular activating system. Focal lower cranial nerve dysfunction. Respiratory and cardiovascular function can be significantly affected early with relative preservation of upper brainstem function such as pupillary light reflexes and vertical eye movements.
Central herniation	Increased pressure in both cerebral hemispheres causing downward displacement of the diencephalon through the tentorium, causing brainstem compression.	**Diencephalic stage:** Withdraws to noxious stimuli, increased rigidity or decorticate posturing; small reactive pupils with preserved oculocephalic and oculovestibular reflexes; yawns, sighs, or Cheyne-Stokes breathing. **Midbrain stage:** Decerebrate posturing or no movement; midposition pupils that may become irregular and unreactive; abnormal or absent oculocephalic and oculovestibular reflexes; hyperventilation. **Pons stage:** No spontaneous motor activity; midposition fixed pupils; absent oculocephalic and oculovestibular reflexes; ataxic respirations.

(Continued)

TABLE 21-8 Herniation Syndromes *(continued)*

Herniation Syndrome	Location	Signs
		Medulla stage: Generalized flaccidity; absent pupillary reflexes and ocular movements; ataxic or slow irregular respirations; death.
Transcalvarial herniation	Increased pressure leads to herniation through a skull defect (traumatic or surgical).	Dysfunction of involved brain.

Studies of children with altered mental status in the intensive care unit and the emergency department have demonstrated that approximately 25% have **subclinical seizures.** Only about half can be detected with a 1-hour EEG recording, so often more prolonged EEG monitoring is required. Prolonged nonconvulsive seizures are associated with poorer prognosis. Antiepileptic medications may successfully terminate these seizures, and consideration should be given to levetiracetam, fosphenytoin, and valproic acid. Benzodiazepines and phenobarbital may reduce blood pressure and respiratory drive, thus worsening hypoxic ischemic brain injury.

Suggested Readings

Pediatric Accident and Emergency Research Group, 2006: The management of a child (aged 0–18 years) with a decreased conscious level. Available at: http://www.nottingham.ac.uk/paediatric-guideline/. Accessed November 2007.

Posner JB, Saper CB, Schiff N: *Plum and Posner's Diagnosis of Stupor and Coma.* 4th ed. New York, Oxford University Press, 2007.

Stevens RD, Bhardwaj A: Approach to the comatose patient. *Crit Care Med* 34(1):31–41, 2006.

22 *Constipation*

Douglas Hoffman

INTRODUCTION

Constipation is **difficult or delayed passage of stool,** often accompanied by a **decrease in the frequency** of bowel movements. Because **normal stool frequency varies** by age from early in life (Table 22-1), no single definition of constipation fits neatly into pediatric practice. Approximately 3% to 5% of pediatric primary care visits in the United States are for constipation. This figure reflects the concern among many parents about bowel dysfunction in childhood. In general, constipation is problematic only when stools are hard and dry, but decreased stool frequency can be an **important clue in identifying potentially life-threatening causes** of constipation such as Hirschsprung disease or infantile botulism.

DIFFERENTIAL DIAGNOSIS LIST

Infectious Causes

Chagas disease
Proctitis
Rectal/perirectal abscess
Salmonellosis
Tetanus
Viral ileus

Pharmacological Causes

Aluminum antacids
Amiodarone
Anticholinergics
Antihistamines
Barium
Benzodiazepines
Beta-blockers
Calcium channel blockers
Calcium supplements
Cholestyramine
Diazoxide
Diuretics
Iron
Laxative, enema, suppository overuse

Mesalamine
Omeprazole
Ondansetron
Opioids
Phenobarbital
Phenothiazines
Phenytoin
Ranitidine
Sucralfate
Tricyclic antidepressants
Ursodiol
Vincristine
Vitamin D intoxication

Toxic Causes

Botulism
Lead

Neoplastic Causes

Pelvic/sacral mass
Polyps
Pregnancy
Spinal cord tumor

TABLE 22-1 Normal Frequency of Bowel Movements

Age	Bowel Movements Per Week[*]	Bowel Movements Per Day[†]
0–3 months of age		
Breast milk	5–40	2.9
Formula	5–28	2.0
6–12 months of age	5–28	1.8
1–3 years of age	4–21	1.4
>3 years	3–14	1.0

Acta Paediatr Scand 78:682–684, 1989.
[*]Approximate mean ± 2 standard deviations.
[†]Mean.
Reprinted with permission from Baker SS, Liptak GS, Colletti RB, et al: Constipation in infants and children: evaluation and treatment. A medical position statement of the North American Society for Pediatric Gastroenterology and Nutrition. *J Pediatr Gastroenterol Nutr* 29, 1999.

Anatomic Causes

Anal atresia
Anal/intestinal stenosis
Anterior displaced anus
Ectopic anus
Gastroschisis
Intestinal bands
Prune belly
Rectal duplication
Rectal prolapse
Rectoperitoneal fistula

Anal Lesions

Fissure
Foreign body
Hemorrhoid
Streptococcal perianal
  dermatitis

Metabolic and Genetic Causes

Adrenal insufficiency
Cystic fibrosis (meconium
  ileus)
Diabetes insipidus
Diabetes mellitus (neuropathy)
Hyperparathyroidism
Hypocalcemia
Hypokalemia
Hypomagnesemia
Hyponatremia
Hypothyroidism
Mitochondrial disease
Multiple endocrine neoplasia 2B
Panhypopituitarism
Pheochromocytoma
Porphyria
Renal tubular acidosis

Functional Causes

Anorexia nervosa
Anxiety disorders
Attention deficit disorder
Cognitive deficit/delay
Depression
Excessive cow's milk intake
Genetic predisposition
Insufficient dietary water
  intake
Introduction to solids
Irritable bowel syndrome
Low fiber intake
Overzealous toilet training
School bathroom avoidance
School entry
Sexual abuse
Stool withholding
Toilet phobia
Underfeeding/malnutrition

Inflammatory and Autoimmune Disorders

Amyloidosis
Celiac disease
Ehlers-Danlos syndrome
Inflammatory bowel disease
Milk protein allergy
Mixed connective tissue
  disease
Scleroderma
Systemic lupus erythematosus

Neurogenic/ Neuromuscular Causes

Cerebral palsy
Down syndrome
Familial dysautonomia
Hirschsprung disease
Intestinal neuronal dysplasia

Intestinal pseudoobstruction
Myelomeningocele
Myotonias
Neurofibromatosis
Spina bifida occulta
Spinal cord injury
Spinal muscular atrophy
Static encephalopathy
Tethered cord
Visceral myopathies

Surgical Causes

Appendicitis
Inflammatory bowel
  disease–induced strictures
Malrotation
Necrotizing enterocolitis
Pyloric stenosis
Volvulus

DIFFERENTIAL DIAGNOSIS DISCUSSION

Like fever or abdominal pain, constipation is a symptom with a broad differential diagnosis. In most cases, constipation is not serious, but one must always consider conditions such as **Hirschsprung disease, neurogenic problems, metabolic disorders,** and **anatomic defects.** Such congenital abnormalities are detected most frequently during infancy, yet the most common presentation of constipation in both infancy and childhood is termed *functional.* The focus here is on functional constipation and Hirschsprung disease.

Functional Constipation

Chronic childhood constipation is often functional (idiopathic, nonorganic) without demonstrable underlying disease. The pediatrician can usually identify functional constipation by **thorough history** and **physical examination** alone. Nearly all constipation seen by the general pediatrician and up to 25% seen by pediatric gastroenterologists is functional.

A number of predisposing factors (see differential diagnosis list) appear to be associated with the onset of functional constipation. Whatever the cause, once constipation is triggered, a **positive feedback–type mechanism** ensues. Retained stool in the distal colon begins to lose water across the intestinal wall. As water is resorbed, fecal motility slows, more water is lost, and the feces harden. **A buildup of desiccated stool causes painful defecation** that leads to **ongoing stool retention.** Over time, the **rectum** and distal colon expand to accommodate the growing fecal mass (acquired megacolon), and the internal anal sphincter, normally tonically contracted, loses tone. Under these conditions, a child's ability to sense rectal fullness diminishes, and he or she may not appreciate the need to defecate. A classic sign of chronic constipation is the large, infrequent (up to 1 week or more) stool that clogs the household plumbing. Encopresis, or involuntary fecal soiling, is for many families a source of tremendous stress. It is a complication of severe functional constipation that occurs when watery stool from the proximal colon leaks around the fecal obstruction, passing involuntarily per rectum. Parents or caretakers often misinterpret encopresis as diarrhea. Severe constipation may also lead to rectal prolapse.

Evaluation

The medical evaluation of constipation must differentiate functional from organic or medication-related causes. In most cases of functional constipation, laboratory tests are unnecessary. Any predisposing factors (i.e., low fiber intake, difficult toilet training), coupled with telltale signs such as tenesmus, infrequent/abnormally large stools, stool-withholding behavior or soiling, strongly suggest the diagnosis. Social stigma caused by excess flatulence and the odor of encopresis is not unusual. Physical examination may reveal palpable stool in the abdomen. The anus should be checked for fissures, hemorrhoids (rare in childhood), surrounding dermatitis, and abnormal position. Digital rectal examination almost always demonstrates abundant stool in the vault. External sphincter tone and anal wink reflex should be intact. A thorough neurologic examination, including inspection of the sacral area for sinuses or tufts of hair, is important.

The clinician must screen for occult blood in all constipated infants or any child with abdominal pain, failure to thrive, intermittent diarrhea, or a family history of either colon cancer or polyps. Abdominal radiographs are useful if the diagnosis is in doubt or if rectal examination cannot be performed. Measurement of abdominal transit time with radio-opaque markers is an option when a patient has infrequent bowel movements but lacks other signs of constipation. In the absence of soiling, a child with normal transit time does not require further evaluation. When there is soiling with a normal transit time, treatment relies on behavioral modification, sometimes with psychological evaluation. Because stool impaction may cause urinary stasis, the need for urinalysis and culture must be weighed.

Referral to a pediatric gastroenterologist is indicated when a constipated child fails therapy or if the physician suspects an organic cause. Tests to consider before referral include serum measurements of thyroid-stimulating hormone, thyroxine, calcium, magnesium, lead, and electrolytes.

Treatment

Management of constipation may be as simple as a **dietary change** for simple constipation or as complex as a program of **cleanout, bowel "retraining,"** and **family education** with close **follow-up. Infants** with simple constipation often do well with **stool softeners** such as **sorbitol-containing juices** (prune, apple, pear), **Karo syrup,** or **barley malt extract** (Maltsupex). A glycerin suppository usually relieves the acutely constipated infant.

> **HINT:** Enemas, mineral oil, and stimulant laxatives are contraindicated in infants.

In **severely constipated children, disimpaction** precedes maintenance therapy. Available agents include **phosphate, saline,** or **mineral oil enemas** and **polyethylene glycol** for **oral lavage.** Cleanout is initiated with a **mineral oil enema** to soften the fecal mass and lubricate the rectal canal. A **hypertonic phosphate enema** is administered **30 minutes later.** A **daily phosphate enema** may be given for up to 5 days to induce evacuation. Tap water, herbal, and soap suds enemas should not be used because they are associated with water intoxication, bowel perforation, and bowel necrosis. Failure to achieve disimpaction at home may require **hospitalization** for polyethylene glycol oral lavage.

Following disimpaction, **maintenance therapy** lasting months and sometimes years is begun. Children should **decrease cow's milk intake** and consume a **balanced diet** including whole grains, fruits, and vegetables. A common maintenance agent is **mineral oil,** a lubricant given in doses of 1 to 3 mL/kg per day. Mineral oil should not be used when there is risk for aspiration (infants, swallowing dysfunction). **Fat-soluble vitamins** in the form of a multivitamin supplement may be given daily at a time when mineral oil is not taken. **Osmotic laxatives** such as lactulose and, more recently, MiraLAX (polyethylene glycol) are often used as maintenance therapy. MiraLAX, given at a dose of 1 g/kg per day, is safe, effective, and palatable but has not yet been well studied in infants. Occasionally, **stimulant laxatives** such as senna or bisacodyl are used for **short-term "rescue" therapy** to avoid recurrent impaction.

Behavioral modification involves **unhurried toilet sitting** for 10 minutes, two to three times a day after meals. A footstool is often helpful in maximizing Valsalva maneuver. Parents should understand the basic pathophysiology of constipation and be taught to provide **consistent positive reinforcement.** Praise for successful toileting and encouragement after soiling is essential. A **simple reward system** such as stickers on a calendar can be effective and provides a useful record for the physician at follow-up. Some evidence indicates that biofeedback may be a valid short-term mode of therapy in chronic constipation.

> **HINT:** Be aware of pseudoconstipation: Some healthy breast-fed infants may normally only produce a bowel movement two or three times a week. Grunting baby syndrome includes infants without evidence of fecal impaction who strain while passing soft stools. It is thought to result from immature coordination between forced evacuation (Valsalva maneuver) and voluntary relaxation of the external anal sphincter.

> **HINT:** Three events in early childhood tend to coincide with the onset of functional constipation: the introduction of solid food in infancy, toilet training, and school entry.

Hirschsprung Disease (Congenital Aganglionic Megacolon)

Hirschsprung disease, the **most common cause of lower intestinal obstruction in newborns, blocks the wave of peristalsis** in aganglionic bowel segments. In many patients the result is **failure to pass stool,** or at best ribbon-like stools, leading to **severe bowel obstruction if undiagnosed.** The incidence is approximately 1 in 5,000 live births. The male-to-female ratio is 4 to 1. Hirschsprung disease is unusual beyond infancy, but the diagnosis should always be **considered in any constipated toddler or school-age child** because the **mortality of resulting enterocolitis is high.** In addition to several rare genetic disorders, there is an association with **Down syndrome, congenital cardiac anomalies,** and **neuroblastoma** in <5% of patients.

Etiology

Hirschsprung disease **originates** sometime during weeks 5 through 12 of **gestation** when primitive neural crest cells fail to migrate fully caudad. Neural crest cells normally participate in the formation of submucosal and myenteric parasympathetic ganglia; thus **incomplete migration** gives rise to **aganglionic intestine** having sustained sympathetic contraction. The aganglionic segment always extends proximally from the internal anal sphincter. Eighty percent of cases are limited to some portion of the **rectosigmoid region.** Much less frequently, aganglionosis of the entire colon with or without some small bowel involvement occurs.

Clinical Features

Infants with Hirschsprung disease often have **delayed passage of meconium.** Ninety-four percent of normal-term newborns pass meconium within 24 hours of birth compared with 6% of infants with Hirschsprung disease. The degree of bowel involvement correlates with the timing of diagnosis. Patients with short-segment disease may not be identified until childhood (or rarely, go undetected into adulthood), whereas those with **more extensive involvement present in infancy** with **bilious vomiting, abdominal distension, failure to thrive,** and **refusal to feed.** On examination, the **abdomen** is often **distended,** and anal **sphincter tone** is usually **increased.** The **rectum** is typically **empty,** and as the examining digit is withdrawn there may be a forceful gush of liquid stool. **Enterocolitis** is a **life-threatening complication** with acute clinical onset. Increased intraluminal pressure from bowel obstruction is thought to mechanically diminish mucosal blood flow—in turn compromising mucosal integrity—allowing **bacteria and fecal toxins into the bloodstream.** Progression is rapid and septic patients are **febrile** with **abrupt onset** of foul-smelling **bloody diarrhea, abdominal distention,** and **bilious emesis.** The mortality rate in advanced enterocolitis approaches 30%.

Laboratory Evaluation

Several diagnostic methods are available but vary in reliability. Absent rectal air on a prone **abdominal radiograph** suggests Hirschsprung disease. An unprepped **barium enema** demonstrates a narrow distal colonic segment that abruptly transitions to dilated bowel. Because it may take several weeks for a neonate's unaffected proximal bowel segment to dilate with stool, a normal barium study can be misleading. Retention of barium for ≥24 hours is an abnormal finding. A **negative barium study requires further investigation.** Anorectal manometry assesses the internal anal sphincter's response to artificial balloon distention. A normal sphincter relaxes under pressure—an aganglionic sphincter either remains contracted or increases its tone. Normal sphincter relaxation obviates the need for biopsy. When manometry results are abnormal, **rectal biopsy samples** obtained and interpreted by experienced practitioners provide definitive diagnosis.

Management

The treatment of Hirschsprung disease is **surgical resection** of the aganglionic bowel with temporary placement of a **diverting ostomy** proximal to the affected segment. The sensitive anoderm is left intact to ensure future continence. Anastomotic stricture occurs in 5% of patients. More than 90% of patients ultimately have normal bowel function. Before surgery, management of enterocolitis in the intensive care setting includes **nasogastric and rectal decompression, antibiotics, and correction of fluid and electrolyte imbalances.**

> **HINT:** In patients with Hirschsprung disease, the rectum is typically empty on digital exam. However, like functional constipation, patients with short-segment aganglionosis may accumulate stool in the vault. Therefore, patients who do not respond to conventional therapy should be referred to a pediatric gastroenterologist.

TABLE 22-2 Comparison of Functional Constipation and Hirschsprung Disease

	Functional Constipation	Hirschsprung Disease
Symptoms as a newborn	Rare	Almost always
Late onset (>3 years)	Common	Rare
Difficult bowel training	Common	Rare
Stool size	Large	Small, ribbonlike
Urge to defecate	Rare	Common
Obstructive symptoms	Rare	Common
Enterocolitis	Rare	Sometimes
Failure to thrive	Rare	Common
Abdominal distention	Rare	Common
Stool in rectal ampulla	Common	None
Barium enema	Copious stool No transition zone	Delayed evacuation Transition zone
Rectal biopsy	Normal	No ganglion cells Increased anticholinesterase staining
Anorectal manometry	Distention of rectum causes relaxation of the internal sphincter	No sphincter relaxation

Neurogenic Bowel Dysfunction

Neurogenic bowel dysfunction occurs in children when diseases such as **myelomeningocele, tethered cord, lipomeningocele,** or **lumbosacral spinal cord tumors** interfere with the normal neurologic control of defecation. Typical findings include a history of spinal cord trauma, weakness or dysesthesia of the lower extremities, fecal incontinence after successful toilet training, or urinary incontinence. Myelomeningocele-spinal dysraphism in the lumbosacral region can cause constipation and megarectum, but these problems more often manifest as **urinary and fecal incontinence.** Spina bifida occulta (failed fusion of the vertebral arches) is a common finding that usually does not interrupt rectal innervation. **Sacral cysts or fistulae** should be **identified in the newborn** nursery and evaluated by **ultrasound.** Management of patients with neurogenic bowel dysfunction depends on the type, severity, and location of the lesion. Children with moderate-to-severe impairment benefit from interdisciplinary collaboration among physicians, occupational therapists, and behavioral or mental health specialists.

Suggested Readings

Abi-Hanna A, Lake A: Constipation and encopresis in childhood. *Pediatr Rev* 19:23–30, 1998.

Abrahamian FP, Lloyd-Still JD: Chronic constipation in children: longitudinal study of 186 patients. *J Pediatr Gastroenterol Nutr* 3:460–467, 1984.

Amiel J, Sproat-Emison E, Garcia-Barcelo M, et al: Hirschsprung disease, associated syndromes and genetics: a review. *J Med Genet* 45(1):1–14, 2008.

Baker SS, Liptak GS, Colletti RB, et al: Evaluation and treatment of constipation in infants and children: evaluation and treatment. Recommendations of the North American Society for Pediatric Gastroenterology, Hepatology and Nutrition. *J Pediatr Gastroenterol Nutr* 43:e1–e13, 2006.

Davidson M, Jugler MM, Bauer CH: Diagnosis and management in children with severe and protracted constipation and obstipation. *J Pediatr* 62:261–275, 1963.

de Vries M, de Vries M: Cultural relativity of toilet training readiness: a perspective from East Africa. *Pediatrics* 60:170–177, 1977.

Felt B, Wise CG, Olson A, et al: Guideline for the management of pediatric idiopathic constipation and soiling. Multidisciplinary team from the University of Michigan Medical Center in Ann Arbor. *Arch Pediatr Adolesc Med* 153:380–385, 1999.

Goyal R, Hirano I: The enteric nervous system. *N Engl J Med* 334: 1106–1115, 1996.

Loening-Baucke V: Encopresis and soiling. *Pediatr Clin North Am* 43: 279–298, 1996.

McClung HJ, Boyne L, Heitlinger L: Constipation and dietary fiber intake in children. *Pediatrics* 96:999–1001, 1995.

Rudolph C, Benaroch L: Hirschsprung disease. *Pediatr Rev* 16:5–11, 1995.

Taubman B: Toilet training and toileting refusal for stool only: a prospective study. *Pediatrics* 99:54–58, 1997.

INTRODUCTION

Cough is one of the most common presenting symptoms in children. The duration of the symptoms determines the level of concern and degree of workup that is warranted. An **acute cough,** lasting <3 weeks, is frequently related to an infectious illness and is often self-limited. This chapter is concerned with **chronic cough,** a cough that persists for ≥3 weeks and suggests a potentially more serious underlying cause. A cough has three components. First, there is an **inspiratory phase,** when the patient takes a deep breath. The inspiratory phase is followed by **closure of the glottis and contraction of the expiratory muscles.** During this phase, the intrathoracic pressure increases. Finally, the **glottis opens,** allowing the previously inspired air to be expelled at a high velocity (about 60 to 70 mph). The purpose of coughing is to shake irritants loose from the airway mucosa and move them proximally (if the irritant is located distally) or expel them (if the irritant is located proximally).

DIFFERENTIAL DIAGNOSIS LIST 🔒

Infectious Causes
Bacterial Infection
  Bacterial pneumonia
  Sinusitis
  Tuberculosis
  Pertussis
  Chlamydia infection
  Mycoplasma infection
Viral Infection
  Upper respiratory tract
    infection
  Viral pneumonia
  Bronchiolitis—respiratory
    syncytial virus infection,
    parainfluenza infection
  Croup
  Influenza
Fungal Infection
  Aspergillosis

Allergic bronchopulmonary
  aspergillosis
Histoplasmosis
Coccidioidomycosis

Toxic (Irritant) Causes
Cigarette smoke
Industrial pollutants
Wood-burning stoves
Cleaning solvents
Perfumes/colognes

Neoplastic Causes
Teratoma
Lymphoma
Leukemia
Metastatic malignancy

Congenital Causes
Pulmonary Malformations
  Bronchogenic cysts

Cystic adenomatoid
malformation
Congenital lobar emphysema
Pulmonary sequestration
Vascular Malformations
Aberrant innominate artery
Double aortic arch
Airway hemangiomas
Gastrointestinal Malformations
Esophageal duplications
Tracheoesophageal fistula

Genetic Causes
Cystic fibrosis
Immotile cilia syndrome

Inflammatory Causes
Asthma
Allergies
Sarcoidosis

Psychosocial Causes
Psychogenic (habitual) cough
Paradoxical vocal cord
dysfunction

Miscellaneous Causes
Pulmonary Disorders
Bronchopulmonary dysplasia-
Laryngotracheobronchomalacia

Foreign body in airway
Bronchiectasis
**Ears, Nose, and Throat
Disorders**
Foreign body in the nose
or ear canal
Postnasal drip
Middle ear effusion
Cardiovascular Disorders
Congestive heart failure
Pulmonary edema
Gastrointestinal Disorders
Gastroesophageal reflux
disease (GERD)
Diaphragmatic or
subdiaphragmatic mass
Foreign body in the
esophagus
Immunologic Disorders
Congenital immunodeficiency
Medications
Beta-blockers (e.g.,
propanolol)
Angiotensin-converting
enzyme inhibitors (e.g.,
captopril, enalapril,
lisinopril)

DIFFERENTIAL DIAGNOSIS DISCUSSION

Asthma

Asthma, the **most common chronic illness in children,** affects 5% to
10% of children in the United States.

Etiology

The underlying cause of asthma is unknown, although airway inflammation is known to be a major component. The triad of **airway inflammation, smooth muscle hyperreactivity,** and **reversible airway obstruction** is
characteristic for patients with asthma.

Numerous triggers can precipitate an asthma flare-up, including upper respiratory tract infections, sinus infections, exercise, exposure to cold air, weather changes, exposure to allergens (e.g., dust, cockroaches, animal dander, pollen, grass, mold, or certain foods such as shellfish or peanuts), exposure to strong odors (e.g., cigarette smoke, strong chemicals, perfumes), and emotional states (e.g., fear, laughing, crying).

Clinical Features

Asthma symptoms are secondary to airway obstruction and increased airway resistance. **Wheezing** is the classic presentation of asthma, but other symptoms include chronic coughing (cough-variant asthma), shortness of breath, and chest pain or tightness.

Evaluation

A detailed history and physical are key to making the diagnosis of asthma. Wheezing, rhonchi, coarse or decreased breath sounds, or a prolonged expiratory phase may be noted on pulmonary examination. Lung sounds can also be entirely normal at the time of examination, even in a patient with a significant history.

Spirometry with a bronchodilator response is used to assess for asthma. In patients with asthma, an obstructive pattern with postbronchodilator normalization is frequently seen. If spirometry is not available, a handheld peak-flow meter can be substituted.

> **HINT:** Pulmonary function testing can be normal in many patients with cough-variant asthma. If asthma is strongly suspected in spite of normal results on pulmonary function testing, provocational testing (e.g., exercise testing, methacholine challenge) may be indicated to help elicit airway hyperreactivity. Exercise testing is specific in patients with exercise-induced asthma, whereas the more sensitive methacholine challenge can detect more subtle degrees of airway hyperreactivity.

Treatment

Proper treatment of asthma entails both pharmacologic and nonpharmacologic modalities. For most patients with asthma, ideal therapy includes the use of a daily anti-inflammatory medication with a bronchodilator given on an as needed basis to treat breakthrough symptoms. Short bursts of oral steroids are helpful for treating acute flare-ups of asthma, although the side effects of long-term use preclude the use of oral steroids as a chronic maintenance medication (except in severe cases).

■ **Anti-inflammatory medications** include mast cell stabilizers (e.g., cromolyn sodium, nedocromil calcium), inhaled steroids (e.g., beclomethasone, triamcinolone, fluticasone, budesonide), and leukotriene inhibitors (e.g., zileuton, zafirlukast, montelukast).

- **Bronchodilators.** β_2-Agonists (e.g., albuterol, terbutaline, pirbuterol) are the most effective and commonly used bronchodilators for rescue therapy. Long acting β_2-agonists (e.g., salmeterol, formoterol) may be used in combination with inhaled steroids (Advair = salmeterol + fluticasone; Symbicort = formoterol + budesonide) to provide improved symptom control and pulmonary function values when inhaled steroids alone prove insufficient at controlling the patient's asthma. Methylxanthine derivatives (e.g., theophylline) and parasympathetic antagonists (e.g., atropine, ipratropium) may also be used (although they are no longer routinely used in children).
- **Nonpharmacologic management** entails patient education (to improve self-management), environmental control and prevention skills (to decrease exposure to asthmatic triggers and the likelihood of developing an asthma attack), and home monitoring with a peak-flow monitor (to assess pulmonary status objectively so that appropriate interventions can be instituted and their effects measured).

Cystic Fibrosis

Etiology

An autosomal recessive disorder, cystic fibrosis is the **most common genetic disease affecting whites.** The gene is located on chromosome number 7 and codes for a transmembrane protein (cystic fibrosis transmembrane conductance regulator protein) that functions as a chloride channel. The most common abnormality is an amino acid defect consisting of the deletion of a phenylalanine (the Δ F508 mutation). The disease is characterized by **multiorgan involvement.** Chronic sinopulmonary infections (facilitated by excess altered mucus production in the respiratory tract), pancreatic insufficiency, and abnormalities of the exocrine glands and reproductive tract are major manifestations. In the lungs, dry, thickened secretions hinder clearance of pulmonary secretions. Impaired clearance, in combination with abnormal colonization with organisms (e.g., *Staphylococcus aureus, Pseudomonas aeruginosa*), lead to the development of bronchiectasis and permanent lung damage.

Clinical Features

Major symptoms include a chronic productive cough, yellow-green sputum, hemoptysis, chest congestion, steatorrhea, poor weight gain, failure to thrive, and meconium ileus or meconium ileus equivalent (intestinal obstruction).

Evaluation

A detailed family history should be obtained as well as growth patterns and stool characteristics. Cardinal features noted on physical examination may include tachypnea, bronchial breath sounds, wheezes, crackles, a prolonged expiratory phase, nasal polyps, upper airway congestion, digital clubbing, reduced height and weight, rectal prolapse, and hepatomegaly and splenomegaly.

The following laboratory studies are indicated:

- **Chloride sweat test.** Pilocarpine is used to stimulate sweat collection. The sweat chloride level is considered to be elevated if >60 mEq/L.
- **Sputum culture.** *P. aeruginosa* and *S. aureus* are the bacterial pathogens most often responsible for the chronic sinopulmonary infections. Other organisms, such as *Burkholderia cepacia, Stenotrophomonas maltophilia,* and *Alcaligenes xylosoxidans,* are also seen and tend to be more resistant to therapy.
- **Complete blood cell (CBC) count.** A CBC should be obtained to rule out anemia and to assess for leukocytosis. Hypersplenism has also been reported (evidenced by leucopenia and thrombocytopenia).
- **Liver function tests** are ordered to assess for hepatobiliary disease and obstruction.
- **Prothrombin time (PT).** A PT should be obtained to assess vitamin K sufficiency.
- **Vitamin A, E,** and **D** levels should be measured to assess for possible fat-soluble vitamin deficiency.
- **Fecal fat analysis.** A 72-hour stool collection should be obtained to assess the degree of pancreatic insufficiency.
- **Oxygen saturation analysis** and **pulmonary function tests** should be performed to assess the degree of pulmonary involvement (arterial blood gas analysis is not necessary in most cases).
- **Genetic testing** is indicated. More than 70% of patients have the Δ F508 mutation.

> **HINT:** All children with recurrent sinopulmonary infections, steatorrhea, growth failure, or asthma who do not respond to appropriate therapy should be tested for cystic fibrosis.

> **HINT:** All siblings of patients with cystic fibrosis should be tested for cystic fibrosis using the chloride sweat test. They should also undergo genetic analysis because they have a 2 in 3 chance of being a carrier (this should be after the proband's genetic mutation has been identified).

Treatment

Therapy is directed toward maintaining optimal pulmonary function and nutritional status.

- **Daily airway clearance** with chest physiotherapy, breathing exercises, and (frequently) nebulized bronchodilators is indicated. The efficacy of mucolytic agents such as Mucomyst is questioned; however, Pulmozyme was demonstrated in clinical studies to improve lung function. Recent studies support the use of hypertonic saline as part of the airway clearance regimen.

- **(Chronic) antibiotic therapy** is frequently used to help suppress the effects of chronic bacterial colonization. Inhaled high-dose tobramycin (TOBI) used on a twice daily schedule given on alternating months as well as azithromycin given on a 3 day per week schedule helped in prospective studies to maintain pulmonary function when compared with placebo.

- **(Acute) antibiotic therapy** is used to treat acute exacerbations of cystic fibrosis. Symptoms of these exacerbations include increased cough and mucus production, wheezing, shortness of breath, decreased exercise tolerance, decreased appetite, weight loss, and general malaise. Oral antibiotics (in combination with increased airway clearance) can often treat these symptoms when they are mild. In cases with more severe symptoms or when oral antibiotics have not been successful, broad-spectrum intravenous antibiotics are required (usually given in the inpatient setting).

- **Pancreatic insufficiency** is treated with the administration of supplemental pancreatic enzymes along with multivitamins (in particular, the fat-soluble vitamins A, D, E, and K). Vitamin K administration is frequently required, especially if the patient takes antibiotics chronically or if the PT is increased (vitamin K should be given intramuscularly if the PT is seriously elevated or if the patient is actively bleeding).

- **Hemoptysis** is a complication usually indicating a severe exacerbation of underlying infection. Treatment is with antibiotics as outlined earlier; however, it may be necessary to withhold chest physiotherapy until the bleeding subsides (12 to 24 hours). Most episodes of hemoptysis manifest as blood streaks and respond to a treatment course of antibiotics. Massive hemoptysis, although rare, is a medical emergency that usually results from erosion of an underlying bronchial vessel into a bronchus. This is frequently treated with bronchial artery embolization.

- **Other major emergencies** in patients with cystic fibrosis include acute intestinal obstruction, massive hemorrhage from esophageal varices, liver failure, pulmonary hypertension, cor pulmonale with cardiac failure, pneumothorax, and chronic hypoxemia.

Sinusitis

Sinusitis, characterized by inflammation and infection of the mucosal lining of the sinuses, is a common cause of chronic cough.

Etiology

In an otherwise healthy host, sinus infections are usually a **complication of upper respiratory tract infections** (i.e., bacterial superinfection following a viral infection). The usual bacterial pathogens include *Streptococcus pneumoniae, Haemophilus influenzae,* and *Moraxella catarrhalis.*

Clinical Features

Sinusitis can present in a variety of ways. Common features include persistent symptoms of an upper respiratory tract infection, chronic cough, a mucopurulent nasal discharge, headaches, and malodorous breath.

Evaluation

The diagnosis can be made clinically, based on the history and physical examination. Physical examination findings may include tenderness over the affected sinus and erythema of the nasal mucosa, with or without a mucopurulent nasal discharge. The physical examination, however, may be normal. Radiographic studies that can aid in the diagnosis include **sinus films** and **computed tomography (CT)** of the sinuses. Opacification of the sinuses, mucosal thickening, or the presence of an air-fluid level are typical findings.

Treatment

The usual treatment for sinusitis is a prolonged course of **antibiotics,** usually lasting 14 to 21 days. Therapy should be directed toward the usual bacterial pathogens. The concomitant use of topical **decongestants** is only recommended for 4 to 7 days. **Surgical drainage** of the sinus is sometimes used in refractory cases.

Bronchiectasis

Bronchiectasis is a condition in which the bronchi are damaged, leading to the development of bronchial dilation with the loss of underlying airway support structures (e.g., cartilage and elastic tissue). Acute or chronic inflammation and recurrent infections are also associated with bronchiectasis. Bronchiectasis is the end result of numerous insults to the lung and can be **reversible** (e.g., cylindrical bronchiectasis) or **permanent** (e.g., saccular bronchiectasis).

Etiology

Some of the more common causes of bronchiectasis include **infection** (e.g., following severe pneumonia caused by *S. aureus, S. pneumoniae,* adenovirus, or influenza virus), **genetic conditions** (e.g., cystic fibrosis, immotile cilia syndrome), **recurrent aspiration events,** or a **retained foreign body.**

Clinical Features

Chronic coughing with excessive sputum production (bronchorrhea) is a cardinal sign of bronchiectasis. In severe cases, hemoptysis and recurrent fevers may also be seen.

Evaluation

- **Physical findings** are related to the extent of the disease. Although the pulmonary examination can be normal early in the course of disease, one is apt to find coarse breath sounds, rhonchi, rales, and expiratory wheezes as the disease progresses. Digital clubbing is also seen in advanced disease.
- **Chest radiographs** typically show thickened bronchial walls in the peripheral lung, although early in the course of disease the films may be normal. Other findings include recurrent atelectasis and localized hyperinflation.
- **Chest CT scans** are more sensitive than radiographs for defining the extent of the disease, especially in patients with milder cases. Typical findings include bronchial wall thickening extending to the periphery, cystic changes in the bronchi, and air-fluid levels in the damaged bronchi.
- **Other studies** may prove useful in the evaluation of the patient with bronchiectasis. These studies depend on the past medical history and can include a sweat test (if cystic fibrosis is to be considered); bronchoscopy (if a foreign body is suspected or if respiratory cultures are desired); an immunologic evaluation (if recurrent pneumonia has occurred); or a pH probe or milk scan (if GERD is suspected).

Treatment

Treatment should be directed toward the underlying cause of the bronchiectasis, if one can be identified.

- **Airway clearance.** Maintenance of good pulmonary toilet is important, regardless of the cause of the bronchiectasis. Aiding in the removal of excessive secretions and preventing superinfection can help prevent further bronchial damage. Aerosolized bronchodilators, chest physiotherapy, and postural drainage promote the removal of excess mucus.
- **Antibiotics.** Oral or intravenous antibiotics may be indicated for patients with acute exacerbations of bronchiectasis exacerbated by a bacterial infection. Chronic prophylactic antibiotic use to prevent exacerbations is controversial and should be determined on a case-by-case basis.
- **Surgery.** In certain patients with well-localized bronchiectasis, surgical removal of the affected lung can be curative. Surgery, however, should only be performed when medical management has failed and the likelihood of disease progression after surgery is minimal.

Immotile Cilia Syndrome

Etiology

Immotile cilia syndrome is an autosomal recessive disease characterized by abnormal function of the cilia. Histologic defects in the cilia may include abnormalities in the dynein arms, defects in the radial spokes connecting the microtubules that form the cilia, and defects in the microtubules themselves.

Clinical Features

Patients with immotile cilia syndrome typically present with recurrent episodes of **otitis media, sinusitis, chronic cough,** and **pulmonary infections.** Physical findings include recurrent otitis media, chronic sinus drainage, nasal polyps, pulmonary findings suggestive of bronchiectasis, and, in more severe cases, digital clubbing (secondary to the bronchiectasis). **Situs inversus** is seen in 50% of cases.

> **HINT:** The triad of sinusitis, bronchiectasis, and situs inversus is referred to as Kartagener syndrome.

> **HINT:** Male infertility secondary to abnormally functioning sperm is common.

Evaluation

Frequently, the diagnosis is made by clinical history and by ruling out other causes. It can be difficult to diagnose the condition definitively. Approaches include (**electron**) **microscopic evaluation** of the cilia (with tissue obtained via nasal mucosa scrapping or tracheal biopsy), examination of the **ciliary beat frequency or waveform** (under light microscopy), and the **saccharin test** (a drop of saccharin is placed in the nose and the length of time it takes the patient to taste the sweetness is measured).

Radiographic findings (chest radiograph or CT scan) are similar to those of cystic fibrosis and bronchiectasis. Sinus films typically show pansinusitis.

Treatment

Treatment is the **same as for bronchiectasis.** Maintaining adequate pulmonary drainage is key to minimizing lung damage. Recurrent otitis media is frequently treated with the placement of myringotomy tubes. Chronic use of antibiotics is controversial.

(Allergic) Rhinitis

Allergic rhinitis is characterized by chronic or recurrent watery nasal discharge and can represent a very common cause of chronic cough.

Etiology

Allergic rhinitis is an IgE-mediated response to agents found in nature. These allergens generate IgE antibodies, which then bind to mast cells. When a sensitized patient is then reexposed to this allergen, it binds to the IgE antibody, which leads to mast cell degranulation. Several chemicals are released from these mast cells, in particular, histamine, which leads to the symptoms described later. Depending on the specific antigen triggering this response, the allergic rhinitis may be seasonal or perennial (throughout the year).

Clinical Features

Allergic rhinitis can present with a variety of symptoms. Common symptoms include rhinorrhea, sneezing, coughing, recurrent throat clearing, allergic shiners, Dennie lines, conjunctivitis, and nasal and ocular itching. Physical examination may reveal pale and boggy nasal turbinates with a watery discharge evident. Cobblestoning of the eyelids and posterior oropharynx along with a postnasal drip are frequently evident.

Evaluation

Although the diagnosis can be made by history, allergy testing can be useful for identifying the specific antigens responsible for these symptoms. Skin testing (simple prick testing) can identify agents to which the patient has been sensitized. A positive skin test correlates well (although not fully) with clinical symptoms. Radioallergosorbent testing (RAST) measures IgE levels to various antigens. Although highly specific, there is not as much correlation between positive RAST testing and clinical symptoms as is seen with positive skin testing, especially with low-level positive RAST values.

> **HINT:** Positive RAST and skin testing identify antigens to which the patient has been exposed and to which they have mounted an IgE-medicated response. One must then clinically correlate these positive test results to the actual clinical symptoms. A positive "allergy test" does not tell you what you are allergic to, just what you are sensitized to.

Treatment

Treatment for allergic rhinitis involves both pharmacologic and non-pharmacologic measures.

■ **Pharmacologic management.** Antihistamines and nasal steroids are the mainstays of pharmacologic therapy. Antihistamines block the effects of the histamine released by mast cell degranulation. The older first-generation antihistamines (i.e., diphenhydramine, hydroxyzine) tend to be sedating, whereas the newer second-generation antihistamines (i.e., loratadine, cetirizine, fexofenadine) do not cross the blood-brain barrier and are nonsedating.

As with asthma therapy, anti-inflammatory agents help stop the inflammatory cascade associated with mast cell degranulation and/or prevent the mast cells themselves from degranulating. Nasal steroids (i.e., triamcinolone, fluticasone, budesonide) are the mainstay of therapy to control the symptoms of allergic rhinitis. Other agents found to be effective in controlling allergic rhinitis include the leukotriene inhibitor montelukast and the mast cell stabilizer (nasally inhaled) cromolyn.

Immunotherapy (commonly referred to as "allergy shots") is also an effective therapy for treating allergies. This is especially useful when antihistamines and nasal steroids are ineffective. It consists of recurrent subcutaneous injections of a particular antigen at increasing concentrations, which desensitizes the body to that particular antigen.

■ **Nonpharmacologic management.** Many nonpharmacologic therapies are available to help control allergies. Avoidance of the specific antigen is very effective at diminishing symptoms. Removing pets from the household (or at least minimizing exposures) can be a useful adjunctive therapy. Control of dust mites can be accomplished by maintaining low humidity in the household, washing bedsheets in hot water, encasing pillows and mattresses in plastic sheets, and removing dust-attracting agents (i.e. stuffed animals, window blinds) from the patient's room. Cleaning up loose food and the use of exterminators can decreases cockroach exposures.

Gastroesophageal Reflux Disease (GERD)

Gastroesophageal reflux disease is discussed in Chapter 82, "Vomiting."

EVALUATION OF COUGH

Patient History

Present Illness

The present illness should be defined:

■ What is the duration of the cough?
■ How frequent is the cough?

TABLE 23-1 Types of Cough

Quality	Likely Diagnosis
Staccato	Pertussis or parapertussis infection
Bark-like (seal-like) or brassy	Croup
Throat clearing	Postnasal drip, possibly secondary to sinusitis or allergies
Foghorn-like and occurring only when awake	Pathognomonic for a psychogenic (habitual) cough

- When does the cough occur (e.g., upon awakening, later in the evening)?
- What does the cough sound like (Table 23-1)?
- Is the cough productive or nonproductive for sputum?

> **HINT:** Children frequently swallow rather than expectorate sputum, making assessment of sputum productivity difficult. If the child is too young to expectorate sputum, examination of any emesis can indirectly assess for sputum production.

- Were there any precipitating events (e.g., infection, choking episode, allergies)?
- Are there any triggers for the cough (Table 23-2)?
- Are there accompanying symptoms (e.g., rhinorrhea, watery eyes, headaches, fever, poor weight gain or weight loss, symptoms of food malabsorption, wheezing)?
- How many school days have been missed?
- Is the cough improving or getting worse?
- What medications is the child currently taking? Angiotensin-converting enzyme (ACE) inhibitors can cause a chronic cough and β_2 antagonists can precipitate bronchospasm in patients with asthma.
- What is the patient's travel history?
- Are other family members ill?

TABLE 23-2 Triggers for Coughing

Trigger	Associations
Cold air, exercise, or upper respiratory tract infections	Asthma
Supine position	Postnasal drip, GERD
Eating	GERD, tracheoesophageal fistula

GERD = gastroesophageal reflux disease

Past Medical History

Important information to be gathered includes the following:

- The patient's birth history
- Information regarding any previous illness or surgery
- Information regarding allergies
- The patient's immunization status

Family History

The patient's parents should be queried about a family history of any of the following disorders:

- Asthma
- Allergies
- Cystic fibrosis
- Emphysema
- Sarcoidosis
- Tuberculosis

Environmental History

An environmental history can sometimes prove useful in identifying the exacerbating factors in patients with a chronic cough, especially if the underlying cause is asthma or allergies. The following are important factors:

- **Home heating system.** Forced-air heating systems that use a duct network can carry dust through the house. Radiator and baseboard heating are much less likely to cause a problem for children with allergies.
- **Wood-burning stoves.** Older stoves often do not burn wood efficiently. The incompletely burned wood releases hydrocarbons that can be a potent, noxious irritant for patients with asthma.
- **Location of the home.** In rural and suburban settings, patients are exposed to numerous aeroallergens, whereas in urban environments, patients are exposed to industrial irritants, dust mites, and cockroaches.
- **Condition of the home.** Dusty homes can aggravate allergies. If the basement is cool and damp, the possibility of mold exposure exists. Older homes, especially in overcrowded urban areas, can have cockroaches, which are recognized as a potent allergen and can lead to poorly controlled allergies and asthma. Construction within the home can expose the child to various noxious irritants, ranging from dust to paint and chemical odors. Mold spores can also be released into the air. For patients with severe dust allergies, removing the carpeting, drapes, blinds, and stuffed animals from the patient's room and encasing the mattress and pillow in plastic may help minimize exposure to dust mites.

- **Cigarette exposure.** Smoking in the home can be a potent trigger for coughing, particularly in children with asthma. Children exposed to cigarette smoke have a higher incidence of asthma, recurrent upper respiratory tract infections, and recurrent sinusitis or otitis media. This cigarette smoke effect can be seen even when the parents do not smoke in direct contact with the child.
- **Pets.** Exposure to pets can be a problem for children with allergies and asthma.
- **Child care.** Recurrent exposure to other children increases the likelihood of the child developing recurrent upper respiratory tract infections.

Physical Examination

The following should be noted on physical examination:

- **General appearance**—height and weight, degree of distress
- **Skin**—eczema, rashes
- **Head, ears, eyes, nose, and throat**—watery eyes, cerumen in the ear, sinus tenderness, nasal discharge, pale or boggy nasal turbinates, post-nasal drip, pharyngeal cobblestoning (i.e., a cobblestone-like appearance to the mucosa that is seen in patients with allergic disease)
- **Lungs**—respiratory rate, chest appearance, breath sounds (rhonchi, rales, wheezes) and their symmetry
- **Heart**—murmur
- **Extremities**—cyanosis, clubbing

> **HINT:** The presence of digital clubbing raises the possibility of a more severe underlying pulmonary problem, such as cystic fibrosis, bronchiectasis, or chronic hypoxia. Clubbing makes asthma a much less likely etiology for the cough.

Laboratory Studies

Selection of laboratory studies is based on a thorough history and physical examination.

Suspected Asthma

- **Pulmonary function testing** can help confirm the diagnosis of asthma by demonstrating reversible obstructive lung disease or significant airway hyperreactivity. This test can be reliably done in children as young as 5 years old.
- **Pulmonary function provocational testing** can be used to assess for airway hyperreactivity in cases with normal pulmonary function values. A decrease of pulmonary function by 20% during a **methacholine challenge** or 15% during an **exercise challenge** is diagnostic of asthma.

Suspected Allergy

- **Diagnostic skin testing** is the most accurate test for determining atopy; skin testing is best done in patients >2 years.
- **CBC with differential.** Eosinophilia suggests an allergic component.
- **IgE level.** Elevation suggests an allergic component.
- **Radioallergosorbent testing (RAST).** RAST is used in the evaluation of allergy but is not as clinically sensitive as skin testing.

Suspected Infection

- **Purified protein derivative (PPD)** is used to rule out tuberculosis (TB). Tine testing is no longer recommended as a screening test. The usual dose of PPD for the Mantoux tuberculin skin test is 5 U given as an intradermal injection.
- **Sputum culture with Gram stain** is indicated for patients who have a productive cough. Acid-fast staining should be done if TB is suspected.

Suspected Immunologic Disorder

A CBC with differential; quantitative IgG, IgA, and IgM levels; functional antibody levels (to assess B lymphocyte function); an anergy panel (to assess T lymphocyte function); and an HIV test are indicated.

Other Disorders

- **Sweat chloride test.** A sweat chloride of >60 mEq/mL is diagnostic of cystic fibrosis.
- α_1**-Antitrypsin (α_1-AT) level.** An α_1-AT level with genetic variants should be obtained in patients with emphysema to rule out α_1-AT deficiency.
- **Angiotensin-converting enzyme (ACE) level.** The ACE level may be elevated in patients with sarcoidosis.

Diagnostic Modalities

- **Radiographic studies.** Radiographs or CT scans of the chest or sinuses may be indicated. A barium swallow should be considered for most infants with chronic cough to rule out GERD, tracheoesophageal fistula, or vascular ring or sling. GERD can also be assessed for by a gastric emptying (milk) scan or a pH probe.
- **Bronchoscopy (with or without lavage)** is useful for inspecting airway anatomy and dynamics, detecting a foreign body, and sampling lung material for culture.

TREATMENT OF COUGH

To treat a chronic cough properly, its underlying cause must be determined. Symptomatic relief, however, should be considered when the cough causes discomfort, interferes with the patient's ability to sleep or perform well in school, and there is otherwise *no specific* therapy available. Symptomatic cough medications fall into three classes: expectorants, antitussives, and mucolytic agents.

- **Expectorants** help moisturize secretions, making it easier for the patient to cough up sputum. The most effective expectorant is water; patients should be advised to drink plenty of fluids. Another effective expectorant is guaifenesin, found in numerous over-the-counter cough and cold preparations.
- **Antitussive agents** fall into two classes: peripherally acting and centrally acting medications. Peripherally acting agents (e.g., diphenhydramine) work by decreasing the sensitivity of the cough receptors in the lung. Centrally acting agents (e.g., codeine, dextromethorphan) act on the cough center located in the medulla. They abate coughing by decreasing the stimulus to cough. Dextromethorphan is as effective as codeine but is not a narcotic and thus not habit forming. Dextromethorphan is available in several over-the-counter cough preparations, usually in combination with antihistamines, expectorants, or both. Codeine is available only with a prescription and can be obtained as a single agent or mixed with other cough and cold preparations. Antitussive agents are not indicated when the child is otherwise well and not bothered by the cough.
- **Mucolytic agents** (e.g., Mucomyst, Pulmozyme) help patients who have thick, tenacious sputum (e.g., patients with cystic fibrosis). These agents help break up the mucus and, with the aid of chest physiotherapy, allow the patient to expectorate sputum more easily.

Suggested Readings

Black P: Evaluation of chronic or recurrent cough. In *Pediatric Respiratory Disease: Diagnosis and Treatment.* Philadelphia, WB Saunders, 1993, 143–154.

Chang AB, Asher MI: A review of cough in children. *J Asthma* 38(4): 299–309, 2001.

de Jongste JC, Shields MD: Cough-2: Chronic cough in children. *Thorax* 58:998–1003, 2003.

Irwin RS, Boulet LP, Cloutier MM, et al.: Managing cough as a defense mechanism and as a symptom. A consensus panel report of the American College of Chest Physicians. *Chest* 114:133S–181S, 1999.

Katcher ML: Cold, cough and allergy medications: uses and abuses. *Pediatr Rev* 17:12–17, 1996.

Wilmott RW: Cough. In *Pediatric Primary Care: A Problem-Oriented Approach.* Edited by Schwartz MW. St. Louis, Mosby, 1997, 216–224.

24 *Cyanosis*

Claudio Ramaciotti and Bradley S. Marino

INTRODUCTION

Cyanosis is a physical sign characterized by a **bluish discoloration of the mucous membranes, skin, and nail beds.** Cyanosis results from **hypoxemia** (decreased arterial oxygen saturation) or **abnormal hemoglobin molecules.** Cyanosis does not become clinically evident until the absolute concentration of deoxygenated hemoglobin is at least 3.5 g/dL. Cyanosis is produced by clinical conditions associated with one or more of the following abnormalities: **intracardiac right-to-left shunting, ventilation-perfusion mismatch in the lungs, impairment of oxygen diffusion in the lungs, alveolar hypoventilation, or decreased affinity of hemoglobin for oxygen.** Factors that influence the degree of cyanosis include the total hemoglobin concentration (related to the hematocrit) *and* factors that affect the O_2 dissociation curve (pH, P_{CO_2}, temperature, and ratio of adult-to-fetal hemoglobin). Cyanosis will be evident sooner (and be more pronounced) under the following conditions: high hemoglobin concentration (polycythemic patient), lower pH (acidosis), elevated P_{CO_2} (lowered respiratory rate), elevated temperature, and elevated ratio of adult-to-fetal hemoglobin. Cyanosis should not be confused with **acrocyanosis** (blueness of the *distal* extremities *only*). Acrocyanosis is caused by peripheral vasoconstriction and is a normal finding during the first 24 to 48 hours of life.

DIFFERENTIAL DIAGNOSIS LIST 🔒

Cardiac
Ductal-Independent
Mixing Lesions
Truncus arteriosus
Total anomalous pulmonary venous return without obstruction
D-transposition of the great arteries [a]
Lesions with Ductal-Dependent Pulmonary Blood Flow
Tetralogy of Fallot with pulmonary atresia [b]

Ebstein anomaly [b]
Critical pulmonic stenosis
Tricuspid valve atresia [b] with normally related great arteries [b]
Pulmonic valve atresia with intact ventricular septum
Heterotaxy
Lesions with Ductal-Dependent Systemic Blood Flow
Hypoplastic left heart syndrome
Interrupted aortic arch

Critical coarctation of the
aorta
Critical aortic stenosis
Tricuspid valve atresia with
transposition of the great
arteries [b]

Pulmonary

Primary Lung Disease
Respiratory distress
syndrome
Meconium aspiration
Pneumonia
Persistent pulmonary hyper-
tension of the newborn
Airway Obstruction
Choanal atresia
Vocal cord paralysis
Laryngotracheomalacia
**Extrinsic Compression
of the Lungs**
Pneumothorax

Chylothorax
Hemothorax

Neurologic

Central nervous system
dysfunction
Drug-induced depression
of respiratory drive
Postasphyxial cerebral
dysfunction
Central apnea
**Respiratory Neuromuscular
Dysfunction**
Spinal muscular atrophy
Infant botulism
Neonatal myasthenia
gravis
Hematologic
Methemoglobinemia
Polycythemia

DIFFERENTIAL DIAGNOSIS DISCUSSION

Methemoglobinemia

Etiology

Methemoglobinemia involves oxidation of the iron within the hemoglobin molecule resulting in reduced oxygen-carrying capacity of blood and
impaired delivery to tissues. Methemoglobin may occur because of hereditary abnormalities of hemoglobin as well as exposures to oxidizing toxins. **Toxic causes** include analgesics (e.g., benzocaine), aniline dyes, some
antimicrobials (e.g., dapsone, sulfonamides), azo compounds, and
nitrites. Young infancy is a period of increased risk for methemoglobinemia, when it has also been described during infections such as gastroenteritis.

Clinical Features

Patients with methemoglobinemia present with **cyanosis** and **abnormal
pulse oximetry** in the presence of a **normal Pao_2** value.

---

[a]A patent ductus arteriosus may improve mixing, especially with an intact ventricular septum.
[b]Most forms.

Evaluation

Bedside diagnosis of methemoglobinemia entails placing a **drop of the patient's blood on a piece of filter paper.** After 30 seconds of exposure to air, normal blood turns red, whereas blood taken from a patient with methemoglobinemia remains **chocolate brown.** Methemoglobin levels are measured as part of a blood gas by **co-oximetry.**

Treatment

Methylene blue given intravenously reduces the abnormal ferric hemoglobin molecule. Methylene blue is usually recommended when the methemoglobin level >20% because lower levels typically resolve with supportive care alone. Methylene blue is contraindicated in patients with glucose-6-phosphate dehydrogenase deficiency because it may cause a severe hemolytic anemia.

EVALUATION OF CYANOSIS

Neonates

Patient History

Important information to obtain from the history includes the following:

- A complete birth history that includes maternal history; prenatal, perinatal, and postnatal complications; history of labor and delivery; history of maternal infection, and neonatal course should be obtained.
- When did the mother's membranes rupture? Early rupture of the membranes predisposes the neonate to infection or sepsis.
- Is there a history of asphyxia?
- What was the baby's gestational age?
- How old was the baby when the first episode of cyanosis occurred? Exactly when the child developed cyanosis is critical because certain congenital heart defects present at birth, whereas others may take as long as 1 month to become evident.

Physical Examination

- **General assessment and vital signs.** The initial physical examination should focus on the vital signs and the cardiac and respiratory examinations, assessing for evidence of right, left, or biventricular congestive heart failure and impending respiratory failure. The infant's body temperature should be noted. If the baby is hypothermic, examination should take place after measures have been taken to warm the patient.
- **Skin color.** Blue or dusky mucous membranes are consistent with cyanosis. Skin color has an impact on the diagnosis; in light-skinned patients, cyanosis is usually noted with an arterial oxygen saturation of <85%; in dark-skinned patients, the arterial oxygen saturation must be even lower.

- **Respiratory examination.** Evaluate for rales, stridor, grunting, flaring, retractions, and evidence of consolidation or effusion on pulmonary examination. An increased respiratory rate, increased heart rate, grunting, nasal flaring, and retractions are signs of respiratory distress. Breath sounds should be documented. Hyperpnea with cyanosis but without signs of respiratory distress is frequently observed in patients with congenital heart defects. Apnea is commonly related to prematurity, intracerebral problems, or medication usage. Tachypnea with nasal flaring, grunting, and intercostal and subcostal retractions often reflects an upper or lower airway disturbance. A high respiratory rate (>80 breaths/minute) is unusual with cardiac lesions that are associated with restricted pulmonary blood flow.

- **Cardiovascular examination.** On cardiovascular examination, the precordial impulse is palpated, and the clinician should evaluate for systolic or diastolic murmurs, the intensity of S_1, S_2 splitting abnormalities, and the presence of an S_3 or S_4 gallop, ejection click, opening snap, or rub. Absence of a heart murmur does not rule out congenital heart disease; severe cyanosis without a heart murmur suggests transposition of the great arteries. Examination of the extremities should focus on the strength and symmetry of the pulses in the upper and lower extremities, evidence of edema, and cyanosis of the nail beds. Hepatosplenomegaly may be consistent with right ventricular or biventricular heart failure.

Laboratory Studies

The goal of the initial evaluation of the cyanotic neonate is to determine whether the cyanosis is cardiac or noncardiac in origin. Preductal and postductal oxygen saturation and four extremity blood pressures should be documented. An electrocardiogram (ECG), chest radiograph, and hyperoxia test should be performed.

Preductal (right extremity) and **postductal** (lower extremity) oxygen saturations are evaluated to assess for **differential cyanosis and reverse differential cyanosis.** Differential cyanosis is present when the oxygen saturation in the right upper extremity is greater than the lower extremities. In the neonatal period, differential cyanosis is observed in patients with persistent pulmonary hypertension of the newborn (PPHN) or left ventricular outflow tract obstruction such as interrupted aortic arch, critical coarctation of the aorta, and critical aortic stenosis, secondary to significant right-to-left ductal shunting. In older patients, differential cyanosis is seen in association with patent ductus arteriosus and pulmonary vascular obstructive disease. When the preductal saturation is lower than the postductal saturation, reverse differential cyanosis is present. Reverse differential cyanosis results from transposition of the great arteries with PPHN or left ventricular outflow obstruction (e.g., critical coarctation of the aorta, interrupted aortic arch, critical aortic stenosis). Oxygenated blood from the pulmonary circulation enters the descending aorta through a patent ductus arteriosus, increasing the postductal oxygen saturation.

Four extremity blood pressure measurements demonstrating a right upper extremity systolic blood pressure at least 10 mm Hg greater than the lower extremity is consistent with arch hypoplasia, coarctation of the aorta, or other lesions with ductal dependent systemic blood flow with a restrictive ductus arteriosus. The chest radiograph is obtained to determine the size of the heart and whether the pulmonary vascularity is increased or decreased. The ECG evaluates the heart rate, rhythm, axis, intervals, forces (atrial dilation, ventricular hypertrophy), and repolarization (abnormal Q wave pattern, ST/T waves, and/or corrected QT interval).

A hyperoxia test should be carried out in all neonates with a resting pulse oximetry reading <95%, visible cyanosis, or circulatory collapse (see Chapter 84, "Cardiology Laboratory"). The hyperoxia test consists of obtaining a baseline right radial (preductal) arterial blood gas measurement with the child breathing room air ($Fio_2 = 0.21$), and then repeating the measurement with the child inspiring 100% oxygen ($Fio_2 = 1.00$). The Pao_2 should be measured directly via arterial puncture, although properly acquired transcutaneous oxygen monitor values are also acceptable. Pulse oximetry measurements are not appropriate for interpretation of the hyperoxia test. A Pao_2 >250 mm Hg in both upper and lower extremities on 100% oxygen essentially rules out cardiac disease. These patients are more likely to have a pulmonary cause for their cyanosis. A Pao_2 between 50 and 150 mm Hg on 100% oxygen suggests a cardiac lesion characterized by complete mixing *without* restricted pulmonary blood flow (see Table 24-1). A Pao_2 <50 mm Hg on 100% oxygen indicates a cardiac lesion with parallel circulation *or* a mixing lesion *with* restricted pulmonary blood flow.

TABLE 24-1 Cyanotic Congenital Heart Diseases (Grouped by Hyperoxia Test Results)

Pao_2 between 50 and 150 mm Hg on 100% oxygen (suggesting a cardiac lesion with complete mixing *without* restricted pulmonary blood flow):
Truncus arteriosus
Total anomalous pulmonary venous connection without obstruction
Hypoplastic left heart syndrome (HLHS) and HLHS variants
Pao_2 <50 mm Hg on 100% oxygen (suggesting a cardiac lesion with parallel circulation or a mixing lesion with restricted pulmonary blood flow):
D-transposition of the great arteries *with* or without ventricular septal defect
Ebstein's anomaly
Tricuspid atresia with normally related great arteries and critical pulmonary valve stenosis or atresia
Tetralogy of Fallot with critical pulmonary valve stenosis or atresia
Pulmonary atresia with intact ventricular septum
Critical pulmonary valve stenosis

The combined results of the preceding tests should point the clinician in the right direction as to the source of the cyanosis and may also suggest a likely diagnosis. If a cardiac cause is deemed likely, an **echocardiogram** and cardiology consultation should be obtained.

A **complete blood count** (CBC) with differential, **blood cultures,** and **urine cultures** should also be obtained. If infection is strongly suspected, a **lumbar puncture** may be indicated. A **serum glucose** level may be appropriate.

Treatment

Cyanotic infants require immediate assessment of **airway, breathing, and circulation,** and **stabilization. Prostaglandin** E_1 (PGE$_1$) administration, via continuous intravenous infusion, should be started in any unstable infant with a strong suspicion of congenital heart disease. In newborns with mixing lesions or defects that have ductal-dependent pulmonary or systemic blood flow, PGE$_1$ acts to maintain patency of the ductus arteriosus until definitive surgical treatment can be accomplished. Rarely, the patient with congenital heart disease may become progressively more unstable after the institution of PGE$_1$ therapy, indicating a defect that has obstructed blood flow out of the pulmonary veins or left atrium. These lesions include: hypoplastic left heart syndrome with restrictive or intact foramen ovale; other variants of mitral atresia with restrictive foramen ovale; transposition of the great arteries with an intact ventricular septum and restrictive foramen ovale; and total anomalous pulmonary venous return with obstruction.

Older Children

Patient History

- What is the onset, duration, and frequency of episodes?
- Is there associated coughing, wheezing, or stridor?
- Were there any precipitating factors?
- Have there been previous episodes?
- What is the child's medication history?
- Have the child's growth and development been normal?
- Has the child had any contact with anyone with an infectious disease?
- What is the child's family history?

Physical Examination

As with infants, the physician should check for signs of impending respiratory or circulatory failure and should be prepared to give ventilatory support.

- **Vital signs** should be documented.
- **Respiratory examination.** Rhinorrhea should be noted, and the patient should be examined for signs of otitis media, pharyngitis, and sinusitis.

Hoarseness, drooling, stridor, and breath sounds (e.g., rales, wheezing) should be noted. If epiglottitis is suspected, the pharynx should not be examined.

- **Cardiovascular examination.** The pulse rate and blood pressure in all four extremities should be documented.

> **HINT:** Clubbing refers to selective bullous enlargement of the distal segments (particularly of the dorsal surface) of the fingers and toes. This enlargement is caused by proliferation of connective tissue. Clubbing may be hereditary, idiopathic, or associated with a variety of disorders, including congenital heart disease, infective endocarditis, pulmonary conditions, and gastrointestinal diseases (e.g., regional enteritis, chronic ulcerative colitis, hepatic cirrhosis). It is usually seen only after the first few months of life. Patients with abnormal hemoglobins that cause cyanosis usually do not have clubbing of the fingers and toes.

Laboratory Studies and Diagnostic Modalities

Appropriate studies may include:

- A CBC with differential and a blood culture
- Arterial blood gas analysis (if the cyanosis is severe)
- Pulmonary function tests
- A chest radiograph

Treatment

Cyanosis in the older child is almost always respiratory or neurologic in origin. Care is supportive and may require intubation and ventilation for respiratory failure that may result from intrinsic lung disease or neurologic disease.

Congenital heart disease patients with tetralogy of Fallot may have attacks of paroxysmal hyperpnea and increased cyanosis that occur spontaneously or are associated with crying, agitation, or defecation. These attacks (**tet spells**) occur most commonly in infants 3 to 18 months of age. Treatment involves delivering 100% oxygen, placing the patient in the knee-chest position, and administering intravenous morphine sulfate, propranolol, or phenylephrine.

Suggested Readings

Dahshan A, Donovan GK: Severe methemoglobinemia complicating topical benzocaine use during endoscopy in a toddler: a case report and review of the literature. *Pediatrics* 117(4):e806–e809, 2006.

Sasidharan P: An approach to diagnosis and management of cyanosis and tachypnea in term infants. *Pediatr Clin North Am* 51(4):999–1021, iv, 2004.

Woods WA, McCulloch MA: Cardiovascular emergencies in the pediatric patient. *Emerg Med Clin North Am* 23:1233–1249, 2005.

25 *Dehydration*

Philip R. Spandorfer

INTRODUCTION

Dehydration is a total body fluid deficit and a cause of hypovolemic shock. It occurs when total fluid loss is greater than fluid intake. It is not a diagnosis in itself but rather a symptom of another process. The most common cause of dehydration brought to medical attention is gastroenteritis. Dehydration can be classified based on the degree of dehydration with <5% representing mild dehydration, 5% to 10% representing moderate dehydration, and >10% representing severe dehydration. If serum electrolytes are assessed, the dehydration can be further classified based on serum sodium. The chapter focuses primarily of dehydration from gastroenteritis.

DIFFERENTIAL DIAGNOSIS LIST 🔒⌀

Increased Output
Gastroenteritis
Vomiting
  Pyloric stenosis
  Appendicitis
  Pancreatitis
  Small bowel obstruction
  Intussusception
  Lower lobe pneumonia
  Pyelonephritis
  Increased intracranial
    pressure
Diarrhea
  Malabsorption
  Inflammatory bowel disease
  Celiac disease
  Cystic fibrosis

Increased insensible losses
  (fever, sweating, hyperventilation, etc.)
Renal losses (diabetic ketoacidosis, diabetes insipidus,
  Bartter syndrome, etc.)

Decreased Intake
Voluntary (pharyngitis, stomatitis, respiratory distress, etc.)
Physical restriction (infant/
  elderly, coma, child abuse, etc.)

Translocation of Fluids
Burns
Hypoproteinemic states
  (ascites, peripheral
  edema, etc.)

DIFFERENTIAL DIAGNOSIS DISCUSSION

Gastroenteritis

Physiology

Under normal physiologic conditions, water comprises 70% of lean body mass in children and adults and 75% in infants. Two thirds of the fluid is intracellular and one third is extracellular. Of the extracellular fluid, 75% is interstitial and 25% is intravascular. Fluid that is lost from the body often has an electrolyte composition similar to plasma. Most of the fluid deficit during the early stages of dehydration is from the extracellular space, but with time, the fluid losses equilibrate and fluid leaves the intracellular space. During the recovery phase, fluid administered to the patient is in the extracellular space and will need time to re-equilibrate with the intracellular space.

Etiology

Gastroenteritis can be caused by viral, bacterial, or parasitic pathogens. The predominant cause in developed countries is viral. Rotavirus is known to cause more serious illness than other viral causes. Worldwide, all children have had at least one episode of rotavirus gastroenteritis by 5 years of age.

Clinical Features

Gastroenteritis typically starts with the acute onset of vomiting, which may be persistent and severe. Clinicians should consider other etiologies in a child presenting with vomiting alone, but the subsequent development of diarrhea may clarify a diagnosis of viral gastroenteritis. The overall course of illness typically lasts about 5 to 7 days.

> **HINT:** The onset of abdominal pain prior to the vomiting should make the clinician consider appendicitis.

Children with dehydration from gastroenteritis may develop electrolyte abnormalities. Approximately one third of patients who are moderately dehydrated have hypoglycemia. These children appear listless. Less commonly, patients have elevated serum sodium. This hypernatremia represents a free water deficit. The sodium acts osmotically to draw water from the cellular compartment extracellularly. This results in a state of intracellular dehydration. The acute manifestations of hypernatremia include early neurologic irritability (e.g., seizures). The degree of dehydration may be more difficult to assess in these children because most of the clinical findings of dehydration are caused by decreased extracellular fluid; one clue may be the presence of "doughy" skin. Conversely, hyponatremia results in intracellular swelling. These patients also may present with neurologic symptomatology, primarily seizures, lethargy, and coma.

Evaluation

Evaluation of dehydration focuses on a thorough history and physical examination. Historical points to consider include possible exposures to other children who have been sick, timing of the symptoms, number of episodes of vomiting and diarrhea, or presence of blood or bile. Exposure to well water, camping, or recent travel may raise the suspicion for an etiology other than viral gastroenteritis. High fever with bloody diarrhea would be concerning for bacterial dysentery.

A thorough physical examination can aide in confirming the diagnosis. The examiner should assess the overall appearance of the child for the presence of lethargy or listlessness that may be associated with dehydration. Other common examination features include an assessment of the urine output, the presence and quality of tear production, the quality of the mucous membranes (moist, tacky, or dry), the capillary refill (measured at the distal fingertip, considered prolonged if >2 seconds in an warm ambient environment), assessment of the skin turgor, assessment of the heart rate and distal pulses, as well as assessment of the fontanelle in the infant. Research on assessing the degree of dehydration has been helpful in creating a framework within which to evaluate a dehydrated patient. A recent meta-analysis presents data that are helpful (Table 25-1). If a finding is present, it may increase the likelihood of dehydration. For example, the likelihood ratio for the presence of prolonged capillary refill is 4.1 with a 95% confidence interval that ranges from 1.7 to 9.8. We can interpret this to mean that if prolonged capillary refill is present, then the

TABLE 25-1 **Signs and Symptoms of the Presence of at Least 5% Dehydration**

Finding	Likelihood Ratio If Present (95% CI)	Likelihood Ratio If Absent (95% CI)
Prolonged capillary refill	**4.1 (1.7–9.8)**	0.57 (0.39–0.82)
Abnormal skin turgor	**2.5 (1.5–4.2)**	0.66 (0.57–0.75)
Abnormal respirations	**2.0 (1.5–2.7)**	0.76 (0.62–0.88)
Sunken eyes	1.7 (1.1–2.5)	**0.49 (0.38–0.63)**
Dry mucous membranes	1.7 (1.1–2.6)	**0.41 (0.21–0.79)**
Cool extremity*	1.5, 18.8	0.89, 0.97
Weak pulse*	3.1, 7.2	0.66, 0.96
Absent tears	2.3 (0.9–5.8)	0.54 (0.26–1.13)
Increased heart rate	1.3 (0.8–2.0)	0.82 (0.64–1.05)
Sunken fontanelle	0.9 (0.6–1.3)	1.1 (0.82–1.54)
Poor overall appearance	1.9 (0.97 to 3.8)	**0.46 (0.34 to 0.61)**

Adapted from Steiner MJ, DeWalt DA, Byerley JS: Is this child dehydrated? *JAMA* 291(22):2746–2754, 2004.

*These findings were only evaluated in two studies and a pooled value was not obtained. The range of the point estimates is presented.

The likelihood ratio (LR) is interpreted such that the likelihood of dehydration would increase if the LR if present is >1.0. Clinically useful values have a LR positive value of ≥2 with a 95% confidence interval (CI) that does not cross 1.0. Furthermore, the LR if absent means the likelihood of dehydration would decrease if the sign was absent. Clinically useful values have a LR negative value of <0.5 and have a 95% CI that does not cross 1.0. The values in bold are the clinically helpful values.

odds of the child having at least 5% dehydration are 4.1 times higher than if prolonged capillary refill was not present. The examination findings in the meta-analysis that significantly increase the likelihood of dehydration include prolonged capillary refill, abnormal skin turgor, and abnormal respiratory pattern. Conversely, some findings if they are absent decrease the likelihood of the patient being 5% dehydrated. For example, the likelihood ratio for the absence of poor overall appearance is 0.46 with a 95% confidence interval that ranges from 0.34 to 0.61. We can interpret this to mean that the odds are less than half as likely for the patient to be at least 5% dehydrated if there is a normal general appearance. The findings that would decrease the likelihood of significant dehydration if they are absent include dry mucous membranes, sunken eyes, and poor overall appearance.

Although helpful, these summary statistics on physical examination findings are often hard to implement clinically. However, one high-quality study of a 10-point dehydration scoring system took a subset of four symptoms and was able to demonstrate that the subset of four findings had the same diagnostic accuracy as the larger 10-point dehydration score presented. The 4-point dehydration score consists of poor overall appearance, absent tears, dry mucous membranes, and delayed capillary refill (Table 25-2). One point is awarded for each feature present. The interpretation is that a score of 0 out of the 4 features represents no dehydration present, 1 of the 4 represents mild dehydration (<5%), 2 of the 4 features represents moderate dehydration (5% to 10%), and a score of 3 or 4 of the 4 features represents severe dehydration (>10%). This 4-point system is a clinically useful score because most practitioners already assess and can easily remember these four features.

Electrolytes

There is no role for the routine evaluation of electrolytes in dehydrated patients. They should be checked as directed by the clinical evaluation, particularly if an unusual history or examination finding suggests an electrolyte abnormality. Electrolytes do not assist in determining if dehydration is present; they are helpful to determine the degree of acidosis present and

TABLE 25-2 **Four-Point Dehydration System**

Overall poor appearance
Absent tears
Dry mucous membranes
Delayed capillary refill

Adapted from Gorelick MH, Shaw KN, Murphy KO: Validity and reliability of clinical signs in the diagnosis of dehydration in children. *Pediatrics* 99(5):E6, 1997.
The patient is assigned one point for each feature present. A score of zero indicates no dehydration present. A score of 1 indicates mild dehydration (<5%). A score of 2 indicates moderate dehydration (5%–10%). A score of 3 or 4 indicates severe dehydration (>10%).

if there is a need for specialized treatment because of hypernatremia or hyponatremia. It is important to appreciate that approximately one third of moderately dehydrated patients are concurrently hypoglycemic.

Treatment

Emergency Treatment

Emergency treatment focuses on identifying and addressing life-threatening issues. The presence of severe dehydration and shock requires aggressive fluid resuscitation. The clinician should place an intravenous line and administer sequential 20 mL/kg boluses of isotonic fluids. Therapy is directed at restoring circulating volume and perfusing vital organs. If there is a need, blood products can be used to restore intravascular volume. After the shock has been addressed, appropriate therapy can be continued.

The fluid deficit can be calculated from the percentage of dehydration present. The fluid lost during gastroenteritis has a specific gravity near 1. Hence the weight loss approximates the fluid deficit. By determining the percent dehydration as discussed previously or if a well and dehydrated weight are known, the fluid deficit can be determined. Five percent of a liter is 50 mL. Hence 5% dehydration requires 50 mL/kg fluid replacement. Likewise, 10% dehydration is 100 mL/kg.

> **HINT:** Mild (<5%) dehydration requires about 50 mL/kg fluid replacement; moderate (5% to 10%) dehydration requires 100 mL/kg fluid replacement.

> **HINT:** The fluid deficit can be administered over a 4-hour period. Therapy can be initiated under medical supervision. If the patient is performing oral rehydration therapy (ORT) well, they can be discharged to home to continue the fluid replacement.

> **HINT:** Ondansetron is helpful in decreasing emesis associated with gastroenteritis. The oral dissolving tablet can be used prior to starting therapy.

Oral Rehydration Therapy

ORT is recommended as the initial therapy of choice by the American Academy of Pediatrics, the World Health Organization, and the Centers for Disease Control and Prevention for mildly and moderately dehydrated children and can even be used for severely dehydrated children. ORT is not simply giving the patient Pedialyte or a sports beverage to drink. That would be considered an oral challenge. Rather, ORT is the frequent administration of small volumes of an appropriate oral rehydration solution on a regular schedule. Although ORT is effective at rehydrating moderately dehydrated children in an emergency department (ED) setting, its use in the United States has been limited. The most frequent obstacles to successful oral rehydration in the ED are false perceptions that oral rehydration is too slow or not a definitive procedure. Physicians and nurses hold these beliefs as frequently as parents. Generally, 5 minutes spent preparing for and describing ORT to the family reduces or eliminates these obstacles. ORT spares the child the pain of an intravenous (IV) line, promotes more direct parental involvement in the management of the child's dehydration, and teaches the parents a skill that can be used for the ongoing illness and the next time the child becomes dehydrated. After starting ORT, frequent reassessments should be made. If the patient is not tolerating the therapy, then an IV line should be started and IV fluids administered. The administration of ondansetron prior to initiating ORT has improved the success rate of ORT to >80%. If a patient is going to fail with ORT, it generally happens early in the treatment process, typically within 30 minutes.

> **HINT:** 10 mL of unflavored Pedialyte administered with a syringe over a 5-minute period is one method of ORT. The volume can be increased as tolerated and the interval can be shortened.

Use of an appropriate oral rehydration solution (ORS) assists in ensuring success. The physiology of ORT uses the passive absorption of water from the intestines using the sodium-glucose cotransport mechanism. This cotransport is maintained even in the case of severe gastroenteritis when there is significant sloughing of the brush border of the small intestine. The optimal stoichiometric carbohydrate (i.e., glucose) to sodium ratio is 1:1. This ratio is maintained by the World Health Organization in their two ORSs (Table 25-3). The original WHO ORS was developed for cholera and has a higher sodium concentration of 90 mEq/L. The WHO has recently manufactured a second ORS that has a reduced sodium concentration of 75 mEq/L. This second ORS is designed for treatment of dehydration from both viral and bacterial gastroenteritis. Other commercial products are designed for the rehydration phase of ORT, specifically Rehydralyte. The more commonly used Pedialyte is actually a maintenance solution and not technically a rehydration solution, however, it is effective at treating mild to moderate dehydration from gastroenteritis. The commercial products have a higher glucose concentration and therefore deviate from the 1:1 ratio of carbohydrate to sodium. Often, children may refuse the ORS because it has a salty taste.

TABLE 25-3 Appropriate Oral Rehydration Solutions

Solution	Sodium (mEq/L)	Potassium (mEq/L)	Chloride (mEq/L)	Base (mEq/L)	Carbohydrate %(mmol/L)	Osmolarity (mmol/L)	Carbohydrate-to-Sodium Ratio
WHO solution (1)	90	20	80	10	2% (111)	311	1:1
WHO solution (2)	75	20	65	10	1.4% (75)	245	1:1
Rehydralyte	75	20	65	30	2.5% (139)	329	2:1
Pedialyte	45	20	35	30	2.5% (139)	269	3:1

TABLE 25-4 Inappropriate Oral Rehydration Solutions

Solution	Sodium (mEq/L)	Potassium (mEq/L)	Chloride (mEq/L)	Base (mEq/L)	Carbohydrate %(mmol/L)	Osmolarity (mmol/L)	Carbohydrate-to-Sodium Ratio
Gatorade	20	3	17	3	4.6% (58)	330	12:1
Coca-Cola	2	<1		13	12%(112)	>600	—
Apple juice	3	32	2	0	12.4% (120)	730	230:1
Chicken broth	250	8	250	0	0	500	—

This tends to occur more commonly in older children or children who are minimally dehydrated. As an alternative in mild dehydration, a sports beverage diluted 1:1 with water may be more palatable. Administration of a saltine cracker would increase the sodium administered for this rehydration technique. Table 25-4 lists the fluids that are not appropriate for rehydration solutions for dehydration from gastroenteritis.

> **HINT:** Syringe administration often helps the child to swallow the ORS despite the salty taste. Children may refuse the ORS when offered in a cup.

ORT may fail. Typical reasons include patient refusal, parental noncompliance with administration recommendations, persistent emesis, and losses greater than the amount of fluid administered. Additionally, children and parents have a hard time staying awake and performing rehydration during the middle of the night. Patients dehydrated from stomatitis or pharyngitis may refuse oral fluid because of pain. Addressing pain in these patients may assist in avoiding IV fluids.

Intravenous Fluid Therapy

If administration of ondansetron and an attempt at ORT was unsuccessful or the patient is severely dehydrated, then IV fluid rehydration is warranted. Current recommendations for IV fluid rehydration focus on goal-directed therapy. Replacement of the fluid deficit and maintaining ongoing losses are the primary goals. Sequential fluid boluses may be required with frequent reassessment to assess for improved perfusion, urine output, continued emesis, and so on. Boluses should be made with isotonic fluids; frequently normal saline or lactated Ringer's solution is used. The bolus volume is 20 mL/kg. Glucose should not be included in the bolus because the amount of glucose in a 20 mL/kg bolus would be two to four times the amount of glucose required for documented hypoglycemia. After the bolus volume has been administered, glucose-containing IV fluid can be started at 1.5 times maintenance. The child should be encouraged to take enteral feeds. Younger children may require hospitalization until they demonstrate adequate oral intake. Older children can be rehydrated in the ED and discharged to home to continue the therapy unless extenuating circumstances require the continued administration of IV fluids.

Electrolyte Abnormalities (See Chapter 32, "Electrolyte Disturbances")

Hypoglycemia is common in dehydrated patients, particularly patients who are moderately dehydrated. ORT addresses the hypoglycemia by providing glucose in the treatment phase. During IV fluid therapy, the practitioner should assess for hypoglycemia as indicated. Treatment for documented hypoglycemia is 0.5 g/kg of glucose. This amount can be easily calculated by using the "rule of 50." Fifty divided by the concentration of dextrose solution to be used (e.g., D5, D10, D25, D50) provides the number of milliliters per kilogram that equal 0.5 g/kg of glucose.

Suggested Readings

Gorelick MH, Shaw KN, Murphy KO: Validity and reliability of clinical signs in the diagnosis of dehydration in children. *Pediatrics* 99(5): E6, 1997.

Harting L, Bellemare S, Wiebe N, et al.: Oral versus intravenous rehydration for treating dehydration due to gastroenteritis in children. *Cochrane Database Syst Rev* 3:CD004390, 2006.

Spandorfer PR, Alessandrini EA, Joffe MD, et al.: Oral versus intravenous rehydration of moderately dehydrated children: a randomized, controlled trial. *Pediatrics* 115(2):295–301, 2005.

Steiner MJ, DeWalt DA, Byerley JS: Is this child dehydrated? *JAMA* 291(22):2746–2754, 2004.

INTRODUCTION

Diabetes mellitus is a disorder of glucose metabolism characterized by **hyperglycemia** caused by insulin deficiency. Diabetes encompasses several clinical syndromes including, but not limited to, **type I diabetes mellitus (T1DM),** characterized by rapid onset, a tendency toward ketoacidosis, and absolute insulin deficiency; and **type 2 diabetes (T2DM),** associated with obesity, insulin resistance, a lesser likelihood of ketoacidosis, and nonabsolute dependence on insulin for survival. Both types of diabetes are associated with the same long-term complications. T1DM affects approximately 1 in 350 children by the age of 18 and is more common in children of European background. T2DM is more commonly seen in African American, Native American, and Latino children, but its prevalence is increasing in all ethnic groups.

DIFFERENTIAL DIAGNOSIS LIST 🔒

Infectious Disorders
Urinary tract infection (UTI)
Gastroenteritis
Pneumonia
Sepsis

Toxic Disorders
Salicylate ingestion
Steroid use
Diuretic use

Endocrine and Metabolic Disorders
Hypercalcemia

Diabetes insipidus
Inborn error of metabolism

Miscellaneous Disorders
Renal glucosuria
Stress hyperglycemia

Psychosocial Disorders
Psychogenic polydipsia
Enuresis

EVALUATION OF DIABETES

Patient History
- **Polyuria, polydipsia,** and **polyphagia** are classic symptoms.
- **Weight loss** and **poor growth** may go undetected.
- **Nausea, vomiting,** and **lethargy** occur as the child's illness progresses to diabetic ketoacidosis (DKA).
- **A precipitating event** (intercurrent illness or stress) often prompts medical attention.

Physical Examination

Physical examination is usually normal early in the course of disease. Later findings can include the following:

- **Signs of dehydration** (e.g., tachycardia, poor skin perfusion, hypotension)
- **Hyperpnea (Kussmaul respirations)**, a sign of metabolic acidosis
- **Fruity odor to the breath**, a sign of ketosis

Laboratory Studies

The diagnosis of diabetes may be made in three ways:

- **Fasting blood glucose** level ≥126 mg/dL.
- **Random blood glucose** level ≥200 mg/dL in the setting of symptoms of diabetes.
- **Two-hour blood glucose** level ≥200 mg/dL during an oral glucose tolerance test.
  - **Urinalysis** reveals glycosuria and may include ketonuria (T1DM).
  - **Glycosylated hemoglobin** is elevated.

Other biochemical parameters may be normal until the development of diabetic ketoacidosis, at which time:

- **Serum electrolyte panel** may reveal hyponatremia (sodium level <136 mEq/L) from hyperglycemia and hypertriglyceridemia, hypokalemia or hyperkalemia (a potassium level of <4.0 mEq/L or >6.0 mEq/L, respectively), or a metabolic acidosis (bicarbonate level <15 mEq/L).
- **Arterial or venous blood gases** may reveal a metabolic acidosis (pH <7.3, partial pressure of carbon dioxide [P_{CO_2}] <35 mm Hg).
- **Complete blood cell count** may reveal elevated white blood cell count even in the absence of infection.

DIFFERENTIAL DIAGNOSIS

- **UTI** and **nocturnal enuresis.** The early signs of diabetes (i.e., polyuria and nocturia) may be mistaken for UTI or nocturnal enuresis. Urinalysis, however, demonstrates the presence of glucose and ketones and the absence of markers of infection.
- **Renal glucosuria** (a condition in which glucose is excreted in the urine at normal blood glucose levels) may be mistaken for diabetes. Diabetes should never be diagnosed by the presence of glucosuria alone: An elevated blood glucose level is required for the diagnosis of diabetes.
- **Other metabolic disorders** may present with acidosis and dehydration, but a history of polyuria, polyphagia, and weight loss with an elevated blood glucose is characteristic of diabetes.

- **Gastroenteritis and surgical abdomen.** The abdominal pain and vomiting of DKA may be mistaken for gastroenteritis or a surgical abdomen, but DKA may be differentiated not only from these disorders but also from other metabolic diseases by the distinct history of polyuria, polydipsia, and a characteristic fruity odor to the breath.
- **Intercurrent febrile illnesses** or the **administration of glucocorticoids** for inflammatory conditions may cause an insulin-resistant state and precipitate hyperglycemia, glucosuria, and even small amounts of ketonuria. These conditions must be differentiated from true diabetes. In patients who do not have diabetes, resolution of the fever and acute illness or discontinuation of the medications should result in normalization of the blood sugar. It is important to go back and determine whether the typical symptoms of polydipsia and polyuria are present: In the absence of these symptoms, the diagnosis of diabetes is less likely. Occasionally, however, a latent case of true diabetes may be discovered. In these cases, the presence of anti-islet cell antibodies or an elevated hemoglobin A1c value may be useful in establishing the proper diagnosis.
- **Asthma** or **pneumonia.** The Kussmaul respirations that occur with progressive acidosis may resemble asthma or pneumonia, but auscultation and radiography reveal clear lung fields.

TREATMENT OF DIABETES

Optimal care requires the efforts of the child, the family, and a team of physicians, nurses, dietitians, and counselors specializing in the treatment of children with diabetes. The physician's primary responsibilities are the **prompt recognition of symptoms** leading to a definitive diagnosis, **referral** to a pediatric diabetes center, and **continued supervision** of the child's medical care. Children with diabetes should attend a multidisciplinary pediatric diabetes center at least every 3 months or more frequently if treatment goals are not being met.

Treatment goals are to maintain blood glucose levels as close to normal as possible, avoidance of severe hypoglycemia, and maintenance of the child's normal physical and psychosocial growth and development. To accomplish these goals, the child must not only take insulin or oral antidiabetic medications but also monitor the blood sugar several times during the day, exercise, and adhere to the prescribed meal plan. Family members should be trained to monitor blood sugars, give insulin, and recognize and treat low blood sugar reactions. **Psychosocial factors are critical** in the management of children with diabetes, and potential problems should be addressed by experienced behavioral or family therapists.

TABLE 26-1 Pharmacokinetics of Common Insulin Preparations

Insulin	Onset	Peak	Duration
Rapid-acting insulin analogs: Lispro (Humalog) Aspart (NovoLog) Glulisine (Apidra)	10–15 min	1–3 hr	3–5 hr
Short acting (regular)	0.5–1 hr	2–4 hr	4–8 hr
Intermediate acting (NPH)	2–4 hr	4–10 hr	10–18 hr
Long-acting analogs: Glargine (Lantus)	2–3 hr	None	24+ hr
Detemir (Levemir)	1 hr	None	Up to 24 hr

Insulin

The goal of diabetes therapy is to maintain the blood glucose levels as close to normal as possible. For the child with T1DM, this means reliance on multiple doses of insulin daily. These may be administered either by subcutaneous injections via syringe or via continuous subcutaneous insulin infusion by a portable wearable pump (insulin pump therapy). In both cases, insulin dosages are used to mimic the body's pattern of basal insulin delivery between meals and overnight, with spikes in insulin release (boluses) for meal-related carbohydrates. Insulin doses must be individually titrated, and even in one individual, insulin needs typically change from day to day because of variations in meals, physical activity, illness, and other factors. Table 26-1 shows the most commonly used insulin preparations. Table 26-2 gives recommended insulin adjustments.

Fixed-dose (**split mix**) insulin regimens are often employed early in the course of diabetes while children and families are still learning to manage the disease. Insulin doses are generally kept constant and given as mixtures of rapid/intermediate acting or rapid/long acting to minimize the number of daily injections. Such regimens typically consist of the following:

- Two-thirds total daily dose before breakfast—one third as rapid acting, two thirds as intermediate acting.
- One-third total daily dose before dinner—half as rapid acting, half as intermediate or long acting (the intermediate- or long-acting insulin can alternatively be given at bedtime).
- Flexible (**basal-bolus**) regimens require more frequent injections than split-mix regimens but are ultimately more effective in controlling both hyperglycemia and hypoglycemia. In these regimens, a fixed dose of long-acting insulin analog is given once or twice daily to provide the basal insulin requirement, and smaller doses of rapid-acting insulin analogs are given with each meal or snack based on the carbohydrate

TABLE 26-2 Adjustments for Fixed-Dose Insulin Regimens*

Blood Glucose	Time	Recommended Action
High	Pre-breakfast	Increase evening intermediate- or long-acting insulin; if this results in nighttime lows, may need to eliminate bedtime snack.
Low	Pre-breakfast	Decrease evening intermediate- or long-acting insulin or increase bedtime snack content.
High	Pre-lunch	Increase morning rapid-acting insulin first; then intermediate acting if needed.
Low	Pre-lunch	Decrease morning rapid-insulin first; then intermediate acting if needed.
High	Pre-dinner	Increase morning intermediate-acting insulin; if this results in midday lows, extra shot of rapid-acting insulin may be needed after school.
Low	Pre-dinner	Decrease morning intermediate-acting insulin.
High	Bedtime	Increase evening rapid-insulin.
Low	Bedtime	Decrease evening rapid-acting insulin.

*For basal-bolus regimens, the long-acting insulin analog is titrated to produce a fasting morning blood glucose level in the target range. Meal bolus doses are titrated to yield normal blood glucose levels at the next meal.

content of the coming meal and the blood glucose level at the time of the meal, for example:

- **At breakfast:** 0.4 to 0.5 U/kg long-acting insulin analog.
- **Before each meal:** 1 U rapid-acting insulin analog for every 15 g of carbohydrate in the coming meal *plus* 1 U for every 100 mg/dL elevation of the blood glucose (BG) level over the target (e.g., 1 extra unit if BG = 200 and target BG = 100).

Insulin pumps have emerged as a preferred means of insulin delivery because of the ability to vary basal and bolus rates easily. Basal rates can be decreased to prevent nighttime or exercise-related hypoglycemia or increased for periods of illness. Bolus doses can be given without the need for a separate injection; and the newer pumps contain software that can determine the proper bolus dose when the current blood glucose level and carbohydrate content of the coming meal are entered.

Insulin injection sites should be rotated among the arms, legs, buttocks, and stomach to avoid lipoatrophy or lipohypertrophy. Insulin pump infusion catheters are commonly inserted in the abdomen or buttocks and should be changed every 2 to 3 days.

Oral antidiabetic medications are not indicated in the treatment of T1DM in children but play an important role in T2DM. The insulin sensitizer **metformin** may be considered the first-line medication if lifestyle interventions such as diet and physical activity are insufficient to normalize blood glucose levels. Metformin may be initiated at a dose of 500 mg daily and increased to a maximum of 1,000 mg twice daily. Common side effects are nausea, anorexia, and gastrointestinal discomfort, which may be lessened if the drug is taken with food and the dose increased gradually. Insulin secretagogues (sulfonylureas and meglitinide analogs) and the other insulin sensitizers (rosiglitazone, pioglitazone) are less commonly used because of the relative scarcity of pediatric data and the side effect of weight gain.

Complications of Insulin Therapy

Hypoglycemia is the most common acute complication of diabetes management. Typical symptoms include hunger, headache, lethargy, dizziness, irritability, confusion, sweating, and tachycardia. Mild symptoms are easily treated with oral glucose (e.g., glucose tablets, orange juice). **Severe hypoglycemia** may lead to seizures and coma. These are treated with glucagon, 1 mg, given intramuscularly. All children with diabetes should carry oral glucose tablets with them at all times and keep glucagon at home. **Recurrent hypoglycemia** should be corrected aggressively.

Intercurrent Illnesses and Diabetic Ketoacidosis

Intercurrent illnesses should be managed with more frequent blood glucose monitoring, and supplementary insulin if needed for hyperglycemia. It should be stressed that children with T1DM always needs insulin, even if they are not eating because of illness; in this instance, the short-acting insulin may be withheld and the long-acting insulin reduced to prevent hypoglycemia. Urine ketones should be monitored as an indication to increase insulin dosages. If blood glucose cannot be maintained in the normal range, intravenous fluids containing dextrose may be necessary. Table 26-3 describes the management of ketosis and DKA.

Monitoring

The goals of **blood glucose monitoring** are to gauge the effectiveness of the current medication regimen and minimize episodes of hypoglycemia. The availability of accurate, easy-to-use home glucose meters has facilitated home monitoring of blood sugars and adjustment of therapy. The blood glucose should be monitored before each meal and before the bedtime snack, with more frequent monitoring when the child is sick, vomiting, or having symptoms of hypoglycemia. Glucose levels 2 to 3 hours after meals may be checked to gauge the effectiveness of meal-dose insulin or in patients not on insulin therapy, to determine whether to initiate insulin. When blood sugar levels are out of the target range, prompt

TABLE 26-3 Guidelines to Treatment of Acute Illness

Mild Illness ("Sick Days")

Insulin

Variable; stress of illness may increase insulin requirements, particularly in presence of fever and ketones; however, smaller more frequent doses may be needed if child is not eating well or vomiting.

Fluids

Increase oral fluid intake to prevent dehydration, reduce hyperglycemia, and clear ketones; sugar-containing fluids preferable if glucose levels are low and child requires more insulin to clear ketones.

Monitoring

More frequent blood glucose monitoring is important during sick days; every 2 to 3 hours for young children or in setting of vomiting or decreased oral intake.

Ketoacidosis (DKA): Glucose >200 mg/dL, pH <7.3, or Bicarbonate <15 mEq/L

Intravenous Fluids

10–20 mL/kg 0.9% saline bolus to restore intravascular volume, then replace deficit slowly over 48 hours using isotonic fluids (0.9% saline).
Nothing by mouth until acidosis corrected (serum HCO_3 =15 mEq/L).

Sodium

Deficit 10 mEq/kg—replace with normal saline in rehydration fluid.

Potassium

Deficit 5–10 mEq/L—start after patient urinates.
If K >4.0, add 40 mEq/L.
If K <4.0, add 60 mEq/L.
Give potassium as 1:1 with potassium chloride to potassium phosphate.

Insulin

0.1 U/kg per hour (the amount of glucose in the intravenous fluids and the rate of insulin infusion should be titrated to lower the blood sugar 50 to 100 mg/dL per hour

modifications should be made to the insulin regimen (see Table 26-2). Urine should also be monitored for ketones during periods of intercurrent illness, fever, vomiting, or when the blood sugar persistently exceeds 240 mg/dL.

Diet

Medical nutrition therapy is central to the management of diabetes in children but differs markedly between T1DM and T2DM. For children with T1DM, knowledge of the carbohydrate content of meals and snacks is important for regulating blood glucose levels. Children on fixed insulin regimens should aim for consistency in carbohydrate content (e.g., 60 to 75 g for each meal, 15 to 20 g for snacks) so that the proper amount of insulin is "matched" for the meal. Children on flexible insulin regimens may vary their meal-related insulin dosages depending on the carbohydrate content of their meal (e.g., 1 U of rapid-acting insulin ____ ingested carbohydrate). For children·with T2DM, in ____ insulin resistance may be a significant factor, adheren ____ designed to promote gradual, sustained weight loss m ____ tant than the actual carbohydrate content. Low-carbohydrate diets are not recommended in children with T1DM; these diets promote weight loss but have not been well studied in children with T2DM.

Exercise

A regular exercise program is important for optimal health and blood sugar control in the child with T1DM, and it is absolutely necessary for management of the child with T2DM. Exercise lowers blood sugar and insulin requirements and improves insulin sensitivity. It is also a useful tool to lower the blood sugar level acutely. Vigorous exercise should be avoided in the presence of ketosis, however.

Psychosocial Factors

The management of diabetes is particularly stressful for the child and whole family unit. Children should be screened regularly for signs of depression, anxiety, and stress. Similarly, because the safe management of a child with diabetes requires responsible care on the part of the adult caretakers in the house, the clinician should also assess parenting skills, coping strategies, and adjustment in the parent, along with parent-child interactions. Referral to a behavioral or family therapist is necessary when problems are identified.

Suggested Readings

Pinhas-Hamiel O, Zeitler P: Clinical presentation and treatment of type 2 diabetes in children. *Pediatr Diabetes* 8(Suppl 9):16–27, 2007.

Silverstein J, Klingensmith G, Copeland K, et al.: Care of children and adolescents with type 1 diabetes: a statement of the American Diabetes Association. *Diabetes Care* 28:186–212, 2005.

Tamborlane WV, Swan K, Sikes KA, et al.: The renaissance of insulin pump treatment in childhood type 1 diabetes. *Rev Endocr Metab Disord* 7:205–213, 2006.

Wolfsdorf J, Glaser N, Sperling MA: Diabetic ketoacidosis in infants, children, and adolescents: a consensus statement from the American Diabetes Association. *Diabetes Care* 29:1150–11599, 2006.

Diarrhea, Acute

Catherine C. Wiley

INTRODUCTION

Acute diarrhea is defined as stools with **increased water content** that occur at **increased frequency** for a period of **<5 to 7 days.** Most cases of acute diarrhea are of infectious (predominantly viral) origin and are self-limited. Approximately 5% of children with acute diarrhea require medical evaluation. The differential diagnostic considerations for acute diarrhea overlap with those for chronic diarrhea (see Chapter 28, "Diarrhea, Chronic").

DIFFERENTIAL DIAGNOSIS LIST 🔒

Infectious Causes
Viruses
  Rotavirus
  Noroviruses
  Enteric adenoviruses
  Enteroviruses
  Astroviruses
  Caliciviruses
  Hepatitis A virus
Bacteria
  Salmonella species
  Shigella species
  Campylobacter species
  Yersinia enterocolitica
  Pathogenic *Escherichia coli*
  Aeromonas
  Clostridium difficile
  Vibrio species
Parasites
  Giardia species
  Cryptosporidium species
  Entamoeba histolytica
  Blastocystis hominis
Parenteral
  Otitis media
  Urinary tract infection (UTI)
  Hepatitis
  Sepsis

Toxic Causes
Foodborne illness
Pharmacologic agents—iron, laxatives, antibiotics
Plant or mushroom toxicity
Household cleaners or soap
Serotonin syndrome
Neonatal drug withdrawal

Metabolic or Genetic Causes
Adrenal insufficiency
Congenital adrenal hyperplasia (CAH)
Hyperthyroidism

Inflammatory Causes
Appendicitis
Inflammatory bowel disease
Eosinophilic gastroenteritis

Anatomic Causes
Intussusception
Partial obstruction

Miscellaneous Causes
Dietary factors—malnutrition, specific food intolerance (e.g., lactose intolerance), overfeeding, sorbitol

Systemic illness—hemolytic uremic syndrome (HUS), Henoch-Schönlein purpura, immunodeficiency

Functional—irritable bowel syndrome

DIFFERENTIAL DIAGNOSIS DISCUSSION

Infectious Diarrhea

Etiology

As noted previously, infectious diarrhea can be **viral, bacterial,** or **parasitic** in origin. Transmission is usually by the fecal-oral route. Adolescents may have diarrhea or proctitis following the sexual transmission of *Neisseria gonorrhoeae, Treponema pallidum, Chlamydia trachomatis,* or herpes simplex virus (HSV).

Clinical Features

Infectious diarrhea most often affects young children, especially those in child care. Children commonly present with crampy abdominal pain, vomiting, and 6 to 10 watery bowel movements per day. Associated symptoms (e.g., fever, vomiting, abdominal pain, rash, joint pain) often support an infectious cause. On examination, the abdomen is usually nondistended and soft, with diffuse tenderness. Bowel sounds may be hyperactive.

Although the clinical syndrome is rarely specific for a particular pathogen, diagnostic clues do exist (Table 27-1). The history may also provide clues regarding the cause:

- There is a **seasonal predilection** for many pathogens; viral infections are more common during the winter, and bacterial infections occur more frequently in the summer.
- The abrupt onset of diarrhea characterized by the passage of more than four stools per day and no vomiting prior to the onset of diarrhea suggests **bacterial enteritis.**
- Bloody diarrhea and fever are seen most commonly in **bacterial enteritis,** although **parasitic** (*Cryptosporidium*) infection should be considered in children with these symptoms who attend child care.
- A **history of contact** with other ill individuals, **child-care attendance, travel,** or certain exposures may provide clues regarding the specific causative agent. For example, *G. lamblia* infection is more common in individuals who drink well water or contaminated water while camping, and *Campylobacter, Salmonella,* and *G. lamblia* can be transmitted through contact with pets. Infectious organisms common to the child-care setting include rotavirus and other viruses, *Giardia, Cryptosporidium, Campylobacter,* and *Shigella* species.

TABLE 27-1 Common Causes of Infectious Diarrhea

Causative Agent	Peak Age	Season	Incubation Period	Fever	Character of Stools
Rotavirus	4 months–3 yr	Winter	1–3 days	Variable	Watery, foul smelling
Noroviruses	School age	Fall–Winter	12–96 hr	Rare	Loose to watery
Salmonella	1 month–2 yr	Summer	8–48 hr	Common	Green, slimy, "rotten egg" odor, occasionally bloody
Shigella	1–5 yr	Summer	1–7 days	Common	Watery, bloody, odorless
Campylobacter	1–5 yr	Summer	1–7 days	Common	Watery; may be bloody
Yersinia	1 month–2 yr	Winter	1–14 days	Common	Mucoid; may be bloody
Giardia lamblia	School age	All year	1–4 wk	Rare	Loose, greasy, pale, and of protracted duration
Entamoeba histolytica	All ages	All year	1–4 wk	Variable	May be mucoid, bloody
Cryptosporidia	1–5 yr	Summer	2–14 days	Common	Watery; may be bloody

- **Swimming** in contaminated water is a common source of exposure to infectious organisms, particularly *Shigella, Giardia, Cryptosporidia*, and *Entamoeba* species and *E. Coli* 0157-H7. Many waterborne parasites are resistant to chlorination.
- *C. difficile* infection occurs predominantly in children who have received **antibiotics** during the preceding 3 weeks.
- **Antacid therapy with H₂ blockers** increases susceptibility to bacterial pathogens.

Evaluation

In most patients with infectious diarrhea, laboratory studies are not required. However, the following studies may be indicated:

- **Serum electrolyte panel.** In children with moderate to severe dehydration (see Chapter 25, "Dehydration," Table 25-3), a serum electrolyte panel may reveal hyponatremia or hypernatremia and significant acidosis, especially if the diarrhea is prolonged. Serum electrolytes may be normal despite significant dehydration.
- A **complete blood cell (CBC) count** may show hemoconcentration caused by dehydration or **bandemia** associated with bacterial enteritis.
- **Stool culture** is generally recommended for hospitalized patients, patients with severe or bloody diarrhea, patients who appear toxic, patients who have been exposed to bacterial enteritis, patients with persistent diarrhea on dietary therapy, patients in child care or institutional settings, and patients with underlying chronic conditions. Some laboratories test for *Campylobacter, Yersinia,* and pathogenic *E. coli* only by special request. *C. difficile* culture and toxin analysis may be helpful in children with antibiotic exposure. (Of note, the asymptomatic carrier rate for *C. difficile* is 30% to 50% in neonates and 3% after 12 months of age.)
- **Serology.** Rotazyme, an enzyme-linked immunoassay for rotavirus, is useful in hospitalized patients, in patients with prolonged illness, and for epidemiologic purposes (e.g., during outbreaks). Identification of *Cryptosporidium* requires use of a modified auramine acid–fast stain or serologic testing.
- **Ova and parasites (O&P).** A stool examination for the presence of O&P should be considered for children who attend child care or who have traveled outside of the country, particularly if the diarrhea is protracted.

Treatment

Antimicrobial agents are not necessary for many patients despite bacterial enteritis. **Antibiotics are contraindicated in some settings.** For example, antibiotic administration may prolong intestinal carriage of *Salmonella* and may increase the risk of HUS in *E. coli* 0157:H7 infection.

- **Campylobacter jejuni.** Erythromycin can be administered orally for 5 to 7 days to reduce fecal shedding, shorten illness, and prevent relapse. Azithromycin is an alternative therapy. In severely ill children, consider intravenous administration of erythromycin, cefotaxime, or an aminoglycoside. Tetracycline is an alternative treatment for children ≥8 years.
- **Shigella.** Most *Shigella* infections do not require treatment. To shorten the duration of illness and reduce contagion, trimethoprim-sulfamethoxazole (TMP-SMX) administered orally or intravenously for 5 days is the treatment of choice. If the organism is sensitive, ampicillin can be used instead. Ceftriaxone and azithromycin are alternatives. Because of the increasing incidence of resistance, antimicrobial susceptibility testing should be performed on all isolates.
- **Salmonella.** Enterocolitis should only be treated in those patients at risk for developing invasive disease, such as infants <3 months, children with hemoglobinopathies (including sickle cell disease), children with malignancies, immunocompromised children (e.g., those with AIDS, those undergoing therapy with immunosuppressive agents, and those with splenic dysfunction), children with cardiac disease at risk for endocarditis, children with *Salmonella typhi* infection, and children with *Salmonella* bacteremia or enteric fever. Antimicrobial susceptibility testing should be performed on all isolates because of the increasing incidence of resistance. If the organism is sensitive to ampicillin or TMP-SMX, one of these agents can be used, with treatment lasting 7 to 14 days. Alternatives are intravenous ceftriaxone or cefotaxime. Neonates and patients with meningitis may require different doses, and patients with osteomyelitis need extended treatment (e.g., for 4 to 6 weeks).
- **Clostridium difficile.** Metronidazole should be administered orally for 7 to 10 days after discontinuing administration of other systemic antimicrobials if possible. Vancomycin can be administered orally for seriously ill patients or for those in whom treatment has failed.
- **Vibrio cholera.** Most *Vibrio* infections do not require treatment. Tetracycline for 3 to 5 days is the treatment of choice in children ≥8 years. TMP-SMX, doxycycline, and cefotaxime are alternative therapies.
- **Enterotoxigenic E. coli.** Treatment is not typically recommended, but TMP-SMX for 3 days may be administered.
- **Enteroinvasive E. coli.** TMP-SMX or ampicillin (if the organism is sensitive) may be used. Azithromycin is an alternative therapy.
- **Giardia lamblia.** Metronidazole (5 to 7 days), tinidazole, or nitazoxanide are the drugs of choice. Furazolidone orally for 7 to 10 days is an alternative therapy.

- *Cryptosporidium.* Nitazoxanide is the agent of choice. This drug has limited efficacy in HIV-infected patients.
- *Entamoeba histolytica.* Metronidazole orally or intravenously for 10 days or tinidazole for 3 days can be administered to patients with symptomatic colitis or extraintestinal disease. Either method of treatment must be followed by iodoquinol administered orally for 20 days or paromomycin for 7 days. Additional agents may be needed in the case of severe or invasive disease. If the patient is asymptomatic, iodoquinol alone is used for 20 days. Alternative treatments for asymptomatic infection are also available.
- *Cyclospora.* TMP-SMX is administered for 7 to 10 days.

Foodborne Illness

Etiology

Foodborne diarrhea may occur secondary to ingestion of an infectious agent or ingestion of a preformed toxin. A number of pathogens may be transmitted in contaminated water or food or via food handlers. Table 27-2 lists the common sources of foodborne diarrhea.

TABLE 27-2 Common Sources of Foodborne Gastroenteritis

Source	Infectious Agent or Toxin
Meat	*Staphylococcus aureus* toxins
	Clostridium perfringens toxin
	Pathogenic *Escherichia coli*
	Campylobacter
	Salmonella
	Aeromonas
Pork chitterlings	*Yersinia enterocolitica, Bacillus cereus*
Poultry	*Salmonella*
	Shigella
	Campylobacter jejuni
Eggs	*Salmonella*
Shellfish	*Salmonella*
	Vibrio cholerae
	Vibrio parahaemolyticus
	Noroviruses
	Caliciviruses
Fish	Ciguatera
	Scombroid
Raw milk	*Salmonella*
	Campylobacter jejuni
	Yersinia enterocolitica
Fried rice, dried fruit, powdered milk	*Bacillus cereus*
Mushrooms	Mushroom toxin
Produce	*Shigella, Aeromonas, Salmonella, E. coli* 0157-H7
Apple cider	*E. coli* 0157-H7

Clinical Features

The **simultaneous, acute onset of gastroenteritis** among individuals who have shared a meal is typical of foodborne illness. These illnesses generally last **<24 hours.** Vomiting is prominent in most food poisonings and usually has its onset prior to diarrhea. The severe vomiting of *S. aureus* toxin illness begins 1 to 6 hours after ingestion of contaminated meat products. Symptoms of *C. perfringens* toxin illness are seen 12 hours after ingestion and typically include secretory diarrhea without vomiting.

> **HINT:** The onset of symptoms the same day as the ingestion suggests that a preformed toxin is the causative agent. Symptoms that begin 24 hours to several days after ingestion suggest enteric pathogens as the cause.

Evaluation

Food poisoning is mainly a clinical diagnosis. Stool cultures may be obtained for detection of enteric pathogens. *C. perfringens* infection may be confirmed by culture of the contaminated food source.

Treatment

Generally, only supportive care is required. Antimicrobial administration is recommended for some enteric pathogens.

Intussusception

Intussusception is discussed in Chapter 9, "Abdominal Pain, Acute."

Hemolytic Uremic Syndrome

HUS is discussed in Chapter 78, "Urine Output, Decreased"

EVALUATION OF ACUTE DIARRHEA

Patient History

The initial patient history aims both to establish **hydration** status and to uncover the **cause of the diarrhea.** The adequacy and type of fluid and solid intake and the urine output should be carefully assessed. In addition, note the size, frequency, and character of the stools (e.g., watery, mucoid, bloody, or foul smelling) and any associated symptoms. For example, the presence of ear pain or dysuria suggests a diagnosis of parenteral diarrhea.

> **HINT:** *Shigella* emits a neurotoxin, and seizures may precede the gastrointestinal symptoms.

Physical Examination

- **Vital signs, level of consciousness, fontanelles, mucous membranes, skin turgor, and capillary refill.** Note signs of dehydration (see Chapter 25, "Dehydration," Table 25-3).
- **Skin.** Note maculopapular rash (seen in viral gastroenteritis, typhoid, and *Shigella* infection), pallor, petechiae, or purpura.
- **Abdomen.** Auscultate for the presence and quality of bowel sounds; then percuss and palpate for tenderness, organomegaly, or masses. Focal tenderness alerts the examiner to consider alternative diagnoses and potential complications of infection.
- **Rectum.** Note focal tenderness; stool can be examined and tested for occult blood.

Laboratory Studies

Laboratory studies are unnecessary for most outpatients with acute diarrhea. If there is a concern about dehydration, testing of **urine specific gravity** may be helpful. In addition, **serum electrolyte analysis** may suggest inadequate fluid replacement (hypernatremic dehydration) or hypotonic fluid replacement (hyponatremic dehydration).

Methylene blue staining of the stool can be used to screen outpatients requiring a bacterial stool culture and may occasionally identify *G. lamblia*. Although the presence of sheets of polymorphonuclear leukocytes suggests bacterial enteritis and the need for bacterial stool culture, the absence of leukocytes does not entirely eliminate the possibility of a bacterial infection. A jar specimen provides a better yield than does a diaper or swab specimen. Viral cultures, stool examination for ova and parasites, and other specialized tests are available to diagnose other organisms but are not typically necessary.

Blood cultures should be obtained if there is suspicion of bacteremia or sepsis.

TREATMENT OF ACUTE DIARRHEA

> **HINT:** Children with diarrhea and no dehydration should continue to be fed age-appropriate diets.

Although children who are severely dehydrated require immediate intravenous fluid replacement, **oral rehydration therapy is the first line of treatment** for all children with mild to moderate dehydration (see also Chapter 25, "Dehydration"). Glucose-electrolyte rehydration solutions contain 75 to 90 mEq/L of sodium, and maintenance solutions contain

40 to 60 mEq/L of sodium. Rehydration with oral rehydration solutions should be performed over 4 to 6 hours. Preliminary research suggests that reduced osmolarity oral rehydration solutions significantly reduce stool volume. **Oral maintenance fluids** can be administered after rehydration, but **age-appropriate foods** should be reintroduced within 24 hours.

> **HINT:** Vomiting is not a contraindication to oral rehydration in the mild to moderately dehydrated patient.

The BRAT (bananas, rice, applesauce, and toast) diet is not recommended. This restricted diet contains inadequate calories and protein to meet nutritional requirements, and its use is associated with greater weight loss than an age-appropriate diet. Proper nutrition helps facilitate mucosal repair after illness. The use of lactose-free formulas and dietary lactose restrictions are not of clear benefit except in the small minority of patients with clinically significant secondary lactase deficiency.

Antidiarrheal medications are not efficacious and are potentially dangerous. They may enhance bacterial proliferation and toxin absorption by promoting reduced gut motility. In addition, they may mask intraluminal fluid loss.

Some studies suggest that bismuth subsalicylate, zinc, and probiotic agents (e.g., *Lactobacillus GG*) may reduce the duration and severity of diarrhea, but confirmation of these findings is needed, and they are not routinely recommended.

APPROACH TO THE PATIENT (FIGURE 27-1)

- **Test a stool sample for the presence of gross or microscopic blood.** The presence of blood should be confirmed using a guaiac reagent test, which excludes dyes, medications, and vegetable matter as the source of red stools. Broken skin must also be excluded as a source of blood.
- **Determine whether the child has recently had antibiotic therapy.** Recent antibiotic therapy in a child with bloody diarrhea suggests the presence of pseudomembranous colitis. Recent antibiotic therapy in a child with nonbloody diarrhea suggests the presence of antibiotic-induced gastroenteritis or *C. difficile* infection without colitis.
- **In an afebrile child with bloody diarrhea,** it is particularly important to rule out intussusception (suggested by lethargy, irritability, an abdominal mass, or currant-jelly stools), HUS (suggested by pallor, petechiae, and oliguria), and Henoch-Schönlein purpura (suggested by purpura, especially of the buttocks and lower extremities).

Figure 27-1 ■ Evaluation of a patient with acute diarrhea
HSP = Henoch-Schönlein purpura; HUS = hemolytic uremic syndrome;
R/O = rule out; RUQ = right upper quadrant.

- Most patients are diagnosed as having **presumed viral gastroenteritis.**
- Rotavirus gastroenteritis is the most common specific cause of severe diarrhea in young children. Immunization with an oral, live attenuated rotavirus vaccine (RotaTeq) in infancy is an important preventive measure and likely to change the epidemiology of acute diarrheal illness significantly in this age group.

Suggested Readings

American Academy of Pediatrics: *2006 Red Book: Report of the Committee on Infectious Diseases,* 27th ed. Elk Grove Village, Il, American Academy of Pediatrics, 2006.

Amieva MR: Important bacterial gastrointestinal pathogens in children: a pathogenesis perspective. *Pediatr Clin North Am* 52:749–777, 2005.

Brown KH, Peerson JM, Fontaine O: Use of nonhuman milks in the dietary management of young children with acute diarrhea: A meta-analysis of clinical trials. *Pediatrics* 93:17–27, 1994.

Centers for Disease Control and Prevention: Managing acute gastroenteritis among children: oral rehydration, maintenance and nutritional therapy. *MMWR* 52(RR-16):1–16, 2003.

Deenehy PH: Acute diarrheal disease in children: epidemiology, prevention, and treatment. *Infect Dis Clin North Am* 19:585–602, 2005.

Fry AM, Braden CR, Griffin PM, et al.: In *Principles and Practice of Infectious Diseases,* 6th ed. Edited by Mandell GL, Bennett JE, Dolin R. Philadelphia, Elsevier, 2005, 1286–1299.

Guerrant RL, Lohr JA, Williams EK: Acute infectious diarrhea. *Pediatr Infect Dis J* 5:353–359, 1986.

Hartling L, Bellemare S, Wiebe N, et al.: Oral versus intravenous rehydration for treating dehydration due to gastroenteritis in children. Cochrane Database Syst Rev 3:CD004390, 2006.

Hoque KM, Binder HJ: Zinc in the treatment of acute diarrhea: current status and assessment. *Gastroenterology* 130:2201–2205, 2006.

Huang DB, White AC: An updated review on *Cryptosporidium* and *Giardia. Gastroenterol Clin* 35:291–314, 2006.

Huebner ES, Surawicz CM: Probiotics in the prevention and treatment of gastrointestinal infections. *Gastroenterology Clin* 25:355–365, 2006.

Lifshitz F (ed): Management of acute diarrheal disease. *J Pediatr* 118: S25–138, 1991.

Northrup RS, Flanigan TP: Gastroenteritis. *Pediatr Rev* 15:461–472, 1994.

Parashar UD, Alexander JP, Glass RI: Prevention of rotaviral gastroenteritis among infants and children. Recommendations of the Advisory Committee on Immunization Practices (ACIP). *MMWR* 55(RR-12): 1–13, 2006.

Sarker SA, Mahalanabis D, Alam NH, et al.: Reduced osmolarity oral rehydration solution for persistent diarrhea in infants: A randomized controlled clinical trial. *J Pediatr* 138:532–538, 2001.

Vanderhoof JA, Young RJ: Pediatric applications of probiotics. *Gastroenterol Clin* 34:451–463, 2005.

Wong CS, Jelacic RL, Habeeb SL, et al.: The risk of the hemolytic-uremic syndrome after antibiotic treatment of *E. coli* 0157:H7 infections. *New Engl J Med* 342:1930–1936, 2000.

28 Diarrhea, Chronic
Andrew Grossman

INTRODUCTION

Stool output of >10 g/kg per day (in infants) or 200 g/kg per day (in children) is defined as diarrhea. Chronic diarrhea is the persistence of loose, frequent stools for >2 to 3 weeks.

Diarrhea can be classified as **secretory, osmotic, inflammatory, or motility related.** Presence of an unabsorbable compound in the lumen of the intestine creates an osmolar load that results in osmotic diarrhea. Secretory diarrhea is caused by an imbalance of water and electrolyte absorption and secretion in the intestine.

> **HINT:** If diarrhea stops when the patient is given nothing by mouth, this is osmotic diarrhea.

DIFFERENTIAL DIAGNOSIS LIST

Infectious Causes
Bacterial, parasitic, or viral infection (see Chapter 27, "Diarrhea, Acute")
Small bowel bacterial overgrowth
Postinfectious enteritis
Necrotizing enterocolitis
Parenteral diarrhea

Toxic Causes
Antibiotics
Laxatives
Mannitol
Motility agents
Chemotherapeutic agents

Neoplastic Causes
Neuroblastoma
VIPoma
Gastrinoma
Lymphoma
Polyposis
Mastocytosis

Metabolic or Genetic Causes
Carbohydrate malabsorption— lactose intolerance, glucosegalactose transporter defect, sucrase isomaltase deficiency
Fat malabsorption—congenital lipase deficiency, pancreatic disease (cystic fibrosis, chronic pancreatitis, Shwachman syndrome), chronic liver disease, congenital bile salt malabsorption, Wolman disease
Protein-losing enteropathy (PLE)—intestinal lymphangiectasia

Celiac disease
Congenital chloride diarrhea
Congenital sodium diarrhea
Acrodermatitis enteropathica
Hyperthyroidism
Hypoparathyroidism
Congenital adrenal hyperplasia
Diabetes
Lipoprotein disorders

Anatomic Causes
Malrotation
Partial small bowel obstruction
Short bowel syndrome
Blind loop syndrome
Fistula
Pyloroplasty
Hirschsprung disease with
  enterocolitis

Dietary Causes
Overfeeding (food or liquid)
Food or milk- or soy-protein
  allergy
Eosinophilic gastroenteritis
Malnutrition
Fructose intolerance

Fiber
Sorbitol

Inflammatory Causes
Inflammatory bowel disease
Severe combined
  immunodeficiency
Immunoglobulin A (IgA)
  deficiency
Autoimmune enteropathy
Hemolytic uremic syndrome
  (HUS)

Psychosocial Causes
Munchausen by proxy
  syndrome

Miscellaneous Causes
Chronic nonspecific diarrhea
  of infancy
Irritable bowel syndrome
Hepatobiliary disorders
  (hepatitis, cholestasis,
  cholecystectomy)
Encopresis
Radiation enteritis
Neonatal drug withdrawal
  syndrome

DIFFERENTIAL DIAGNOSIS DISCUSSION

Chronic Nonspecific Diarrhea of Infancy

Chronic nonspecific diarrhea of infancy (also known as **toddler's diarrhea** or **irritable colon syndrome of childhood**) is the most common cause of diarrhea in children between **6 months and 3 years of age.**

Etiology

The cause is unclear. The disorder may be related to **increased bowel motility** or **low intake of fat and fiber,** or it may follow a bout of **infectious gastroenteritis.**

Clinical Features

Patients pass **3 to 10 loose stools per day,** usually diminishing in frequency in the evening. The child has a good appetite and appropriate weight gain, although undigested food particles are visible in the stool.

Evaluation

The diagnosis is **by exclusion** of other causes. Workup for infection and malabsorption are negative. A stool heme workup is also negative. Clinically, a history of **excessive intake of juices** and a **diet low in fat and fiber** in a child who is thriving supports the diagnosis.

Treatment

The child's consumption of fruit juice and **excessive fluids should be restricted,** and consumption of **dietary fat and fiber** should be **increased.** Reassure parents that the problem will resolve by the time the child is 2 to 3 years of age.

> **HINT:** Remember the *four* Fs: fruit juice, fluids, fat, and fiber.

Infectious Enteritis

Infectious enteritis is the **most common cause** of **chronic diarrhea.** Gastrointestinal infections are **usually acute** and resolve in approximately **2 weeks,** but sometimes they can persist for as long as **2 months.** Viral gastroenteritis in an infant can be prolonged as a result of the slow healing of the intestinal mucosa. In addition, infections tend to last longer than usual in immunocompromised patients.

Etiology

Common **bacterial causes** of chronic diarrhea include *Salmonella, Shigella, Yersinia enterocolitica, Campylobacter,* enteroadherent *Escherichia coli, Aeromonas, Clostridium difficile,* and *Plesiomonas.* **Parasitic causes** include *Giardia lamblia, Cryptosporidium, Entamoeba histolytica,* and *Isospora.* Rotavirus, adenovirus, and norovirus are common **viral causes.**

> **HINT:** Herpes virus, *Mycobacterium avium-intracellulare, Blastocystis hominis,* Microsporidia, and fungi can cause chronic diarrhea in immunocompromised patients. They usually present with recurrent or prolonged infections.

Clinical Features

- *Y. enterocolitica* **infection** involves the terminal ileum and can mimic inflammatory bowel disease or appendicitis. It is more common in patients whose normal bowel flora has been changed secondary to antibiotic therapy.

- *E. histolytica* infection can cause colitis. Blood, mucus, or both are seen in the stool, and patients have a fever.
- *Giardia lamblia* infection is usually asymptomatic but may manifest with bloating, abdominal pain, anorexia, chronic diarrhea, and failure to thrive (see Chapter 10, "Abdominal Pain, Chronic").

Evaluation

A **stool sample** should be obtained for **bacterial and viral culture.** The laboratory should be instructed to culture for all of the most commonly implicated bacteria and viruses. Stool samples for **rotazyme** (an enzyme-linked immunoassay for rotavirus) and assays for *C. difficile* **toxins A and B** should also be obtained. **Three stool specimens** should be submitted for **ova and parasites (O&P) analysis.**

Treatment

If the cause is **bacterial,** treatment is with the appropriate **antibiotic** (see Chapter 27, "Diarrhea, Acute"). **Giardiasis** is treated with **furazolidone, metronidazole,** or **quinacrine** (see Chapter 10, "Abdominal Pain, Chronic"). **Nutritional supplementation** may be required for patients with **viral** diarrhea and **immunocompromised patients.**

C. difficile Colitis (pseudomembranous colitis, antibiotic-induced colitis)

C. difficile colitis is discussed in Chapter 34, "Gastrointestinal Bleeding, Lower."

Parenteral Diarrhea

Etiology

Extraintestinal infection (e.g., upper respiratory tract infection, urinary tract infection [UTI], otitis media, mastoiditis, sinusitis, pneumonia) may be associated with diarrhea. Diarrhea may also be one of the symptoms **associated with other systemic infections** (e.g., toxic shock syndrome, Rocky Mountain spotted fever). The pathogenesis of the diarrhea is unknown.

Clinical Features

The patient may be **otherwise asymptomatic** (e.g., in the case of UTI), or he may have a **range of symptoms** related to the primary illness.

Evaluation

The diagnosis is based on **clinical suspicion.** An appropriate workup for the suspected primary illness should be performed. In an otherwise asymptomatic child, a **urine culture** is necessary.

Treatment

Treatment of the primary illness results in resolution of the diarrhea.

Postinfectious Enteritis

Etiology

In children, infectious gastroenteritis is usually uncomplicated; however, in infants (especially those with a borderline nutritional status), severe mucosal damage may follow an infectious gastroenteritis. The mucosal damage results in disaccharidase deficiency (most commonly lactase deficiency).

Clinical Features

Long after the infectious process has been resolved, the patient experiences intractable watery diarrhea and nutritional compromise, manifested as failure to thrive. Rarely, evidence of vitamin and mineral deficiency is seen.

Evaluation

The diagnosis is made on the basis of clinical suspicion. In some patients, a lactose breath test may be appropriate.

Treatment

Temporary avoidance of dairy products and introduction of a lactose-free formula or an elemental formula are needed to allow the brush borders of the small intestine to heal.

Celiac Disease (Gluten-Sensitive Enteropathy)

Etiology

Gluten-sensitive enteropathy is a hereditary type of malabsorption that is caused by a permanent inability to tolerate gluten, which is present in wheat, oat, barley, and rye. Gliadin, the offending protein, causes severe atrophy of the small intestinal mucosa. This disease is increasingly recognized in all cultures and is thought to affect approximately 1% of the U.S. population.

Clinical Features

Symptoms usually start approximately 1 month after gluten is introduced to the diet. Common manifestations include apathy and irritability, anorexia, vomiting, chronic diarrhea, steatorrhea, abdominal distension, clubbing of the fingers, and malnutrition with symptoms and signs related to nutrient deficiency.

Evaluation

The patient should be **screened for IgA antiendomysial antibodies and IgA anti-transglutaminase antibodies.** However, IgA deficiency must be excluded. IgA antigliadin antibodies result in a very high false-positive rate, and this screening test is generally not used for celiac disease.

Treatment

Complete removal of gluten from the diet and replacement with corn, rice, or potato starch results in resolution of the symptoms. Complete recovery of the intestinal mucosa is expected in 1 to 2 years.

Encopresis

Etiology

Patients with **chronic constipation and impaction** may present with chronic diarrhea as a result of encopresis, or **continuous leakage of loose stool around the hard stool.** In patients with **Hirschsprung disease,** diarrhea is usually **secondary to enterocolitis.**

Clinical Features

The patient has a **history of constipation.** On **abdominal examination,** hard stool may be **palpated,** and on **rectal examination,** the **vault is dilated** and **filled with hard stool.**

Evaluation

An **abdominal radiograph** confirms the diagnosis, which is based on clinical suspicion.

Treatment

Treatment entails **evacuation of the bowel** with **multiple enemas. Stool softeners** or an osmotic medication should be prescribed for **several months,** and **diet** and **behavioral modification** should take place. Patients with **Hirschsprung disease** require **surgery** for definitive treatment.

Fat Malabsorption

Etiology

Fat digestion and absorption is a complex process. **Lipase** (a pancreatic enzyme), **bile acid secretion** (to help with micellar solubilization), an intact **intestinal brush border** (to facilitate micelle absorption), intact β lipoprotein metabolism, and an intact **transport mechanism** (to carry the chylomicron to the lymphatics) all play a role. A **defect in any of these steps** may result in fat malabsorption.

Clinical Features

Fat malabsorption is manifested with **diarrhea (bulky, greasy stools), failure to thrive,** and signs and symptoms related to **fat-soluble vitamin deficiency** (e.g., rickets, night blindness, neurologic signs, bleeding tendency).

Evaluation

Fat malabsorption caused by pancreatic insufficiency is suggested by a low concentration of **fecal elastase.** Definitive diagnosis of fat malabsorption requires a **72-hour stool collection** for measurement of fecal fat, which must be compared to dietary fat intake. The workup for the cause of fat malabsorption is extensive, and referral to a **gastroenterologist** is recommended.

Treatment

The **underlying cause** must be identified and treated if possible. All patients with fat malabsorption require **additional calorie intake** to compensate for the excessive fat loss. **Medium-chain triglyceride (MCT)–based formulas** are often preferred. Because MCTs have a smaller molecular weight and higher water solubility than long-chain triglycerides, they are absorbed directly into the portal blood. Patients with fat malabsorption also require **fat-soluble vitamin supplementation.**

Carbohydrate Malabsorption

Etiology

The absorption of carbohydrates involves **amylase** (a pancreatic enzyme); **lactase, isomaltase,** and **sucrase** (intestinal brush border enzymes); and an intact **transport system.** The most common type of carbohydrate malabsorption is **lactase deficiency** (see Chapter 10, "Abdominal Pain, Chronic"). Congenital carbohydrate malabsorption is rare but has to be considered in the differential diagnosis of diarrhea in a young infant.

Clinical Features

In general, carbohydrate malabsorption syndromes are manifested with **failure to thrive, osmotic diarrhea** (often voluminous and watery), **abdominal cramps, increased flatulence,** and **borborygmi.**

Evaluation

Detection of reducing substances or a **stool pH <5.0** is indicative of carbohydrate malabsorption. Definitive diagnosis of disaccharidase deficiencies can be made by a specific **hydrogen breath test** or measurement of enzyme activity from **small bowel biopsy.**

Treatment

Symptoms usually resolve with complete **removal of the offending carbohydrate** from the diet. **Supplying the deficient enzyme** may be helpful (e.g., lactase for lactose intolerance).

Protein Malabsorption

Diseases that involve the gastrointestinal mucosa (e.g., Crohn disease) or obstruct lymphatic drainage of the gastrointestinal tract can cause **protein-losing enteropathy (PLE)**. **Primary intestinal lymphangiectasia** is a congenital disorder associated with abnormally dilated lymphatics that results in chronic loss of albumin, immunoglobulins, and other proteins. It is also associated with loss of lymphocytes through the gastrointestinal tract.

Clinical Features

Patients may present with signs and symptoms that reflect the **underlying cause, chronic diarrhea, failure to thrive, edema,** or **recurrent infection.**

Evaluation

Patients have **hypoalbuminemia, hypoproteinemia, abnormal immunoglobulins,** and they may have **lymphocytopenia.** Hypocalcemia and **decreased serum iron and copper levels** occur secondary to the loss of binding proteins. Before making the diagnosis of PLE, **urinary loss of albumin must be ruled out.** Increased stool α_1-antitrypsin (α_1-AT) is the **definitive** means of diagnosing PLE.

Treatment

The **primary cause** of the PLE should be identified. Patients require a **diet that is rich in protein and MCT oil.**

Allergic Enteropathy

Allergic enteropathy is discussed in Chapter 34, "Gastrointestinal Bleeding, Lower."

Inflammatory Bowel Disease

Inflammatory bowel disease is discussed in Chapter 34, "Gastrointestinal Bleeding, Lower."

EVALUATION OF CHRONIC DIARRHEA

A detailed **history** and **physical examination** can obviate the need for laboratory evaluation in some cases.

Patient History

- Onset and duration of the diarrhea
- Stool pattern and aggravating or alleviating factors
- Quality of stool—color; odor; consistency; volume; presence of blood, mucus, or undigested food
- Presence of fever and associated symptoms
- A history of gastroenteritis, constipation, or recurrent pneumonia before the onset of chronic diarrhea
- Dietary history (4 "Fs"—fiber, fluid, fat, fruit juice)
- Recent travel or exposure to infections
- Medication history
- Pertinent family history

Physical Examination

The following should be noted on examination:

- **General appearance**—hydration status, weight and height, growth chart
- **Skin**—edema, jaundice, pallor, eczematous rash, bruising, clubbing
- **Lungs**—wheezing, rales
- **Abdomen**—tenderness, mass (stool, abscess, tumor, enlarged organs)
- **Rectum**—evidence of perianal disease, rectal prolapse, Hirschsprung disease, constipation

Laboratory Studies

Initial screening studies may include:

- A serum electrolyte panel
- Liver function tests
- Complete blood count with differential and erythrocyte sedimentation rate
- Celiac disease panel
- Stool sample for occult blood
- Stool samples for culture, *C. difficile* toxin A and B assay, and O&P
- Urinalysis and urine culture
- Stool electrolytes, anion gap, osmolarity

Depending on the suspected diagnosis, additional studies may be indicated:

- **Carbohydrate malabsorption**—stool pH (<5.0), reducing substance (positive)
- **Fat malabsorption**—72-hour fecal fat; sweat chloride test; prothrombin time (PT, prolonged); vitamin E and vitamin D levels (may be decreased)
- **PLE**—stool α_1-AT (increased), hypoalbuminemia, lymphopenia, hypogammaglobulinemia
- **Small bowel disease**—d-xylose test (abnormal)

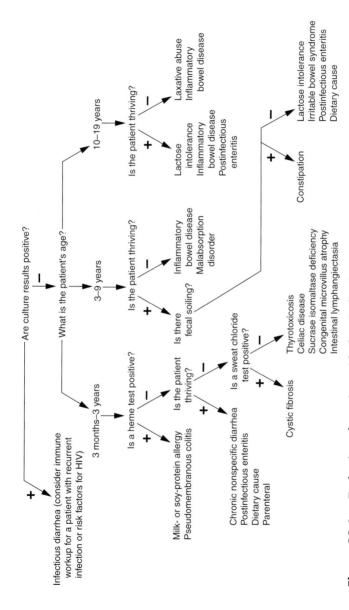

Figure 28-1 ■ **Evaluation of a patient with chronic diarrhea**
Most patients are diagnosed as having presumed viral gastroenteritis.

TREATMENT OF CHRONIC DIARRHEA

The underlying cause of the diarrhea must be identified and treated.

- Consultation with a nutritionist is advisable for patients with disorders such as malabsorption, celiac disease, or allergic enteropathy.
- For patients who are not vomiting, an oral glucose electrolyte solution can be given to correct fluid, electrolyte, and acid-base imbalances. Patients may be started on a lactose-free or an elemental formula later, depending on the cause and severity of the diarrhea.
- Unstable or malnourished patients should be admitted for stabilization and nutritional rehabilitation. Reinitiation of feeding in a malnourished patient may result in refeeding syndrome, which is manifested by an acute drop in serum potassium, phosphate, magnesium, and calcium levels secondary to the sudden intracellular shift of these elements. If these electrolyte abnormalities are not corrected in a timely manner, cardiopulmonary compromise and death may result. All electrolyte imbalances must be corrected before initiation of feeding to prevent refeeding syndrome. A continuous drip of a diluted formula is started, and gradually the rate and concentration are increased while monitoring the patient's electrolytes and calcium, phosphate, and magnesium levels.
- Total parenteral nutrition may be required for those with severe malnutrition who cannot tolerate feeding.
- Additional nutritional supplementation (e.g., zinc, iron, vitamins) may be required.

APPROACH TO THE PATIENT (FIGURE 28-1)

Suggested Readings

Baldassano RN, Liacouras CA: Chronic diarrhea, a practical approach for the pediatrician. *Pediatr Clin North Am* 38(3):667–686, 1991.

Guerrant RL, Bobak DA: Bacterial and protozoal gastroenteritis. *New Engl J Med* 325:327–340, 1991.

Hanauer SB: Inflammatory bowel disease. *N Engl J Med* 334:841–848, 1996.

Heitlinger LA, Lebenthal EB: Disorders of carbohydrate digestion and absorption. *Pediatr Clin North Am* 35:239–255, 1988.

Hyams JS, Stafford RJ, Grand RJ, et al.: Correlation of the lactose breath test, intestinal morphology and lactase activity in young children. *J Pediatr* 97:609–612, 1980.

Picarelli A, Sabbatella L, Di Tola M, et al.: Celiac disease diagnosis in misdiagnosed children. *Pediatr Res* 48(5):590–592, 2000.

Smith MM, Lifshitz F: Excess fruit juice consumption as a contributing factor in nonorganic failure to thrive. *Pediatrics* 93(3):438–443, 1994.

Vanderhoof JA: Chronic diarrhea. *Pediatr Rev* 19(12):418–422, 1998.

Walker-Smith JA, Guandalini S, Schmitz J, et al.: Revised criteria for the diagnosis of celiac disease. *Arch Dis Child* 65:909–911, 1990.

Chapter	**29**	***Drowning***
		Kathy N. Shaw and Mercedes M. Blackstone

INTRODUCTION

Terminology

Historically, the terminology used to describe drowning events has been somewhat confusing. The World Congress on Drowning has suggested that the **term "drowning" be uniformly applied** to describe any process in which there is respiratory impairment from submersion in a liquid medium, regardless of outcome. Inconsistent terms such as "near drowning," "wet drowning," and "dry drowning" should be abandoned. Similarly, there is no need to distinguish freshwater or saltwater drownings because it makes little difference in the management of the patient. Water temperature at the time of drowning is significant because children who drown in very cold water ($<5°C$) may have a better prognosis. Drowning usually results in either **severe permanent brain damage or prompt complete recovery.**

Epidemiology

Nationally, drowning is **second only to motor vehicle accidents** as the most common cause of death caused by nonintentional injury in children <19 years. **Males of all ages** drown at higher rates than females. The **highest rate** of drowning is seen in **children 1 to 4 years** of age. In California, Arizona, and Florida, drowning is the leading cause of death in this age group. The vast majority of deaths in this age group occur in **residential swimming pools. Infants** are most likely to drown in **bathtubs,** and these drownings are sometimes the result of **abuse or neglect.** A second peak in drowning deaths occurs in the **teen and young adult** age groups in bodies of **fresh water,** with the highest rate in black males. These deaths are often associated with drug and alcohol use and other risk-taking behaviors.

Most drownings are **preventable.** Passage of legislation that requires proper pool fencing, limits alcohol access at public pools and beaches, and demands pool owners to be proficient in cardiopulmonary resuscitation (CPR) could significantly reduce morbidity and mortality rates. Preventive counseling for parents should also be provided.

Pathophysiology

- **Pulmonary injury** results from poor surfactant function and increased capillary permeability. Alveolar injury and pulmonary edema lead to hypoxemia as a result of an altered ventilation-perfusion ratio and intrapulmonary shunting. Hypercapnia occurs as a result of apnea or hypoventilation but is usually readily corrected with the use of ventilation during resuscitation. The persistent hypoxemia and the effects of anoxic-ischemic cell injury (i.e., cytotoxic edema, cellular disruption) are the primary management issues.

- **Central nervous system injury,** including cerebral edema and increased intracranial pressure, is a secondary result of global anoxic-ischemic injury. It is not reversible. Hypothermia may actually protect the brain by causing a decrease in metabolic demand, but this is true only if the hypothermia occurred at the time of the near drowning in extremely cold water.

- **Cardiac injury and dysrhythmias** are usually caused by postresuscitation myocardial dysfunction from acidosis and hypoxemia. In conjunction with intravascular depletion, all of these factors can lead to persistent shock.

EVALUATION OF DROWNING AND NEAR DROWNING

Patient History

The **duration of submersion, temperature of the water,** presence of **cyanosis or apnea at the scene, performance of CPR** at the recovery scene, and **amount of time that elapsed until CPR** was initiated are all important historical points that influence prognosis and management (Table 29-1). One should also inquire about the possibility of a **diving**

TABLE 29-1 Prognostic Indicators of Poor Neurologic Outcome in Near-Drowning Victims*

At the Scene

Submersion time >4–10 min
Delay in beginning CPR
Resuscitation >25 min

In the Emergency Department

Necessity for CPR
Fixed, dilated pupils
pH <7.0
GCS score <5

After Initial Resuscitation

Persistent GCS score <5
Persistent apnea
Persistent lack of spontaneous, purposeful movements within 24 hr

*Applies to victims of warm water near drownings only. Hypothermic victims of cold water near drownings may have a better prognosis.
CPR = cardiopulmonary resuscitation; GCS = Glasgow coma score

injury, alcohol use, or a past history of a seizure disorder or underlying cardiac dysrhythmia.

Physical Examination

During the physical examination, particular attention should be paid to assessment of vital signs (including the temperature) and to the neurologic and respiratory examinations. Performing neurologic and respiratory examinations at periodic intervals is an extremely important component of managing near-drowning victims.

Pupillary response and the Glasgow coma score (GCS) (see Chapter 21, "Coma," Table 21-1) should be assessed serially to determine the extent of anoxic-ischemic injury and the patient's response to resuscitation attempts. The child who presents in asystole with fixed, dilated pupils and a GCS score of <5 generally has a poor prognosis unless he responds fairly rapidly to resuscitation efforts or he has a core temperature of <32°C following a very-cold-water near drowning. In children with a GCS score of >5 at presentation, the outcome is generally good. Unfortunately, neurologic damage as a result of near drowning cannot be reversed.

Careful attention is paid to the respiratory examination, even in an alert, active child without obvious respiratory distress. Close monitoring for signs of respiratory involvement (in the form of serial examinations) is crucial, even for the initially asymptomatic child. Signs of lower respiratory involvement (e.g., the use of accessory muscles, tachypnea, cough, wheezing, rales, nasal flaring) may be delayed for minutes to hours, and the injury is usually progressive.

Laboratory and Imaging Studies

- Serial pulse oximetry should be used to detect early signs of pulmonary involvement that are not clinically detectable (e.g., oxygen desaturation of <95%).
- Electrolyte values are rarely abnormal. Respiratory or metabolic acidosis may be present and should be corrected.
- Anticonvulsant levels in victims with seizure disorders should be assessed.
- Electrocardiographic monitoring is indicated for the severely affected patient or for a patient in whom a cardiac electrophysiologic conduction delay (e.g., a prolonged QT interval) may have precipitated unconsciousness, leading to the drowning episode.
- Toxicology screens, including an ethyl alcohol level measurement, may be indicated.
- Chest radiography is indicated following intubation or if there are signs of lower airway involvement.
- Cervical spine films are indicated for victims of high-impact events.

HINT: Initial pulse oximetry and chest radiographs are often normal in drowning victims with brief periods of submersion. As such, even well-appearing drowning victims should be monitored in the emergency department for 6 to 8 hours.

APPROACH TO THE PATIENT

Resuscitation

The **prognosis** of drowning victims is directly related to the duration of the **hypoxic-ischemic injury** and the **adequacy of the initial resuscitation.** Therefore, a **brief, well-executed resuscitation effort** with initiation of **advanced cardiopulmonary life support** measures, if necessary, should be made as information is gathered regarding the accident, the patient's core temperature, and the response to therapy. Resuscitation should be initiated **in all apneic and pulseless victims,** but it should only be **continued for prolonged periods** in victims of a **cold-water near drowning** and then only until the **patient's core temperature exceeds 32°C.** The goal of therapy is to **prevent further anoxic-ischemic injury.**

The **gag reflex** should be assessed to determine whether the child can protect his or her own airway. In diving accidents, the possibility of a **neck injury** should be considered, and the neck should be **immobilized.** The **airway** should be **suctioned** and properly positioned to ensure air entry. See Figure 29-1 for how to manage the airway and breathing of near-drowning victims.

HINT: The Heimlich maneuver (with the victim's head turned sideways) should be used only if foreign matter is obstructing the airway, and it should never be used if cervical trauma is suspected.

Intubation is required if the child is apneic, if she is in severe respiratory distress, if the administration of >50% oxygen is required to maintain an arterial oxygen tension of >60 mm Hg, or if the protective reflexes are missing because of obtundation. The **stomach** should be **emptied of water** by means of a nasogastric tube once the airway is protected. **Assisted ventilation** (e.g., bag-valve-mask ventilation) is initiated if necessary. Use of the **Sellick maneuver** during initial ventilation may assist in the prevention of aspiration. With this technique, an assistant applies anteroposterior pressure to the cricoid cartilage to compress the esophagus against the cervical vertebrae. In children with severe hypoxemia, the most effective treatment is **continuous positive airway pressure,** which helps improve ventilation-perfusion matching in the lungs.

Figure 29-1 ■ Management of the airway and breathing in a near-drowning victim

ABG = arterial blood gases; BVM = bag-valve-mask; CPAP = continuous positive airway pressure; CPR = cardiopulmonary resuscitation; C-spine = cervical spine; CXR = chest radiograph; ICU 5 intensive care unit; O₂ = oxygen; O₂ sat = oxygen saturation; Pao₂ = arterial oxygen tension

Children who show signs of **lower respiratory involvement** should be admitted and closely **monitored** for the development of **progressive respiratory failure.** Children who required no resuscitation and are **asymptomatic** upon arrival at the emergency department should be **observed and monitored** for any signs of respiratory impairment for a minimum of **6 to 8 hours** before discharge.

Circulation

The victim should be assessed for **adequacy of circulation.** If a pulse cannot be felt, chest compressions should be started (but not if the patient is still in the water). An intravenous line should be started and **normal saline** given in 20 mL/kg aliquots if there are signs of poor perfusion. Poor perfusion usually occurs only in children with severe ischemic injury or pulmonary edema and in those who require mechanical ventilation. Children with **respiratory distress** should receive intravenous fluids at **1.5 times** the maintenance requirement.

Restoration of Core Temperature

In a child who has experienced cold-water near drowning, it may be necessary to use a **low-reading thermometer** to obtain the core temperature. The child's **wet clothing** should be **removed** immediately, and the child should be dried and warmed. If the child's core temperature is **32°C to 35°C,** active external warming should be started using a heating blanket or radiant warmer. A patient with a core temperature of <32°C requires **internal warming,** which entails gastric and bladder lavage with warm fluid and the administration of heated aerosolized oxygen and intravenous fluids. In severe cases of icy-water drownings, **peritoneal dialysis or hemodialysis, mediastinal irrigation,** or **cardiac bypass** may be used if the technique is available.

> **HINT:** The popular saying "A drowning victim is not dead until he is warm and dead" applies only to hypothermia patients who were immersed in cold water, not to those who are hypothermic because they have been asystolic for an extended period of time following a warm-water drowning.

Suggested Readings

Brenner RA: Prevention of drowning in infants, children, and adolescents. *Pediatrics* 112(2):440–445, 2003.

Brenner RA, Trumble AC, Smith GS, et al.: Where children drown, United States, 1995. *Pediatrics* 108(1):85–89, 2001.

Burford AE, Ryan LM, Stone BJ, et al.: Drowning and near-drowning in children and adolescents: a succinct review for emergency physicians and nurses. *Pediatr Emerg Care* 21(9):610–616; quiz 7–9, 2005.

Hwang V, Shofer FS, Durbin DR, et al.: Prevalence of traumatic injuries in drowning and near drowning in children and adolescents. *Arch Pediatr Adolesc Med* 157(1):50–53, 2003.

Ibsen LM, Koch T: Submersion and asphyxial injury. *Crit Care Med* 30(11 Suppl):S402–408, 2002.

Idris AH, Berg RA, Bierens J, et al.: Recommended guidelines for uniform reporting of data from drowning: the "Utstein style." *Circulation* 108(20):2565–2574, 2003.

Jacinto SJ, Gieron-Korthals M, Ferreira JA: Predicting outcome in hypoxic-ischemic brain injury. *Pediatr Clin North Am* 48(3):647–660, 2001.

Lavelle JM, Shaw KN: Near drowning: is emergency department cardiopulmonary resuscitation or intensive care unit cerebral resuscitation indicated? *Crit Care Med* 21(3):368–373, 1993.

Lavelle JM, Shaw KN, Seidl T, et al.: Ten-year review of pediatric bathtub near-drownings: evaluation for child abuse and neglect. *Ann Emerg Med* 25(3):344–348, 1995.

Meyer RJ, Theodorou AA, Berg RA: Childhood drowning. *Pediatr Rev* 27(5):163–168; quiz 9, 2006.

Modell JH: Drowning. *N Engl J Med* 328(4):253–256, 1993.

Peden MM, McGee K: The epidemiology of drowning worldwide. *Inj Control Saf Promot* 10(4):195–199, 2003.

Quan L, Kinder D: Pediatric submersions: prehospital predictors of outcome. *Pediatrics* 90(6):909–913, 1992.

Rosen P, Stoto M, Harley J: The use of the Heimlich maneuver in near drowning: Institute of Medicine report. *J Emerg Med* 13(3):397–405, 1995.

Salomez F, Vincent JL: Drowning: a review of epidemiology, pathophysiology, treatment and prevention. *Resuscitation* 63(3):261–268, 2004.

Shaw KN, Briede CA: Submersion injuries: drowning and near-drowning. *Emerg Med Clin North Am* 7(2):355–370, 1989.

Suominen P, Baillie C, Korpela R, et al.: Impact of age, submersion time and water temperature on outcome in near-drowning. *Resuscitation* 52(3):247–254, 2002.

Watson RS, Cummings P, Quan L, et al.: Cervical spine injuries among submersion victims. *J Trauma* 51(4):658–662, 2001.

30

Ear, Painful

Christine S. Cho
Susan C. Kim (Second Edition)

INTRODUCTION

Diseases that produce ear pain are some of the most common maladies of childhood. Most cases of otalgia are caused by **acute otitis media**. **Otitis externa** is also commonly seen, especially during the summer months.

DIFFERENTIAL DIAGNOSIS LIST

External Ear Pain

Infectious Causes
  Otitis externa (swimmer's ear)
  Infected preauricular sinus
  Herpes simplex virus infection
  Herpes zoster
  Auricular cellulitis
  External canal abscess
Neoplastic Causes
  Neoplasms of the external auditory canal
Traumatic Causes
  Frostbite, burns, lacerations
  Hematoma or seroma
Miscellaneous Causes
  Foreign body, cerumen impaction

Middle and Inner Ear Pain

Infectious Causes
  Acute otitis media
  Myringitis
  Mastoiditis
Neoplastic Causes
  Rhabdomyosarcoma, lymphoma
  Histiocytosis X

Traumatic Causes
  Traumatic perforation
  Barotrauma
Inflammatory Causes
  Otitis media with effusion
Miscellaneous Causes
  Eustachian tube dysfunction
  Cholesteatoma

Referred Pain

Infectious Causes
  Dental abscess
  Stomatitis, aphthous ulcer
  Sinusitis
  Cervical lymphadenitis
  Pharyngitis or tonsillitis
  Retropharyngeal abscess
  Peritonsillar abscess
  Infected branchial cyst
  Parotitis
  Meningitis
Neoplastic Causes
  Neoplasms of the jaw, oropharynx, nasopharynx, larynx, facial nerve, or central nervous system
Traumatic Causes
  Oral cavity, pharyngeal, laryngeal, or esophageal trauma or foreign body

Miscellaneous Causes
  Erupting teeth
  Impacted teeth
  Migraine

Temporomandibular joint
  dysfunction or arthritis
Bell palsy

DIFFERENTIAL DIAGNOSIS DISCUSSION

Acute Otitis Media

Etiology

Acute otitis media is an infection of the middle ear space that occurs when the **eustachian tube obstructs** and a buildup of fluid in the middle ear (**effusion**) gets **infected by nasopharyngeal secretions.** Obstruction can result from **infection, allergy, enlarged adenoids, decreased eustachian tube stiffness,** or **inefficient tube opening.** The most common pathogens are (in order of frequency) *Streptococcus pneumoniae,* nontypeable *Haemophilus influenzae,* and *Moraxella catarrhalis.* With the advent of the heptavalent pneumococcal conjugated vaccine, the incidence of otitis media from *S. pneumoniae* is decreasing; however, the long-term impact of the vaccine has yet to be established. Table 30-1 lists some risk factors associated with acute otitis media.

Clinical Features

Symptoms of acute otitis media may include **otalgia, fever, irritability (from the pain), vomiting, diarrhea, hearing loss, anorexia,** and **otorrhea.** It is common for the patient to have a preceding upper respiratory infection.

> **HINT:** Parents commonly state that they are concerned about an ear infection because their child is "pulling on their ears." Although many children with otitis media rub or pull at their ears, this is not a specific sign of the disease.

TABLE 30-1 Risk Factors for Acute Otitis Media

Child-care attendance
Passive cigarette smoke exposure
Bottle propping
Formula fed (as opposed to breast fed)
Male
Winter season
First episode of acute otitis media <6 months of age
Siblings in the home
Sibling with recurrent acute otitis media

Helix

Antihelix

Tragus

Entrance to
ear canal

Mastoid
process

Lobule

Figure 30-1 ■ Anatomy of the Ear

Evaluation

To facilitate examination of the tympanic membrane, the clinician should **properly position the child** in the parent's arms, lap, or on the examining table **as well as manipulate the ear** (i.e., pull the pinna posteriorly and superiorly and push the tragus forward by applying traction to the skin in front of the ear). See Figure 30-1 for ear anatomy. If necessary, **remove cerumen** with a curette or by irrigation with water (however **irrigation is contraindicated** when a **perforated tympanic membrane** is suspected).

In acute otitis media, the tympanic membrane is **opaque or cloudy, bulging, red,** and has **decreased mobility.**

> **HINT:** Tympanic membrane erythema alone is not a reliable indicator of acute otitis media. A red tympanic membrane can also be caused by a viral upper respiratory tract infection, by crying, or by efforts to remove cerumen.

Tympanic membrane mobility should be **assessed** using **tympanometry** or **pneumatic otoscopy,** which involves applying positive and negative pressure to the tympanic membrane with a rubber bulb connected by a tube to the otoscope.

> **HINT:** To perform pneumatic otoscopy, use the largest speculum that fits comfortably in the auditory meatus and fits the speculum tightly to the ear canal.

Laboratory evaluation is usually not necessary. Some clinicians do recommend that **febrile infants** with acute otitis media who are <12 **weeks** undergo a full **sepsis evaluation.**

Treatment

Many patients who have physical findings consistent with the diagnosis of otitis media recover without treatment, and antibiotics afford only small improvement in symptom relief. **Some experts recommend withholding antibiotic treatment** for 48 to 72 hours and focusing on treatment of pain.

> **HINT:** In addition to diagnosing the cause of the ear pain, it is important to treat the pain. Acetaminophen or ibuprofen (for children >6 months) provides adequate pain control for most patients. Anesthetic otic drops are also useful but should be avoided if a perforation is suspected.

Initially withholding antibiotics helps curtail the emergence of resistant organisms and **does not increase the incidence of complications** such as mastoiditis or meningitis. However, some studies suggest using antibiotics in **children <2 years of age** and in those with **bilateral otitis media** shows more significant **benefit in relief of symptoms.** A wait-and-see approach can still be used but more judiciously in these circumstances.

First-line therapy includes the following:

- **High-dose amoxicillin** (80 to 90 mg/kg per day divided two or three times a day for a total of 10 days) should be used as first-line therapy in most children. **Twice-a-day dosing improves adherence** over three-times-a-day treatment. An increased dose of amoxicillin is used to overcome moderately **resistant strains of *S. pneumoniae.*** The following increases the risk of resistant organisms:
  - Children <2 years of age
  - Recent beta-lactam use
  - Exposure to child care
  - Communities with a high incidence of resistant organisms
- **Amoxicillin** (45 mg/kg per day) can be used in limited circumstances. Most communities have a high incidence of resistant *S. pneumoniae;* however, local bacteriologic data should be used to tailor initial antibiotic choice.

- A **5- to 7-day course** may be sufficient for children >2 years of age.
  - **Cephalosporins or azithromycin** may be used in patients who are allergic to penicillin. Given the 10% to 25% incidence of cephalosporin allergy in penicillin-allergic patients, the decision to use cephalosporins should be based on individual factors, including severity of the allergy.

With appropriate antimicrobial therapy, most children experience **symptomatic improvement within 48 to 72 hours.** If a patient does not respond fully to amoxicillin, the cause of the otitis may be viral or there may be bacterial resistance.

The choice of a **second-line antibiotic** depends on the suspected mechanism of resistance. *H. influenzae* and *M. catarrhalis* produce beta lactamase, therefore **amoxicillin-clavulanate** or a **second-generation cephalosporin** may be used. *S. pneumoniae* alters penicillin binding-proteins; therefore **high-dose amoxicillin** (80 to 90 mg/kg per day) is recommended if not used initially. **Amoxicillin-clavulanate or cephalosporins,** including **intramuscular ceftriaxone,** may be effective against resistant strains. **Intramuscular ceftriaxone** is not recommended for routine treatment of otitis media. It may be considered **when oral therapy is impossible** or when appropriate **first- and second-line therapy** for *S. pneumoniae* **has already failed.** When used for treatment of resistant organisms, ceftriaxone, 50 mg/kg, should be given for a total of three doses.

> **HINT:** The tympanic membrane does not return to normal appearance for 6 to 12 weeks. Many times when the ear is examined shortly after an episode of otitis media, the tympanic membrane may appear dull and pink when it is in the healing phase and not infected.

Infants **<4 weeks** who present with fever and/or irritability and acute otitis media should be **hospitalized** for **intravenous antibiotic administration,** pending cultures of the blood, urine, and cerebrospinal fluid. **Well-appearing, afebrile infants <4 weeks** may be treated **cautiously as outpatients** with **careful follow-up.**

Prevention

Some **controversy** surrounds the administration of **preventive antibiotics** because of the risk of accelerated bacterial resistance and the marginal benefit of prophylaxis found in some clinical trials.

Children who have **repeated cases of otitis media** may need **evaluation for myringotomy.** However, the short- and long-term benefits must be weighed because there is question as to the value of tympanostomy tube placement.

Otitis Media with Effusion

Etiology

Otitis media with effusion (i.e., a **middle ear effusion without** the **clinical manifestations** of acute otitis media) is usually either an **extension** of an **upper respiratory tract infection** or a **sequela** to an episode of acute otitis media.

> **HINT:** When otitis media with effusion follows properly treated acute otitis media, it usually represents the beginning of resolution of the infection (as opposed to persistent infection).

Clinical Features

Most children are **asymptomatic,** although some complain of fullness in the ear, hearing loss, and, less commonly, tinnitus and vertigo.

Evaluation

Otoscopy often reveals a retracted tympanic membrane with **decreased mobility.** Laboratory evaluation is not necessary.

Treatment

Most cases of otitis media with effusion **clear spontaneously** without active treatment. The management of otitis media with effusion is undergoing reevaluation. Studies from Europe and the United States show little long-term effect from **insertion of ventilation tubes.** Likewise, treatment with **antibiotics** may have some short-term beneficial effects, but the effect does not last when compared with patients not treated with antibiotics. Each case has to be individualized, but the main strategy continues to be **patient observation** for infection and speech difficulties.

> **HINT:** Decongestants and antihistamines have not been proven effective in the treatment of acute otitis media or otitis media with effusion.

Otitis Externa (Swimmer's Ear)

Etiology

Otitis externa, **an infection of the ear canal** and **external surface of the tympanic membrane,** results from **chronic irritation** as a result of **excessive moisture** in the ear canal. **Trauma** or **foreign bodies** in the ear canal can also precipitate otitis externa.

Diffuse otitis externa is most commonly caused by *Pseudomonas aeruginosa* and *Staphylococcus aureus* (which can also cause **abscesses** in the ear canal). Less commonly, *Enterobacter aerogenes, Proteus mirabilis, Klebsiella pneumoniae,* streptococci, and *Staphylococcus epidermidis* can be implicated, and, rarely, fungi and herpes virus causes acute otitis externa.

Clinical Features

The initial symptom of otitis externa is **pruritus** of the auditory canal leading to **ear pain.** The pain **worsens with touching or movement** of the ear and **during chewing.**

> **HINT:** Recent history of swimming is a common risk factor for the development of otitis externa. Swimming in water with higher bacteriologic counts increases the risk for otitis externa.

Evaluation

Patients may report **purulent drainage,** and **otorrhea** is often noted in the ear canal on examination. The canal appears **erythematous** and **edematous,** and the ear is **tender** to palpation or manipulation.

Treatment

Initial management consists of **removing the debris** from the affected ear—wiping the ear canal with a dry cotton swab usually suffices, but occasionally gentle suction is needed. An **antibiotic otic suspension** or combination **antibiotic and corticosteroid otic** preparation should be instilled in the affected ear three to four times daily for up to 10 days. If a perforated tympanic membrane is suspected, corticosteroids are contraindicated. If the canal is particularly edematous, a wick of cotton or gauze should be inserted into the canal to facilitate medication entry. Patients should be advised **to avoid swimming** during treatment. Failure to respond to **two courses of treatment** or the presence of **severe inflammation** should prompt referral to an **otolaryngologist.**

Prevention

In susceptible patients, prevention of otitis externa entails **abstaining from swimming** or placing **2% acetic acid solution in each ear canal after swimming** or bathing.

Foreign Bodies

Etiology

Foreign bodies rank **second to inflammatory and infectious disorders** of the ear as causes of otalgia. Solid nonorganic objects are most commonly seen, although live insects can also enter the ear canal.

Treatment

Most foreign bodies can be **gently removed** with an ear curette or otologic forceps. **Insects should be killed** before attempting removal (e.g., with mineral oil, microscope immersion oil, or alcohol). If the object cannot be removed with an ear curette or otologic forceps, **irrigation** of the ear canal with **water at body temperature** is often effective. The stream of water should be directed toward the edge of the foreign body in an attempt to push it toward the external meatus. **Inability to remove the foreign body** necessitates referral to an **otolaryngologist** for removal.

> **HINT:** If the foreign body is vegetable matter, irrigation should not be attempted because the vegetable matter can swell and occlude the ear canal.

Acute Mastoiditis

Etiology

Acute mastoiditis is one of the **most serious complications of acute otitis media.** Infection of the mastoid air cells in the temporal bone poses a risk because it is contiguous with the posterior and middle cranial fossae, the sigmoid and lateral sinuses, the facial nerve, and the semicircular canals. Although all cases of acute otitis media are characterized by concomitant inflammation of the mucosal lining of the mastoid air cells, clinically significant mastoiditis occurs when the **passageway from the middle ear to the mastoid becomes obstructed.** Acute mastoiditis is most commonly caused by *S. pneumoniae, H. influenzae,* and *M. catarrhalis,* but *Streptococcus pyogenes, S. aureus, Pseudomonas aeruginosa,* and anaerobic organisms may also be involved.

Clinical Features

Patients with acute mastoiditis present with **persistent otalgia** and **fever.** Otoscopy usually reveals a **bulging, red, poorly mobile tympanic membrane; purulent drainage** (through a perforation in the membrane) may be visible. **Edema** and **erythema** can be seen **over the mastoid bone,** obliterating the postauricular crease and **causing the characteristic downward and forward displacement of the pinna.** The mastoid region is **tender** to palpation.

Evaluation

A **computed tomography (CT) scan** of the temporal bone reveals **inflammation and destruction of the mastoid.** If the tympanic membrane is perforated, the canal should be cleaned of debris and fresh pus should be obtained for culture.

Treatment

Broad-spectrum **intravenous (IV) antibiotic therapy** covering the most common organisms should be initiated and later narrowed according to culture results when available. A third-generation cephalosporin can be initiated as first-line therapy; however, if cephalosporin-resistant *S. pneumoniae,* anaerobes, or methicillin-resistant *S. aureus* are considered potential pathogens, antibiotics should be tailored accordingly. An **otolaryngologist** should be consulted, as **mastoidectomy** may be necessary if there **is poor response to IV antibiotics.** Placement of **ventilating tubes** may be appropriate to ensure continued drainage.

Trauma

Etiology

- **External ear injuries** can be caused by athletic injuries, falls, direct blows to the ear, earrings that tear through the lobe, burns, or frostbite.
- **Middle and inner ear injuries.** The ear canal can be injured by objects used to scratch the ear or to remove cerumen. Traumatic perforation of the tympanic membrane is most commonly caused by poking an object into the ear canal, but trauma to the head and barotrauma can also cause tympanic membrane perforation. Barotrauma occurs when the eustachian tube is obstructed and changes in ambient pressure cannot be transmitted to the middle ear cavity. The increased ambient pressure is transmitted to the vessels of the middle ear mucosa, creating mucosal edema. The pressure differential between the mucosa and the middle ear cavity causes rupture of the mucosal vessels, bleeding into the middle ear, and possibly perforation.

Evaluation

A history of ear trauma may be elicited. The **external ear** should be **examined for hematomas or seromas,** which appear as smooth blue masses on the lateral auricle and obscure its natural contour. **Microscopic examination** of the tympanic membrane is necessary in patients with suspected traumatic tympanic membrane perforations to ensure that the edges of the perforation do not enter the middle ear cavity. Cholesteatoma formation can occur as a complication if the edges of the ruptured tympanic membrane protrude into the middle ear.

Treatment

For **external ear injuries,** immediate evacuation of hematomas and seromas of the auricle is necessary to prevent cartilage damage. Use of epinephrine should be avoided when lacerations of the pinna are sutured because epinephrine causes vasoconstriction and may lead to tissue necrosis.

For a **perforated tympanic membrane,** clean perforations (i.e., those in which the edges do not enter the middle ear cavity) usually heal spontaneously within 2 to 3 weeks. The perforation should be kept clean and dry. A patient with a traumatic perforation that does not heal in 3 weeks or one who experiences vertigo, sensorineural hearing loss, or facial nerve paralysis must be referred to an otolaryngologist.

Barotrauma should be treated with antibiotics to prevent infection of the middle ear hemorrhagic effusion. Patients with barotrauma and acute sensorineural hearing loss or vertigo, and those with barotrauma injuries that do not heal, require prompt referral to an otolaryngologist.

Suggested Readings

American Academy of Family Physicians, American Academy of Otolaryngology-Head and Neck Surgery, American Academy of Pediatrics Subcommittee on Otitis Media with Effusion: Clinical practice guideline: otitis media with effusion. *Pediatrics* 113(5): 1412–1429, 2004.

American Academy of Pediatrics and American Academy of Family Physicians Subcommittee on Management of Acute Otitis Media: Clinical practice guideline: diagnosis and management of acute otitis media. *Pediatrics* 113(5):1451–1465, 2004.

Bhetwal N, McConaghy JR: The evaluation and treatment of children with acute otitis media. *Prim Care* 34:59–70, 2007.

Spiro DM, Tay KY, Arnold DH, et al.: Wait-and-see prescription for the treatment of acute otitis media: a randomized controlled trial. *JAMA* 296(10):1235–1241, 2006.

INTRODUCTION

Edema refers to the demonstrable accumulation of an excessive amount of fluid in the **extravascular interstitial space** of the body. The balance of Starling forces between plasma and the interstitium normally favors the net filtration of fluid from the capillary lumen into the interstitial space. This fluid is then collected by the lymphatic system and returned to the circulation via the thoracic duct. Edema occurs **when the rate of filtration of fluid from the capillaries increases beyond the capacity of the lymphatics to remove it or when lymphatic function is impaired.** Increased hydrostatic and oncotic pressure gradients across the capillary wall or an increase in capillary wall permeability favors the formation of edema. Edema may be **localized or generalized.**

Localized edema is found in diseases of the lymphatic system, in diseases associated with venous obstruction, and in conditions associated with increased permeability of the capillary wall (e.g., infection, burns, trauma, allergic reactions). **Allergic reaction** is the **most common cause** of localized edema **in childhood.**

Generalized edema usually develops secondary to increased protein losses, decreased protein production, or heart failure. **Minimal-change nephrotic syndrome (MCNS)**, although uncommon (with an incidence of about 2 in 100,000 children per year), **accounts for most cases** of generalized edema.

DIFFERENTIAL DIAGNOSIS LIST

Many diseases cause localized or generalized edema; they may be classified according to pathophysiologic mechanism.

Increased Capillary Permeability

Allergic Causes
Insect bites
Contact dermatitis
Drug or food allergy

Infectious Causes
Cellulitis
Scarlet fever
Epstein-Barr virus
Roseola
Sepsis—bacterial, viral, fungal

Vasculitic or Rheumatologic Causes
Serum sickness
Henoch-Schönlein purpura
Systemic lupus erythematosus (SLE)
Dermatomyositis
Mucocutaneous lymph node syndrome
Rheumatoid arthritis

Miscellaneous Causes
Burns

Hereditary angioneurotic
edema

Vitamin E deficiency in
premature infants

Sickle cell anemia hand-
foot syndrome
(dactylitis)

Thyroid dysfunction
(hypothyroidism more
than hyperthyroidism)

Angioedema secondary to
use of medications (e.g.,
angiotensin-converting
enzyme inhibitors)

Systemic inflammatory
response syndrome

Decreased Plasma Oncotic Pressure (Hypoproteinemia)

Renal Causes

Nephrotic syndrome

Nephrotic syndrome with
nephritis

Preeclampsia

Hepatic Causes

Cirrhosis/liver failure

Hepatitis

Congenital fibrosis

Metabolic disorders (e.g.,
galactosemia)

Gastrointestinal Causes

Protein-losing enteropathy

Cystic fibrosis

Celiac disease

Enteritis with malabsorption

Miscellaneous Causes

Protein-calorie malnutrition
(kwashiorkor)

Severe iron-deficiency
anemia

Beriberi

Increased Hydrostatic Pressure

**Local or Systemic Venous
Hypertension**

Venous compression

Venous thrombosis

Compartment syndrome

Congestive heart failure

Pericardial effusion and
tamponade

Constrictive pericarditis/
restrictive cardiomyopathy

Cirrhosis/liver failure

Increased Plasma Volume

Excessive iatrogenic intravenous fluid

Renal failure

Glomerulonephritis

Medications (e.g., nons-
teroidal anti-inflammatory
drugs, calcium channel
blockers, minoxidil,
diazoxide, corticosteroids)

Pregnancy

Premenstrual

**Impaired Lymphatic Drainage
or Increased Interstitial
Oncotic Pressure**

Hereditary disorders
(e.g., Milroy disease)

Congenital disorders
(e.g., Turner syndrome)

Protozoal infections
(e.g., filariasis)

Trauma

Neoplasia—obstruction
secondary to primary or
metastatic disease, surgical
lymph node resection

DIFFERENTIAL DIAGNOSIS DISCUSSION

This differential diagnosis discussion is limited to **causes of generalized edema.**

Nephrotic Syndrome

Etiology

The nephrotic syndrome, characterized by the **onset of edema with massive proteinuria, hypoalbuminemia, and hypercholesterolemia,** may be a manifestation of **numerous clinical entities.** The edema forms **secondary to decreased oncotic pressure** (hypoalbuminemia) **and increased salt and water reabsorption by the kidneys. In primary nephrotic syndrome,** the disease is confined to the **kidney,** whereas **secondary nephrotic syndrome** occurs during the course of a **systemic illness.**

- **Causes of primary nephrotic syndrome** in children include MCNS, congenital nephrotic syndrome, focal segmental glomerulosclerosis, membranoproliferative glomerulonephritis, membranous nephropathy, and crescentic glomerulonephritis.
- **Secondary nephrotic syndrome** may occur in association with vasculitides (e.g., Henoch-Schönlein purpura), SLE, malignant lymphomas (e.g., Hodgkin disease), or infectious diseases (e.g., quartan malaria, hepatitis B and C, HIV).

Nephrotic syndrome during infancy requires special consideration; it may be congenital or caused by intrauterine infections such as congenital syphilis.

Clinical Features

MCNS accounts for **>75% of cases** of nephrotic syndrome in children. It is **twice as common in boys** as in girls, and onset most commonly occurs between the ages of **2 and 7 years.** Patients usually present with **edema** and **decreased urine volume.** Blood pressure is rarely elevated and **hematuria,** present in a minority of patients, is usually microscopic.

The **onset of edema** associated with nephrotic syndrome is usually **insidious and fluctuates;** the fluid characteristically appears in the dependent portions of the extremities or in distensible tissues (e.g., eyelids, scrotum, or labia).

> **HINT:** The early periorbital edema in children with nephrotic syndrome may be erroneously attributed to and treated as an allergic reaction.

> **HINT:** Remember that although these children do not appear dehydrated, their intravascular volume may be decreased, and they are at increased risk for hypovolemic shock in the setting of vomiting or diarrhea.

Evaluation

Acceptable clinical criteria for confirmation of significant proteinuria include urinary protein losses at a rate of **40 mg/m² per hour** or a **urine protein-to-urine creatinine ratio** (Upr:Ucr) that **exceeds 1.0** in a randomly collected specimen. A ratio of <0.15 is normal, a ratio of >1.0 suggests nephrotic-range proteinuria, and a ratio of >2.5 is diagnostic of nephrotic syndrome.

Children usually develop edema when the serum albumin level falls below 2.7 g/dL. The **hemoglobin level may be increased** secondary to hemoconcentration, and the **erythrocyte sedimentation rate is increased**. **Mild prerenal azotemia** may be present secondary to reduced intravascular volume. Unless severe hypovolemia is present, the glomerular filtration rate is normal in patients with MCNS. **Hypercholesterolemia** occurs secondary to increased lipoprotein synthesis and urinary losses of lipases.

Children with nephrotic-range proteinuria, hypoalbuminemia, edema, and hypercholesterolemia have nephrotic syndrome. Their evaluation should include investigation of **possible infectious or systemic causes** based on the history and physical examination. **Syphilis** should be **ruled out** in **patients <6 months.**

Complications

The main complication of nephrotic syndrome is infection, including upper and lower respiratory tract infection, cellulitis, and peritonitis with encapsulated organisms such as *S. pneumoniae*. Patients with nephrotic syndrome are also at increased risk for venous and arterial thrombosis.

> **HINT:** Intestinal wall edema causes abdominal pain, but the physician must always think about primary peritonitis and deep venous thrombosis in the nephrotic patient with abdominal or flank pain.

Treatment

Corticosteroids are the first-line treatment. MCNS is characterized by responsiveness to corticosteroid therapy—treatment with glucocorticoids and a low-salt diet usually results in remission of the renal disease with prompt diuresis and resolution of the edema.

HINT: Patients with nephrotic syndrome who fail to respond to steroid therapy and children with an atypical clinical presentation for MCNS require a renal biopsy to rule out focal segmental glomerulosclerosis, membranous glomerulopathy, and membranoproliferative glomerulonephritis, which demonstrate a more variable response to therapy and may progress to renal failure.

- **Salt restriction** helps minimize the edema.
- **Albumin (25 g/dL) infusions and diuretic administration** may be necessary for patients with severe edema. However, these agents should be used with caution to avoid intravascular depletion and pulmonary edema.
- **Angiotensin-converting enzyme inhibitors and angiotensin receptor blockers** may exert a renoprotective effect in patients with steroid-resistant nephrotic syndrome.
- **Alkylating agents.** Further immunosuppression with an alkylating agent (e.g., cyclophosphamide, chlorambucil) may be necessary in patients who do not respond to glucocorticoids or who become glucocorticoid dependent.
- **Calcineurin inhibitors (e.g., cyclosporine, tacrolimus) and mycophenolate mofetil** have been used to treat children with steroid-resistant nephrotic syndrome; however, their efficacy remains unproven.

Acute Postinfectious Glomerulonephritis

Acute poststreptococcal glomerulonephritis is discussed in Chapter 39, "Hematuria."

Congestive Heart Failure

Etiology

Increased systemic venous pressure is a prerequisite for the development of **cardiac edema** because the venous back pressure is critical in the alteration of the transcapillary filtration pressure. Decreased effective intravascular volume also leads to a neurohumoral cascade that promotes renal sodium and water reabsorption. Congestive heart failure may occur **secondary to congenital heart disease, myocarditis,** or **cardiomyopathy.**

Clinical Features

In children, the signs and symptoms of congestive heart failure are similar to those seen in adults; however, **edema is a mild finding** and most often seen in severely decompensated patients. The edema is first noted on the backs of the hands or feet or in dependent areas.

Children may present with fatigue, dyspnea on exertion, decreased exercise tolerance, anorexia, abdominal pain, or cough. More specific and worrisome signs and symptoms include: **dyspnea, orthopnea, basilar** rales, hepatomegaly, cyanosis, and **cardiomegaly.** In **infants,** symptoms of congestive heart failure include **feeding difficulties, tachypnea, diaphoresis,** and **labored respiration;** edema is frequently not detected clinically.

Evaluation

Evaluation is directed toward **identifying the underlying cardiac disease.** The **auscultatory findings** (e.g., gallop rhythm, murmur) are produced by the basic lesion and may help identify the underlying cause. **Echocardiography** delineates structural abnormalities and assesses myocardial function.

Treatment

Therapy is primarily aimed at management of the underlying heart disease. Supportive management strategies may include **diuretics** (to decrease the excessive salt and water load), afterload-reducing agents, and **inotropic medications** to improve the contractile performance of the heart.

Cirrhosis

Cirrhosis is discussed in Chapter 16, "Ascites."

Protein-Calorie Malnutrition (Kwashiorkor)

Etiology

Kwashiorkor, the most **prevalent form of malnutrition** in the world, is a clinical syndrome that results from **severely deficient protein and calorie intake.** The resultant **hypoalbuminemia** reduces the colloid osmotic pressure, leading to edema.

Clinical Features

Initial signs (e.g., lethargy, irritability) are nonspecific. Patients with advanced cases demonstrate **edema, poor growth, poor stamina, decreased muscle mass, dermatitis,** and **increased susceptibility to infection.** Failure to gain weight may be masked by edema, which is often present in internal organs before it can be identified in the hands or face.

Evaluation

A **decrease in the serum albumin level** is the most **characteristic** laboratory finding. The **hemoglobin level** and **hematocrit** are usually **low.** Height may be normal or retarded, depending on the chronicity of the illness.

Treatment

Restoration of nutritional status can be achieved by **frequent feedings with high-protein, high-energy formulas.** The initial treatment should provide average energy and protein requirements, followed by a **gradual increase to 1.5 times the energy and 3 to 4 times the protein requirements.**

The resolution of the edema may initially result in no change in weight or in weight loss.

EVALUATION OF EDEMA

Patient History

The following information should be sought:

- Was the onset of the edema acute or insidious?
- What are the associated symptoms (e.g., dark urine, suggestive of nephritis; respiratory distress, suggestive of congestive heart failure; diarrhea, suggestive of a gastrointestinal disorder)?
- Is there a history of a sore throat or cutaneous rash?
- Is there a history of recurrent localized edema associated with abdominal pain (suggestive of hereditary angioneurotic edema)?

Physical Examination

The first determination to make is whether the edema is **localized or generalized.** Findings in patients with **localized edema** may include **pruritus** or **urticaria** (associated with an allergic reaction); **tenderness, erythema, or fever** (associated with cellulitis); or **localized pronounced swelling** (associated with insect bites, especially those near the eyelids). If the patient has **fixed localized edema** (especially of an **extremity**), **lymphatic obstruction** should be considered (Figure 31-1).

Generalized edema is frequently associated with a **significant underlying disease.** The initial physical examination should include careful attention to the **cardiovascular system,** the **abdomen,** and the **skin.**

Laboratory Studies

The following studies may be indicated for the evaluation of generalized edema:

- Urinalysis
- Serum albumin level
- Complete blood count, erythrocyte sedimentation rate, C-reactive protein, prothrombin time
- Specific serologic tests (guided by clinical findings)
- Serum electrolytes, blood urea nitrogen, and creatinine level
- Serum cholesterol level
- Brain natriuretic peptide level (for heart failure)

> **HINT:** The critical step in the laboratory evaluation of edema is to test the urine for evidence of significant proteinuria (i.e., urinary protein losses that exceed 40 mg/m^2 per hour or a Upr:Ucr ratio that exceeds 1.0).

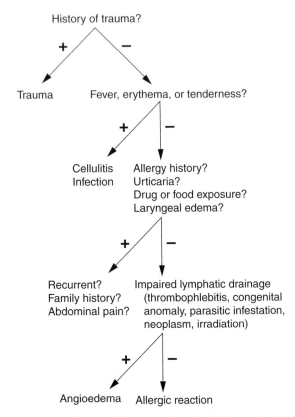

Figure 31-1 ■ Differential diagnosis for physical examination findings in a patient with localized edema

TREATMENT OF EDEMA

In patients with generalized edema, **treatment of the primary disease** usually results in **resolution of** the edema. The mainstay of edema therapy consists of **salt restriction** and **diuretics**, although in patients with MCNS (the most common cause of generalized edema) diuretic therapy is **rarely necessary**. It is often **not necessary to treat the edema before** establishing the **diagnosis**.

APPROACH TO THE PATIENT (FIGURE 31-2)

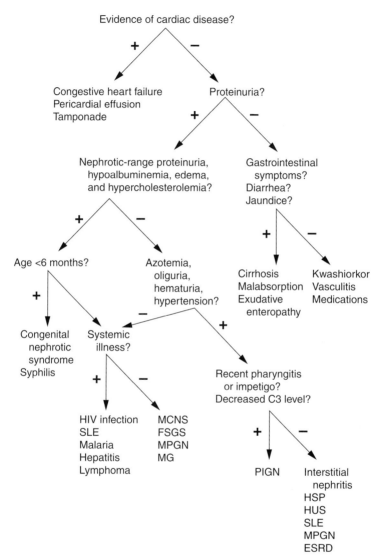

Figure 31-2 ■ Approach to the patient with generalized edema
C3 = complement; ESRD = end-stage renal disease; FSGS = focal segmental glomerulosclerosis; HSP = Henoch-Schönlein purpura; HUS =
hemolytic uremic syndrome; MCNS = minimal-change nephrotic syndrome; MG v membranous glomerulopathy; MPGN = membranoproliferative glomerulonephritis; PIGN = postinfectious glomerulonephritis;
SLE = systemic lupus erythematosus.

Suggested Readings

Andreucci M, Federico S, Andreucci VE: Edema and acute renal failure. *Semin Nephrol* 21(3):251–256, 2001.

Cho S, Atwood JE: Peripheral edema. *Am J Med* 113:580–586, 2002.

Eddy AA, Symons JM: Nephrotic syndrome in childhood. *Lancet* 362(9384):629–639, 2003.

Farkas H, Varga L, Széplaki G, et al.: Management of hereditary angioedema in pediatric patients. *Pediatrics* 20(3):e713–e722, 2007.

Fenton M, Burch M: Understanding chronic heart failure. *Arch Dis Child* 92(9):812–816, 2007.

Hisano S, Hahn S, Kuemmerle NB, et al.: Edema in childhood. *Kidney Int Suppl* 59:S100–S104, 1997.

Hodson EM, Habashy D, Craig JC: Interventions for idiopathic steroid-resistant nephrotic syndrome in children. *Cochrane Database Syst Rev* 2:CD003594, 2006.

Hodson EM, Willis NS, Craig JC: Corticosteroid therapy for nephrotic syndrome in children. *Cochrane Database Syst Rev* 4:CD001533, 2007.

Kaplan BS, Meyers KEC: *Pediatric Nephrology and Urology: The Requisites in Pediatrics*. Philadelphia, Elsevier Mosby, 2004.

Martin P-Y, Schrier RW: Renal sodium excretion and edematous disorders. *Endocrinol Metab Clin North Am* 24:459–479, 1995.

Rosen FS: Urticaria, angioedema, anaphylaxis. *Pediatr Rev* 13:387–390, 1992.

DIFFERENTIAL DIAGNOSIS LIST

Sodium imbalance
Potassium imbalance
Calcium imbalance
Magnesium imbalance

Phosphate imbalance
Metabolic acidosis
Metabolic alkalosis

DIFFERENTIAL DIAGNOSIS DISCUSSION

Hypernatremia

Etiology

Hypernatremia is a serum sodium level >150 mEq/L. The causes of hypernatremia fall into four major categories:

- **Water loss** is by far the most common cause of hypernatremia. Usually sodium loss is involved as well, but the water loss exceeds the sodium loss. Major causes of water loss include diarrhea, vomiting, or both with inadequate fluid intake; diabetes insipidus (see Chapter 77, "Urinary Frequency and Polyuria"); increased evaporative water loss (e.g., from radiant warmers or fever); and renal disease with urinary concentrating defect.
- **Excess sodium intake** is frequently iatrogenic and results from orally or intravenously administered sodium chloride or sodium bicarbonate.
- **Inadequate water intake** can result from an impaired thirst mechanism, an inability to swallow, or a lack of access to water.
- **Essential hypernatremia** is rare in childhood and results from defective osmoreceptors.

Clinical Features

The signs and symptoms of hypernatremia vary among individuals and partially depend on the magnitude of the sodium concentration and the rate of change. Signs and symptoms are **nonspecific** and include irritability, lethargy, a harsh "cerebral" cry, increased deep tendon reflexes, seizures, and, occasionally, focal neurologic signs.

Evaluation

Hypernatremic states, especially when associated with water loss, involve significant shifts of fluid from the intracellular space, with relative sparing of the extracellular fluid (ECF). Nevertheless, the physical examination should **focus on ECF volume assessment.** The adequacy of the intravascular compartment can be determined by evaluating the peripheral pulses,

TABLE 32-1   Assessment of Hypernatremia

Underlying Cause	ECF Volume	Urine Output	Urine Sodium	Specific Gravity
Sodium excess	Increased	Normal or increased	Increased	High
Water loss (DI)	Decreased	Increased	Decreased	Low
Sodium and water loss (water more than sodium)	Normal or decreased	Decreased	Increased	High

DI = diabetes insipidus; *ECF* = extracellular fluid

perfusion, temperature, and capillary refill time. The adequacy of the interstitial compartment can be ascertained by evaluating the skin turgor, tears, and mucous membranes.

Laboratory studies include serum electrolytes; glucose, calcium, blood urea nitrogen (BUN), and creatinine levels; and urinalysis, urine osmolarity, sodium, and creatinine.

Table 32-1 summarizes the findings suggestive of the various underlying mechanisms of hypernatremia.

Treatment

Significant **intravascular volume compromise or shock** should be **treated promptly** and independently of the serum sodium concentration by administering normal saline in amounts adequate to restore pulses and perfusion. Initially, a bolus of 20 mL/kg should be administered rapidly (over 20 to 30 minutes). The child should be reassessed and additional fluid given as needed.

After the patient with hypernatremic dehydration is stabilized, an attempt should be made to **reduce the serum sodium level slowly,** generally at a rate of approximately 0.5 mEq/L/hour and no greater than 15 mEq/L in a 24-hour period. Administering intravenous fluids consisting of one-third normal saline and spreading the administration of maintenance and deficit fluids evenly over 48 hours is recommended, even though calculated sodium needs are usually less (i.e., approximately 2 mEq/kg, which would require only a eighth to a fourth normal saline to replete). The use of very hypotonic fluids, especially when given rapidly, can lead to intracellular water shift, cell swelling, and cerebral edema.

In patients with **severe total body sodium excess,** judicious use of fluids, with or without furosemide administration, dialysis, or both, is recommended (under the guidance of a nephrologist).

Hyponatremia

Etiology

Hyponatremia is defined as a serum sodium level of <130 mEq/L. All causes of hyponatremia can be considered to be dilutional, depletional, or both (Table 32-2).

TABLE 32-2 Causes of Hyponatremia

Dilutional Hyponatremia

Water intoxication (excess ingestion or iatrogenic administration)
Edema-associated states
   Congestive heart failure
   Nephrotic syndrome
   Renal failure
   Hepatic failure
   Neuromuscular blockade (e.g., pancuronium-induced)
Excess antidiuretic hormone (ADH)* (nonedematous state)
   Exogenous administration
   Syndrome of inappropriate antidiuretic hormone (SIADH)
Reset osmostat
Hyperglycemia

Depletional Hyponatremia

Renal sodium wasting (e.g., Fanconi syndrome)
Adrenal sodium wasting (e.g., adrenal insufficiency)
CAH (21-hydroxylase deficiency)
Diuretic therapy
Osmotic diuresis (e.g., glucosuria)
Gastrointestinal fluid losses with hypotonic replacement
Excessive perspiration associated with large sodium loss (e.g., cystic fibrosis)

*Conditions associated with increased ADH or an ADH-like effect and hyponatremia include pain, vomiting, central nervous system disorders (e.g., trauma, infection, neoplasia), intrathoracic conditions (e.g., infection, mechanical ventilation), and some drugs (e.g., narcotics, barbiturates, carbamazepine, nonsteroidal anti-inflammatory agents [NSAIDs], cyclophosphamide, vincristine).
CAH = congenital adrenal hyperplasia

- **Dilutional hyponatremia.** The total body water is generally expanded and is increased relative to total body sodium.
- **Depletional hyponatremia.** There is a decreased (or normal) amount of total body water and a sodium deficit, in which the sodium loss exceeds the water loss.
- **Pseudohyponatremia.** Sodium is not distributed throughout the serum and its concentration is artificially lowered. Causes of pseudohyponatremia include hyperlipidemia and hyperproteinemia.

Clinical Features

As with hypernatremia, the signs and symptoms are variable, nonspecific, and depend on both the severity of the hyponatremia and the rapidity with which it developed. Findings include lethargy, weakness, encephalopathy, and seizures.

Evaluation

Because depletional hyponatremia is associated with a water shift to the intracellular fluid (ICF) compartment, careful assessment and prompt restoration of the ECF **and intravascular volume** are critical.

Useful **laboratory studies** include serum electrolytes; glucose, BUN, creatinine, albumin, and cholesterol levels; serum cortisol, with and

Figure 32-1 ■ Narrowing the differential diagnosis for the underlying cause of hyponatremia
ADH = antidiuretic hormone

without adrenocorticotropic hormone (ACTH) stimulation, and ACTH levels (if adrenal insufficiency is suspected); and **urinalysis** to evaluate urine sodium and creatinine. A random urine sample permits calculation of the fractional excretion of sodium (FE_{Na}), which can be useful when the urine sodium concentration is borderline (e.g., 19 to 21 mEq/L):

$$FE_{Na} = [U_{Na} \times P_{Cr}] / [U_{Cr} \times P_{Na}] \times 100\%$$

Figure 32-1 demonstrates how the differential for the specific cause of the hyponatremia can be narrowed on the basis of urine output and urine sodium excretion.

Therapy

- **Compromised intravascular volume.** When indicated, the intravascular volume should be restored promptly with the administration of isotonic saline. A reasonable initial fluid volume is 20 mL/kg, given rapidly intravenously over 20 to 30 minutes. Additional isotonic fluid boluses may be indicated after reassessing the patient.
- **Sodium deficit.** The sodium deficit should be calculated and measures taken to restore the sodium level. The sodium deficit can be calculated as follows:

$$Na^+ \text{ deficit (mEq)} = 0.6 \times wt \text{ (kg)} \times (\text{desired } Na^+ - \text{observed } Na^+)$$

When a rapid increase in the serum sodium level is required (e.g., with hyponatremia-induced seizures), 3% saline (which contains 0.5 mEq/mL of sodium) should be administered. Care should be taken not to over-correct hyponatremia. The goal is to prevent or reverse symptoms. In general, in acute hyponatremia, the sodium level should be corrected to 125 mEq/L or to a level slightly higher than that associated with symptoms. Overzealous correction, especially of chronic hyponatremia, can lead to neurologic deterioration (osmotic demyelinization syndrome or central pontine myelinolysis).

- **Severe hyperglycemia.** Hyponatremia may be associated with severe hyperglycemia as a result of transcellular fluid shifts. The fluid shifts are caused by the osmotic effect of the hyperglycemia. The following formula can be used to calculate the expected sodium concentration after hyperglycemia has been resolved:

$$\text{Final } Na^+ \text{ (mEq/L)} = \text{measured } Na^+ + 0.016 \text{ [glucose (mg/dL)} - 100]$$

- **Acute edematous states.** In hyponatremic patients with acute edematous states secondary to hypoalbuminemia, it is essential not to restrict water intake because intravascular volume may be compromised. It is more important to restrict sodium intake to prevent further edema.
- **Adrenal insufficiency.** If adrenal insufficiency is suspected, hydrocortisone (50 mg/m^2) should be given as an initial bolus intravenously, followed by a hydrocortisone drip or doses given every 6 hours. Mineralocorticoid maintenance using fludrocortisones is ultimately required.

HINT: Syndrome of inappropriate ADH (SIADH) is an uncommon syndrome in pediatric patients, but it should be considered when hyponatremia occurs in the absence of volume depletion, edema, or renal insufficiency, or in association with certain drugs (Table 32-2). The diagnosis is based on the excretion of urine that is not maximally dilute and is >1.5 times a serum osmolality that is <280 mOsm/kg. Under most circumstances, a reliable estimate of the serum osmolality can be obtained by doubling the serum sodium level (mEq/L) and adding 10. In patients with hyperglycemia or azotemia, the serum osmolality can be calculated as follows:

$$2 \times Na \text{ (mEq/L)} + \text{glucose}/18 + \text{BUN}/2.8$$

Treatment consists of restricting fluid intake to slightly less than the total of the estimated insensible water loss plus the urine output, the sum of which usually approximates two thirds of maintenance fluids. The condition is usually transient in children, and chronic measures are not required.

TABLE 32-3 Drugs Associated with Hyperkalemia

Potassium-sparing diuretics (spironolactone, triamterene, amiloride)
Potassium supplements (e.g., potassium chloride)
Potassium-containing penicillins
Stored blood
Cyclosporine
Nonsteroidal anti-inflammatory drugs (NSAIDs)
Heparin
Angiotensin-converting enzyme (ACE) inhibitors
β-adrenergic blockers
Chemotherapeutic agents

Hyperkalemia

Etiology

Hyperkalemia is defined as a serum potassium level >5.5 mEq/L. There are four major underlying mechanisms:

- **Transcellular potassium shifts** are the most common cause of hyperkalemia in childhood. Shifts of potassium from the ICF to the ECF can be associated with metabolic acidosis, β-adrenergic blockade, strenuous exercise, insulin deficiency, and hyperkalemic periodic paralysis.

> **HINT:** The presence of acidosis does not always account for the hyperkalemia and may lead to failure to recognize and treat another cause.

- **Increased potassium intake** can result from potassium supplements, drugs containing potassium (e.g., potassium penicillins), salt substitute use, and blood transfusions (stored blood).
- **Decreased renal excretion of potassium** can result from renal failure, certain drugs (Table 32-3), type 4 renal tubular acidosis (RTA), mineralocorticoid deficiency, or mineralocorticoid resistance. Types of mineralocorticoid deficiency include adrenal insufficiency, congenital adrenal hyperplasia (CAH), hyporeninemic hypoaldosteronism, and primary mineralocorticoid deficiency. Mineralocorticoid resistance may be a transient condition in the newborn or caused by obstructive nephropathy or pseudohypoaldosteronism.
- **Increased endogenous cellular release of potassium** is associated with hypoxic or toxic cell death, burns, intravascular hemolysis, rhabdomyolysis, and acute tumor lysis syndrome.

Clinical Features

Symptoms of hyperkalemia are neither predictably present nor specific. They include muscle weakness, decreased deep tendon reflexes, ileus, anorexia, tingling of the mouth and extremities, malaise, and tetany.

Evaluation

A **serum electrolyte panel** should be obtained. Cardiac changes are usually seen when the potassium level exceeds 6.0 mEq/L and are more likely with a rapidly increasing potassium level. Cardiotoxicity is increased with concomitant hyponatremia or hypocalcemia.

> **HINT:** Spurious hyperkalemia may be seen with hemolyzed specimens, significant thrombocytosis, or extreme leukocytosis. Because heelstick samples, which are commonly obtained in infants, frequently result in hemolyzed specimens, increased potassium values are common and need immediate verification (by repeating the test) if treatment is considered. Venipuncture with a ≥22-gauge needle is preferred when possible to avoid damaging erythrocytes.

An **electrocardiogram** (ECG) should be obtained to assess for cardiac changes associated with hyperkalemia, commonly manifested as tall, "tented" T waves (especially in the precordial leads) and prolonged PR intervals or a widened, prolonged QRS complex. Late life-threatening ECG changes include flattened P or T waves (or both) with ST segment depression, a sine wave pattern, and tachyarrhythmias or bradyarrhythmias.

Indications for serious concern and instituting treatment include the following:

- A potassium value >7.0 mEq/L
- A rapidly increasing potassium concentration
- A clinical state in which the potassium level is expected to continue to increase (e.g., rhabdomyolysis)
- The presence of renal failure
- Symptoms of hyperkalemia

Treatment

If the verified potassium level is high or there are hyperkalemic signs and symptoms, emergency measures should be initiated. Table 32-4 summarizes the options for the management of hyperkalemia.

> **HINT:** Sodium bicarbonate and calcium salts are incompatible in intravenous solutions.

> **HINT:** Increased potassium excretion can be achieved with the use of furosemide, even in children with significant renal impairment.

TABLE 32-4 Treatment of Hyperkalemia

Agent	Indication	Mechanism of Action	Dose	Side Effects/Potential Problems
10% calcium gluconate	ECG changes	Stabilizes membranes	1 mg/kg IV over 5–10 min	Hypercalcemia
Sodium bicarbonate	ECG changes or very high K⁺ level	Shifts K⁺ to intracellular compartment	1 mg/kg IV over 5–10 min	Sodium load
Glucose plus insulin	ECG changes or very high K⁺ level	Shifts K⁺ to intracellular compartment	0.25–0.5 g/kg glucose plus 0.3 U insulin/g glucose over 30–60 min	Hyper- or hypoglycemia
Albuterol (β-agonist)	ECG changes or very high K⁺ level	Shifts K⁺ to intracellular compartment	1.25–2.5 mg by nebulizer	Tachycardia
Kayexalate resin	To remove K⁺ from body	K⁺ binds to resin in gut	1 g/kg PO or PR in 50%–70% sorbitol	Constipation
Furosemide	Symptomatic hyperkalemia	Enhances urinary K⁺ excretion	1–2 mg/kg IV	May not be enough renal function to be effective
Hemodialysis or peritoneal dialysis	No renal function	Removes K⁺ in dialysate	—	Risks associated with dialysis
Exchange transfusion	ECG changes or very high K⁺ level	Donor blood must be washed and have had most K⁺ removed	Double volume	Risks associated with exchange transfusion

ECG = electrocardiogram; IV = intravenous; K⁺ = potassium; PO = orally; PR = parenterally

TABLE 32-5 Drugs Associated with Hypokalemia

Drugs Associated With Increased Renal Loss

Aminoglycoside toxicity
Amphotericin B
Cisplatin
Penicillins in high doses
Corticosteroids
Diuretics (except for potassium-sparing ones)

Drugs Associated With Increased Cellular Uptake of Potassium

Terbutaline
Epinephrine
β-Adrenergic agents (e.g., albuterol)
Theophylline toxicity
Barium toxicity
Insulin

Hypokalemia

Etiology

Hypokalemia is defined as a serum potassium level <3.5 mEq/L. There are five major underlying mechanisms:

- **Severely limited nutrition** (e.g., anorexia nervosa)
- **Increased gastrointestinal losses** (e.g., vomiting, diarrhea, cathartic abuse)
- **Increased skin losses** (e.g., excessive perspiration, burns)
- **Increased renal losses**—Fanconi syndrome, RTA, Bartter syndrome, diuretic therapy, osmotic diuresis (e.g., glucosuria), hyperaldosteronism, CAH, 11-β-hydroxysteroid dehydrogenase deficiency (or inhibition with natural licorice ingestion), Liddle syndrome, Gitelman syndrome (magnesium-losing tubulopathy), excess adrenocorticotropic hormone (ACTH), drugs (Table 32-5), magnesium depletion, and chloride depletion
- **Transcellular potassium shifts**—alkalosis (metabolic and respiratory), excess insulin, hypokalemic periodic paralysis, and certain drugs (Table 32-5)

> **HINT:** The administration of intravenous glucose, especially in high concentrations, may worsen hypokalemia by stimulating insulin release, which increases cellular uptake of potassium.

Clinical Features

Signs and symptoms of hypokalemia, as in other electrolyte disturbances, are multiple, variable, and nonspecific.

- **Neuromuscular signs** include weakness, paralysis, tetany, ileus, ureteral aperistalsis, lethargy, confusion, autonomically mediated hypotension, and rhabdomyolysis.

- Cardiovascular signs include bradyarrhythmias and tachyarrhythmias.
- Renal and metabolic abnormalities include impaired renal concentrating capacity and polyuria, chronic nephrotoxicity, and impaired insulin secretion.

Evaluation

Laboratory studies should include a serum electrolyte panel; serum calcium, magnesium, and glucose levels; and urinalysis to evaluate urine

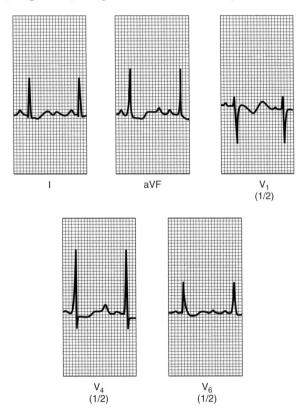

Figure 32-2 ■ Characteristic electrocardiogram (ECG) pattern in a patient with hypokalemia
These tracings are from a 4-year-old with nephrotic syndrome. Note the prominent U waves in all leads with ST segment depression and T wave inversion in leads I, aVF, V_4, and V_6. (Reprinted with permission from Garson A, Jr: Electrocardiography. In The Science and Practice of Pediatric Cardiology, 2nd ed. Edited by Garson A, Jr, Bricker JT, Fisher D, et al. Baltimore, Williams & Wilkins, 1998, 772.)

potassium and creatinine (to calculate the fractional excretion of potassium, FE_K). Hyperglycemia may occur. Other tests (e.g., aldosterone assessment) should be ordered if a specific disorder is suspected on the basis of the history and physical examination.

An **ECG** should also be obtained. ECG changes are seen with severe potassium deficit (i.e., usually <2.5 mEq/L). In addition, hypokalemia increases susceptibility to digitalis toxicity. Potential changes include T-wave flattening, U waves, which give the appearance of a long corrected QT interval (QTc), ST segment depression, and prolonged PR intervals (Figure 32-2).

Therapy

Potassium deficits frequently occur with other abnormalities (e.g., calcium, magnesium, and chloride depletion) and cannot be completely corrected until the accompanying deficits are repaired.

Potassium replacement for hypokalemia should be via the oral route whenever possible, although **oral potassium supplements** may cause gastric irritation, vomiting, or may be nonpalatable to a young child. Table 32-6 summarizes available oral preparations. A normal diet usually provides potassium in excess of daily maintenance requirements (2 to 3 mEq/kg). Foods rich in potassium include dried fruits, bananas (1.5 mEq/inch), tomatoes, and most other fruits. Prune juice and orange juice provide 16 mEq and 12 mEq of potassium per 8 ounces, respectively.

Patients with severe or symptomatic hypokalemia should receive **potassium intravenously** at a rate of no greater than 0.3 to 0.5 mEq/kg per hour. Because most of the body's potassium is not in the ECF, the serum potassium concentration may not reflect (and does not permit calculation of) the total potassium deficit. Serum potassium level and acid-base status must be followed closely when repairing deficits. Potassium should not be administered intravenously until it is certain that the patient is not anuric.

TABLE 32-6 Oral Potassium Supplements		
Preparation	**Formulation**	**Potassium Supplied**
Potassium phosphate	Tablet	1.1, 2.3, or 3.7 mEq
Potassium chloride	Extentabs	10 mEq
	Powder packet	20 mEq
	Effervescent tablets	20 mEq
	Liquid	20 mEq
Potassium citrate	Tablets, crystals, or syrup	1 mEq/mL (Polycitra) or 2 mEq/mL (Polycitra-K)
Potassium gluconate	Liquid	20 mEq/15 mL

> **HINT:** In the intravenous administration of potassium, concentrations of ≥40 mEq/L are irritating to small peripheral veins and often result in pain or loss of access site. Administration of high concentrations (>60 mEq/L) through a central line does not cause pain but is potentially dangerous, and benefits must be weighed against the risk of development of fatal arrhythmias. Children should be monitored carefully and continuously.

> **HINT:** In acute metabolic acidosis, the serum potassium level may be increased owing to extracellular shift while the total body potassium level is diminished. A rule of thumb is that a 0.1 decrease in pH acutely results in an increase in potassium level of 0.7 mEq/L.

Hypercalcemia

Etiology

Hypercalcemia is defined as a serum calcium level >11 mg/dL or an ionized calcium level >5.0 mg/dL. Hypercalcemia reduces renal blood flow and, as a result, decreases the glomerular filtration rate (GFR); increases sodium, potassium, and magnesium excretion; decreases renal concentrating capacity; and leads to metabolic acidosis. Causes of hypercalcemia include:

- **Enhanced vitamin D activity**—excess vitamin D administration, increased endogenous vitamin D sensitivity or activity (such as occurs in idiopathic infantile hypercalcemia, sarcoidosis, certain malignancies, and neonatal fat necrosis)
- **Skeletal disorders of calcium deposition or mobilization**—hyperparathyroidism, immobilization hypercalcemia, hypophosphatasia, vitamin A intoxication, skeletal dysplasias, and metastatic bone disease
- **Renal disorders**—hypocalciuric hypercalcemia, thiazide diuretic therapy, rhabdomyolysis with acute myoglobinuric renal failure
- **Miscellaneous causes**—milk-alkali syndrome, severe hypophosphatemia, blue diaper syndrome (tryptophan transport defect), excessive intravenous calcium administration, hypothyroidism or hyperthyroidism

Clinical Features

The onset and severity of symptoms vary among individuals, but generally symptoms are more severe the higher the serum calcium level. Symptoms are uncommon at levels <12 mg/dL. Levels of >16 mg/dL are life threatening and should be treated as an emergency.

Hypercalcemia that is renal in origin is characterized by polyuria, polydipsia, and signs of renal insufficiency, nephrocalcinosis, and nephrolithiasis.

Nonrenal hypercalcemia can cause a variety of symptoms:

- **General**—fatigue, weakness, anorexia
- **Gastrointestinal**—nausea, vomiting, constipation, xerostomia, symptoms of pancreatitis
- **Central nervous system**—headache, drowsiness, apathy, apnea (infancy)
- **Skin and mucous membranes**—pruritus, conjunctivitis
- **Musculoskeletal**—myalgias, arthralgias, bone pain, hypotonia
- **Cardiovascular**—hypertension, short QT interval, arrhythmias, heart block

Evaluation

Laboratory studies should include total and ionized calcium levels; a serum electrolyte panel; serum phosphorus, alkaline phosphatase, magnesium, urea, creatinine, total protein, and albumin levels; and an intact or aminoterminal assay for parathyroid hormone (PTH). **Other studies,** such as vitamin D levels (25 OH vitamin D and 1, 25 dihydroxy vitamin D), should be chosen based on clinical suspicion.

Calcium excretion can be assessed using a 24-hour urine collection (normal is <4 mg/kg per day) or, more quickly, by determining the calcium-to-creatinine ratio from a random sample. (Normal is <0.2 for children >6 years. Normal newborn values are up to 0.86.)

Therapy

Dehydration should be corrected, **hydration status** should be closely monitored, and **intravascular volume** should be maintained. If possible, the underlying cause of the hypercalcemia should be identified and removed. Calcium excretion should be maximized via saline diuresis and the use of loop diuretics.

Other therapies (e.g., steroids, calcitonin, mithramycin, bisphosphonates, chelators) may be indicated, depending on the specific disorder responsible for the hypercalcemia. These therapies should be used under the direction of a nephrologist or endocrinologist.

Hypocalcemia

Etiology

Hypocalcemia is defined as a serum calcium level <9.0 mg/dL (7.0 mg/dL in newborns) or an ionized calcium level <4.8 mg/dL (4.0 mg/dL in newborns). Causes include:

- Hypoalbuminemia (total calcium is decreased, but ionized calcium usually remains normal)
- Hyperphosphatemia
- Renal failure
- Hypocalcemia of the newborn, early (within 72 hours of birth) or late (5 to 7 days after birth)

- Hypoparathyroidism
- Pseudohypoparathyroidism
- Exchange transfusion
- Vitamin D–deficient rickets
- Vitamin D–dependent rickets
- Pancreatitis
- Hypomagnesemia

Clinical Features

The following signs and symptoms may be seen, especially with a reduced ionized calcium level:

- Muscle weakness, fasciculations, or both
- Numbness and tingling in extremities
- Cramps
- Hyperreflexia
- Positive Chvostek and Trousseau signs
- Tetany
- Seizures

Evaluation

Laboratory studies should include those recommended for the evaluation of hypercalcemia. Ionized calcium level determinations may be useful in assessing a child with hypocalcemia; unfortunately, this test is frequently unavailable in hospital laboratories, and it can be unreliable. A prolonged QTc interval may be seen on ECG (Figure 32-3).

Treatment

The decision to treat is based on the presence of symptoms, the calcium concentration, and the cause of hypocalcemia. Table 32-7 summarizes the commonly used calcium preparations.

Oral therapy is indicated only for correction of **chronic and mildly symptomatic states.** Maintenance calcium needs are not precisely known but generally considered to be 20 to 50 mg/kg per day of elemental calcium. In patients with hyperphosphatemia, therapy includes the use of phosphate binders (either calcium- or aluminum-containing salts). When indicated, vitamin D therapy increases absorption of calcium from the gastrointestinal tract and increases phosphaturia. Calcitrol and paricalcitol are available to treat the secondary hyperparathyroidism associated with chronic renal failure.

Patients with **severe symptoms** (e.g., seizures) require 10 to 20 mg/kg elemental **calcium administered intravenously and slowly.** The child must be monitored for bradyarrhythmias. Extravasation of calcium

A V_1 B V_1

Figure 32-3 ■ (*A*) Corrected QT (*QTc*) interval in a healthy newborn. (*B*) Prolonged QTc interval in a patient with hypocalcemia *(Reprinted with permission from Garson A, Jr: Electrocardiography. In The Science and Practice of Pediatric Cardiology, 2nd ed. Edited by Garson A, Jr, Bricker JT, Fisher D, et al. Baltimore, Williams & Wilkins, 1998, 746.)*

into the subcutaneous tissues may cause serious skin sloughs. Treatment with hyaluronidase should be considered for these patients.

> **HINT:** Hypomagnesemia frequently accompanies hypocalcemia, so the magnesium level should always be measured. If it is low in a child with apparent symptoms of hypocalcemia, the magnesium level should be corrected.

Hypermagnesemia

Etiology

Hypermagnesemia is defined as a serum magnesium level >2.5 mEq/L. Mechanisms include excess intake (almost always accompanied by significant renal insufficiency) and decreased renal excretion (seen with a

TABLE 32-7 Commonly Used Calcium Preparations

Preparation	Elemental Calcium Content	Route
Calcium gluconate (10%)	1 mL = 9 mg = 0.45 mEq	Intravenous
Calcium chloride (10%)	1 mL = 27 mg = 1.36 mEq	Intravenous
Calcium glubionate	1 mL = 23 mg = 1.12 mEq	Oral

glomerular filtration rate [GFR] <10 mL/minute, hypothyroidism, and familial hypocalciuric hypercalcemia). Sources of excess magnesium intake include magnesium-containing antacids, laxatives, or enemas; high-dose intravenous magnesium administration; and, in newborns, prepartum administration of large amounts of magnesium sulfate to the mother.

Clinical Features

Signs and symptoms, including decreased deep tendon reflexes, weakness, confusion, lethargy, and hypotension, relate to adverse effects on neuromuscular transmission and usually first appear when the magnesium level exceeds 7 mEq/L.

Evaluation

It is important to assess the GFR and the calcium concentration because hypocalcemia worsens the signs and symptoms of hypermagnesemia.

Therapy

The source of the increased magnesium level must be discovered and removed. **Continuous heart rate and blood pressure monitoring** are indicated for patients with magnesium levels >5 mEq/L. If the patient has symptoms, or if the magnesium level is >7 mEq/L, **intravenous administration of calcium** is indicated to decrease the serum magnesium level temporarily. In patients with severe hypermagnesemia and renal insufficiency, **peritoneal dialysis or hemodialysis** may be required.

Hypomagnesemia

Etiology

Hypomagnesemia is defined as a serum magnesium level <1.5 mEq/L and is frequently seen in association with hypocalcemia and hypokalemia. Rarely, hypomagnesemia is caused by dietary insufficiency. More common causes include increased gastrointestinal losses, increased renal excretion, and redistribution (Table 32-8).

> **HINT:** The association of hypomagnesemia with hypocalcemia and hypokalemia is common but confusing. In some situations, a cause-and-effect relationship may be in place. For example, hypomagnesemia leads to hypocalcemia as a result of diminished PTH secretion or decreased responsiveness of bone to PTH. Likewise, hypomagnesemia increases renal potassium loss. In other situations, a shared cause (e.g., aminoglycoside toxicity) accounts for the overlap. Attempts to treat one of these deficiencies without recognizing the presence of another will not be successful.

TABLE 32-8 Causes of Hypomagnesemia

Increased Gastrointestinal Losses

Small bowel disease or inflammation
Fat malabsorption (including cystic fibrosis)
Laxative abuse
Protein-calorie malnutrition
Gluten sensitivity
Gastroenteritis or chronic diarrhea

Increased Renal Losses

Primary renal tubular magnesium wasting (Gitelman syndrome)
Postobstructive diuresis
Recovery phase of acute renal failure
Diuretic therapy
Hypokalemic states
Hyperaldosteronism
Drugs (aminoglycosides, amphotericin, cyclosporine)
Hypoparathyroidism or hyperparathyroidism
Renal tubular acidosis
Hyperthyroidism

Redistribution

Refeeding, total parenteral nutrition
Pancreatitis
"Hungry bone" syndrome

Clinical Features

The signs and symptoms of hypomagnesemia are sometimes difficult to separate from those associated with concomitant electrolyte disturbances. Clinical features of hypomagnesemia include weakness, tremors, anorexia, lassitude, and, rarely, seizures.

Evaluation

Laboratory studies should include a serum electrolyte panel and serum calcium, phosphorus, alkaline phosphatase, and PTH levels.

An ECG may reveal associated cardiovascular problems, such as tachycardia (sinus or nodal), premature beats (supraventricular or ventricular), and changes similar to those seen in hypokalemia (i.e., flat, broad T waves; prolonged PR and QT intervals). Patients with hypomagnesemia also have increased susceptibility to digitalis toxicity.

Treatment

Therapy of symptomatic hypomagnesemia entails the administration of **magnesium sulfate** (25 to 50 mg/kg intravenously via a slow drip or every 4 to 6 hours intramuscularly). The patient must be monitored for hypotension.

TABLE 32-9 Normal Phosphorus Values	
Age	**Normal Phosphorus Value (mg/dL)**
Newborn	4.8–8.2
1–3 yr	3.8–6.5
4–11 yr	3.7–5.6
12–15 yr	2.9–5.4
15+	2.7–4.7

Prevention involves ensuring an adequate supply of magnesium in the diet or in parenteral fluids. Normal requirements are approximately 4 mg/kg per day (0.3 mEq/kg per day). Oral magnesium supplements frequently produce diarrhea and should be used with caution in children with renal insufficiency.

Hyperphosphatemia

Etiology

The normal phosphorus values vary according to age (Table 32-9). Causes of hyperphosphatemia include:

- **Renal failure** (usually associated with a GFR <50 mL/minute)
- **Increased renal tubular reabsorption**—hypoparathyroidism, pseudo-hypoparathyroidism
- **Increased phosphate intake**—cow's milk in infants, phosphate-containing enemas
- **Increased endogenous phosphate release**—tumor lysis syndrome
- **Most hypocalcemic states**

Clinical Features

Hyperphosphatemia is almost always accompanied by hypocalcemia, and signs and symptoms are related to the latter.

HINT: A serious complication of hyperphosphatemia is metastatic or ectopic calcification in vessel walls and tissues. The risk is greatly increased when the calcium and phosphorus product exceeds 70.

Evaluation

Appropriate laboratory studies include those for the assessment of calcium disorders as well as those that allow determination of renal function and assessment of the urine creatinine and phosphate level.

Assessment of the urine creatinine and phosphate level allows determination of tubular reabsorption of phosphate (TRP):

$$\text{TRP} = 1 - (U_{Phos}/P_{Phos})/(U_{Cr}/P_{Cr}) \times 100\%$$

Normal is a TRP >80%.

Treatment

Phosphate intake must be restricted and an **oral phosphate binder** (e.g., calcium carbonate, aluminum-containing salts) should be administered. Calcium carbonate is the preferred agent; a reasonable starting dose is 1 g with each meal, titrated thereafter as indicated. Chronic phosphate binding therapy is with sevelamer (Renagel). It is effective and well tolerated. Aluminum salts should never be used chronically because of the neurotoxicity of aluminum accumulation.

Phosphate excretion should be maximized by **saline diuresis** if renal function is normal. In patients with severe renal insufficiency, either **peritoneal dialysis or hemodialysis** may be effective.

Hypocalcemia should be corrected, if possible.

Hypophosphatemia

Etiology

Table 32-9 lists the normal phosphate values. Hypophosphatemia can result from hypercalcemic states, decreased phosphate intake, binding of phosphate in the gastrointestinal tract (e.g., antacid abuse), or increased renal phosphate loss (e.g., hyperparathyroidism, Fanconi syndrome, hypophosphatemic rickets).

Clinical Features

Symptoms and signs generally do not occur until the phosphorus level is <1.5 mg/dL. Clinical features include muscle weakness, rhabdomyolysis, bone pain, arthralgias, hemolytic anemia, anorexia, nausea, and vomiting.

Evaluation

Appropriate laboratory studies include those for the assessment of calcium disorders as well as those that allow determination of renal function and assessment of the urine creatinine and phosphate level.

Treatment

The underlying condition should be treated or removed. If possible, the **accompanying hypercalcemia** should be treated. Often, treatment of the hypercalcemia resolves the hypophosphatemia.

If necessary, **phosphate** should be administered to increase the serum phosphorus level to 2.0 mg/dL. Phosphate should be given at a rate of

TABLE 32-10 Causes of Metabolic Acidosis

Normal Anion Gap

Gastrointestinal loss of bicarbonate
  Diarrhea
  Drainage of intestinal fluid (e.g., ileostomy, nasojejunal tube drainage)
Administration of acid
  Total parenteral nutrition (e.g., amino acids)
Acute extracellular fluid expansion (e.g., following the rapid administration of intravenous fluids)
Renal loss of bicarbonate or failure to secrete net acid
  Renal tubular acidosis
  Therapy with carbonic anhydrase inhibitors (e.g., acetazolamide)

Wide Anion Gap

Renal failure
Ketoacidosis
  Diabetes mellitus
  Starvation
Lactic acidosis
Other organic acidosis (e.g., methylmalonic acidemia)
Intoxications (e.g., methanol, salicylates, ethylene glycol)

15 to 20 mg/kg per day, either orally or intravenously. It is important to ensure that the patient's renal function is normal before administering phosphate. The intravenous administration of phosphate is **contraindicated in the presence of hypercalcemia** because it may lead to the development of metastatic calcifications.

Metabolic Acidosis

Etiology

Metabolic acidosis is defined as any state that reduces the serum bicarbonate concentration to less than the normal range of 24 to 26 mmol/L.

Metabolic acidosis may be accompanied by either a normal anion gap (hyperchloremic metabolic acidosis) or a wide anion gap. Table 32-10 summarizes the causes of metabolic acidosis.

Renal tubular acidosis (RTA) is a group of disorders in which hyperchloremic metabolic acidosis occurs because of excess renal tubular loss of bicarbonate, failure to excrete dietary net acid, or both. The many causes of RTA (Table 32-11) can be categorized according to the type: **type 1** (distal or classic) RTA, **type 2** (proximal) RTA, or **type 4** (hyperkalemic) RTA. Table 32-12 summarizes the characteristics of each of these types of RTA.

Clinical Features

Signs and symptoms of metabolic acidosis are nonspecific, variable, and generally overshadowed by the illness or disorder leading to the acidosis.

TABLE 32-11 Selected Causes of Renal Tubular Acidosis

Type 1 (Distal or Classic) RTA

Idiopathic
  Sporadic
  Inherited (autosomal dominant or recessive)
Associated with renal disease
  Obstructive nephropathy
  Reflux nephropathy
  Postrenal transplant
Associated with disorders causing nephrocalcinosis
  Medullary sponge kidney
  Hyperparathyroidism
  Hypervitaminosis D
Associated with systemic disease
  Sickle cell disease
  Marfan syndrome
  Ehlers-Danlos syndrome
  Hereditary elliptocytosis
  Wilson disease
Associated with autoimmune disorders
  SLE
  Sjögren syndrome
  Polyarteritis nodosa
  Hypergammaglobulinemia
Associated with drug toxicity
  Amphotericin B
  Lithium

Type 2 (Proximal) RTA

Idiopathic or isolated
  Sporadic
  Inherited (autosomal dominant)
Associated with Fanconi syndrome*
Associated with systemic disease
  Cystinosis
  Lowe (oculocerebrorenal) syndrome
  Galactosemia
  Glycogen storage disease
  Hereditary fructose intolerance
  Tyrosinemia
  SLE and other autoimmune disorders
Associated with toxins
  Drugs (e.g., aminoglycosides, chemotherapeutic agents)
  Heavy metals
Associated with renal disorders
  Nephrotic syndrome
  Medullary cystic disease
  Renal venous thrombosis
  Renal transplant rejection
Associated with carbonic anhydrase deficiency
  Congenital (sporadic or familial)
  Drug-induced (acetazolamide)

Type 4 (Hyperkalemic) RTA

Associated with renal disease
Diabetic nephropathy

(Continued)

TABLE 32-11 Selected Causes of Renal Tubular Acidosis (*continued*)

Type 4 (Hyperkalemic) RTA

Obstructive nephropathy
Hyporeninemic hypoaldosteronism[†]
Associated with aldosterone deficiency
    Addison disease
    Chronic adrenal suppression
    Congenital adrenal hyperplasia (21-hydroxylase defect)
Associated with aldosterone resistance
    Pseudohypoaldosteronism
    Transient resistance (in newborns)
Associated with drugs
    Spironolactone
    Triamterene
    Amiloride
Chloride shunt (excess reabsorption of chloride)

[*]Fanconi syndrome is characterized by generalized proximal tubular dysfunction.
[†]Type 4 RTA may be found with any chronic tubulointerstitial nephritis.
RTA = renal tubular acidosis; *SLE* = systemic lupus erythematosus

Isolated metabolic acidosis (e.g., RTA) is occasionally associated with anorexia and vomiting. Hyperventilation, an almost immediate compensatory response to metabolic acidosis, is often, but not always, apparent.

Evaluation

The serum bicarbonate concentration is virtually equivalent to the total carbon dioxide value reported with serum electrolytes. The first step in the evaluation of a low bicarbonate level is to **calculate the anion gap:**

$$\text{Anion gap} = (Na^+) - [(Cl^-) + (HCO_3^-)]$$

TABLE 32-12 Characteristics of Renal Tubular Acidosis

	Type 1	Type 2	Type 4
Renal function?	Normal	Normal	Normal or decreased
Failure to thrive?	Yes	Yes	Yes
Polyuria or polydipsia?	Yes	Yes	No
Potassium level?	Normal or low	Normal or low	Elevated
Bicarbonate leak?	Usually	Significant	Small
Urine maximally acid?	No (pH >6)	Yes (below serum threshold)	Yes
Nephrocalcinosis or nephrolithiasis?	Yes	No	No
Fanconi syndrome?	No	Often	No
Osteomalacia or rickets?	Rarely	If Fanconi syndrome is present	No

The normal gap is 12, with a range of 8 to 16.

- If the **anion gap is normal,** a history of diarrhea or other gastrointestinal losses should be sought. If there is none, an accurate (meter) pH determination using a freshly voided urine sample transported in an airtight container should be obtained, and evaluation for RTA should be undertaken.
- If the **anion gap is >16,** the source of the unexplained anion should be considered. For example, the possibility of lactic acidosis or diabetic ketoacidosis (DKA) must be excluded. Although the history is helpful, several laboratory studies may be useful as well. A blood gas analysis should be obtained to assess the pH and arterial carbon dioxide tension ($Paco_2$) to determine the degree of compensation or the presence of a mixed acid-base disturbance. A blood ammonia level and evaluation of urine for organic acids may be helpful.

 HINT: Not all low serum bicarbonate levels indicate metabolic acidosis. Fingerstick carbon dioxide levels are often spuriously low because of prolonged exposure of the blood to air. Decreased bicarbonate concentrations may occur as compensation for chronic respiratory alkalosis.

HINT: Metabolic acidosis may occur with a normal bicarbonate value in children with mixed metabolic acid-base disturbances. For example, an infant with bronchopulmonary dysplasia who is receiving furosemide chronically (metabolic alkalosis) may develop severe diarrhea (metabolic acidosis) and have a normal bicarbonate concentration. Mixed disturbances involving metabolic acidosis may be detected by the delta-delta, that is, the difference between the delta anion gap (observed minus normal) and the delta of the serum bicarbonate. Delta-deltas more than and less than zero usually indicate mixed disorders.

HINT: A change in the bicarbonate concentration of 10 mmol/L is expected to lead to a change in pH of 0.15 in the same direction.

Therapy

Treatment should be directed at correcting or removing the cause of the acidosis (e.g., insulin administration in a patient with DKA). Because the lungs permit the removal of volatile acid as carbon dioxide, it is important to ensure **adequate ventilation.**

Alkali therapy is controversial and usually not indicated in the treatment of acute acidosis. In chronic acidosis, **alkali therapy** may help prevent both growth failure and the use of the skeleton as a buffer, which can lead to calcium loss. **Bicarbonate therapy** may be started at 2 mEq/kg per day and may be increased as needed to normalize the bicarbonate level. (The normal serum bicarbonate level is 22 to 24 mmol/L.) In patients with renal bicarbonate loss, up to 20 mEq/kg per day of bicarbonate may be required. Commonly used oral alkalinizing agents in children include the following:

- **Polycitra syrup,** which provides 2 mEq/mL of bicarbonate, 1 mEq/mL of sodium, and 1 mEq/mL of potassium
- **BICITRA solution,** which provides 1 mEq/mL of bicarbonate and 1 mEq/mL of sodium
- **Shohl solution (citric acid and sodium citrate),** which supplies 1 mEq/mL bicarbonate
- **Sodium bicarbonate tablets,** which supply 650 mg of bicarbonate (8 mEq/tablet)

Metabolic Alkalosis

Etiology

Metabolic alkalosis is defined as any state that increases the serum bicarbonate concentration to greater than the normal level of 24 to 26 mmol/L.

Metabolic alkalosis is often divided into two categories: **chloride sensitive** or **chloride resistant** (Table 32-13). Chloride-sensitive metabolic alkalosis is associated with a decreased extracellular fluid volume, and the urinary chloride level is <10 mEq/L. Chloride-resistant metabolic alkalosis is associated with a urinary chloride level >20 mEq/L.

TABLE 32-13 Causes of Metabolic Alkalosis

Chloride Sensitive

Vomiting or nasogastric suction
Chronic diuretic therapy
Chloride-deficient diet
Cystic fibrosis (increased skin loss of chloride)
Congenital chloride diarrhea (autosomal recessive)

Chloride Resistant

Alkali administration (e.g., antacid therapy)
Acute diuretic therapy
Hypokalemic state
Mineralocorticoid excess
Compensation for respiratory acidosis
Bartter syndrome
Liddle syndrome

Clinical Features

As with metabolic acidosis, signs and symptoms are generally those of the underlying disorder. Sudden, severe metabolic alkalosis may result in diminished ionic calcium levels, leading to hypocalcemic cramps or tetany.

Evaluation

The physical examination should focus on assessment of the ECF volume status.

Laboratory studies should include a serum electrolyte panel; serum urea and creatinine levels; and urine electrolyte levels, including chloride. In some children, a sweat chloride determination is indicated.

> **HINT:** There may be mixed metabolic acidosis and alkalosis occurring together, and the measured bicarbonate concentration may be normal.

> **HINT:** Metabolic alkalosis and frank alkalemia may occur if long-standing respiratory acidosis is corrected suddenly (e.g., with mechanical ventilation). This condition is called posthypercapnic alkalosis.

Treatment

If there is volume contraction, **hydration status** should be restored with normal saline. If present, **hypokalemia** should be corrected. Diuretic therapy should be discontinued, if possible, or given intermittently. Alkali therapy should be discontinued.

Suggested Readings

Adrogue HJ, Modios NE: Hypernatremia. *New Engl J Med* 342(20):1493–1499, 2000.

Chon JC, Scheinmann JI, Roth KS: Renal tubular acidosis. *Pediatr Rev* 22(8):277–286, 2001.

Evans KJ, Greenberg A: Hyperkalemia: a review. *J Intensive Care Med* 20(5):272–290, 2005.

Kraut JA, Madias NE: Serum anion gap: its uses and limitations in clinical medicine, *Clin J Am Soc Nephrol* 2(1):162–174, 2007.

Marks KH, Kilav R, Naveh-Many T, et al.: Calcium, phosphate, vitamin D, and the parathyroid. *Pediatr Nephrol* 10(3):364–367, 1996.

Moritz ML, Ayus JC: Preventing neurological complications from dysnatremias in children: *Pediatr Nephrol* 20(12):1687–1700, 2005.

Ruth JL, Wassner SJ: Body composition: salt and water. *Pediatr Rev* 27(5):181–187, 2006.

Schwaderer AL, Schwartz GJ: Back to basics: acidosis and alkalosis. *Pediatr Rev* 25(10):350–357, 2004.

33 *Fever*

Elizabeth R. Alpern and Louis M. Bell

INTRODUCTION

Fever is the abnormal elevation of body temperature. It is a **nonspecific sign** of disease. The significance of fever lies in its indication of disease processes. Fever is defined as a core body temperature ≥38.0°C (100.4°F). However, the clinically relevant defined cutoff point of an abnormally elevated temperature is based on a particular child's risk for infection. Fever in neonates or in immunocompromised patients is defined as ≥38.0°C (100.4°F) and in older children as 38.5°C (101°F) to 39.0°C (102°F).

Body temperature is usually measured by **rectal thermometry** in infants and young children and by **sublingual thermometry** in older children and adolescents. Because temperature may vary in different areas of the body, tympanic, temporal artery, and pacifier thermometers may not correlate with rectal measurements in young children.

Because fever is an indication of disease, the most important management and therapeutic measures are to determine the underlying cause of the fever (e.g., infection, inflammation, neoplasm). When the underlying disease is treated appropriately, the fever can be managed with antipyretics as needed to make the child comfortable.

DIFFERENTIAL DIAGNOSIS LIST

Infectious Causes

Systemic
  Sepsis
  Occult bacteremia
  Viral syndrome
  Tickborne infections (Lyme disease, Rocky Mountain spotted fever)
CNS
  Meningitis
  Encephalitis
Respiratory Tract
  Upper respiratory tract infection
  Pharyngitis/tonsillitis
  Retropharyngeal abscess

Otitis media
Croup
Sinusitis
Pneumonia
Bronchiolitis
Abdominal/Pelvic
  Gastroenteritis
  Appendicitis
Genitourinary
  Urinary tract disease
  Pelvic inflammatory disease
  Tubo-ovarian abscess
Musculoskeletal
  Osteomyelitis
  Septic arthritis

Cutaneous
  Cellulitis
  Abscess
Miscellaneous
  Adenitis
  Orbital cellulitis
  Fever of unknown origin

Toxicologic Causes
  Salicylates
  Cocaine
  Amphetamine
  Anticholinergics
  Malignant hyperthermia

Neoplastic Causes
  Leukemia
  Lymphoma

Inflammatory Causes
  Acute rheumatic fever
  Systemic lupus erythematosus
  Juvenile rheumatoid arthritis
  Kawasaki disease
  Inflammatory bowel disease
  Serum sickness
  Drug and immunization
    reactions

Miscellaneous Causes
  Heat stroke
  Thyrotoxicosis
  Dehydration
  Prolonged seizures
  Factitious

EVALUATION OF COMMON PRESENTATIONS

Infant Less Than 2 Months of Age

Well-appearing infants (0 to 60 days of age) with a fever (≥38.0°C [100.4°F]) but without an identifiable source of infection are at risk for **occult serious bacterial infections.** These young infants may have only vague or nonspecific signs and symptoms of illness that do not indicate the severity of potential infection.

History
- High risk—**prematurity, perinatal complication, immunocompromised state (sickle cell disease, HIV), exposure to recent antibiotics, steroids, surgery**
- Low risk—**full-term gestation, uncomplicated prenatal course**

Physical Examination
Physical examination should concentrate on identifying infections that are more common in neonates, such as meningitis, herpes simplex virus encephalitis, omphalitis, pneumonia, and pyelonephritis.

Screening Tests
Table 33-1 presents the low-risk criteria for three published screening protocols.

TABLE 33-1 Low-Risk Screening Criteria

	Philadelphia Protocol	Boston Protocol	Rochester Criteria
History/Physical examination	Normal	Normal	Normal
WBC count	5,000–15,000/mm³	<20,000/mm³	5,000–15,000/mm³
Differential	Band-to-neutrophil ratio <0.2		Absolute band count ≤1,500/mm³
Urinalysis	<10 WBC/hpf	<10 WBC/hpf	<10 WBC/hpf
CSF	<8 WBC/hpf	<10 WBC/hpf	
CXR	Normal	Normal	
Stool	If symptoms: negative blood and few WBC on smear		If symptoms: <5 WBC/hpf
Social	Readily available transportation and phone	Readily available transportation and phone	Readily available transportation and phone
Negative predictive value (for SBI) of screen	100%	94.6%	98.9%
Treatment option if low risk	Home without antibiotics and follow-up in 24 hr	Home with Ceftriaxone IM and follow-up in 24 hr	Home without antibiotics and follow-up in 24 hr

CSF = cerebrospinal fluid; CXR = chest X-ray; hpf = high-power field; IM = intramuscular; SBI = serious bacterial infection; WBC = white blood cell.

Management

The management of febrile infants is determined by age, history, and screening tests. Figure 33-1 presents the management options.

Children 2 Months to 24 Months of Age

Occult bacteremia is the presence of pathogenic bacteria in the blood of a well-appearing febrile child (usually defined as ≥39.0°C [102°F]) who lacks a focal bacterial source of infection. The current risk of occult bacteremia in an immunized child is approximately 1% to 2%. This risk increases with increasing temperature or a white blood cell count. Occult bacteremia carries a risk of **progression to focal infection, meningitis, or sepsis.** The degree of this risk depends on the etiology of the bacteremia. In a population immunized with the *Haemophilus influenzae* B vaccine and the conjugate pneumococcal vaccine, the risk of serious adverse outcome is extremely low. In this population, the most common bacterial isolate causing occult bacteremia is still *Streptococcus pneumoniae*, which usually resolves spontaneously.

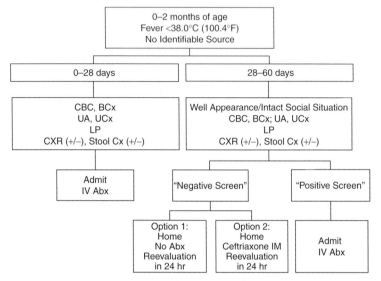

Figure 33-1 ■ Management of febrile infants less than 2 months of age. BCx = blood culture; CBC = complete blood cell count; CSF = cerebrospinal fluid; Cx = culture;
CXR = chest X-ray; IM = intramuscularly; IV Abx = intravenous antibiotics; LP = lumbar puncture; UA = urinalysis; UCx = urine culture.

History

An **immunocompromised state** (e.g., long-term steroid use, oncologic processes, acquired or inborn immunodeficiencies, sickle cell anemia, congenital heart disease) or the presence of an **indwelling medical device** (e.g., ventriculoperitoneal shunts, indwelling catheters) puts a child at increased risk of invasive bacterial infection. The child's **immunization history** is also important. The newly licensed pneumococcal conjugate vaccine has significantly decreased the risk of bacteremia and other invasive pneumococcal diseases. Prior antibiotic use may mask presenting signs or symptoms of focal bacterial infections and should be noted.

Physical Examination

Any sign of focal **bacterial infection** (e.g., pneumonia, abscess, urinary tract infection) or **pathognomonic viral illness** (e.g., varicella, stomatitis) guides diagnosis and treatment plans appropriate for that particular infection. However, the well-appearing child without focal infection should be evaluated for occult infections such as occult bacteremia or occult urinary tract infection. Children with **nonspecific viral syndromes** and **otitis media** are also at risk for occult bacteremia.

TABLE 33-2 Risk Factors for Urinary Tract Infections	
Girls	**Boys**
Temperature ≥39°C (102°F) Fever ≥2 days Caucasian Age ≤1 yr Lack of other focal source of infection	Age ≤ 6 months Uncircumcised penis Lack of other focal source of infection

Screening Tests

- **Blood culture** is the gold standard for diagnosing occult bacteremia. Some authorities advocate the white blood cell (WBC) count for use as a risk stratification measure when considering expectant antibiotic therapy for the child at risk for occult bacteremia. However, because of the low incidence of occult bacteremia, this screening test has significant limitations. A WBC count ≥15,000/mm^3 has a positive predictive value of <5%.

- **Chest radiographs** are indicated in children with significant respiratory symptoms or persistent tachypnea.

- **Urinalysis and culture** are helpful for those children with dysuria, foul-smelling urine, prior history of urinary tract infection, urinary tract abnormality, or other risk factors for occult urinary tract infections (UTIs). See Table 33-2 for risk factors associated with occult UTIs in young children.

Management

Reevaluation in 24 to 48 hours is imperative if the diagnosis of occult bacteremia is suspected. Controversy exists regarding whether presumptive therapy for children at risk for the development of occult bacteremia is indicated. Two meta-analyses have failed to show a significant difference in risk of meningitis in children with occult bacteremia who are treated with antibiotics.

Suggested Readings

Alpern ER, Alessandrini EA, Bell LM, et al.: Occult bacteremia from a pediatric emergency department: current prevalence, time to detection, and outcome. *Pediatrics* 106:505–511, 2000.

Alpern ER, Henretig FM: Fever. In *Textbook of Pediatric Emergency Medicine*, 4th ed. Edited by Fleisher GR, Ludwig S. Philadelphia, Lippincott, Williams & Wilkins, 2000.

Bulloch B, Craig WR, Klassen TP: The use of antibiotics to prevent serious sequelae in children at risk for occult bacteremia: a meta-analysis. *Acad Emerg Med* 4:679–683, 1997.

Carstairs K, Tasnen D, Johnson AS, et al.: Pneumococcal bacteremia in febrile infants presenting to the emergency department before and after the introduction of the heptavalent pneumococcal vaccine. *Ann Emerg Med* 49:772–777, 2007.

Gorelick MH, Shaw KN: Clinical decision rule to identify febrile young girls at risk for urinary tract infection. *Arch Pediatr Adolesc Med* 154:386–390, 2000.

Jaskiewicz JA, McCarthy CA, Richardson AC, et al.: Febrile infants at low risk for serious bacterial infection—an appraisal of the Rochester criteria and implications for management. *Pediatrics* 94:390–396, 1994.

Lee GM, Harper MB: Risk of bacteremia for febrile young children in the post-*Haemophilus influenzae* type b era. *Arch Pediatr Adolesc Med* 152(5):624–628, 1998.

Rothrock SG, Harper MB, Green SM, et al.: Do oral antibiotics prevent meningitis and serious bacterial infections in children with *Streptococcus pneumoniae* occult bacteremia? A meta-analysis. *Pediatrics* 99(3):438–444, 1997.

Shaw KN, Gorelick MH: Urinary tract infection in the pediatric patient. *Pediatr Clinic North Am* 46(6):1111–1124, 1999.

Whitney CG, Farley MM, Hadler J, et al.: Decline in invasive pneumococcal disease after the introduction of protein-polysaccharide conjugate vaccine. *N Engl J Med* 348:1737–1746, 2003.

34 *Gastrointestinal Bleeding, Lower*

Chris A. Liacouras

INTRODUCTION

The presence of **blood in the gastrointestinal tract is always abnormal.** Blood in the stool can occur in several forms: **hematochezia** (bright red blood on the stool), **"currant-jelly" stools** (thickened brick-red blood on the stool), **melena** (dark or black stools), or **occult bleeding** (normal-appearing stools that test positive by Hemoccult or guaiac testing).

Blood acts as a cathartic that decreases intestinal transit time. Therefore, hematochezia usually signifies colonic disease (i.e., bleeding from a site between the distal colon and the terminal ileum), but it may be the result of profuse proximal gastrointestinal tract bleeding. Melena usually signifies profuse upper intestinal bleeding (proximal to the terminal ileum), whereas currant-jelly stools commonly occur as a result of an active Meckel diverticulum or intussusception. Normal-appearing stools that test positive for blood suggest slow gastrointestinal tract bleeding. Table 34-1 lists causes of bloody stools by site.

> **HINT:** Rapid upper gastrointestinal tract bleeding should always be considered in any child with first-time bloody stools, and a nasogastric tube should be passed.

DIFFERENTIAL DIAGNOSIS LIST

The following are common causes of hematochezia and melena.

Infectious Causes

Bacterial Infection
  Salmonella
  Shigella
  Campylobacter
  Yersinia
  Enterohemorrhagic
    Escherichia coli
  Aeromonas
  Plesiomonas
  Clostridium difficile
Parasitic Infection
  Entamoeba histolytica
  Balantidium coli
  Necator americanus
    (hookworm)
  Strongyloides stercoralis
  Ascaris lumbricoides
Viral Infection
  Adenovirus
  Rotavirus
  Cytomegalovirus
  HIV

Neoplastic Causes
  Leiomyoma

Lymphoma
Adenocarcinoma
Carcinoid

Traumatic Causes

Anal fissure
Foreign body
Sexual abuse

Congenital or Vascular Causes

Meckel diverticulum
Enteric duplication
Arteriovenous malformation (AVM)
Hemangioma
Hemorrhoids
Rectal varices
Esophageal varices (rapid flow)
Hirschsprung enterocolitis

Inflammatory Causes

Juvenile polyps

Polyposis syndromes
Inflammatory bowel disease
Lymphonodular hyperplasia
Necrotizing enterocolitis
Milk- or soy-protein allergy
Eosinophilic gastroenteritis
Graft-versus-host disease
Vasculitis (systemic lupus erythematosus)

Miscellaneous Causes

Rapid upper gastrointestinal bleeding
Intussusception
Volvulus
Solitary rectal ulcer
Coagulopathy
Thrombocytopenia
Anticoagulant drug therapy
Henoch-Schönlein purpura
Hemolytic uremic syndrome

TABLE 34-1 Causes of Bloody Stools by Site

Site	Cause
Nasopharynx	Epistaxis, gum disease, oral or nasal trauma, tonsillectomy, adenoidectomy
Esophagus	Esophageal stricture, esophagitis, ulcer, varices, eosinophilic enteritis, graft-versus-host disease (GVHD)
Stomach	Gastritis, ulcer, foreign body, vascular anomaly, tumor, duplication, polyp, infection
Duodenum	Ulcer, celiac disease, malrotation, vascular anomaly, postviral enteritis, parasitic infection
Small bowel	Inflammatory bowel disease, celiac disease, volvulus, malrotation, necrotizing enterocolitis, infection, Henoch-Schönlein purpura, duplication, Meckel diverticulum, vascular anomaly, tumor, eosinophilic enteritis
Colon	Polyp, inflammatory bowel disease, infection, Hirschsprung disease, trauma, sexual abuse, hemorrhoid, tumor, hemolytic uremic syndrome, Henoch-Schönlein purpura, milk-protein or soy-protein allergy, rectal varices, intussusception, volvulus, fissure, solitary rectal ulcer, foreign body, vascular anomaly, GVHD

TABLE 34-2 Foods and Drugs Mimicking Blood in the Stool

False Hematochezia	False Melena	False Heme-Positive Stools
Foods that contain red dye	Spinach	Red meat
Juice	Blueberries	Cherries
Candy	Licorice	Tomato skin
Kool-Aid	Purple grapes	Iron supplements
Jell-O	Chocolate	
Tomatoes	Grape juice	
Beets	Bismuth subsalicylate	
Cranberries	Iron supplements	

> **HINT:** Certain foods, drugs, and occurrences (e.g., factitious menstrual bleeding, hematuria, swallowed maternal blood) can mimic blood in the stool and must be ruled out (Table 34-2).

DIFFERENTIAL DIAGNOSIS DISCUSSION

> **HINT:** Lower gastrointestinal tract bleeding in children is most often caused by infection. Bacterial infections often present with acute abdominal pain, fever, and bloody diarrhea.

C. difficile Colitis (Pseudomembranous Colitis, Antibiotic-Induced Colitis)

Etiology

The toxins produced by *C. difficile* have **cytotoxic effects** on the colonic mucosa. Although *C. difficile* colitis is usually associated with an imbalance of the gastrointestinal flora **following the administration of broad-spectrum antibiotics** (e.g., clindamycin, amoxicillin, cephalosporin), it can develop in patients with **underlying intestinal disorders** (e.g., inflammatory bowel disease) and those who have undergone **recent abdominal surgery.** *C. difficile* can also cause disease in **young infants** (secondary to an increase in intestinal colonization), **institutionalized patients** (as a result of cross-infection), and, sporadically, in otherwise healthy patients.

> **HINT:** Antibiotic-induced colitis commonly occurs within 2 weeks of introducing the drug.

Clinical Features

C. difficile is associated with a **wide variety of clinical symptoms**. Patients may be **asymptomatic**, or they may experience **frequent, painful, bloody diarrhea**, a sign of severe, life-threatening colitis. Typically, children present with abdominal pain and bloody, mucus-streaked, foul-smelling, watery stools that occur at frequent intervals. Some patients may be **dehydrated**.

Evaluation

C. difficile-induced colitis should be suspected whenever a patient presents with bloody diarrhea. **Fresh stool specimens** (transported on ice or frozen) should be collected and evaluated for the presence of *C. difficile* toxins A and B. In patients with persistent bloody diarrhea and a negative microbiologic evaluation, **colonoscopy** should be performed. Colonoscopy often reveals the classic mucosal pseudomembrane formation (raised yellow plaques).

Treatment

Therapy varies depending on the severity of symptoms. Mild cases may be self-limited and usually respond to the **discontinuation of the inciting antibiotic**. Patients with features of more severe colitis are treated with either **oral metronidazole or vancomycin** (see Chapter 27, "Diarrhea, Acute"); symptoms usually resolve within 3 to 5 days. Dehydrated patients require **intravenous fluids** and the short-term introduction of clear liquids.

Recurrent episodes may occur following cessation of therapy; in this situation, repeat treatment and further evaluation for other underlying systemic disorders (e.g., inflammatory bowel disease) are indicated.

Meckel Diverticulum

Etiology

Meckel diverticulum, the **most common** of all **congenital gastrointestinal anomalies**, occurs in 1% to 3% of all infants. The diverticulum is derived from a congenital remnant of the embryonic yolk sac that originates from the antimesenteric border of the intestine. This abnormality is typically located within 2 feet (60 cm) of the ileocecal valve. The diverticulum commonly contains ectopic gastric tissue, which can cause **peptic ulceration** (manifested as painless bright red or currant-jelly rectal bleeding).

 HINT: Enteric duplications (intestinal cysts) originate from the mesenteric border of the bowel and, like a Meckel diverticulum, can also contain ectopic gastric tissue and manifest with hematochezia or currant-jelly bleeding.

Clinical Features

Intermittent, painless rectal bleeding in a 2-year-old child is the most common presentation. A small percentage of patients may present with massive life-threatening rectal bleeding.

Bowel obstruction (secondary to internal herniation or intussusception of the enteric diverticulum) can lead to abdominal pain and bilious vomiting.

Evaluation

The diagnosis is made either via a **Meckel scan,** a specific nuclear medicine test that uses a radioisotope to identify gastric mucosa, or by a **nonspecific tagged red blood cell scan** that identifies sites of rapid gastrointestinal bleeding. Routine abdominal radiographs and contrast studies are almost never useful for making the diagnosis of a Meckel diverticulum.

Treatment

Surgical excision is performed in all cases of documented Meckel diverticulum.

Colonic Polyps

Etiology

Most juvenile polyps are **inflammatory** in origin. **Polyposis syndromes,** which may involve a few polyps or hundreds of polyps, are typically **genetic** in origin and include inflammatory, hamartomatous, and adenomatous changes. The presence of **five or more polyps** usually carries an **increased risk of cancer.**

Clinical Features

Painless hematochezia in a child between 2 and 10 years of age is the typical presentation. Juvenile polyps are the most common cause of painless hematochezia in children who have no evidence of perianal or rectal trauma. Other common presentations include **tenesmus, mucus-streaked stools, and rectal (or polyp) prolapse** through the rectum. Rarely, intussusception occurs secondary to a lead point (e.g., a colonic polyp or Meckel diverticulum). Juvenile polyps are usually palpable on rectal examination. As many as 30% of children may develop an **iron-deficiency anemia.**

Evaluation

In the past, barium enemas were used to diagnose colonic polyps; however, because stool retention secondary to improper bowel preparation may hide polyps and the present treatment of choice is polypectomy,

colonoscopy is now the preferred diagnostic tool. In addition to allowing visualization of the entire colon (thus identifying the exact cause and all possible polyps), colonoscopy allows the endoscopist to treat the problem by performing a polypectomy.

Treatment

In the past, conservative therapy consisted of observation with the hope that the polyp would auto-amputate. However, currently, **colonoscopy with polypectomy** is recommended to eliminate the source of bleeding, to identify the presence of other polyps, and to identify the type of polyp so that future management of the patient can be determined.

Inflammatory Bowel Disease

Etiology

Inflammatory bowel disease is an **idiopathic, multifactorial inflammatory condition** of the alimentary tract.

- **Crohn disease** may occur in both the upper and lower gastrointestinal tract and results in chronic intestinal inflammation associated with severe mucosal damage, transmural wall thickening, serosal induration, granuloma formation, fistula and abscess formation, intestinal strictures, and perforation. The terminal ileum is the most common site of involvement, although the disease may "skip" to noncontiguous areas.
- **Ulcerative colitis** is confined to the colon and rectum and typically causes severe mucosal destruction without transmural involvement. Unlike Crohn disease, ulcerative colitis is continuous along the lower gastrointestinal tract, although the rectum may be spared.

> **HINT:** Toxic megacolon, a potential complication of ulcerative colitis, is a true surgical emergency and should be ruled out promptly.

Clinical Features

Children with inflammatory bowel disease usually present with **fever, bloody diarrhea, weight loss, and crampy abdominal pain.** Associated systemic abnormalities in inflammatory bowel disease include growth failure, arthralgias, arthritis, skin lesions (pyoderma gangrenosum, erythema nodosum), perianal disease (rectal abscess, skin tags, or fistula formation), ophthalmologic abnormalities (episcleritis and uveitis), mouth sores, and hepatobiliary disease. Many children with Crohn disease develop an **iron-deficiency anemia** and a **secondary lactase deficiency.**

> **HINT:** Profuse rectal bleeding, hypogastric pain, tenesmus, and frequent diarrhea usually suggest ulcerative colitis, whereas right lower quadrant pain, weight loss, failure to thrive, and perianal disease typify Crohn disease.

Evaluation

- The **physical examination** may reveal abdominal tenderness that is usually focal in the lower quadrants and signs of systemic involvement (e.g., mouth sores, joint involvement, erythema nodosum, pyoderma gangrenosum, perianal disease).
- **Laboratory studies** such as a complete blood count (CBC), erythrocyte sedimentation rate (ESR), chemistry panel, and lactose breath test are useful for determining the biochemical abnormalities associated with inflammatory bowel disease. Patients with inflammatory bowel disease usually have an elevated ESR, hypoalbuminemia, and an elevated white blood cell (WBC) count.
- **Colonoscopy with biopsy** is the test of choice for diagnosing ulcerative colitis and Crohn disease. The diagnosis may be made by visual inspection of the intestinal mucosa (aphthous ulcers and mucosal damage) or by biopsy (granulomas, crypt abscesses, and mucosal inflammation).
- **Upper gastrointestinal small bowel follow-through contrast studies** are useful for assessing small bowel (terminal ileal) disease.

Treatment

The prognosis depends on aggressive treatment of exacerbations, but aggressive intervention with nutritional support is equally important.

- **Corticosteroids** are the first line of therapy for patients with moderate to severe disease. The recommended dosage (1 to 2 mg/kg per day) is tapered over 4 to 8 weeks, depending on the clinical response. Immunosuppressive agents (e.g., 6-mercaptopurine, azathioprine, cyclosporin A) are used in children who have an increased risk for complications from steroid treatment, who require prolonged steroid use, or who are refractory to other treatment regimens.
- **Oral salicylate derivatives,** which help heal the intestinal mucosa, are the mainstay of treatment. In the past, sulfasalazine (50 to 100 mg/kg per day) was used for patients with mild to moderate exacerbations. Folic acid (1 mg/day) was administered concurrently because sulfasalazine competitively inhibits folate absorption. 5-Aminosalicylic acid (5-ASA), the active component, is minimally absorbed and thus acts directly on the mucosa as an anti-inflammatory agent. Recently, mesalamine, which does not require coliform bacteria to metabolize itself to 5-ASA, has been used. The dose is 30 to 70 mg/kg per day.

- **Antibiotics** are effective for patients with perianal disease and mucosal inflammation. Metronidazole, used when evidence of bacterial overgrowth, fistulae, or perianal disease exists, has been effective against anaerobes but also has anti-inflammatory properties.
- **Surgical intervention,** such as resection with colectomy and eventual endorectal pull-through, is useful in patients with ulcerative colitis. Surgery should be avoided, however, in children with Crohn disease unless abscess, fistula, toxic megacolon, perforation, acute obstruction, or uncontrolled bleeding exist.

As an adjunct to therapy, **nutritional support** is paramount to achieve optimal growth. Special issues, such as deficiencies in trace elements (e.g., zinc, magnesium, and calcium), protein-losing enteropathy (PLE), and fat malabsorption resulting in vitamin A, D, E, and K deficiency, must be addressed. An oral elemental diet, total parenteral nutrition, or both are the primary modes of nutritional support for these patients. The goal is to provide at least 125% to 140% of the recommended daily allowance for calories and protein.

Because of the chronicity of this disease, **psychological support** is vital. It is important to teach adaptive responses to the illness, rather than enabling maladaptive responses to progress.

Hirschsprung Enterocolitis

Etiology

Hirschsprung disease is caused by a **congenital absence of ganglion cells** (see Chapter 22, "Constipation"). An associated enterocolitis occurs secondary to poor colonic motility, stagnation of fecal material in the rectum, and breakdown of the mucosal barrier.

Clinical Features

Although Hirschsprung enterocolitis is **uncommon,** the possibility should be considered in any infant with **rectal bleeding** who has **abdominal distention, foul-smelling diarrhea, a history of delayed meconium passage, constipation, fever, and sepsis.** There may also be evidence of intestinal obstruction.

Evaluation

A **barium enema** (unprepped—to prevent dilation of the colonic transition zone) may suggest the diagnosis. Often, a submucosal or full-thickness **rectal biopsy** (demonstrating absence of ganglion cells and hypertrophied nerve bundles) is required to confirm the diagnosis.

Treatment

Infants with suspected Hirschsprung enterocolitis should be placed on **nothing by mouth** and administered **fluids and broad-spectrum antibiotics intravenously.** A **nasogastric tube** should be inserted to decompress the proximal bowel. **Surgical correction** is required to remove the aganglionic bowel segment and to relieve the intestinal obstruction.

Milk-Protein or Soy-Protein Allergy

Etiology

Milk-protein or soy-protein allergy is the **most common immunologic cause of gastrointestinal bleeding** in infants. The most common explanation for milk-protein allergy is that it is caused by an antigen-induced, IgE-mediated reaction with subsequent mast cell activation and eosinophilic infiltration of the intestinal mucosa.

Clinical Features

Many children have a history of rhinitis, bronchospasm, and coughing.

There are several clinical manifestations, including an **immediate hypersensitivity reaction**, a **delayed systemic reaction** (characterized by a rash and headache), and a **gastrointestinal reaction** that occurs several days later. Infants most commonly present with bloody, mucus-streaked **diarrhea, abdominal pain, weight loss, and vomiting.** Patients may also have signs of **anaphylaxis** (e.g., urticaria, bronchospasm, hypotension).

Peripheral eosinophilia is often present.

> **HINT:** Approximately 20% of infants with milk-protein allergy are also allergic to soy, and 1% may also be allergic to most simple foods.

Evaluation

The diagnosis is usually made on the basis of the **clinical history.** Although a strict placebo-controlled **food challenge test** is the only way to make a definitive diagnosis, food elimination can often strongly suggest the offending agent. Helpful diagnostic tests include a **Wright stain of the stool** (to reveal stool eosinophils) **or endoscopy,** which may demonstrate eosinophilic infiltration of the intestinal mucosa.

Treatment

Treatment consists of **removing the offending antigen** from the diet. In infants, this disorder typically resolves by 2 years of age. Older children who develop food allergies often require a lifetime of avoidance.

Eosinophilic Enteritis

Etiology

Idiopathic eosinophilic gastroenteritis is a rare disorder caused by eosinophilic tissue infiltration and mast cell activation without known antigenic stimulation. Three forms exist: **mucosal infiltration** (vomiting, diarrhea, PLE), **muscular infiltration** (gastric outlet obstruction), and **serosal infiltration** (ascites without other intestinal symptoms). Common sites of involvement include the gastric antrum, esophagus, and colon. Eosinophilic enteritis can produce **severe esophagitis, gastritis, duodenitis, or all three.**

Clinical Features

Patients present with **nausea, vomiting, abdominal pain, and upper or lower gastrointestinal bleeding. Hematemesis** results from mucosal infiltration, which promotes an inflammatory response. Other clinical findings include **diarrhea, weight loss, failure to thrive, ascites, and peripheral edema.**

Laboratory findings include **peripheral eosinophilia, iron-deficiency anemia, elevated serum IgE levels, and hypoalbuminemia** (secondary to PLE).

Evaluation

Initial evaluation includes searching for evidence of mucosal malabsorption using the D-**xylose absorption test** and performing **radiographic contrast studies,** which may show small bowel edema and ulceration. Definitive diagnosis can be made by **endoscopy with biopsy.**

Treatment

Treatment involves **supportive care, dietary manipulation,** and the administration of **corticosteroids** (in severe cases) and **oral cromolyn sodium.** Long-term care should be coordinated by a pediatric gastroenterologist.

Intussusception

Intussusception is discussed in Chapter 9, "Abdominal Pain, Acute."

EVALUATION OF LOWER GASTROINTESTINAL BLEEDING

Patient History

- **Travel history.** The travel history may suggest an infectious cause.
- **Events suggesting upper gastrointestinal tract trauma.** A recent history of epistaxis, nasogastric or gastrostomy tube placement, retching (suggestive of a Mallory-Weiss tear), surgery (e.g., tonsillectomy, adenoidectomy), or caustic ingestion may explain melena or heme-positive stools.
- **Medication history.** Melanotic stools can be caused by drug-induced gastritis, for example from nonsteroidal anti-inflammatory agents or salicylates. In addition, certain drugs can mimic blood in the stool (see Table 34-2).

Physical Examination

- **Perianal and digital rectal examinations** should always be performed in children with hematochezia to look for anal fissure, hemorrhoids, rectal trauma, foreign bodies in the rectum, and signs of sexual abuse (e.g., cutaneous bruising, anal tears, labial or penile irritation).
- **Abdominal palpation** may reveal hepatosplenomegaly, which suggests portal hypertension and possible varices.
- **Cutaneous examination** may reveal hemangiomas (suggestive of an alimentary AVM), purpura on the buttocks and lower extremities (consistent with Henoch-Schönlein purpura), or erythema nodosum and pyoderma gangrenosum (seen in children with inflammatory bowel disease).

Laboratory Studies

Stool culture and testing for WBCs is always indicated for a child who presents with bloody diarrhea.

Diagnostic Modalities

Upper gastrointestinal endoscopy and colonoscopy are the most important tests for the diagnosis of gastrointestinal bleeding and may be therapeutic. Table 34-3 summarizes other diagnostic modalities and their indications.

TABLE 34-3 Useful Diagnostic Tests for Evaluation of Gastrointestinal Bleeding

Test	Indication
Meckel scan	Identification of a Meckel diverticulum or intestinal duplication
Tagged red blood cell scan	Identification of a site of rapid intestinal bleeding
Colonoscopy	Evaluation of hematochezia or colonic disease
Upper endoscopy	Evaluation of causes of upper gastrointestinal bleeding proximal to the ligament of Treitz
Angiography	Identification of vascular causes of gastrointestinal bleeding
Barium enema	Identification of anatomic abnormalities of the colon (Hirschsprung disease, intussusception, stricture, mass)
Upper gastrointestinal series	Identification of anatomic and inflammatory abnormalities of the esophagus, stomach, and small intestine
Enteroclysis	Used when enhancement of the mucosal detail of the small intestine is required
Abdominal radiograph	Identification of foreign body, intestinal obstruction, mucosal edema (thumbprinting)

TREATMENT OF LOWER GASTROINTESTINAL BLEEDING

Lower gastrointestinal bleeding can be life threatening. Patients with persistent, rapid bleeding or associated dizziness, fatigue, or severe abdominal pain require immediate evaluation and stabilization:

- Orthostatic vital signs and a CBC should be obtained as soon as possible.
- Patients with hypotension or anemia should receive intravenous fluids and blood products (when necessary).
- A plain abdominal radiograph is useful for revealing intestinal obstruction or perforation.
- In patients with significant lower gastrointestinal bleeding, a nasogastric tube should be placed to decompress the bowel and to determine the severity and origin of the bleeding (e.g., from the stomach or esophagus).
- The patient should be admitted under the care of a pediatric gastroenterologist.

Suggested Readings

Brown RL, Azizkhan RG: Gastrointestinal bleeding in infants and children: Meckel's diverticulum and intestinal duplication. *Semin Pediatr Surg* 8(4):202–209, 1999.

Feldman M, Friedman LS, Brandy LJ: *Sleisenger and Fordtran's Gastrointestinal and Liver Disease: Pathophysiology, Diagnosis, Management.* Philadelphia, WB Saunders, 2006.

Fox VL: Gastrointestinal bleeding in infancy and childhood. *Gastroenterol Clin North Am* 29(1):37–66, v, 2000.

Hoffenberg EJ, Sauaia A, Maltzman T, et al.: Symptomatic colonic polyps in childhood: not so benign. *J Pediatr Gastroenterol Nutr* 28(2): 175–181, 1999.

Lee KH, Yeung CK, Tam YH, et al.: Laparoscopy for definitive diagnosis and treatment of gastrointestinal bleeding of obscure origin in children. *J Pediatr Surg* 35(9):1291–1293, 2000.

Saulsbury FT: Henoch-Schönlein purpura in children. Report of 100 patients and review of the literature. *Medicine* 78(6):395–409, 1999.

Treem WR: Gastrointestinal bleeding in children. *Gastrointest Endosc* 4:75, 1994.

Walker WA, Goulet O, Kleinman RE, et al.: *Pediatric Gastrointestinal Disease*, 4th ed. Hamilton, On, BC Decker, 2004.

Wyllie R, Hyams JS: *Pediatric Gastrointestinal Disease: Pathophysiology, Diagnosis, Management,* 3rd ed. Philadelphia, WB Saunders, 2005.

Gastrointestinal Bleeding, Upper

Chris A. Liacouras

INTRODUCTION

The presence of hematemesis usually suggests that the site of bleeding is proximal to the ligament of Treitz. Common sites of upper gastrointestinal tract bleeding are summarized in Table 35-1.

DIFFERENTIAL DIAGNOSIS LIST

Infectious Causes
Bacterial gastritis—
  Helicobacter pylori infection
Viral infection—
  cytomegalovirus, varicella,
  herpes, adenovirus
Fungal esophagitis or gastritis

Toxic Causes
Drugs—nonsteroidal
  anti-inflammatory drugs
  (NSAIDs), aspirin, steroids
Caustic substances
Alcohol gastritis

Neoplastic Causes
Zollinger-Ellison syndrome
Leiomyoma
Leiomyosarcoma

Traumatic Causes
Mallory-Weiss tear
Epistaxis
Oropharyngeal trauma
  (e.g., postsurgical trauma)
Nasogastric or gastric tube
  trauma
Foreign body

Congenital or Vascular Causes
Enteric duplication
Dieulafoy ulcer
Arteriovenous malformation
Esophageal or gastric
  varices

Inflammatory Causes
Gastric or duodenal ulcer
Esophagitis (reflux or
  chemical)
Gastritis (caustic or
  chemical)
Duodenitis
Eosinophilic gastritis

Miscellaneous Causes
Hemobilia
Graft-versus-host disease
Swallowed maternal
  blood
Pulmonary disease
  (hemoptysis)
Factitious bleeding
  (Munchausen by proxy
  syndrome)

TABLE 35-1 Causes of Hematemesis by Site

Site	Cause
Oropharynx	Epistaxis
	Mouth-/nose-/throat-surgery trauma
	Foreign body
Esophagus	Esophagitis
	Esophageal stricture
	Mallory-Weiss tear
	Infection
	Foreign body
	Esophageal varices
Stomach	Ulcer
	Gastritis (drug, infection, caustic ingestion)
	Eosinophilic enteritis
	Graft-versus-host disease
	Vascular abnormality
	Varices duplication
	Tumor
	Gastric polyps
Duodenum	Ulcer
	Eosinophilic enteritis
	Hemobilia

DIFFERENTIAL DIAGNOSIS DISCUSSION

Mallory-Weiss Tear

Etiology

A Mallory-Weiss tear is a **linear mucosal tear of the distal esophagus** that occurs as a result of **forceful vomiting or retching.**

Clinical Features

Bloody streaks are seen in the vomitus.

Evaluation

Mallory-Weiss tears, which are not visible on radiographs, are diagnosed using **upper endoscopy.** Initially, the tear appears as a **vertical, linear red streak;** after healing, it is seen as a **white streak** with surrounding erythema.

Treatment

Most patients can be managed in the outpatient setting because Mallory-Weiss tears usually **resolve spontaneously.** In severe cases, hospital observation is indicated. Rarely, blood transfusion, vasopressin therapy, or balloon tamponade may be necessary.

Esophagitis

Etiology

Esophagitis (**inflammation of the esophageal mucosa**) can be caused by acid or bile reflux, viral or *H. pylori* infection, inflammation, allergy, or caustic ingestions. Esophagitis may cause vomiting, or it may result from disorders that promote delayed gastric emptying and vomiting.

Clinical Features

Typically, patients with esophagitis experience **heartburn, chest pain, water brash** (sour taste in the mouth), or **vomiting and regurgitation. Blood-streaked emesis** occurs in patients with severe or untreated esophagitis.

In infants with reflux esophagitis, parents may notice pooled bloody secretions on the infant's bedding. In older children with esophagitis, bloody emesis is usually associated with epigastric or chest pain and a history of frequent regurgitation and a "sour taste" in the mouth.

Evaluation

Upper endoscopy, the test of choice when esophagitis is suspected, allows inspection of the esophageal mucosa and biopsy of the esophagus to determine the cause of the inflammation and the degree of histologic involvement.

Contrast radiography is often useful for determining the anatomic configuration of the upper gastrointestinal tract. This study is most valuable for ruling out other causes of upper gastrointestinal bleeding (e.g., gastric or duodenal ulcer disease, esophageal strictures, esophageal or gastric varices).

Treatment

The treatment of esophagitis depends on its cause.

- **Acid reflux esophagitis** is treated with a combination of prokinetic agents (e.g., metoclopramide) and gastric acid blockers.
- **Inflammatory esophagitis** requires the use of protective agents, such as sucralfate, and treatment of the underlying inflammatory process (e.g., Crohn disease, allergic esophagitis) with corticosteroids or food elimination.
- **Strictures** necessitate dilation.
- **Infectious esophagitis** is treated with antimicrobials.

Gastritis

Etiology

Gastritis (**inflammation of the gastric mucosa**) can be classified as primary or secondary:

- **Primary gastritis** results when acid or bile causes direct mucosal damage.
- **Secondary gastritis** is either a complication of another disease process (e.g., severe burns, systemic illness, Henoch-Schönlein purpura) or is caused by an offending agent (e.g., ingested drugs or corrosives, infections).

Clinical Features

Epigastric pain and vomiting are the most common symptoms of gastritis in children. The pain often occurs during, or just after, meals, and the patient often complains of nausea and early satiety. Small amounts of fresh blood or "coffee ground" material may be seen in the vomitus.

Evaluation

In children, radiographic contrast studies often do not have the sensitivity necessary to show gastritis. Upper endoscopy is a more valuable tool; the gastric mucosa can be directly visualized and biopsies can be obtained to determine the cause of the gastritis.

Treatment

Although it is important to identify and treat the specific cause of the gastritis, a generalized treatment approach is usually necessary initially. Acid-blocking medications (e.g., antacids, H_2 blockers) are required to raise the gastric pH above 4.0. Drugs (e.g., aspirin, NSAIDs) should be eliminated. Patients with major hemorrhage require fluid resuscitation and transfusion.

Gastric or Duodenal Ulcer

Etiology

Gastric or duodenal ulcers may result from infection (*H. pylori*), increases in hormones (Zollinger-Ellison syndrome), increased gastric acidity, or direct injury (drugs, caustic ingestion, foreign body). In addition, the development of ulcers is associated with several systemic diseases, including sickle cell disease, cystic fibrosis, and asthma.

> **HINT:** Gastric ulcers are more common in children <6 years, whereas duodenal ulcers occur more frequently in older children.

Clinical Features

Major symptoms include upper gastrointestinal bleeding, abdominal pain, vomiting, anorexia, syncope or dizziness (secondary to anemia), weight loss or failure to thrive, and heartburn. The pain can awaken the child at night or in the early morning and usually occurs after meals. Symptoms of ulcer disease have often been present for as long as 2 years prior to diagnosis.

Evaluation

Although an upper gastrointestinal contrast study can confirm the diagnosis in up to 50% of patients, upper endoscopy remains the most efficacious test. Upper endoscopy allows identification of the ulcer, determination of the cause (via a biopsy), and, in some cases, treatment (e.g., cauterization in the case of acute bleeding).

> **HINT:** When the ulcers are multiple or recurrent, disorders such as Zollinger-Ellison syndrome or antral G cell hyperplasia should be considered.

Treatment

Routine medical therapy consists of **gastric acid suppression** (with antacids, H_2 blockers, and proton pump inhibitors) and **mucosal protection** (with sucralfate). **Infectious causes and systemic diseases should be treated** to prevent recurrences.

Profuse bleeding may require endoscopy with **electrocautery; surgery** is indicated in the rare case of intractable bleeding or perforation.

Esophageal or Gastric Varices

Etiology

Varices occur **secondary to portal hypertension caused by chronic liver disease, vascular obstruction** (Budd-Chiari syndrome), **or portal vein obstruction** (cavernous transformation, thrombosis). The portal hypertension and subsequent vascular shunting cause the development of varices (esophageal, gastric, and rectal) and abdominal caput medusae. Increased vascular pressure results in elevated wall tension, thinning of the blood vessel wall, and, eventually, vascular rupture.

Clinical Features

Painless, profuse vomiting of bright-red blood is often the first sign of bleeding varices. Approximately 25% of children with varices have had no prior diagnosis and present with hematemesis.

Patients may have **signs of liver disease** (e.g., jaundice, palmar erythema, spider angiomas). Almost all patients with varices have palpable **splenomegaly.**

Evaluation

An **abdominal examination** is revealing because most children with varices have evidence of either hepatomegaly or splenomegaly. There may be **laboratory evidence of liver disease** (e.g., elevated transaminases). Although radiographic studies may provide some additional information—for example, a contrast study can show the outline of the varices and an abdominal ultrasound can detect associated liver disease and the direction of blood flow in the portal system—**upper gastrointestinal endoscopy** is the most accurate method of diagnosing varices.

Treatment

Bleeding varices are an **absolute medical emergency.** The patient must be admitted to a **pediatric intensive care facility** and placed in the care of a **pediatric gastroenterologist.** Upper gastrointestinal endoscopy is indicated for diagnosis and treatment (**sclerotherapy or variceal banding**).

EVALUATION OF UPPER GASTROINTESTINAL BLEEDING

Patient History

- Is there a history of prolonged retching or recent stress?
- Could the child be swallowing blood as a result of epistaxis, tonsillectomy or adenoidectomy, trauma to the teeth or gums, or trauma from foreign objects or nasogastric tube insertion?
- Has the child eaten any food that may resemble blood in the vomitus?
- Does the child's medication history include NSAIDs or aspirin (which can cause gastritis) or steroids (which can cause gastric ulcers)?

Physical Examination

- The **nares, mouth, and throat** of any child who presents with hematemesis should be carefully examined.
- The child's **fingernails** should be inspected for evidence of dried blood because digital manipulation of the nose is the most common cause of nosebleeds in children. A negative rectal examination for occult blood should alert the physician to the possibility that epistaxis is responsible for the blood in the vomitus.
- **Hepatosplenomegaly or isolated splenomegaly** almost always occurs in conjunction with portal hypertension and varices.
- **Freckles over the lips and under the axilla** may suggest Peutz-Jeghers syndrome with gastric polyps.

Diagnostic Modalities

Upper gastrointestinal endoscopy and contrast studies are useful for discovering the cause of hematemesis. Although an upper gastrointestinal contrast study occasionally shows pathognomonic esophageal findings, **upper endoscopy with biopsy and culture** is the study of choice.

For children who have recurrent bleeding episodes and for whom endoscopy or contrast studies have been negative, **nuclear medicine bleeding scans** may be useful. The patient must be actively bleeding at the time of the test.

TREATMENT OF UPPER GASTROINTESTINAL BLEEDING

The first step in the management of a patient with upper gastrointestinal tract bleeding is to provide supportive care:

- Obtain vital signs and manage the airway, breathing, and circulation.
- Place a large-bore intravenous line.
- Obtain a complete blood cell count, type and cross-match, serum electrolyte panel, and blood urea nitrogen and creatinine levels.
- Administer crystalloid (normal saline) or a blood transfusion (if necessary).
- Place a nasogastric tube to irrigate the stomach.
- Place a deep venous line for central venous pressure measurement (if indicated).
- Obtain the patient's history and evaluate for prior bleeding episodes or chronic disease.
- Consult a pediatric gastroenterologist.

In addition to supportive care, acute medical management entails the **intravenous administration of vasopressin or octreotide** to promote vasoconstriction of bleeding blood vessels. These medications are extremely useful in children with active esophageal or gastric varices and ulcers. Patients given vasopressin or octreotide should be monitored in an **intensive care setting** and should be in the care of a **pediatric gastroenterologist.**

Other medical treatments include **endoscopy with sclerotherapy or electrocautery** and **balloon tamponade. Surgery** is indicated for patients with uncontrolled bleeding in whom medical treatment has failed.

APPROACH TO THE PATIENT

The **first episode** of upper gastrointestinal tract bleeding in children should always be **treated as a medical emergency.** Once the patient is stabilized, a careful history and physical examination should be performed to determine the cause of the bleeding.

Suggested Readings

Chawla S, Seth D, Mahajan P, et al.: Upper gastrointestinal bleeding in children. *Clin Pediatr* 46(1):16–21, 2007.

Feldman M, Friedman LS, Brandy LJ: *Sleisenger and Fordtran's Gastrointestinal and Liver Disease: Pathophysiology, Diagnosis, Management.* Philadelphia, WB Saunders, 2006.

Molleston JP: Variceal bleeding in children. *J Pediatr Gastroenterol Nutr* 37(5):538–545, 2003.

Polin RA, Ditmar MF: *Pediatric Secrets,* 4th ed. Philadelphia, Hanley & Belfus, 2005.

Treem WR: Gastrointestinal bleeding in children. *Gastrointest Endosc* 4:75, 1994.

Walker WA, Goulet O, Kleinman RE, et al.: *Pediatric Gastrointestinal Disease,* 4th ed. Hamilton, On, BC Decker, 2004.

Wyllie R, Hyams JS: *Pediatric Gastrointestinal Disease: Pathophysiology, Diagnosis, Management,* 3rd ed. Philadelphia, WB Saunders, 2005.

36 *Goiter*
Craig Alter and Marta Satin-Smith

INTRODUCTION

Goiter (**enlargement of the thyroid gland**) arises under a variety of clinical circumstances. Morbidity from an enlarged thyroid ranges from that associated with carcinoma, or a tender gland, to simple cosmetic effects. The majority of children who present with a goiter have normal hormone levels.

DIFFERENTIAL DIAGNOSIS LIST

Infectious Causes
Acute suppurative thyroiditis
Subacute thyroiditis

Toxic Causes
Environmental goitrogens
Lithium carbonate
Amiodarone
Iodide-containing drugs

Neoplastic Causes
Thyroid adenoma
Papillary carcinoma
Follicular carcinoma
Medullary carcinoma
Anaplastic carcinoma (adults)
Thyroid-stimulating hormone (TSH)-secreting adenoma
Nonthyroid carcinomas—lymphoma, teratoma, hygroma

Congenital Causes
Agenesis (absent gland)
Ectopic gland (e.g., lingual)
Unilateral agenesis
Dyshormonogenesis
Thyroxine (T_4) resistance

Metabolic Causes
Iodine deficiency

Inflammatory Causes
Chronic lymphocytic thyroiditis (CLT, Hashimoto thyroiditis)
Graves disease (acquired and neonatal)

Miscellaneous Causes
Simple colloid goiter (adolescent goiter)
Multinodular colloid goiter
Thyroglossal duct cyst

DIFFERENTIAL DIAGNOSIS DISCUSSION

Chronic Lymphocytic Thyroiditis (Hashimoto Thyroiditis)

Etiology

CLT, an autoimmune condition, is the **most common cause of goiter** in the pediatric population. Its incidence is **highest in adolescent girls,** with a female-to-male ratio of 2:1.

TABLE 36-1 Signs and Symptoms of Hypothyroidism and Hyperthyroidism

Hypothyroidism	Hyperthyroidism
Goiter in some patients	Goiter, bruit over thyroid
Lethargy, slow speech	Nervousness, restless sleep
Cold skin, decreased sweating	Sweating, heat intolerance
Bradycardia	Palpitation, tachycardia
Weakness	Fatigue, weakness
Anorexia	Increased appetite
Weight gain	Weight loss
Constipation	Increased stool frequency
Stiff, aching muscles	Tremor of hands and tongue
Edema of face and eyelids	Exophthalmos, lid lag
Dry, coarse skin	Increased skin pigmentation
Hair loss with increased coarseness	Fine hair
Poor growth	Accelerated growth
Delayed puberty and tooth eruption	Poor school performance
	Moodiness or irritability

Clinical Features

Some patients with CLT present for medical examination with symptoms of **hypothyroidism** (Table 36-1). Most have enlargement of the gland without systemic complaints. Rarely, patients with CLT show symptoms of **hyperthyroidism**. These children **progress toward hypothyroidism** over a period of months. The **thyroid gland** itself **is diffusely enlarged** (although possibly with **asymmetry**), **mobile, nontender,** and **firm.** It usually has a granular or pebbly texture but can be smooth. However, in the most severe cases of hypothyroidism and CLT, the thyroid is often so **degenerated** that it is not easily palpable. Enlargement of the thyroid in CLT may be caused by lymphocytic infiltration or stimulation by the increased TSH. A goiter due to increased TSH stimulation typically decreases with treatment.

There is a **family history** of thyroid disease in 30% to 40% of patients with CLT. Histologic findings include infiltration of the gland with plasma cells and lymphocytes, parenchymal atrophy, and eosinophilic degeneration of acini.

Evaluation

Laboratory studies should include assessment of T_4 and/or free T_4, TSH, and **antithyroglobulin and antithyroperoxidase antibodies.** Table 36-2 shows normal values of thyroid function studies. In children with CLT, thyroid function tests indicate either a **euthyroid state** (no abnormalities), **compensated hypothyroidism** (normal level of T_4 with increased TSH), or **hypothyroidism** (low level of T_4 with mildly increased TSH). **One or both of the antithyroid antibodies is present** in 90% to 95% of patients with CLT.

TABLE 36-2 Normal Thyroid Hormone Levels*

Parameter	Normal Finding
T$_4$	
Total	5.5–12.8 µg/dL (prepubertal)
	4.9–13 µg/dL (pubertal)
Free	0.8–2.2 ng/dL (prepubertal)
	0.8–2.3 ng/dL (pubertal)
T$_3$	119–218 ng/dL (prepubertal)
	80–185 ng/dL (pubertal)
TSH	0.6–5.5 uU/mL (prepubertal)
	0.5–4.8 uU/mL (pubertal)

T_3 = triiodothyronine; T_4 = thyroxine; *TSH* = thyroid-stimulating hormone.
*Results from LabCorp and Esoterix assays; other assays may differ slightly.

These antibodies represent the immunologic response to the presence of elements of thyroid tissue in the bloodstream and are not the cause of the thyroiditis.

Treatment

If the child is euthyroid at presentation and again at 6 months, yearly monitoring of T$_4$ and TSH is indicated. **Thyroid hormone replacement** is indicated for the treatment of overt hypothyroidism and occasionally for compensated hypothyroidism accompanied by a significantly enlarged gland. Initial doses of **sodium l-thyroxine** at 100 µg/m^2 of body surface area or 2 to 5 µg/kg per day should be **adjusted after 4 to 6 weeks** of therapy to keep T$_4$ and TSH levels in the normal, or low normal, range. Shrinkage of the goiter may not occur if the inflammation is long standing and the fibrosis is extensive. Once an appropriate dose of sodium l-thyroxine is established, **biannual follow-up** is necessary to ensure compliance and appropriate growth. Some may require more frequent laboratory studies.

Spontaneous remission occurs in up to 30% of adolescents. It is acceptable to discontinue hormone replacement therapy when growth is completed to ascertain whether spontaneous remission has occurred.

Simple Colloid Goiter

Etiology

Simple colloid goiter (**adolescent goiter**) is the **second most common** cause of nontoxic thyroid enlargement in the pediatric population. Its cause is uncertain, although an autoimmune cause is a possibility. There is often a **family history** of goiter.

Clinical Features

There is **diffuse enlargement** of the thyroid gland in **asymptomatic adolescents.** The gland is enlarged and usually softer and more homogeneous than in chronic lymphocytic thyroiditis. **Nodularity** may develop after several years, even in those patients in whom regression has occurred.

Evaluation

There are usually **no antithyroid antibodies,** and the T_4 **and TSH levels are normal.** Some patients have an increased level of thyroid growth-stimulating antibodies in their serum, which suggests this may be a mild form of autoimmune disease.

Treatment

Treatment with sodium l-thyroxine is not required. In many cases, the goiter **resolves with time.**

Graves Disease

Etiology

Graves disease, a **multisystem autoimmune disorder,** is the **most common cause of hyperthyroidism** in the pediatric population. The incidence in males and females is equal in infancy and early childhood, with a female predominance occurring in adolescence. In Graves disease, elaboration of an immunoglobulin G1 antibody stimulates the TSH receptor, resulting in hyperfunctioning follicular cells with **increased production and release of thyroid hormone.** Other antibodies, including thyroid growth-stimulating antibody, may contribute to enlargement of the gland. Exophthalmos in Graves disease may be caused in part by a collagen-stimulating antibody.

Clinical Features

Graves disease presents with signs of **hyperthyroidism** and **thyromegaly. Exophthalmos** is occasionally present and, rarely, dermopathy. Children with hyperthyroidism caused by Graves disease often are brought to medical attention because of **worsening school performance** and a **change in behavior** (emotional lability and irritability). The majority of symptoms of hyperthyroidism (see Table 36-1) are caused by stimulation of the sympathetic nervous system resulting from increased levels of thyroid hormones.

Evaluation

On physical examination, the thyroid gland is symmetrically **enlarged, smooth,** and **nontender.** The texture is soft to firm, and the size is variable, but the severity of the hyperthyroid correlates with the size of the gland. Graves disease is rare in a child without a **goiter.** The child is usually **tachycardic** with a widened pulse pressure and an active precordium. A **vascular bruit** may be heard over the gland. **Proptosis with stare** and **upper lid lag** is noted in many cases; however, the eye disease

TABLE 36-3 Laboratory Findings in Graves Disease

Parameter	Finding Suggestive of Graves Disease
Total T_4	Levels increased
Free T_4	Levels increased
T_3	Levels increased
TSH	Significantly suppressed and often undetectable
Thyroid-stimulating immunoglobulin	Elevated
Thyroid antibodies	
Antithyroglobulin antibody	May be detectable but rarely increased to the degree seen in CLT; if levels are very high, consider the possibility of CLT
Antithyroperoxidase antibody	May be detectable but rarely increased to the degree seen in CLT; if levels are very high, consider the possibility of CLT
[123]I uptake study	Increased uptake of the isotope at 6 and 24 hr postadministration is supportive of Graves disease (decreased uptake is seen in CLT and subacute thyroiditis). A focal area of increased iodine uptake implies a hot nodule.

CLT = chronic lymphocytic thyroiditis; [123]I = iodine-123; T_3 = triiodothyronine; T_4 = thyroxine; TSH = thyroid-stimulating hormone

in children rarely reaches the severity seen in adults. Dermopathy, caused by an accumulation of mucopolysaccharide in the skin and subcutaneous tissue, is uncommon in children.

Table 36-3 shows the laboratory and radiologic studies that support the diagnosis of Graves disease and help distinguish it from other causes of hyperthyroidism.

Treatment

There are three main approaches to the management of Graves disease: **antithyroid medications, iodine-131 (^{131}I) ablation therapy,** and **subtotal thyroidectomy.** In general, medical management with **medications should be the first intervention,** followed by either ablation with ^{131}I or surgery. The mainstays of long-term medical treatment in children are the **thioamide derivatives,** propylthiouracil (PTU) and methimazole. These medications inhibit the organification of iodide, thus blocking the synthesis (but not the release) of thyroid hormone. β-Blocking agents are used as adjuvant treatment to control symptoms when long-term therapy is initially introduced; they may be discontinued when the thyroid disease is well controlled. Side effects of the medication include skin rash, pruritus, and, rarely, agranulocytosis. If a **child on PTU or methimazole** presents with a **severe sore throat,** a complete blood cell count should be obtained.

Thyroid Storm (Thyroid Crisis)

Etiology

Thyroid storm is a **medical emergency**. A very rare condition, it typically occurs in individuals who have **preexisting hyperthyroidism** and who are **undertreated or noncompliant**. Infection, trauma, and surgical procedures are the most common precipitating events. Pneumococcal sepsis is occasionally found. The release of large amounts of thyroid hormone leads to a **hypermetabolic state** with **excessive thermogenesis** and **significant fluid losses**. **Increase in temperature** can be extreme.

Clinical Features

Children with thyroid storm show **fever, rapid tachycardia, tremor, nausea and vomiting, diarrhea, dehydration,** and **delirium or coma**. Occasionally, patients have a true **toxic psychosis**. The markedly increased cardiac workload can lead to **congestive heart failure**.

Treatment

Treatment of thyroid storm includes the **immediate administration of β-blocking agents** to suppress the activity of the sympathetic nervous system. Next, **hydration** must be achieved, and appropriate measures must be taken to **lower the body temperature slowly**. Propylthiouracil (6 to 10 mg/kg per day, divided, every 8 hours) is administered orally. Subsequently, **iodide treatment** to rapidly terminate the release of thyroxine is administered in the form of Lugol iodide, 5 drops every 8 hours, or sodium iodide, 125 to 250 mg/day intravenously over 24 hours.

Acute Suppurative Thyroiditis

Etiology

A **fistula tract** may have formed between the **left pyriform sinus of the pharynx** and the **left lobe of the thyroid gland**. Because of high endogenous levels of iodine, the thyroid gland is inherently resistant to bacterial infection. However, **infections** do occur and **must be treated promptly** to prevent abscess formation.

Clinical Features

Patients present with the rapid onset of **anterior neck pain** associated with **dysphagia, pharyngitis, mandibular pain,** and a **hoarse voice;** fever; and signs of **systemic toxicity**. The thyroid itself is **exquisitely tender and nonmobile** and may have areas of fluid. The **pain increases with neck extension**.

Evaluation

Organisms identified by means of needle biopsy include *Streptococcus pyogenes, Staphylococcus aureus, Streptococcus pneumoniae,* anaerobes, fungi, and parasitic organisms. Marked leukocytosis and an increased sedimentation rate are the most consistent laboratory findings. Thyroid function tests usually are normal, but a transient increase in T_4 levels can occur. Nuclear medicine scanning with iodine-123 (^{123}I) demonstrates decreased uptake of the isotope.

Treatment

Antibiotic treatment should be tailored to the suspected organism. Areas of abscess may require **surgical drainage. β-Blocking drugs** can be used if signs of transient thyrotoxicosis develop. Recovery without residual thyroid disease is the natural course.

Subacute Thyroiditis

Etiology

Subacute thyroiditis is a **self-limited inflammation** of the thyroid gland that most often is associated with, or follows, a **viral illness.** Viral agents implicated include mumps virus, adenovirus, coxsackievirus, influenza virus, Epstein-Barr virus, and enteric cytopathic human orphan virus. The incidence is the same in boys and girls.

Clinical Features

It can be **difficult to distinguish between subacute and acute** suppurative thyroiditis. Patients present for treatment with **fever** and **anterior neck pain.** The **area over the thyroid** may be **warm and erythematous.** The thyroid is usually tender and **enlarged.** Signs and symptoms of **hyperthyroidism** develop because of the release of stored hormone from the inflamed gland. These symptoms can persist for 1 to 4 weeks and can be followed by a 2- to 9-month period of hypothyroidism.

Evaluation

Free and total T_4 and triiodothyronine (T_3) levels are increased in the majority of patients with subacute thyroiditis for a period of **several weeks.** Most patients do not develop antithyroid antibodies. As in acute suppurative thyroiditis, an ^{123}I scan demonstrates decreased **uptake of isotope.**

Treatment

Treatment includes the administration of **nonsteroidal anti-inflammatory drugs** and a beta-blocker. In severe cases, the use of **corticosteroids** may be indicated. Typically, full recovery of thyroid function occurs. If **hypothyroidism** develops, it is usually transient, but it **should be treated.**

Congenital Goiter

Etiology

Most cases of newborn goiter are caused by **inborn defects of thyroid hormone metabolism** (dyshormonogenesis). Most of these defects are inherited as autosomal recessive traits. These defects include the following:

- Abnormal iodide trapping or organification
- Iodotyrosine deiodinase defect
- Defects in thyroglobulin synthesis, transport, or processing

A second cause of congenital goiter is the **maternal ingestion of goitrogenic agents** during pregnancy, leading to a transient congenital hypothyroidism in the infant. Treatment of maternal hyperthyroidism with PTU or methimazole usually does not cause congenital hypothyroidism unless very high doses are used (>150 mg/day of PTU).

Evaluation

In dyshormonogenesis, free and total T_4 levels **may be normal or low** while the **TSH is elevated.** [123] I scanning usually reveals an **enlarged gland** with **abnormal isotope uptake.**

Treatment

As with other causes of congenital hypothyroidism, infants with dyshormonogenesis need treatment with **sodium l-thyroxine** (10 µ/kg per day) to ensure the normal T_4 levels needed for central nervous system development.

Infants with **presumed transient hypothyroidism** can be **followed closely** without treatment for **2 weeks.** If the T_4 level remains low and the TSH level is elevated, then treatment should be started and continued for the first 2 years of life while the brain thyroid-dependent myelinization occurs.

EVALUATION OF GOITER

Patient History

The major goals during the initial history are to determine if a child has signs or symptoms of **hypothyroidism or hyperthyroidism** (see Table 36-1). The **rapidity of enlargement** of the gland may allow one to focus on an **acute process** (e.g., suppurative thyroiditis) as opposed to a **chronic problem** (e.g., CLT). In the case of a **solitary nodule or unilateral enlargement,** exposure to **radiation** either for treatment of a medical condition or accidental **exposure should be determined.** A family history of thyroid disease and/or autoimmune tendency should be elicited. Because the incidence of thyroid carcinoma in Belarus has increased dramatically following the Chernobyl nuclear accident, children adopted from this area need to be screened carefully.

> **HINT:** Review of systems at each visit should include whether the child has polyuria and polydipsia to screen for early diabetes mellitus. Fatigue in a child with thyroid disease can be caused by inadequately treated hypothyroidism but also new-onset diabetes mellitus.

Physical Examination

- **Vital signs.** Heart rate and blood pressure findings are important in both hypothyroid and hyperthyroid states.
- **Growth.** Poor overall growth may be the first sign of hypothyroidism associated with CLT. Obesity with normal linear growth argues against hypothyroidism as the cause of the increased weight. Accelerated growth is common in hyperthyroidism.
- **Neurologic examination.** Restlessness, tremor, exophthalmos, and hyperreflexia are common features of hyperthyroidism. In contrast, decreased energy and delayed relaxation phase of deep tendon reflexes are common findings in hypothyroidism.
- **Thyroid examination.** Careful palpation and measurement of the gland is performed with the examiner standing behind a seated or standing patient. The size and texture of the gland, symmetry of enlargement, associated lymphadenopathy, and any tenderness should be noted.

Laboratory Studies

Laboratory studies are guided by the history and physical examination findings. They commonly include **evaluation of T_4 and/or free T_4, TSH,** and **thyroid antibodies** (thyroglobulin and peroxidase). In cases of suspected hyperthyroidism, T_3 must also be measured because children occasionally manifest predominantly T_3 toxicosis. Elevations in total T_4 are seen in states of increased binding such as in pregnancy and use of oral birth control pills with an associated increase in thyroid-binding globulin. Free T_4 assays may be affected by certain medications such as antiseizure therapies. Free T_4 by equilibrium dialysis would be an appropriate alternative if one is suspicious of an interfering substance.

Treatment

If an individual with goiter is found to be hypothyroid or hyperthyroid, appropriate treatment with sodium l-thyroxine or antithyroid medications as outlined previously should be initiated. The case of a euthyroid patient is less clear; for example the presence of antibodies with normal

T4 and TSH may not require thyroid hormone replacement. Instead, close monitoring of thyroid function every 3 to 6 months is an acceptable alternative.

Suggested Readings

Alter CA, Moshang T: Diagnostic dilemma: the goiter. *Pediatr Clin North Am* 88:567–578, 1991.

American Academy of Pediatrics, Rose SR; Section on Endocrinology and Committee on Genetics, American Thyroid Association, Brown RS; Public Health Committee, Lawson Wilkins Pediatric Endocrine Society, Foley T, Kaplowitz PB, Kaye CI, et al.: Update of newborn screening and therapy for congenital hypothyroidism. *Pediatrics* 117(6):2290–2303, 2006.

Foley TP: Hypothyroidism. *Pediatr Rev* 25(3):94–100, 2004.

Jaruratanasirikul S, Leethanaporn K, Khuntigij P, et al.: The clinical course of Hashimoto's thyroiditis in children and adolescents: 6 years longitudinal follow-up. *J Pediatr Endocrinol Metab* 14:177–184, 2001.

Jaruratanasirikul S, Leethanaporn K, Suchat K: The natural clinical course of children with an initial diagnosis of simple goiter: a 5-year longitudinal follow-up. *J Pediatr Endocrinol Metab* 13:1109–1113, 2000.

LaFranchi SH, Austin J: How should we be treating children with congenital hypothyroidism? *J Pediatr Endocrinol Metab* 20(5):559–578, 2007.

Reiners C, Demidchik YE: Differentiated thyroid cancer in childhood: pathology, diagnosis and therapy. *Pediatr Endocrinol Rev* 1(Suppl 2):230–235; discussion 235–236, 2003.

Rivkees SA: The treatment of Graves' disease in children. *J Pediatr Endocrinol Metab* 19(9):1095–1111, 2006.

Thyroid Internet Textbook. Available at: http://www.thyroidmanager.org/thyroidbook.htm.

INTRODUCTION

Head injury in children accounts for more than 600,000 emergency department visits, 95,000 hospitalizations, and 7,000 deaths per year. The highest injury rates are found in children <4 years. Brain injuries can be subdivided into primary and secondary injuries. Primary injuries occur as a result of a direct force to the brain. These injuries are usually irreversible. Fatal or irreversible injury is usually a sequela of neuronal cell death and vascular disruption during the first few milliseconds of impact. Another irreversible cause of morbidity is the shearing of the white matter tracts as a result of an acceleration-deceleration injury. Secondary brain injuries result from subsequent pathophysiologic changes. **The only injuries that are reversible with therapy are those with secondary effects on the brain and blood vessels, such as cerebral edema and impaired glucose and oxygen delivery to the neurons.**

DIFFERENTIAL DIAGNOSIS LIST

Focal Injuries
   Scalp lacerations
   Hematoma
   Cerebral contusion
   Fractures

Diffuse Injuries
   Concussion syndrome
   Diffuse axonal injury
   Increased intracranial
      pressure (ICP)

DIFFERENTIAL DIAGNOSIS DISCUSSION

Scalp Lacerations

Scalp lacerations are common findings in patients with head injuries. Blood loss can be extensive, especially in infants and young children. The physician should carefully assess the depth **of the wound** and evaluate it for **retained foreign bodies.** In addition, the **integrity of the galea aponeurotica** (a tendinous sheath located just above the periosteum) should be evaluated; some clinicians suture this layer separately to control bleeding. Finally, the physician should search for **skull fractures or "step-offs"** (dents).

Hematoma

Hematoma caused by head injury may exist outside of the confines of the skull (e.g., cephalohematoma, subgaleal hematoma), or inside the skull (e.g., epidural or subdural hematoma). **Intracranial lesions** may require **neurosurgical intervention**, whereas **extracranial lesions** rarely require any treatment other than **supportive care.**

Cephalohematoma

Newborn infants commonly incur a cephalohematoma, in which blood collects between the periosteum and the table of the skull and is therefore prevented from spreading past the midline. This type of injury is common in traumatic deliveries.

Subgaleal Hematoma

A posttraumatic, well-circumscribed "lump" on an older child's head usually represents a subgaleal hematoma.

Epidural and Subdural Hematomas (Table 37-1)

Epidural hematomas are less often associated with underlying brain injury than are subdural hematomas.

TABLE 37-1 Epidural Versus Acute Subdural Hematoma

	Epidural Hematoma	Subdural Hematoma
Common mechanism	Blunt direct trauma, frequently to parietal region	Acceleration-deceleration injury
Etiology	Arterial or venous	Venous (bridging veins below dura)
Incidence	Uncommon	Common
Peak age	Usually >2 yr	Usually <1 yr Peak at 6 months
Location	Unilateral Commonly parietal	75% Bilateral Diffuse, over cerebral hemispheres
Skull fracture	Common	Uncommon
Associated seizures	Uncommon	Common
Retinal hemorrhages	Rare	Common
Decreased level of consciousness	Common	Almost always
Mortality	Rare	Uncommon
Morbidity in survivors	Low	High
Clinical findings	Dilated ipsilateral pupil, contralateral hemiparesis Period of lucidity prior to acute decompensation and rapid progression to herniation	Decreased level of consciousness Irritability, lethargy
Onset	Acute	Acute (within 24 hr), subacute (within 1 day to 2 wk), or chronic (after 2 wk)
Findings on computed tomography	Convex "lens-shaped" cerebral hemisphere	Concave, diffusely surrounding cerebral hemisphere

Cerebral Contusions and Lacerations

Cerebral contusions can occur as a **coup injury** (at the contact location) or as a **contrecoup injury** (rebounding, on the opposite side). A cerebral contusion commonly manifests as **posttraumatic epilepsy.**

Cerebral lacerations usually result from **penetrating injury** to the brain or from a **depressed skull fracture.** Clinical manifestations are more often a result of the associated concussion and the underlying brain injury than of the focal lesions themselves. These lesions can be visualized on computed tomography (CT) scans.

Skull Fractures

Up to 29% of children with head injury may have skull fractures.

Linear Skull Fractures

Linear skull fractures comprise 75% to 90% of all skull fractures. **Usually no treatment is necessary.** However, if the fracture is located over a vascular structure (e.g., the middle meningeal artery), there is an increased incidence of epidural hemorrhage. Diastatic ("growing") fractures can develop when meninges get caught between the bone edges and continue to separate them.

Basilar Skull Fractures

Basilar skull fractures typically occur in the **petrous portion of the temporal bone.** Potential findings on physical examination of a patient with a basilar skull fracture include the following:

- "Raccoon" eyes (ecchymosis below the eyes)
- Battle sign (ecchymosis at the mastoid)
- Hemotympanum (blood behind the eardrum)
- Cerebrospinal fluid (CSF) otorrhea or rhinorrhea
- Cranial nerve dysfunction, especially involving the seventh and eighth cranial nerves

Depressed Skull Fractures

Depressed skull fractures can sometimes be diagnosed clinically, by palpation of the depression of the skull underneath a hematoma, or radiographically, using tangential views of the skull or a CT scan. **Surgical elevation** may be necessary **if the fracture extends past the inner table of the skull.**

Concussion Syndromes

Concussion syndromes are diagnosed when blunt head injury results in a transient impairment in awareness and responsiveness. According to the American Academy of Neurology, concussions are trauma-induced alterations in mental status that may or may not be associated with loss of consciousness. The **symptoms can last from seconds to hours.** Some patients complain of persistent headaches, dizziness, and subtle differences in memory, anxiety level, and sleep patterns lasting a few weeks after head injury.

Diffuse Axonal Injury

Diffuse axonal injury occurs when nerve fibers are sheared on initial impact. Patients exhibit **persistent functional neurologic deficits** (e.g., a prolonged comatose state) without obvious radiographic abnormalities. Diffuse axonal injury is associated with high morbidity and mortality rates.

Increased Intracranial Pressure

Increased ICP **affects the delivery of oxygen and substrate to the brain tissue.** An increase in one component of the intracranial contents (i.e., blood, CSF, or tissue) necessitates a decrease in another component because, under normal conditions, the sum of these compartments in the cranial vault remains constant. Therefore, if the ICP increases to more than the normal limit (15 mm Hg), small changes in the volume of the intracranial contents result in large changes in ICP. The **brain tissue and blood vessels** become **increasingly compressed,** disrupting cerebral blood flow or causing herniation of brain tissue through the dural reflections.

- **Herniation of the uncal portion of the temporal lobe** through the tentorium disrupts the parasympathetic fibers of the third cranial nerve, resulting in ipsilateral pupillary dilation and contralateral motor deficits. In diffuse injury, the uncal herniation and, therefore, the pupillary and motor deficits, can be noted bilaterally.
- **Herniation of the brainstem** is frequently a premorbid event. Compression of medullary autonomic structures affects heart rate, respirations, and level of consciousness. Cushing's triad, resulting from increased ICP and consisting of hypertension, bradycardia, and irregular respirations, is a classic finding. Decerebrate posturing may also be noted. However, serious sequelae can ensue even if the child has not experienced this constellation of findings.

APPROACH TO THE PATIENT

Stabilization

Initial priorities for any severely injured child are **protection of the airway, maintenance of adequate tissue perfusion,** and **rapid assessment of neurologic status.** Although the primary injury to the brain is irreversible, the secondary injury may be minimized in the acute care setting.

Airway

Upper airway obstruction is initially managed with proper **adjustment of the head, neck, and mandible** to clear the soft tissues and tongue away from the airway. Examination of the cervical spine is considered part of the airway evaluation. Before undertaking radiographic and clinical examination of the cervical spine, a **cervical collar** should be used with side immobilization, or manual immobilization should be provided.

Breathing

The head trauma victim with a clear upper airway but decreased breath sounds may have one of many injuries:

- Pneumothorax
- Pulmonary contusion
- Flail chest
- Central nervous system depression

Circulation

Lack of brain perfusion can lead to irreversible neuronal cell damage. **The cerebral perfusion pressure equals the mean arterial pressure minus the ICP.** Therefore, the goal of management is to normalize the mean arterial pressure while minimizing ICP.

Shock should be dealt with aggressively in the trauma patient, regardless of concern about increased ICP. Shock must be addressed as if it is hypovolemic shock until proven otherwise; it cannot be presumed to be secondary to spinal cord injury (neurogenic shock). The administration of crystalloid (e.g., normal saline or lactated Ringer's solution) or colloid (e.g., whole blood) should be based on the patient's heart rate, skin perfusion, and urinary output.

Assessment of Neurologic Disability

The **Glasgow coma scale (GCS) score** should be obtained (see Chapter 21, "Coma," Table 21-1), and the **pupils** and **gag reflex** should be evaluated relatively early to determine the presence of brain herniation as well as the need for endotracheal intubation. The GCS score is a prognostic tool for patients with head trauma (Table 37-2).

TABLE 37-2 Factors Associated with a Poor Outcome in Children With Head Injury

Age <2 yr
Glasgow coma scale (GCS) score <5
Subdural hematoma
Decerebrate or flaccid posture
Coma >24 hr

Management of Increased ICP

- **Hyperventilation** reduces the "blood" portion of the cerebral vault by constricting the cerebral vessels; however this leads to decreased cerebral perfusion and may result in iatrogenic ischemia in an already traumatized brain. For the latter reason, prophylactic hyperventilation after traumatic brain injury is no longer recommended. The arterial carbon dioxide tension ($Paco_2$) should be maintained at or slightly above approximately 35 mm Hg. Mild hyperventilation ($Paco_2$ 30 to 35 mmHg) is an option in patients with persistently increased ICP refractory to sedation, analgesia, CSF drainage, or hyperosmolar therapy.

- **Hyperosmolar therapy** is thought to reduce the "tissue" portion of the intracranial vault by drawing water out of the brain. Mannitol (0.5 to 1.0 g/kg intravenously as a bolus) or hypertonic saline (3% saline, 0.1 to 1.0 mL/kg per hour as a continuous infusion) are two agents that may be used for this purpose. The presence of hypotension or hypovolemia is a relative contraindication to the use of hyperosmolar agents.

- **Maintenance of normal intracranial pressure** is also facilitated by elevating the head to 30°, correcting systemic hypotension with fluid resuscitation, and taking measures to stop seizure activity, if present.

Further Evaluation

Patient History

A brief history of the **events preceding and subsequent to the traumatic episode** should be obtained, focusing on the timing and mechanism of injury, duration of unconsciousness, presence of amnesia, neurologic assessment at the scene, and any preexisting medical conditions.

Physical Examination

A **secondary survey** should follow soon after the primary survey and include a close inspection of the head, torso, abdomen, genitalia, and extremities. It is important to examine the head for lacerations, depressions, contusions, or signs of basilar skull fracture.

In the comatose patient, a **normal oculovestibular response** implies that the cranial nerve pathways most proximal to the brainstem (i.e., the third, sixth, and eighth cranial nerves) are intact and that, by association, the neighboring brainstem is functional. Performance of this test can be delayed until after the secondary survey is completed.

The **oculocephalic ("doll's eye") reflex** should not be evaluated in patients who might have a cervical spine injury.

Diagnostic Modalities

A skull fracture is a relatively good indicator of intracranial injury in children <2 years. Patients with a skull fracture have up to a 400-fold increased risk of intracranial injury. Children <2 years, especially those with a hematoma over the parietal area, may therefore benefit from **skull radiographs** (which are quicker to obtain, do not require sedation, and are associated with a much lower radiation dose) as an indicator of whether or not to obtain a CT scan. When a **CT scan** of the head is required to investigate the possibility of intracranial lesions, it is not necessary to obtain skull radiographs. CT of the head is indicated for patients with these characteristics:

- Persistently altered level of consciousness (GCS <15)
- Clinical neurologic deterioration
- Persistent focal neurologic deficit
- Parietal skull fracture (middle meningeal location) or evidence of any other significant skull fracture (e.g., basilar skull fracture)
- Persistent vomiting
- Significant mechanism of injury
- History of amnesia or loss of consciousness (often considered in the decision to obtain a head CT; however these factors are not clearly associated with intracranial bleeding)

Management of Complications

Posttraumatic seizures develop in a small percentage of patients who have experienced head trauma. In the acute setting, a **benzodiazepine** should be administered because of its rapid onset of action. **Phenytoin** should be used as a second antiepileptic agent in this setting. Patients with cerebral contusions on CT scan may receive phenytoin initially to prevent rather than treat seizures.

- **Early-onset posttraumatic seizures** (occurring within 1 week of injury) often accompany cerebral lacerations and contusions. Twenty percent of these patients experience late seizures, but the condition rarely progresses to epilepsy.
- **Late-onset posttraumatic seizures** (developing >1 week after injury) are associated with seizures that persist for the next few years in 50% of patients.

TREATMENT OF HEAD TRAUMA

Severe Head Trauma

Treatment consists of **head CT scan** and **management of intracranial pressure** as needed. Patients with "severe" head trauma include those with these characteristics:

- Abnormal neurologic examination
- Persistent seizures

- GCS score ≤14
- Depressed or basilar skull fracture

Moderate Head Trauma

Treatment consists of **12 to 24 hours of observation.** CT of the head may be considered. Patients with "moderate" head trauma include those with a history of amnesia or a brief loss of consciousness but a normal neurologic examination. Patients with persistent or worsening headache, vomiting, or reported seizure activity are also considered to have moderate head injury.

Mild Head Trauma

For the head trauma to be considered "mild," the patient must never have lost consciousness and must have a normal neurologic examination and no reported amnesia. **Skull radiographs** should be considered for the asymptomatic child <2 years with a significant scalp hematoma and an infant <2 to 3 months with a moderate or high-impact mechanism. Other patients can be **observed at home** by a reliable caretaker. The caretaker should bring the patient back to the emergency department if any of the following conditions develop:

- A headache that worsens or is unrelieved by acetaminophen
- Frequent vomiting or vomiting beyond 8 hours postinjury
- Change in behavior or gait
- Vision problems
- Fever or stiff neck
- Evidence of clear or bloody fluid draining from the nose or ear
- Difficulty in awakening from sleep
- Seizures
- Bleeding that is unrelieved by the application of pressure for 5 minutes

Suggested Readings

Adelson PD, Bratton SL, Carney NL, et al.: Guidelines for the acute medical management of severe traumatic brain injury in infants, children and adolescents. *Pediatr Crit Care Med* 4:S1–S71, 2003.

American Academy of Pediatrics Committee on Quality Improvement: The management of closed head injury in children. *Pediatrics* 104: 1407–1415, 1999.

Kirkwood MW, Yeates KO, Wilson, PE: Pediatric sport-related concussion: a review of the clinical management of an oft-neglected population. *Pediatrics* 117:1359–1368, 2006.

Oman JA, Cooper RJ, Holmes JF, et al.: Performance of a decision rule to predict need for computed tomography among children with blunt head trauma. *Pediatrics* 117:e238–e246, 2006.

Schutzman SA, Barnes P, Duhaime AC, et al.: Evaluation and management of children younger than two years old with apparently minor head trauma: proposed guidelines. *Pediatrics* 107:883–993, 2001.

Schutzman SA, Greenes DS: Pediatric minor head trauma. *Ann Emerg Med* 37:65–74, 2001.

Thiessen ML, Woolridge DP: Pediatric minor closed head injury. *Pediatr Clin North Am* 53:1–26, 2006.

38 *Headache*
Nicholas S. Abend

INTRODUCTION

Headaches are reported by children as young as toddlers, and the incidence increases throughout childhood and adolescence, by which time 20% report occasional head pain. Headaches may be classified as primary or secondary (Table 38-1). Primary headaches are diagnosed based on groupings of symptoms and signs; they include migraine, tension-type, and cluster headaches. In secondary headache, the headache is symptomatic of an underlying intracranial or medical condition. It may be useful to classify the headache in terms of time course (Figure 38-1). In acute headache, there is a single episode of headache pain without prior headaches. In acute recurrent headache, there are stereotyped headaches separated by headache-free periods. In chronic progressive headache, there is a gradual but inexorable increase in headache. In chronic nonprogressive headache, there is constant steady headache.

DIFFERENTIAL DIAGNOSIS LIST

Acute Headache
Intracranial hemorrhage (subarachnoid, intraparenchymal, subdural, epidural)
Hydrocephalus
Vasculitis
Meningitis/encephalitis
Intracranial hypertension
  Primary (Pseudotumor cerebri)
  Secondary (i.e., sinovenous thrombosis)
Intracranial hypotension
Arterial ischemic stroke
Neoplasm
Hypertension
Ventricular shunt malfunction
Toxins (e.g., carbon monoxide, lead)

Sinusitis, pharyngitis, otitis media
First migraine, tension-type, or cluster headache
Dental or temporomandibular joint dysfunction

Acute Recurrent Headache
Migraine or tension-type headaches
Episodic intracranial hypertension (i.e., ventricular tumor)

Chronic Progressive Headache
Neoplasm
Intracranial hypertension (primary or secondary)

Neoplasm

Abscess

Epidural or subdural
hemorrhage

Vascular malformation

Toxins (carbon monoxide,
lead)

Chronic Nonprogressive Headache

Chronic daily headache

Medication overuse headache

New daily persistent headache

Psychosomatic

Postconcussion syndrome

DIFFERENTIAL DIAGNOSIS DISCUSSION

> **HINT:** An acute onset severe headache requires urgent evaluation because specific and rapid therapy may be required. A chronic progressive headache is suggestive of an expanding intracranial lesion and requires neuroimaging evaluation.

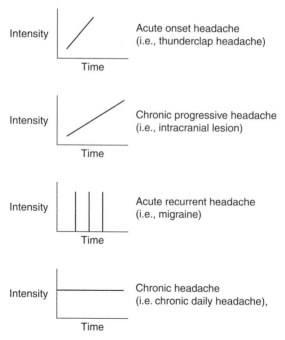

Figure 38-1 ▪ Temporal patterns of headache.

(Adapted from Rothner AD: The evaluation of headaches in children and adolescents. Semin Pediatr Neurol 2:109–118, 1995.)

TABLE 38-1 Simplified International Classification of Headache Disorders

Primary Headache

Migraine
Migraine without aura
Migraine with aura
Hemiplegic migraine (familial or sporadic)
Basilar-type migraine
Childhood periodic syndromes that are commonly precursors of migraine
  Cyclic vomiting, abdominal migraine, benign paroxysmal vertigo of childhood
Retinal migraine
Complications of migraine
  Chronic migraine, status migrainosus, migrainous infarction
Tension headache
  Episodic or chronic
Trigeminal autonomic cephalalgias
  Cluster headache
  Paroxysmal hemicrania (episodic or chronic)
  Short-lasting unilateral neuralgiform headache attacks with conjunctival
  injection and tearing (SUNCT)
Chronic headaches
  New daily persistent headache
  Medication overuse headache
  Transformed migraine or tension headache
  Hemicrania continua
Other
  Exertional, cough, stabbing, hypnic, primary thunderclap

Secondary Headache

Acute and chronic posttraumatic headache
Headache attributed to intracranial hematoma (traumatic or nontraumatic)
Headache attributed to head or neck trauma
Headache attributed to cranial or cervical vascular disorders
Acute ischemic cerebrovascular disorder
Unruptured vascular malformation
Headache caused by arteritis
Cerebral venous thrombosis
High cerebrospinal fluid (CSF) pressure
Low CSF pressure
Noninfectious inflammatory disorder
Headache attributed to neoplasm
Epileptic seizures
Headache due to Chiari type I malformation
Headache associated with substance abuse or withdrawal
Intracranial infection
Systemic infection
Hypoxia and or hypercapnia
Dialysis headache
Hypertension
Hypothyroidism
Fasting
Headache or facial pain associated with disorder of cranium, neck, eyes, ears, nose,
  sinuses, teeth, mouth

Acute Thunderclap Headache

Thunderclap headache (or sudden severe headache onset) is uncommon, but recognition and accurate diagnosis of this headache are important because there is often a **serious underlying brain disorder** that requires specific and urgent therapy. These include subarachnoid hemorrhage, parenchymal hemorrhage, sinovenous thrombosis, intracranial infection, arterial dissection, pituitary apoplexy, intracranial hypotension, and intermittent hydrocephalus. After a history and physical examination, diagnostic testing often begins with a **noncontrast head computed tomography** (CT) that demonstrates acute blood as a bright signal. If subarachnoid hemorrhage is strongly suspected, and the head CT is nondiagnostic, then **lumbar puncture** (with two tubes sent for cell count, to differentiate between subarachnoid blood and a traumatic tap) should be performed. Lumbar puncture is indicated with **opening pressure** in the relaxed lateral decubitus position if intracranial hypertension or hypotension is suspected. Generally, neuroimaging is indicated prior to lumbar puncture because mass lesion may pose the **risk of herniation** with lumbar puncture. Magnetic resonance imaging (MRI) is also indicated if arterial dissection, sinovenous thrombosis, or tumor is suspected. Only after appropriate evaluation can more benign etiologies be diagnosed including first or severe migraine or tension headache, cluster headache, or exertional headache.

Migraine Headache

Migraine is the most common primary headache disorder in children. Pediatric migraine is defined as **five or more attacks** of headache that **last 1 to 72 hours** (which is shorter than required in adult criteria), with a throbbing or pulsatile quality, moderate to severe intensity, bilateral or unilateral in the frontal or temporal regions, exacerbated by or causing avoidance of routine physical activity, associated with nausea and/or emesis, light and sound sensitivity (which may be inferred from behavior), and often a need to sleep. A family history of migraine is often present. Migraine without aura is most common. Migraine with **aura** refers to fully reversible visual, sensory, or language symptoms that generally develop over 5 minutes and last from 5 to 60 minutes. Migraine is a clinical diagnosis, but **neuroimaging** is indicated to evaluate for other etiologies of acute focal signs such as stroke if there are atypical features or with the first aura, especially without the association of a typical migraine headache. Patients may be instructed to keep a **headache diary** to characterize the headaches and to identify precipitating factors. Attention to these details may identify dietary triggers (e.g., chocolate, cheese, nitrate-containing foods such as processed meats, monosodium glutamate), excessive caffeine, or analgesic overuse that may result in chronic headache. Children should be encouraged to obtain adequate sleep/nutrition/exercise and allowed to sleep in a quiet dark room at headache onset.

If headaches are infrequent and the child can accurately identify the headache onset, then **abortive medications** may be indicated. These include ibuprofen, acetaminophen, metoclopramide, and the triptan medications. In addition to traditional tablets, some triptans are available in disintegrating tablet preparation (rizatriptan) and nasal spray (sumatriptan). Proper instruction is required for the nasal spray because it is used differently than typical nasal sprays (don't tilt head back and don't inhale). Triptans are contraindicated if there is history suggesting cerebral ischemia (complicated migraine), cardiac disease, hypertension, or recent use of ergot medications. **Prophylactic medications** may be indicated if headaches are frequent (more than one per week), chronically disabling, or abortive medications are inadequate. Commonly used daily drugs include antidepressants (amitriptyline, nortriptyline), anticonvulsants (topiramate, valproic acid, gabapentin), beta-blockers (propranolol), or calcium channel blockers (verapamil). Treatment is titrated up as needed, and the goal is to reduce headache frequency over several weeks to months. Although some of these medications are approved for prevention of headaches in older children and adolescents, most treatment is anecdotal and off label. There are few studies to guide treatment of **status migrainosus,** but there is clinical experience with dihydroergotamine protocols (generally with metoclopramide to reduce nausea), intravenous metoclopramide or prochlorperazine, intravenous valproic acid, and intravenous steroids.

> **HINT:** Triptans are contraindicated in the setting of focal neurological signs.

Tension Headache

Tension headaches may last from 5 minutes (which is shorter than required in adults) to 7 days. They are usually bilateral with a pressing/tightening quality of pain, mild to moderate in severity, not aggravated by routine physical activity (as versus migraine), and unassociated with other features of migraine. They may be episodic or chronic (if >15 per month). There have been few studies of treatment, but antidepressants (amitriptyline), relaxation training, and biofeedback may be useful.

Trigeminal Autonomic Cephalgias

Cluster headache and the trigeminal autonomic cephalgias consist of repetitive attacks of intense headache that is often excruciating, unilateral, and boring in character accompanied by prominent **cranial parasympathetic** signs and symptoms such as conjunctival injection and tearing, eyelid edema, nasal congestion and rhinorrhea, facial sweating, and miosis ipsilateral to the headache. Migrainous features such as nausea and photophobia may occur. Attack frequency and duration varies in the different syndromes.

Cluster headache attacks generally last 15 to 180 minutes, occur every other day to 8 times per day, and often occur in clusters separated by attack free periods. Attacks lasting 5 seconds to 4 minutes occurring 5 to 200 times per day occur in short-lasting unilateral neuralgiform headache attacks with conjunctival injection and tearing (**SUNCT**). Attacks lasting 2 to 30 minutes and occurring up to 5 times per day constitute **paroxysmal hemicrania**. Although rare, accurate diagnosis is important because specific treatments are available. Indomethacin relieves attacks in paroxysmal hemicrania (and hemicrania continua described later). Oxygen and triptans may relieve cluster headache, and prophylactic medications may include verapamil, lithium, valproic acid, and topiramate.

Chronic Daily Headache

Some children have headaches that are present >15 days per month. Most of these children had episodic headaches that increased in frequency and eventually became chronic, although occasionally headaches may be chronic from the onset (new daily persistent headache). Suggested risk factors for transformation from episodic to chronic include headaches more than one to three times per month, obesity, and medication overuse. **Medication overuse** headache is defined by frequent medication use (>10 to 15 times per month) and may occur with over-the-counter analgesics, triptans, ergots, and opioids. Medications may be changed to longer acting formulations to reduce symptoms of withdrawal, but treatment requires detoxification with elimination of offending medications. Associated psychiatric conditions (e.g., anxiety, mood disorders, and somatoform disorders) are common and must be treated in addition to tapering the overused medication. Hemicrania continua may result in chronic headache with mild associated parasympathetic signs and is relieved with indomethacin.

Pseudotumor Cerebri

Pseudotumor cerebri, or idiopathic elevated intracranial pressure (ICP), typically presents with headache. Initially the headache is position dependent, worse when lying supine or upon awakening in the morning, and improves when upright. However, this position dependence may become less prominent with more long-standing headache. Many patients demonstrate **papilledema** owing to pressure-related axoplasmic stasis in the optic nerves. Other symptoms include transient visual obscurations, horizontal diplopia (caused by VI nerve palsy with elevated ICP). Diagnosis is by lumbar puncture performed in the lateral decubitus position in a relaxed or sedated child. Headache often resolves dramatically after removal of cerebrospinal fluid (CSF), but this improvement is temporary because CSF is continuously produced several times over every day. The diagnosis of idiopathic intracranial hypertension requires eliminating other etiologies such as sinovenous thrombosis (most children should undergo MRI/magnetic resonance venography), medication exposure (tetracycline and related compounds including retinoic acid and vitamin A, growth hormone, steroid hormone withdrawal), and endocrine disease (recent weight gain, hypoparathyroidism, Addison disease). **Secondary causes** are common in children, and the most frequent etiologies are otitis media, viral infections, and predisposing medications. Initial measurement and tracking of **visual fields** is important because permanent vision loss may occur, and rapidly progressive vision deterioration may be an indication for optic nerve sheath fenestration. Secondary etiologies must be treated appropriately. Weight loss is important if there has been recent weight gain. Weight loss and a low salt diet may be sufficient in cases where papilledema is absent or mild. Diuretic medications such as acetazolamide or furosemide may be provided if papilledema is moderate or headache is worsening. Optic nerve sheath fenestration or lumbar-peritoneal drainage is reserved for cases in which papilledema is severe and visual loss is progressive despite medical management.

> **HINT:** Visual fields must be followed carefully in all patients with pseudotumor cerebri because there is a risk of permanent visual loss that can be prevented by medical treatment or surgical intervention including optic nerve sheath fenestration.

TABLE 38-2 Useful Headache Questions

When did your headache start?
Did it start in a split second or start slowly?
Is there a history of head trauma?
What were you doing when your headache started?
Was this a sudden first headache?
Have you had headaches like this before?
How often do you get headaches?
Are your headaches getting worse or more frequent than they used to be?
Do you have the same kind of headaches all the time or do you have different types of headaches?
How often do you get a headache?
How long do your headaches last?
What do your headaches feel like?
How intense are your headaches?
Are there any signs that a headache is going to start?
Do you get nausea, vomiting, dizziness, numbness, weakness with the headache?
Do you get eye or nasal tearing with the headache?
What makes your headache better or worse?
Do you have to stop your activity when you have a headache?
Is there a trigger that causes you to get a headache?
Are you taking any medicines for your headache and how often do you take these medications?
Do you have any other health problems?
Does anyone else in your family get headaches?

Psychological Comorbidities

Many of the primary headaches including migraine and tension-type headaches, and especially chronic headaches, are associated with psychological comorbidity including depression and anxiety, and the treatment plan must address these issues. Treatment may involve medication, psychological counseling, biofeedback, or relaxation training.

EVALUATION OF THE PATIENT

Table 38-2 lists useful questions to help evaluate the type of headache as well as the time course. Physical examination is important because focal signs suggest a secondary etiology of headache.

- Head circumference—enlarging head suggests an intracranial lesion.
- Cranial nerve (CN) II (optic nerve)
  - Papilledema suggests elevated intracranial pressure
  - Visual fields may be reduced with elevated ICP
- Extraocular movements. Deficits suggest a brainstem lesion:
  - Oculomotor nerve (CN III) palsy may present with pupil dilation owing to disruption of parasympathetic fibers and oculomotor palsy (eye looks out and down) and suggests compressive lesions including herniation of acute onset
  - Trochlear nerve (CN IV) palsy presents with head tilt and chin tuck and may occur with head trauma or brainstem lesions
  - Abducens nerve (CN VI) palsy presents with head turn or horizontal diplopia; abnormalities suggest elevated intracranial pressure or brainstem lesions.
- Strength, tone, reflex, and sensory abnormalities suggest focal lesions.
- Cerebellar signs suggest a posterior fossa lesion that may result in elevated ICP, including hydrocephalus.

Table 38-3 lists the indications for neuroimaging.

TABLE 38-3 Indications to Consider Neuroimaging

Acute headache
Worst headache of life
Thunderclap headache
Chronic-progressive pattern
Focal neurologic symptoms or signs
Papilledema
Unvarying headache location
Meningeal signs
Headache on awakening or that wakes child from sleep
Age <5 years or inability to provide clear history

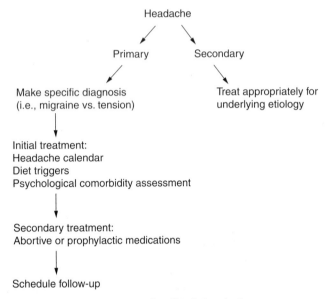

Figure 38-2 ■ Management of pediatric headache.

APPROACH TO THE PATIENT

See Figure 38-2.

TREATMENT

Appropriate treatment depends on the underlying etiology of the headache or the specific primary headache diagnosis.

Suggested Readings

Lewis D, Ashwal S, Hershey A, et al.: Practice parameter: pharmacological treatment of migraine headache in children and adolescents. *Neurology* 63:2215–2224, 2004.

Lewis DW: Pediatric migraine. *Pediatr Rev* 28(2):43–53, 2007.

Lewis DW, Gozzo YF, Avner MT: The "other" primary headaches in children and adolescents. *Pediatr Neurol* 33:303–313, 2005.

Ramadan NM, Olesen J: Classification of headache disorders. *Sem Neurol* 26(2):157–162, 2006.

INTRODUCTION

Hematuria, the medical term for the presence of blood in the urine, is a common pediatric problem. Gross hematuria is clearly visible, whereas microscopic hematuria is defined by the presence of five or more red blood cells (RBCs) per high-power field (hpf) on at least three occasions over a 3-week period in a spun urine sample. The incidence of gross hematuria among children presenting to an emergency department is 1.3 in 1,000, whereas 1% to 2% of school-age children have microscopic hematuria in two or more urine samples. All children should have a screening urinalysis at school entry (4 to 5 years of age) and during adolescence (11 to 21 years of age).

Gross hematuria of glomerular origin usually presents as brown, tea-colored, or cola-colored urine, whereas gross hematuria from the lower urinary tract reveals itself as pink or red urine. Other substances besides blood can cause discolored urine. Microscopic hematuria is generally first detected on a dipstick test but should be confirmed by microscopic examination of a spun sediment of urine (see Table 39-1).

DIFFERENTIAL DIAGNOSIS LIST

Infections
Bacterial, viral (adenovirus), tuberculosis

Structural abnormalities
Congenital anomalies
Polycystic kidneys
Trauma
Vascular anomalies—angiomyolipomas, arteriovenous malformations
Tumors

Hematologic
Sickle cell trait/disease
Coagulopathies—hemophilia, renal vein thrombosis

Hypercalciuria and Nephrolithiasis
Exercise
Medications
Penicillins, polymyxin, sulfa-containing agents, anticonvulsants, warfarin, aspirin, colchicine, cyclophosphamide, indomethacin, gold salts

Glomerular Disorders
Immunoglobulin A (IgA) nephropathy—*recurrent, gross hematuria*
Alport syndrome
Benign familial hematuria

Acute poststreptococcal glomerulonephritis	Rapidly progressive glomerulonephritis
Lupus nephritis	**Others**
Membranoproliferative glomerulonephritis (MPGN)	Dyes (Table 39-1)
Henoch-Schönlein purpura (HSP)	Loin pain-hematuria syndrome
Membranous nephropathy	Urethrorrhagia

DIFFERENTIAL DIAGNOSIS DISCUSSION

Urinary Tract Infection

Children with bacterial infections often present with dysuria, fever, burning on micturition, and increased urinary frequency or urgency. Adenoviral cystitis presents with painful gross hematuria. Urine analysis by dipstick is typically positive for nitrites (Gram-negative organisms) and leukocyte esterase and reveals white blood cells on microscopic examination.

Trauma

Traumatic injury to the urogenital tract is frequently seen with blunt force trauma and may be **life threatening,** depending on the severity of injury.

> **HINT:** The presence of hematuria with minimal traumatic injury is highly suggestive of anatomic abnormalities of the kidney such as polycystic kidney disease.

Hematuria associated with renal trauma requires evaluation by **computed tomography (CT) scan, renal ultrasound,** or **intravenous pyelography (IVP)**.

TABLE 39-1 Causes of Discolored Urine	
Dark yellow or orange urine	Concentrated urine
	Rifampin, Pyridium
Brown or black urine	Bile pigment
	Methemoglobinemia
	Homogentisic acid, thymol, melanin, tyrosinosis, alkaptonuria
	Alanine, cascara, resorcinol
Red or pink urine	Red blood cells, hemoglobin/myoglobin
	Benzene, chloroquine, deferoxamine, phenazopyridine, phenolphthalein
	Beets, blackberries, red dye
	Urates

> **HINT:** When traumatic injury to the lower urinary tract is suspected, any imaging study involving placement of urethral or bladder catheters should be ordered only after urologic consultation.

Treatment is directed on the basis of severity of injury. Most renal contusions or lacerations can be managed **conservatively;** however, significant lacerations of the kidney or injury to the collecting system or lower urinary tract may require **emergent surgical intervention.**

Malignancy

Wilms tumor accounts for >90% of childhood malignancies that arise from the urogenital tract. Other tumors include renal cell carcinoma, mesoblastic nephroma, rhabdomyosarcoma, hemangioma, and sarcomas. Wilms tumor typically presents as an **abdominal mass with or without associated abdominal pain.** Microscopic hematuria is found in about 50% of patients at presentation, but gross hematuria is unusual. Hematuria as a sole presenting feature of Wilms tumor is exceedingly rare.

Up to 80% of patients with **tuberous sclerosis** may develop hematuria associated with hemorrhage from renal angiolipomas. Renal medullary carcinoma should be considered in patients with sickle cell trait.

Hematologic Causes

Hematuria is a common manifestation of **sickle cell hemoglobinopathy.** Affecting patients with either sickle cell disease or sickle cell trait, it is thought to be caused by sickling and sludging of RBCs in the renal medulla. Typically occurring in **adolescent males,** it can be precipitated by **trauma, exercise, dehydration,** or **infection. Papillary necrosis** is also seen with severe dehydration and renal infarction.

> **HINT:** Hematuria, both gross and microscopic, is a common complication in patients with sickle cell trait.

Hematuria, in sickle cell disease, is commonly **painless** and can range from microscopic to severe gross hematuria. Hematuria is rarely the sole finding in a patient with a coagulopathy. However, coagulopathies should be investigated in patients without another source for painless, gross hematuria and a history of bruising/bleeding or a family history of a bleeding diathesis.

Hypercalciuria

Hypercalciuria occurs in states of both **hypercalcemia** and **eucalcemia**. In eucalcemic patients, the most common cause is idiopathic; other causes include immobilization, Cushing syndrome, distal renal tubular acidosis, and Bartter syndrome. Disorders associated with hypercalcemia include hyperparathyroidism, vitamin D intoxication, hypophosphatasia, tumors, and immobilization bone resorption.

Idiopathic hypercalciuria typically presents with **asymptomatic microscopic hematuria**. As with secondary forms of hypercalciuria, these patients can also present with gross hematuria, renal colic, and dysuria.

The initial screening test for hypercalciuria is a **urine calcium-to-creatinine (Ca:Cr) ratio** on a spot urine sample. A ratio >0.2 in older children and adults is highly suggestive of hypercalciuria. Normal values are higher in infants and young children. Confirmation should be obtained by **24-hour urine collection** with an excretion of >4 mg/kg per 24 hours. **Serum chemistries,** including calcium, phosphorus, magnesium, urine pH, and renal function, should also be obtained. A detailed **family history** for stone disease, diet history, and evaluation of medications and nutritional supplements should be sought.

> **HINT:** Hypercalciuria is the most common metabolic abnormality found in patients with renal calculi.

Urolithiasis

Stone disease typically presents with **grossly bloody urine and renal colic**. Presentation with microscopic hematuria, penile pain, and passage of the stone or gravel may also be seen.

A family history of stone disease is frequently noted, particularly in older patients. **Renal ultrasound** or **spiral CT scan** should be considered. If a stone is suspected, **blood chemistries** including calcium, phosphorus, magnesium, uric acid, and creatinine should be performed. **Urine pH** and **24-hour urine collections** for calcium, cystine, oxalate, phosphorus, and uric excretion should be obtained. However, in young children this is difficult. Attempts should be made to **recover the stone** or gravel for analysis of mineral content.

> **HINT:** Simple radiographs can detect kidney stones if the stone is radioopaque (calcium, oxalate, cystine, or struvite). Urate stones are radiolucent and not seen by plain film.

Management of these patients is twofold. Pain management should be optimized. Surgical intervention or lithotripsy is indicated in cases of urinary obstruction or recurrent stones with superimposed urinary tract infections. Once the cause has been determined, therapy to **prevent stone recurrence** can be implemented, which includes increased fluid intake to ensure dilute hypotonic urine, dietary manipulation, and drug therapy in some cases.

Medications

Microscopic hematuria related to drug exposure is not uncommon. Although some of these medications are commonly used in pediatrics, most are not (see differential diagnosis list). **Cyclophosphamide** is frequently associated with gross hematuria that can be severe in some cases.

Loin pain-hematuria syndrome

This syndrome is described by recurrent episodes of **pain in the lower abdomen** with gross or microscopic hematuria usually occurring in women between 20 and 40 years of age. It can, however, occur in younger patients where no cause is determined. The **diagnosis is one of exclusion** after investigating for infection, tumor, stone disease, or trauma. There is often an associated **psychological component.** The "nutcracker syndrome," or an anatomic anomaly with compression of the left renal vein by the aorta and superior mesenteric artery, may also present with loin pain. Treatment generally entails adequate **pain control.**

Urethrorrhagia

Urethrorrhagia typically presents with **terminal hematuria,** bloody spots in the underwear, in boys between **4 and 17 years of age.** The mean age of presentation is 10 years old. Dysuria is present in nearly 30% of patients. It can be recurrent, but resolution usually occurs in nearly 92% with an average time course of 10 months (2 weeks to 3 years). Other causes of gross hematuria should be ruled out. Treatment is restricted to **watchful waiting.** Urethral stricture can be caused by cystoscopy; therefore, such procedures should be avoided.

Alport Syndrome

Alport syndrome is a **hereditary nephritis** associated with **sensorineural hearing loss.** Eighty-five percent of cases are transmitted as an X-linked dominant trait. The primary genetic defect involves the gene for collagen 4A5.

Alport syndrome presents with intermittent or persistent **microscopic hematuria or episodic gross hematuria.** In children, both **ocular defects** (anterior lenticonus and macular lesions) and high-frequency **sensorineural hearing loss** can be found.

Alport is strongly suggested by a **family history of chronic renal failure associated with hearing loss.** Diagnosis is confirmed by **renal biopsy.** Genetic analysis is available on a research basis, and family screening can be considered.

Benign Familial Hematuria

Benign familial hematuria is transmitted in an autosomal dominant fashion, although other patterns of transmission are reported. This disorder is defined by the familial occurrence of persistent **hematuria without proteinuria, hearing loss, or progressive renal disease.**

This is a diagnosis primarily of **exclusion** based on **family history.** Evaluation of parents' urine may be necessary to consider this diagnosis, which can be confirmed by **renal biopsy** that shows thin basement membranes in many patients.

Glomerulonephritis

Glomerulonephritis (Table 39-2) can be categorized according to serum complement (C3) levels at presentation. Usually present is some combination of gross hematuria (often tea- or cola- colored), proteinuria, hypertension, RBC casts, renal dysfunction, and oligoanuria. The most common

TABLE 39-2 Distinguishing Features of Glomerular and Nonglomerular Hematuria

Feature	Glomerular	Nonglomerular
History		
Burning on micturition		Urethritis, cystitis
Systemic complaints	No edema, fever, pharyngitis, rash, arthralgias	Fever with UTI; pain with calculi.
Family history	Deafness in Alport syndrome, renal failure	Usually negative, except with calculi.
Physical Examination		
Hypertension	Often	Unlikely
Edema	Sometimes present	No
Abdominal mass	No	Wilms tumor, polycystic kidneys
Rash, arthritis	SLE, HSP	No
Urine Analysis		
Color	Brown: tea- or cola- colored	Bright red or pink
Proteinuria	Often	No
Dysmorphic RBCs	Yes	No
RBC casts	Yes	No
Crystals	No	May be informative

HSP = Henoch-Schönlein purpura; *RBC* = red blood cells; *SLE* = systemic lupus erythematosus; *UTI* = urinary tract infection forms of nephritis are **acute poststreptococcal glomerulonephritis (APSGN)** and **IgA nephropathy.** An unusual form of glomerular disease noted for its acuity at presentation is **rapidly progressive glomerulonephritis (RPGN)** with worsening renal function. This form can be associated with renal vasculitis, IgA nephropathy, APSGN and HSP.

APSGN typically presents 10 to 14 days after an upper respiratory infection with β-hemolytic streptococci or, in some cases, an episode of impetigo. IgA nephropathy is commonly associated with a viral prodrome 1 to 3 days before the development of grossly bloody urine.

All patients with suspected glomerulonephritis should have a complete blood count, antistreptolysin O (ASO) and streptozyme, C3, antinuclear antibody (ANA) where indicated, blood chemistries including renal function studies, and a microscopic urinalysis performed. The presence of **RBC casts in the urine is diagnostic of a glomerulonephritis.** Renal biopsy may be indicated in some instances.

> **HINT:** Although ASO titers can remain elevated for up to 6 months following an episode of APSGN, C3 levels should return to normal within 6 to 8 weeks after presentation; a persistently low C3 level is suggestive of membranoproliferative glomerulonephritis (MPGN)

The treatment of acute poststreptococcal nephritis is largely **supportive.** Careful attention to **fluid and electrolyte balance** is essential. **Urine output** should be optimized and diuretics may be needed. **Blood pressure should be carefully monitored and treated aggressively.** Treatment of other forms of glomerulonephritis includes immunosuppressive therapy.

EVALUATION OF HEMATURIA (FIGURES 39-1 THROUGH 39-3)

> **HINT:** Gross hematuria should be evaluated as soon as possible. Additionally, if proteinuria and/or red cell casts are absent, a renal ultrasound should be performed to exclude a malignancy.

Patient History

A **complete and thorough history** is essential to guiding the diagnostic evaluation of hematuria. The following information should be obtained:

- Previous episodes of gross hematuria or UTI
- Pattern of hematuria (initial, terminal)
- History of recent upper respiratory tract infections, sore throat, or impetigo

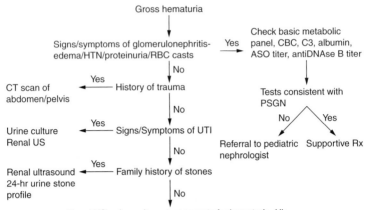

ASO-anti-streptolysin 0 titer;

Figure 39-1 ■ Evaluation of the pediatric patient with gross hematuria
ASO = antistreptolysin O titer; C3 = third component of complement;
CBC = complete blood count; CT = computed tomography; Hb =
hemoglobin; HTN = hypertension; PSGN = poststreptococcal glomer-
ulonephritis; RBC = red blood cells; Rx = prescription; US = ultrasound;
UTI 5 urinary tract infection

- Dysuria, frequency, voiding patterns, fever, weight loss, abdominal or
  flank pain, skin lesions
- Trauma or foreign body
- Drug, dietary, and vitamin or nutritional supplements
- Family history of renal disease including dialysis and transplant,
  hematuria, urolithiasis, sickle cell disease, coagulation disorders,
  hearing loss
- Travel to developing countries

Physical Examination

The examination of the patient should focus on the following:

- Blood pressure
- Edema
- Rash or purpura
- Arthritis
- Abdominal mass
- Ocular defects
- Genitourinary abnormalities

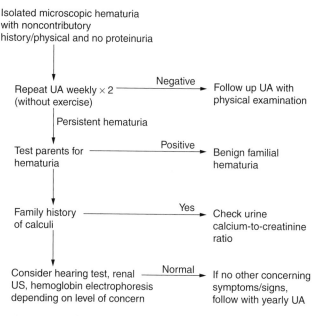

Figure 39-2 ■ Evaluation of the pediatric patient with isolated microscopic hematuria
UA = urinalysis; US = ultrasound

Laboratory Evaluation

The diagnostic evaluation of hematuria should be guided by findings on history and physical examination and may include the following:

- Fresh urinalysis with microscopic examination of sediment for RBCs, crystals, and casts
- Serum electrolytes—blood urea nitrogen, creatinine, calcium, phosphorus, uric acid
- Complete blood count with platelets
- Complement studies
- ASO/Streptozyme
- ANA
- Urine culture
- Urine Ca:Cr ratio or 24-hour urine calcium excretion
- Urinary excretion of cystine, oxalate, phosphorus, citrate, and urate

Diagnostic Modalities

Radiographic imaging is always indicated for evaluation of gross hematuria in the absence of RBC casts and proteinuria. **Ultrasound evaluation**

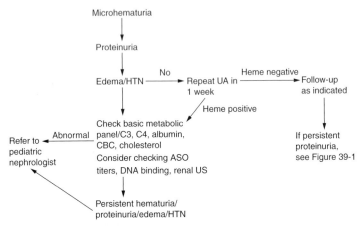

Figure 39-3 ■ Evaluation of the pediatric patient with microscopic hematuria and other findings
ASO = antistreptolysin O titer; C3 = third component of complement; C4 = fourth component of complement; CBC = complete blood count; HTN = hypertension; UA = urinalysis; US = ultrasound

of the kidneys and bladder may demonstrate the presence of tumors, urinary obstruction, renal stones, or evidence of renal parenchymal disease. Small stones or abnormalities of the collecting system, however, may be missed by ultrasound. **IVPs** or magnetic resonance urograms are useful for delineating the anatomic structure of the collecting systems as well as for defining functional obstructions. CT scans also provide valuable anatomic information, in addition to information about the presence of stones, tumors, or obstructions. Additional studies such as nuclear scans, cystoscopy, angiography, or renal biopsy should be considered in consultation with a subspecialist.

TREATMENT OF HEMATURIA

The treatment of hematuria is driven by the underlying pathophysiology and is in large part **conservative.** Hematuria with concurrent proteinuria, hypertension, renal failure, trauma, or severe hemorrhage may indicate the need for more **aggressive investigation and therapy.**

Suggested Readings

Diven SC, Travis LB: A practical primary care approach to hematuria in children. *Pediatr Nephrol* 14:65–72, 2000.
Feld LG, Meyers KE, Kaplan BS, et al.: Limited evaluation of microscopic hematuria in pediatrics. *Pediatrics* 102(4):E42, 1998.

Feld LG, Waz WR, Perez LM, et al.: Hematuria: an integrated medical and surgical approach. *Pediatr Clin North Am* 44(5):1191–1210, 1997.

Lieu TA, Grasmeder HM III, Kaplan BS: An approach to the evaluation and treatment of microscopic hematuria. *Pediatr Clin North Am* 38(3):579–592, 1991.

Mahan JD, Turman MA, Menster MI: Evaluation of hematuria, proteinuria, and hypertension in adolescents. *Pediatr Clin North Am* 44(6):1573–1589, 1997.

Meyers KEC: Evaluation of hematuria in children. *Urol Clin North Am* 31(3):559–573, 2004.

Roy S III: Hematuria. *Pediatr Ann* 25(5):284–287, 1996.

INTRODUCTION

Hemolysis is **increased red blood cell (RBC) destruction with compensatory increased RBC production.** The patient with hemolysis usually presents with symptoms of **anemia and hyperbilirubinemia.** However, chronic hemolysis may be an incidental finding when a complete blood count (CBC) is obtained for other reasons.

The causes of hemolysis can be classified as intrinsic or extrinsic. **Intrinsic causes** are abnormalities that occur within the RBC (i.e., changes that involve the RBC membrane, enzymes, or hemoglobin). **Extrinsic causes** involve damage to normal RBCs by any external process. A second classification system categorizes the causes of hemolysis according to whether **RBC destruction occurs intravascularly or extravascularly** (Table 40-1). A third classification is according to whether the cause of hemolysis is inherited or acquired.

DIFFERENTIAL DIAGNOSIS LIST 🔓

RBC Membrane Abnormalities

Hereditary spherocytosis (HS)
Hereditary elliptocytosis (HE)
Hereditary pyropoikilocytosis
Infantile pyknocytosis
Paroxysmal nocturnal hemoglobinuria

Enzyme Defects

Embden-Meyerhof pathway defects—pyruvate kinase deficiency
Nucleotide metabolism defects—pyrimidine-5-nucleotidase deficiency
Hexose monophosphate shunt defects—glucose-6-phosphate dehydrogenase (G6PD) deficiency

Hemoglobin Disorders

Hemoglobinopathies—hemoglobin S, C, D, E
Thalassemia syndromes—α-thalassemia, β-thalassemia
Unstable hemoglobin syndromes—congenital Heinz-body hemolytic anemia, hemoglobin M disease

Alloimmune Causes

Hemolytic disease of the newborn
Hemolytic transfusion reaction

Autoimmune Causes

Warm-Reactive Antibodies
Idiopathic
Neoplastic causes
Immunodeficiency

TABLE 40-1 Intravascular and Extravascular Causes of Hemolysis

Intravascular Hemolysis

Disseminated intravascular coagulation (DIC)
Hemolytic uremic syndrome
Burns
Acute hemolytic transfusion reactions
Organ graft rejection
Prosthetic heart valves
Hemangiomata
March hemoglobinuria
Drugs
Venoms
Infections
Acute G6PD deficiency
Paroxysmal nocturnal hemoglobinuria

Extravascular Hemolysis

Alloimmune hemolysis
Autoimmune hemolysis
Red blood cell (RBC) membrane abnormalities
RBC enzyme abnormalities
Hemoglobinopathies
Thalassemia syndromes

G6PD = glucose-6-phosphate dehydrogenase

Infectious Causes
Viruses (e.g., cytomegalo-
  virus, hepatitis, influenza,
  coxsackievirus, HIV)
Bacteria (e.g., *Streptococcus,*
  Escherichia coli,
  Salmonella typhi)
Postimmunization (e.g.,
  diphtheria-tetanus-
  pertussis, polio, typhoid
Toxic Causes
Antibiotics—penicillin,
  cephalothin, tetracycline,
  rifampin, sulfonamides
Phenacetin
5-Aminosalicylic acid
Quinine and quinidine
Insulin
Lead

Chlorpromazine
Collagen Vascular Disease
Systemic lupus erythematosus
Scleroderma
Juvenile rheumatoid arthritis
Polyarteritis nodosa
Dermatomyositis
Cold-Reactive Antibodies
Infectious Causes
Mycoplasma
Epstein-Barr virus (EBV)
HIV
Neoplastic Causes
Lymphoproliferative disease

Nonimmune Causes
Microangiopathic hemolytic
anemia
Hypersplenism

Toxic Causes
  Drugs (e.g., vitamin K, phenacetin, sulfones, benzenes, phenylhydralazine)
  Lead
  Venoms

Infectious Causes
  Viruses (EBV, hepatitis)
  Bacteria (*Clostridium*) *perfringens, E. coli, Streptococcus*
  Parasites (malaria, histoplasmosis)

DIFFERENTIAL DIAGNOSIS DISCUSSION

Hereditary Spherocytosis

Etiology

HS, the most common **inherited RBC membrane defect,** is most often seen in patients of **northern European descent.** Genetic mutations in genes encoding RBC skeletal proteins lead to skeletal protein anomalies, membrane instability, and subsequent **hemolytic anemia** in affected individuals. Although HS is inherited in an autosomal dominant fashion, 10% to 25% of all cases are sporadic.

Clinical Features

The clinical severity depends on the severity of the hemolysis, which can be **mild to severe,** and on the degree of compensation by the patient. The classic clinical presentation of hemolytic anemia is **jaundice, pallor, and splenomegaly.** Patients may have hypersplenism, gallstones, worsening red cell destruction (hyperhemolysis) with infections, and transient red cell aplasia primarily caused by human parvovirus B19. Half of patients have a history of **neonatal hyperbilirubinemia.**

Evaluation

The **peripheral blood smear** shows an **increased** number of **spherocytes** (i.e., small, round, dark-staining RBCs that lack central pallor). The mean corpuscular hemoglobin concentration is frequently elevated. Reticulocytosis is present. The **osmotic fragility test** demonstrates decreased resistance to osmotic lysis as compared with normal RBCs. The direct antibody test (DAT), often used to distinguish autoimmune hemolytic anemia, is negative.

Treatment

Treatment of HS is **supportive.** Although transfusion of RBCs may be necessary for acute exacerbation of anemia, only a small number of patients depend on **RBC transfusions. Splenectomy** is used to decrease the extravascular red cell destruction and should be considered in children with poor growth or increased RBC transfusion requirements.

Hereditary Elliptocytosis

Etiology

HE, more common in people of African or Mediterranean descent, is caused by genetic mutations that lead to red cell cytoskeleton instability. Like HS, HE is **inherited** in an autosomal dominant pattern, but sporadic mutations are not as common.

Clinical Features

Most children with HE are **asymptomatic,** but they may present for evaluation with a transient aplastic episode or a hyperhemolytic episode.

Evaluation

The **peripheral blood smear** reveals >15% elliptocytes (i.e., elongated, cigar-shaped, or oval RBCs). The peripheral blood smear in normal patients may contain up to 15% elliptocytes.

The differential diagnosis of HE includes **iron-deficiency anemia.**

Treatment

Splenectomy is curative but is not indicated unless anemia is profound.

G6PD Deficiency

Etiology

G6PD deficiency, **inherited** in an X-linked pattern, is the most common enzyme deficiency of the hexose monophosphate shunt. Affected patients are either heterozygous males or homozygous females. There is an increased incidence of G6PD deficiency in people of **African and Mediterranean descent.** Affected children may have **drug-induced hemolysis** or a **chronic hemolytic process.**

Medications and substances that can induce hemolysis in G6PD-deficient patients include acetanilid, doxorubicin, methylene blue, naphthalene, nitrofurantoin, primaquine, pamaquine, and sulfa drugs.

Clinical Features

Presentation depends on the type of G6PD deficiency variant inherited.

- **Patients with the African variant** of G6PD deficiency rarely present for evaluation with neonatal jaundice or chronic hemolytic anemia. They are usually identified when they present for evaluation following drug (or other substance) exposure. Drug-induced hemolysis can be severe, involving the acute onset of pallor, malaise, scleral icterus, dark urine, and abdominal or back pain.
- **Patients with the Mediterranean variant** of G6PD deficiency usually have a more severe form of G6PD deficiency and may present for evaluation with signs and symptoms of neonatal hyperbilirubinemia, chronic hemolytic anemia, or drug-induced hemolysis.

Evaluation

If G6PD deficiency is suspected, a **blood sample** should be sent for analysis of G6PD enzyme activity. **"Bite"** or **"blister"** cells (RBCs with small outpouchings or blisters on the outer rim) may be identified on the peripheral blood smear. Genetic testing is also available and included in the newborn screen in some states.

Treatment

Drug-induced intravascular hemolysis is **self-limited and reversible** when the offending drug is discontinued. Children with **chronic hemolysis** may require **RBC transfusions** for exacerbations of anemia characterized by cardiovascular compromise.

Sickle Cell Disease

Etiology

Hemoglobin S (Hb S) is the predominant hemoglobin in the group of **genetic disorders** that encompass sickle cell disease (SCD). Hb S is an abnormal hemoglobin caused by a single nucleotide base substitution: Valine replaces glutamic acid in the sixth position of the β globin chain, resulting in structural changes in the RBC membrane. SCD variants include SCD-SS, SCD-SC, SCD-S β-thalassemia, and others. Sickle cell disease is inherited in a recessive fashion with homozygous and compound heterozygous forms.

Clinical Features

Patients with SCD disorders have **hemolytic anemia** and **vaso-occlusive complications** and are at **increased risk for infection**. People with **sickle cell trait** are generally **asymptomatic** but may have occasional hematuria. Currently, most patients are identified through **newborn screening** for hemoglobinopathies. Others, not identified as newborns, present with signs and symptoms of SCD complications:

- **Infection.** Children with SCD, especially those <3 years, are at increased risk for the development of bacterial infections as a result of splenic hypofunction and other immunologic abnormalities. *Streptococcus pneumoniae* is the most commonly implicated microorganism; however, meningococcal organisms, *Haemophilus influenzae*, *E. coli*, *Salmonella* species, and *Staphylococcus aureus* are common pathogens in patients with SCD as well. Pneumococcal sepsis can be rapidly fatal in these patients, despite the use of penicillin prophylaxis and immunization with polyvalent pneumococcal vaccines.
- **Osteomyelitis.** Patients with SCD are at increased risk for osteomyelitis; therefore, any child with SCD, bone pain, and fever or

soft tissue swelling should be evaluated for the presence of osteomyelitis. The most common organisms causing osteomyelitis in this patient population are *Salmonella* and *S. aureus*. It is difficult to discriminate between osteomyelitis and a vaso-occlusive episode in the child with SCD. Evaluation should include radiographic studies and orthopedic evaluation.

- **Stroke.** Children with SCD, particularly types SS and S β-thalassemia, may develop hemorrhagic or infarctive strokes. The clinical presentation includes seizures, hemiplegia, difficulty speaking, or a change in mental status; however, subtle intermittent neurologic symptoms or severe headaches may indicate neurologic complications as well. Transcranial Doppler (TCD) ultrasonography screening identifies young children and adolescents who are at increased risk for infarctive stroke.

- **Acute chest syndrome (ACS),** classically defined as a new infiltrate on chest radiograph, is one of the leading causes of morbidity and mortality in patients with SCD. The cause of ACS may be multifactorial in an individual patient and includes infection, pulmonary vascular damage, infarction, and cytokine release.

- **Painful episodes,** the most common complications of SCD, are unpredictable and often progressive. The exact pathophysiology is unknown but may be related to occlusion and damage of the microvasculature, leading to organ ischemia and infarction.

- **Splenic sequestration** is one of the leading causes of death in children with SCD. These children develop hypovolemic shock as the result of the loss of large volumes of blood into the spleen. Although the spleen in children with SCD-SS has usually autoinfarcted by the time the patient reaches 8 years of age, children with SCD-SC and SCD-S β-thalassemia can present with splenic sequestration at any age. Acute splenic sequestration episodes are characterized by splenic enlargement with evidence of hemoglobin levels below baseline and increased reticulocyte counts. Mild to moderate thrombocytopenia may also occur. Any child who has had one episode of splenic sequestration is at increased risk for another.

- **Priapism** is a prolonged, painful penile erection and can occur in boys and men with SCD at any age. Priapism may be sustained over a long period of time or may be "stuttering" in nature (i.e., characterized by recurrent episodes within short periods of time).

- **Transient aplastic episode** (see also Chapter 57, "Pallor (Paleness)"). Any patient with chronic hemolytic anemia can experience aplastic episode (i.e., a transient arrest in erythropoiesis characterized by the acute onset of pallor, frequently following a viral illness). Human parvovirus B19 infection is the most common cause. The anemia is often severe and reticulocyte counts are usually <2%.

Evaluation

Important historic information to obtain from patients with SCD includes the following:

- Specific disease phenotype or genotype
- Baseline hemoglobin and reticulocyte counts
- Past disease complications
- Dates of last transfusion and related complications

Appropriate laboratory tests in a child suspected of having SCD include a hemoglobin electrophoresis, CBC, and reticulocyte count.

Treatment

- **Suspected infection.** Any child with SCD and fever should be considered bacteremic or septic until proven otherwise. Blood cultures should be obtained promptly and parenteral antibiotics strongly considered, particularly in children with severe disease phenotypes (SS, S β-thalassemia).
- **Stroke.** Children at high risk for stroke based on abnormal TCD results should receive regular red cell transfusions to maintain a HbS% <30 because this significantly lowers initial stroke rates. Exchange transfusions are recommended for patients with acute strokes to decrease further cerebral damage. In children who have had a stroke, chronic transfusion therapy is strongly recommended to decrease the high risk of recurrent stroke.
- **ACS.** Because the underlying cause is often unclear, supportive care should include antibiotics, analgesics, aggressive pulmonary toilet, and supplemental oxygen as needed. Transfusion therapy is beneficial but the clinical indications are not standardized. However, any child who is experiencing hypoxia or significant difficulty in breathing should receive an RBC transfusion, either simple or exchange.

> **HINT:** Any patient who has experienced an episode of ACS is at increased risk for recurrence. This risk may be decreased with hydroxyurea therapy or chronic transfusion therapy.

- **Painful episode.** Care is directed at pain control and close monitoring of patients for other disease complications and side effects of medications. Musculoskeletal pain can be managed acutely with analgesics and nonpharmacologic therapies (e.g., heat and relaxation). Dehydration should be avoided; ACS may be prevented by ambulation and frequent incentive spirometer use. Hydroxyurea (HU), an antimetabolite medication, has decreased painful episodes in patients with SCD-SS and SCD-S β-thalassemia. However, HU therapy is best prescribed and monitored by a pediatric hematologist.

- **Splenic sequestration.** If transfusions are necessary, it is important acutely to transfuse small aliquots of RBCs because the spleen releases the patient's RBCs as the sequestration episode resolves. Long-term management of these children is controversial; however, splenectomy or a chronic transfusion program should be considered for children who have experienced a life-threatening episode or repeated episodes requiring multiple transfusions.
- **Priapism.** If untreated, impotence may result. Initial management includes the use of intravenous hydration and analgesia. A urologist should be consulted, particularly if urinary retention develops or if detumescence does not occur promptly despite medical management.
- **Transient aplastic episode.** Because most children have human parvovirus infections, hospitalized patients should be admitted to single rooms with contact and respiratory isolation. No pregnant caretakers should be permitted in the room. Children with congestive heart failure require RBC transfusion.

Hemoglobin C

Etiology

Hemoglobin C (Hb C) disease, an inherited hemoglobinopathy, results from a substitution of lysine for glutamic acid in the sixth position of the β-polypeptide chain. Variants of Hb C with α- and β-thalassemia exist as well.

Clinical Features and Evaluation

Patients with **homozygous disease** usually have **mild chronic hemolytic anemia with splenomegaly**, and the **peripheral blood smear** shows a marked number of **target cells**. Patients with **Hb C trait** are **asymptomatic**.

Hemoglobin E

Etiology

Hemoglobin E (Hb E) is a common hemoglobin variant, particularly in the **Asian population**. Variants of Hb E with α-thalassemia and β-thalassemia exist as well.

Clinical Features and Evaluation

Patients with **homozygous Hb E** have **mild hemolytic anemia with a mean corpuscular volume (MCV)** that is usually **<70 fL and target cells on the peripheral blood smear**. Patients with **Hb E trait** are **asymptomatic**.

Thalassemia

Etiology

The thalassemia syndromes represent a group of **inherited disorders** caused by **decreased or absent** synthesis of the α or β **human globin chains**.

The thalassemia syndromes occur more frequently in **Mediterranean, Asian, and African populations.** Because of unbalanced globin chain synthesis, unstable hemoglobin complexes are produced. Precipitation of the unpaired globin chains and subsequent RBC membrane damage cause **premature RBC lysis,** which leads to **hemolytic anemia** and a compensatory **increase in RBC production** in affected individuals.

Clinical Features of α-Thalassemia

There are four clinical classifications of the α-thalassemias:

- **One α gene mutation.** These patients, the silent carriers of α-thalassemia, have no clinical symptoms, a normal hemoglobin level, and a normal MCV.
- **Two α gene mutations.** Patients with α-thalassemia trait, caused by two α gene mutations, have mild microcytic hypochromic anemia. Because the degree of microcytosis is out of proportion to the degree of anemia, the likelihood of iron-deficiency anemia as a possible diagnosis is diminished.
- **Three α gene mutations.** Hemoglobin H (Hb H) disease, caused by three α gene mutations, is characterized by moderate to severe microcytic hypochromic anemia. The excess β chains form tetramers, a fast-migrating hemoglobin (seen on hemoglobin electrophoresis) referred to as "Hb H." Hemoglobin Bart's or γ globin chain tetramers can also be present in neonates with Hb H disease or α-thalassemia trait. In Hb H disease, anemia may be severe, with hemoglobin values ranging from 3 to 4 g/dL. Hemolytic episodes may be exacerbated by fever or infection.
- **Four α gene mutations.** Hydrops fetalis is caused by mutations of all four α genes. These infants fail to produce α globin in utero. They are severely anemic, develop congestive heart failure, and are usually stillborn unless treatment is initiated in utero.

Clinical Features of β-Thalassemia

The β-thalassemia syndromes are categorized according to three levels of clinical severity:

- **Thalassemia minor** (β-thalassemia trait). Patients are asymptomatic and have mild hypochromic anemia.
- **Thalassemia intermedia.** Patients have mild to moderate hypochromic anemia and are not transfusion dependent.
- **Thalassemia major** (**Cooley anemia**). Patients have severe hypochromic microcytic anemia (characterized by hemoglobin levels of 3 to 4 g/dL) and are transfusion dependent. Anemia develops frequently within the first 2 years of life, and patients may present for evaluation with pallor, lethargy, and hepatosplenomegaly. Bony expansion, a sign of heightened intramedullary hematopoiesis, may be found on physical examination.

Evaluation

Patients with **thalassemia major** may be diagnosed by **newborn screening for hemoglobinopathies. Hemoglobin A may be low to absent.** For all patients suspected to have thalassemia, a **CBC** should be obtained from the patient and both parents. If **microcytic anemia** is present in either parent or both parents, then **hemoglobin electrophoresis studies** should be obtained.

α- and β-**Thalassemia trait** must be **distinguished from iron-deficiency anemia** because all patients with these disorders may have an MCV <75 fL. In patients with β-thalassemia trait, the MCV would be disproportionately low for the mild degree of anemia seen if the anemia were caused by iron deficiency, and the RBC mass would be increased.

- The red blood cell distribution width index is increased in iron deficiency but normal in thalassemia trait.
- Hemoglobin electrophoresis shows an increased amount of Hb A2, Hb F, or both in patients with β-thalassemia trait but not in those with α-thalassemia trait or iron deficiency.

Iron-deficiency anemia and β-thalassemia trait can coexist and make diagnosis difficult. After treatment for iron deficiency, if the MCV remains low, then diagnostic studies for thalassemia traits should be pursued.

Treatment

Transfusion therapy in thalassemia major is directed at treating the anemia as well as suppressing endogenous RBC production. **Splenectomy** may be indicated in patients with an increasing need for RBC transfusions, in patients with significant growth retardation, or in patients in whom hypersplenism is associated with a worsening of the anemia.

Hemolytic Disease of the Newborn (Isoimmune Hemolytic Anemia)

Etiology

Hemolytic disease of the newborn results from **maternal sensitization to fetal RBC antigens** that differ from her own.

- **In Rh hemolytic disease,** the Rh(D)-negative mother (previously exposed to the D antigen through pregnancy or transfusion) may produce anti-D. During each subsequent pregnancy, transplacental passage of maternal antibody may cause fetal hemolysis.
- **No previous exposure is necessary for ABO hemolytic disease** because anti-A and anti-B are naturally occurring isohemagglutinins. ABO incompatibility is the most common cause of hemolytic disease of the newborn, but Rh incompatibility is associated with the most severe hemolysis in the fetus or the newborn.

■ Hemolytic disease of the newborn can also develop when the mother lacks one of the so-called minor blood group antigens (C, E, Kell, Duffy, or Kidd) that the fetus has inherited from the father.

Clinical Features

Newborns with hemolytic disease of the newborn present for evaluation with **varying degrees of illness,** depending on the degree of anemia. Clinical manifestations result from the rate of RBC destruction and the degree of compensation. Newborns have **jaundice and anemia,** usually within the first 24 hours of life. Anemia may cause **congestive heart failure,** and, if the anemia is severe in utero, **hydrops fetalis** may develop. Neonates with hydrops fetalis usually die shortly after birth. **Hyperbilirubinemia** can also be severe and can lead to **kernicterus.**

Delayed anemia can occur in neonates who have been recognized as having isoimmune hemolytic anemia during the first few days of life or in those with mild hemolysis that was undetected initially. Hemoglobin levels may fall to 4 to 6 g/dL within the first 4 to 6 weeks of life.

Evaluation

If the patient's mother is Rh negative and the father is Rh positive, then the infant is at risk for the development of hemolysis. The **Rh-negative mother** should be **screened routinely for the presence of anti-D** during gestation and should receive **RhoGAM** (anti-D immune globulin) in the last trimester of pregnancy, prophylactically at termination of pregnancy, or postpartum.

Antibody bound to the surface of the neonate's RBCs can often be demonstrated using a **Direct antiglobulin test (DAT),** although a negative DAT does not rule out isoimmune hemolytic disease. The **maternal serum should be tested** for the presence of a specific antibody that may cause the hemolysis.

Treatment

Treatment is directed at reducing severe unconjugated hyperbilirubinemia and correcting severe anemia. **Exchange transfusion** should be considered if the hemoglobin level is <12 g/dL and falling within the first 24 hours of life or if the serum bilirubin level is >20 mg/dL within the first 24 hours of life. **Phototherapy** and **hydration** for hyperbilirubinemia may be the only treatments necessary.

Details regarding the management of women at risk for carrying a fetus with Rh disease can be found in standard obstetrics textbooks. Routine immunization of mothers at risk has succeeded in decreasing the incidence of Rh hemolytic disease of the newborn in the United States.

> **HINT:** If the neonate has type O blood or is Rh negative, he is not at risk for development of major blood group incompatibility. However, he may still be at risk for development of minor blood group incompatibility.

Acute and Delayed Hemolytic Transfusion Reactions

Etiology

Acute hemolytic transfusion reactions result when a **recipient with pre-formed antibodies receives an ABO-incompatible RBC transfusion.** These **life-threatening reactions** are usually caused by the **misidentification** of the donor or recipient of the blood for transfusion and thus are avoidable. Delayed hemolytic transfusion reactions (DHTRs) occur 7 to 14 days following a RBC transfusion. These reactions are caused by the presence of preformed antibodies to **minor blood group antigens** in previously transfused patients.

Clinical Features

Patients with acute hemolytic transfusion reactions develop **fever, chills, and tachycardia** commensurate with the volume of blood that has been transfused. Increased scleral icterus, dark urine, and back pain are frequent clinical features at the time of DHTR diagnosis.

Evaluation

The **urine dipstick test** results may be positive for the **presence of heme** with an **absence of RBCs.** Laboratory findings include a **positive DAT** in both kinds of hemolytic transfusion reactions. **Disseminated intravascular coagulation (DIC) and renal failure** may develop.

Treatment

The first intervention when an acute hemolytic transfusion reaction is suspected is to **stop the blood transfusion.** Treatment should include **aggressive intravenous hydration** and the use of **diuretics** to prevent fluid overload. **Alkalinization** may be considered to prevent renal failure. Intravenous gammaglobulin and steroids are used to decrease the hemolysis associated with DHTRs. Cautious reexposure to red cell units is advised. Repeat transfusion should be considered only in patients with cardiovascular compromise.

Autoimmune Hemolytic Anemia

Etiology

Autoimmune hemolytic anemia (AIHA), which may be **idiopathic or secondary,** can cause **acute, life-threatening anemia** in the pediatric population. The idiopathic diagnosis is the more common in the pediatric population because specific causes are difficult to identify. Secondary AIHA may be caused by warm-reactive or cold-reactive antibodies and may result from infection, malignancy, collagen vascular diseases, drugs, or toxins.

Clinical Features

Children with AIHA may have a **sudden onset of pallor, fever, scleral icterus, and dark urine.** However, a more insidious onset of AIHA may be seen, particularly in children >10 years. **Splenomegaly** is usually present on physical examination. The course of the disease varies from a limited single short episode to a more prolonged illness, with relapses associated with infections.

Evaluation

Laboratory findings include **normochromic, normocytic anemia with spherocytes** seen on **peripheral blood smear,** as well as **reticulocytosis.** Hyperbilirubinemia is present. The **DAT is usually positive;** however, a negative DAT does not eliminate the possibility of AIHA. Childhood AIHA is usually mediated by IgG. The presence of hemolysis with IgM may be associated with *Mycoplasma* or EBV infection.

Treatment

Treatment is directed at **cardiovascular support** and **decreasing the amount of RBC destruction. Prednisone** (2 mg/kg per day) is given orally if the child is stable, or the equivalent dose in a parenteral form can be given. **Urine output should be maintained** to avoid renal failure.

RBC transfusions should be avoided unless hypoxia or cardiovascular compromise is present because severe hemolytic transfusion reactions can occur. **If RBC transfusion is necessary,** the "least incompatible" donor unit of blood should be used. The **first 15 mL of blood should be administered under very close observation.** The urine should be checked for the presence of hemoglobin, and the plasma layer of a spun hematocrit should be checked for a pink tinge consistent with hemolysis.

Microangiopathic Hemolytic Anemia

Etiology

Microangiopathic hemolytic anemia is associated with a variety of conditions, including **DIC, prosthetic heart valves, cardiac disease** (e.g., coarctation of the aorta, severe valvular disease, endocarditis), **hemolytic uremic syndrome, thrombotic thrombocytopenic purpura, severe burns, march hemoglobinuria, renal transplant rejection, and hemangiomata.**

Clinical Features

The degree of anemia is **variable.** Thrombocytopenia may or may not be present, and **reticulocytosis** is usually present. DIC may occur.

Evaluation

The peripheral blood smear shows **prominent RBC fragments,** such as helmet cells and schistocytes.

Treatment

Treatment should be directed at the **underlying cause.**

EVALUATION OF HEMOLYSIS

History and Physical Examination

A well-focused history and physical examination can direct the physician in ordering appropriate tests and making a diagnosis (Table 40-2).

TABLE 40-2 Clinical Evaluation of Pediatric Patients with Suspected Hemolytic Anemia

Question	If the Answer is "Yes," Consider . . .
History	
Is the patient a neonate?	Hemolytic disease of the newborn
Has the child had previous episodes of scleral icterus or dark urine, particularly with intercurrent illnesses?	Chronic (versus an acute) hemolytic process
Is the patient currently taking medications or has he received medications recently?	G6PD deficiency or drug-induced hemolysis, depending on the type of medications and the ethnic background of the child
Are there mothball products in the household?	G6PD deficiency
Has the patient participated in very strenuous exercise recently, such as running a marathon?	March hemoglobinuria
Does the patient have cardiac disease or prosthetic heart valves?	Microangiopathic hemolytic anemia
Has the patient had a recent severe diarrheal illness or viral prodrome?	HUS and chronic hemolytic anemia
Is the patient an African-American?	G6PD deficiency, thalassemia, SCD
Is the patient of Mediterranean descent?	G6PD deficiency, thalassemia
Has the patient had a blood transfusion recently? Is the patient on a chronic transfusion protocol?	Acute or delayed hemolytic transfusion reaction, particularly if the patient is chronically transfused
Is there a family history of gallstones or splenectomy in early childhood? Is there a family history of anemia?	Chronic hemolytic anemia, inherited
Physical Examination	
Is there scleral icterus, jaundice, and splenomegaly?	Hemolytic anemia
Is there evidence of maxillary hyperplasia, towering forehead, or other evidence of bone marrow expansion?	Chronic hemolytic process

G6PD = glucose-6-phosphate dehydrogenase; SCD = sickle cell disease

> **HINT:** Some patients with congenital hemolytic anemias present for evaluation during transient aplastic episodes without histories suggestive of chronic hemolysis.

Laboratory Studies

At minimum, the initial laboratory evaluation should include a CBC and **reticulocyte count.** Lactate dehydrogenase, aspartate aminotransferase, and indirect bilirubin levels are often high in hemolytic states with a low serum haptoglobin. Review of the peripheral blood smear for spherocytes, schistocytes, and increased polychromasia is very **important.** A DAT can be revealing when RBC destruction is caused by antibody production against erythrocytes (e.g., in AIHA or hemolytic disease of the newborn).

> **HINT:** Three common conditions are frequently mistaken for hemolytic anemia: hemorrhage, recovering bone marrow (e.g., seen after chemotherapy or viral illness), and partially treated nutritional deficiencies. The reticulocyte count is often increased with evidence of anemia; however, this finding is not related to intrinsic or extrinsic causes of hemolysis.

APPROACH TO THE PATIENT (FIGURE 40-1)

TREATMENT OF HEMOLYSIS

Generally, treatment for hemolytic anemia is directed toward **managing cardiovascular compromise** and **treating the underlying cause** in patients with acquired disease.

Splenectomy

Splenectomy should be considered for children with **congenital hemolytic anemia** to reduce RBC transfusion requirements and to manage complications of hypersplenism (e.g., poor growth). All children who have had their spleens removed are at **greater risk for development of an infection,** particularly with *S. pneumoniae, H. influenzae, Neisseria meningitidis,* or *E. coli.* The risk of infection is greater after splenectomy in young children, particularly in those <4 years and in those who have underlying conditions associated with increased risk of infection. Immunizations against *H. influenzae, S. pneumoniae,* and *N. meningitidis* are recommended before splenectomy. Prophylactic use of oral penicillin is effective in reducing the incidence of bacterial sepsis.

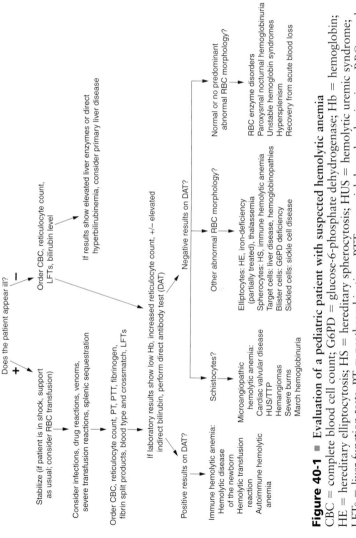

Figure 40-1 ■ Evaluation of a pediatric patient with suspected hemolytic anemia

CBC = complete blood cell count; G6PD = glucose-6-phosphate dehydrogenase; Hb = hemoglobin; HE = hereditary elliptocytosis; HS = hereditary spherocytosis; HUS = hemolytic uremic syndrome; LFTs = liver function tests; PT = prothrombin time; PTT = partial thromboplastin time; RBC = red blood cell; TTP = thrombotic thrombocytopenic purpura

Chronic Transfusion

Children with chronic hemolytic anemia, particularly children with β-thalassemia major or SCD with severe complications, often require frequent transfusions (i.e., every 3 to 6 weeks), either to maintain the hemoglobin level above a certain value or to keep the percentage of Hb S below a certain value. Complications of frequent blood transfusions include iron overload, RBC alloimmunization, and viral infection. Iron overload is treated with chelation therapy, usually with oral chelators such as deferasirox, parenteral chelators such as deferoxamine preparations, or exchange transfusions in appropriate patients with SCD.

Complications of Chronic Hemolytic Anemia

Generally, the complications of chronic hemolytic anemias are related to increased RBC destruction, increased RBC production, and anemia. These complications include folic acid deficiency and gallstones as a result of increased RBC turnover, splenomegaly as a result of increased RBC entrapment and extramedullary hematopoiesis, and transient aplastic episode.

Suggested Readings

Cohen AR: Pallor. In *Textbook of Pediatric Emergency Medicine*, 3rd ed. Edited by Fleisher GR, Ludwig S. Baltimore, Williams & Wilkins, 1993, 388–396.

Segel GB: Anemia. *Pediatr Rev* 10:77–88, 1988.

Stewart CL, Tina LU: Hemolytic uremic syndrome. *Pediatr Rev* 14:218–224, 1993.

Hemoptysis

Laura T. Mulreany
Michael P. Mulreany (Third Edition)

INTRODUCTION

Hemoptysis includes the **expectoration of blood-streaked sputum,** as well as **gross bleeding** from the airways and lung. Spitting or coughing up of blood may occur in many bronchopulmonary diseases, the most common being infection. Although bleeding of more than a few streaks is uncommon in children, **massive hemoptysis** (loss of >8 mL blood/kg or 300 mL blood/24 hours) is a **life-threatening condition** requiring immediate evaluation and therapy. Bleeding from the nasopharynx or the gastrointestinal tract may be mistaken for hemoptysis.

> **HINT:** Patients with massive hemoptysis most likely have a single focus of bleeding.

DIFFERENTIAL DIAGNOSIS LIST

Infectious Causes
Bacterial Infection
  Pneumococcus
  Staphylococcus
  Meningococcus
  Group A *Streptococcus*
  Mycoplasma
  Bordetella pertussis
  Pseudomonas
  Leptospirosis
Viral Infection
  Influenza virus
  Varicella-zoster virus
  Hepatitis B virus
  HIV
Fungal Infection
  Aspergillus
  Histoplasma
  Coccidioides
  Blastomyces

Parasitic Infection
  Visceral larva migrans
  Filariasis
  Toxoplasmosis
  Hydatidosis
Arthropod Infestation
  Hemorrhagic fevers

Toxic Causes
Cocaine
Penicillamine
Trimellitic anhydride
Radiologic contrast
  medium
Smoke inhalation
Radiation exposure
Insecticide inhalation

Neoplastic Causes
Benign Chest Masses
  Hemangiomas

Angiomas—angiokeratoma diffusum, spider angioma
Bronchogenic cysts
Pulmonary sequestration
Inflammatory pseudotumor
Enteric cysts
Malignant Chest Masses
Bronchial carcinoid tumor
Bronchial adenoma (premalignant)
Sarcoma
Teratoma
Metastatic lesions—sarcoma, Wilms tumor, osteogenic sarcoma

Traumatic Causes
Foreign body
Lung contusion
Repeated direct suctioning

Congenital or Vascular Causes
Arteriovenous malformation or fistula—hereditary hemorrhagic telangiectasia
Systemic vasculitis—periarteritis nodosa, Henoch-Schönlein purpura, hypersensitivity angiitis)
Pulmonary capillary hemangiomatosis

Cardiac Causes
Congestive heart failure
Myocarditis
Congenital pulmonary vein stenosis—pulmonary veno-occlusive disease
Tetralogy of Fallot with pulmonary atresia and multiple collaterals
Pulmonary arterial stenosis
Mitral stenosis with left atrial hypertension

Metabolic or Genetic Causes
Cystic fibrosis

Inflammatory Causes
Connective Tissue and Immune-Related Disorders
Goodpasture syndrome—pulmonary renal disease
Wegener granulomatosis
Systemic lupus erythematosus
Immune complex-mediated glomerulonephritis
Progressive systemic sclerosis
Behçet syndrome

Psychosocial Causes
Munchausen by proxy syndrome

Miscellaneous Causes
Pulmonary Disorders
Bronchiectasis
Primary ciliary dyskinesia
Pulmonary hemosiderosis
Allergic bronchopulmonary aspergillosis
Chronic or recurrent aspiration
Pulmonary embolism
Pulmonary infarction
Hematologic Disorders
Consumption coagulopathy
Incompatible blood transfusion
Bleeding disorders—hemophilia A and B, von Willebrand disease
Sickle cell disease and acute chest syndrome
Bone marrow transplant
Other Disorders
Celiac disease
Ehlers-Danlos
Catamenial hemoptysis

DIFFERENTIAL DIAGNOSIS DISCUSSION

> **HINT:** An inhaled foreign body must always be considered in any child with hemoptysis.

> **HINT:** Pneumonia, bronchitis, lung abscess, and laryngotracheitis can be associated with hemoptysis.

Cystic Fibrosis

Cystic fibrosis is the most common nontraumatic cause of pulmonary hemorrhage in the United States and is discussed in Chapter 23, "Cough."

Bronchiectasis

Bronchiectasis is discussed in Chapter 23, "Cough."

Pulmonary Hemosiderosis

Etiology

Hemosiderosis may be primary or secondary.

- **Primary hemosiderosis.** Primary idiopathic hemosiderosis involves bleeding into the lungs, of unknown cause, and is a diagnosis of exclusion. The classification is as follows:
  - Isolated
  - With cardiac or pancreatic involvement
  - With glomerulonephritis (Goodpasture syndrome)
  - With sensitivity to cow's milk and milk-protein allergies (Heiner syndrome)
- **Secondary hemosiderosis** can result from cardiac disease, collagen vascular disease or systemic vasculitis, bleeding disorders, or granulomatosis.

Clinical Features

Patients may present with acute episodes of cough, dyspnea, and wheezing but also may present with chronic fatigue, pallor, and even failure to thrive. Recurrent pneumonia with associated iron-deficiency anemia should also promote consideration.

Typically, the child appears ill (i.e., **lethargic, pale, tachypneic, tachycardic**) and is usually afebrile. The pallor results from **anemia,** which is caused by recurrent subclinical bleeding. **Sputum is frequently rust colored;** frank hemoptysis is less common as a presentation. **Infiltrates** on a chest radiograph may be **diffuse** and fluffy. **Increased work of breathing, decreased breath sounds, and crackles** may be noted on physical examination.

Evaluation

The diagnosis is confirmed by demonstrating **macrophages containing hemosiderin.** A macrophage sample may be obtained via **gastric lavage** (performed three times in the morning before the patient has risen from the supine position) or via **bronchoscopy with bronchoalveolar lavage.**

> **HINT:** Primary idiopathic hemosiderosis is a diagnosis of exclusion and requires a comprehensive workup, including evaluation for immunologic, infectious, and cardiac causes. Milk-protein precipitin values should be obtained for any child with pulmonary hemorrhage of unknown cause.

Treatment

Blood transfusions may be required in the acute phase. Conventional therapy includes prednisone (2 mg/kg per day for 4 to 6 weeks, tapered over 1 to 2 months in an attempt to wean the patient completely or to at least achieve an every-other-day regimen). **Azathioprine or cyclophosphamide** is used for patients who do not respond to steroid therapy or in place of steroids.

Children who test **positive for milk precipitin values** should be placed on a **non-casein-based diet.** Although some children respond, many do not.

Goodpasture Syndrome

A pulmonary-renal immune complex disorder, Goodpasture syndrome is characterized by **deposits of antiglomerular basement membrane (anti-GBM) antibodies in the kidneys and lungs.** Circulating anti-GBM antibodies are also found in the **serum.** The disorder is most common in **young white boys. Hemoptysis,** along with cough and dyspnea, is common and may occur prior to the development of renal disease. Isolated pulmonary disease often responds to corticosteroids, but renal involvement may also require plasmapheresis or dialysis.

Wegener Granulomatosis

Characterized by **vasculitis with granuloma formation,** Wegener granulomatosis involves both the **upper and lower respiratory tracts and the kidney.** The cause is unknown. Wegener granulomatosis is distinguished by necrotizing lesions of the upper and lower respiratory tract and necrotizing glomerulonephritis. The **sinuses, nasal septum, and nasopharynx** are usually involved. The disorder may present with nasal and sinus congestion, arthritis or arthralgia, and skin lesions in addition to cough and hemoptysis. **Massive hemoptysis** may be the presenting symptom and is secondary to **necrotizing pneumonitis** in the lower respiratory tract. **Acute glomerulonephritis** and **renal failure** usually precede the pulmonary manifestations, and radiographic abnormalities may be noted prior to the development of respiratory symptoms. Treatment involves prolonged high-dose corticosteroids and cyclophosphamide, and relapses may be seen.

EVALUATION OF HEMOPTYSIS

Patient History

A careful history is important to rule out an exogenous agent or an underlying pulmonary disorder. A description of the **color of the blood,** the **duration of the bleeding,** and the **amount of blood** is helpful in defining the severity of the condition and making a specific diagnosis. Prior history of pulmonary symptoms or illnesses, as well as general symptoms of fatigue or malaise, pallor, exercise intolerance, or poor growth, should be reviewed.

> **HINT:** It is important to distinguish hemoptysis (coughing of blood) from hematemesis (vomiting of blood). In hematemesis, the blood is often brown and has a low pH as a result of contact with gastric acid. Care must also be taken to differentiate hemoptysis from epistaxis, oral or nasopharyngeal bleeding, and bleeding caused by tonsillitis or gingivitis.

> **HINT:** The main features of alveolar hemorrhage, apart from hemoptysis, are shortness of breath, anemia, hypoxemia, and diffuse pulmonary densities on a chest radiograph.

Physical Examination

The physician should first ensure that the patient's **vital signs and hemodynamic status** are stable prior to any further evaluation. The upper and lower respiratory system should be examined fully, and one might note crackles or wheezing on auscultation. A cardiac examination may reveal a murmur or signs of heart failure. Hepatomegaly and/or splenomegaly may be noted. Features of **systemic illnesses** (e.g., connective tissue disorders, vasculitides) should be sought, with attention to examinations of the skin and extremities. Specific findings that may be suggestive of the cause include the following:

- **Putrid sputum** suggests the presence of a lung abscess or bronchiectasis.
- **Acute pleuritic chest pain** raises the possibility of pulmonary embolism or another pleura-based lesion (e.g., abscess, fungal cavity, vasculitis).
- **Localized wheezing** occurs with an intramural lesion (e.g., foreign body, tumor).
- **Pleural rub** suggests the presence of pleural disease.
- **Clubbing** and **chronic hypoxemia** suggest the presence of a chronic pulmonary or cardiac disorder (e.g., cystic fibrosis, bronchiectasis, cyanotic congenital heart disease).
- **Pallor** may not be noticeable in severe anemia.

Laboratory Studies

A **complete blood count with differential, coagulation studies,** and **sputum culture** and **Gram stain** should be obtained in all patients with significant hemoptysis (more than a few teaspoons). Blood typing and cross-matching should be done if significant blood loss is considered. Stools should be guaiac tested.

Other laboratory studies are ordered according to clinical suspicion for a particular condition. These studies may include the following:

- **Urinalysis, urine microscopy,** and **serum blood urea nitrogen and creatinine levels** (pulmonary-renal disorder)
- **Erythrocyte sedimentation rate, complement, antinuclear antibodies, and rheumatoid factor** (vasculitis and connective tissue disorders)
- **Immunoglobulin E (IgE) level and eosinophil count** (Heiner syndrome, autoimmune disorders)
- **Serum anti-GBM antibody level** (Goodpasture syndrome)
- **Serum c-antineutrophil cytoplasmic autoantibody** (Wegener granulomatosis)
- **Bacterial, viral, fungal, and parasitic cultures** (infection identification)
- **Purified protein derivative analysis** (tuberculosis)
- **Chloride sweat test** (cystic fibrosis)
- **Endomysial IgA** (celiac disease)

Other Diagnostic Modalities

- **Chest radiograph.** A chest radiograph should be obtained for all patients with significant hemoptysis or clinical distress. The acute radiographic changes are usually diffuse and bilateral, often sparing the apices and costophrenic angles. Chronically, more nodular or reticulonodular densities may be seen. Unilateral hyperlucency may indicate a radiolucent foreign body; in that case, a lateral decubitus film should be evaluated for paradoxical asymmetry.
- **High-resolution computed tomography (HRCT) of the chest with contrast** is more sensitive and specific than a chest radiograph for

demonstrating the alveolar pattern in an intrapulmonary bleed. HRCT is also helpful in diagnosing sequestration and locating anomalous vessels. Pulmonary fibrosis may be seen in chronic or recurrent disease.

- **Magnetic resonance imaging and magnetic resonance angiography** are valuable for detecting neoplasia and anomalous vasculature.
- **Pulmonary function testing** may reveal both obstructive (early) and restrictive (later) lung disease.
- **Radionuclide scanning** with technetium-99m-labeled sulfur colloid can detect perfusion defects caused by emboli and may be helpful in detecting a localized bleeding site.
- **Laryngoscopy** or **bronchoscopy** (or both) can differentiate upper from lower respiratory tract bleeding and focal from diffuse bleeding. These modalities can also localize the bleeding to a particular bronchopulmonary segment. A rigid scope should be used for patients with severe bleeding because it enables the physician to ventilate the patient (if necessary), to control the airway, and to provide definitive treatment in some cases. A flexible scope is better suited for diagnostic purposes, lavage, and obtaining samples for culture.
- **Bronchoalveolar lavage** can be used for definitive cultures, and staining for hemosiderin-laden macrophages.
- **Lung biopsy** may be indicated if the workup is negative (consistent with idiopathic or primary pulmonary hemosiderosis) and suspicion of an underlying condition still exists.
- **Echocardiography** may allow exclusion of an underlying cardiac disorder.
- **Cardiac catheterization and angiography** can help delineate the bronchial and pulmonary vasculature, localize an isolated bleeding vessel, define the underlying cause (dilated tortuous bronchial vessels, increased number of vessels, bronchopulmonary anastomosis), and evaluate hemodynamics (in congenital heart disease and suspected pulmonary hypertension). Angiography can include treatment (coiling of collateral vessels) and guide surgical resection in large-vessel diffuse disease.

TREATMENT OF HEMOPTYSIS

In most cases, hemoptysis is self-limited and not life threatening. Definitive treatment, after stabilization, is directed at causative agents and underlying disorders if found.

Stabilization

An **aggressive approach** in an **intensive care setting** is indicated when a massive hemorrhage occurs. An airway must be **established immediately.** (Aspiration of blood and asphyxia are more likely to kill the patient than is exsanguination.) **Supplemental oxygen** should be used for hypoxemia.

One should be prepared to use **intubation and mechanical ventilation** for both airway maintenance and management of hypoxemia and respiratory failure. **Hypovolemia** requires **fluid resuscitation, blood transfusion, or both.** Acidosis requires the administration of **fluids** (e.g., 0.9% normal saline, lactated Ringer's solution) and blood.

Infants with intrapulmonary bleeding almost always have concomitant **left-sided heart failure with pulmonary edema** and may require **positive-pressure ventilation** with **positive end-expiratory pressure, pressor administration** (e.g., dopamine, dobutamine, epinephrine), and **fluid restriction** (except for blood transfusion, when necessary).

Termination of Bleeding

Methods of terminating bleeding include the following. The effectiveness of conservative therapy is well established and is the mainstay except for in cases of massive hemoptysis.

- **Bronchoscopic lavage** of a segment of the lung with iced saline can be successful in some cases but is rarely used.
- **Endobronchial tamponade.** A balloon-tipped catheter is placed in the affected bronchus, inflated, and left in place for 24 hours.
- **Selective embolization** of the bronchial or pulmonary vessels with catheter-introduced coils is an effective way of stopping persistent or recurrent bleeding.
- **Electrocoagulation** is found to be useful by some authors.
- **Selective intubation** of a main bronchus with a cuffed tube may be useful in unilateral bleeding.
- **Surgical resection** of the focus of bleeding may provide definitive treatment in isolated bleeding segments or vascular anomalies.
- **Endobronchial thrombin and intravenous vasopressin** are newer therapies.

> **HINT:** A major pitfall in dealing with hemoptysis is to ascribe recurrent episodes of hemoptysis to a previously established diagnosis, such as chronic bronchiectasis or bronchitis. Failing to search for an underlying diagnosis may result in missing a serious but potentially treatable condition.

Suggested Readings

Barben JU, Ditchfield M, Carlin JB, et al.: Major haemoptysis in children with cystic fibrosis: a 20-year retrospective study. *J Cyst Fibros* 2(3):105–111, 2003.

Batra PS, Holinger LD: Etiology and management of pediatric hemoptysis. *Arch Otolaryngol Head Neck Surg* 127(4):377–382, 2001.

Boat TF: Pulmonary hemorrhage and hemoptysis. In *Kendig's Disorders of the Respiratory Tract in Children,* 7th ed. Edited by Chernick V, Boat TF, Wilmott RW, et al. Philadelphia, WB Saunders, 2006, 676–685.

Godfrey S: Pulmonary hemorrhage/hemoptysis in children. *Pediatr Pulmonol* 37(6):476–484, 2004.

Sidman JD, Wheeler WB, Cabalka AK, et al.: Management of acute pulmonary hemorrhage in children. *Laryngoscope* 111(1):33–35, 2001.

Susarla SC, Fan LL: Diffuse alveolar hemorrhage syndromes in children. *Curr Opin Pediatr* 19:413–320, 2007.

Hepatomegaly

Nicholas Tsarouhas and Paula Agosto

INTRODUCTION

Hepatomegaly, an enlarged liver, is an important clue to a variety of systemic pathological conditions. Alternatively, it may herald disease of the liver itself. **Palpation** is the most common technique used to diagnose hepatomegaly. A palpable liver, however, does not necessarily denote hepatomegaly. In a normal child, the liver edge usually is palpable 1 to 2 cm below the right costal margin in the right midclavicular line. In an infant, the liver edge may be palpable 2 to 3 cm below the costal margin. Although a liver palpable beyond these parameters suggests hepatomegaly, the **liver span is a more reliable indicator.** The liver span is ascertained by percussing the upper edge and by palpating or auscultating the lower edge. **Auscultation** is performed by placing the stethoscope below the xiphoid and "scratching" superiorly from the right lower quadrant until the lower edge of the liver causes a change in the transmitted sound. In the neonate, the normal liver span is 4 to 5 cm; in older children, the span reaches 7 to 8 cm in boys and 6 to 7 cm in girls.

DIFFERENTIAL DIAGNOSIS LIST

Infectious Causes
Viral Infections
  Benign viral infection
  Hepatitis (types A to E)
  Epstein-Barr virus (EBV)
    infection (mononucleosis)
  Cytomegalovirus (CMV)
    infection
  AIDS
Bacterial Infections
  Sepsis
  Liver abscess
  Ascending cholangitis
  Cat-scratch disease
  Brucellosis
  Rocky Mountain spotted
    fever
  Ehrlichiosis
  Tuberculosis

  Syphilis
  Leptospirosis
Other Infections
  Malaria
  Toxoplasmosis
  Babesiosis
  Histoplasmosis
  Amebiasis
  Ascariasis
  Toxocariasis
  Echinococcosis
  Schistosomiasis

Hematologic Causes
  Hemolytic anemia (e.g.,
    sickle cell anemia)
  Thalassemia
  Erythroblastosis fetalis

Neoplastic Causes

Hepatoblastoma
Hepatocellular carcinoma
Hemangioendothelioma
Hemangioma
Adenoma
Hamartoma
Leukemia
Lymphoma
Neuroblastoma
Wilms tumor
Other metastatic disease

Vascular Causes

Congestive heart failure
Constrictive pericarditis
Budd-Chiari syndrome

Anatomic Causes

Extrahepatic
  Biliary atresia
  Biliary hypoplasia
  Bile duct stenosis or stricture
  Choledochal cyst
  Cholelithiasis
  Tumors (hepatic, biliary, pancreatic, duodenal)
Intrahepatic
  Alagille syndrome
  Intrahepatic biliary duct hypoplasia or paucity

Traumatic Causes

Laceration
Hematoma
Traumatic cyst

Metabolic and Genetic Causes

Wilson disease (hepatolenticular degeneration)
α_1-Antitrypsin (α_1-AT) deficiency
Hemochromatosis (primary or secondary)
Cystic fibrosis
Zellweger (cerebrohepatorenal) syndrome
Mitochondrial disease
Progressive familial intrahepatic cholestasis syndromes (types 1 to 3)
Congenital hepatic fibrosis/ autosomal recessive polycystic kidney disease
Dubin-Johnson syndrome
Amino acid metabolism defects
Tyrosinemia
Urea cycle disorders
Methylmalonic acidemia
Homocystinuria
Carbohydrate metabolism defects
Galactosemia
Hereditary fructose intolerance
Glycogen storage diseases (types I to IX), examples include
  Von Gierke disease
  Pompe disease
Lipid metabolism defects
Fatty acid oxidation disorders
Hyperlipoproteinemia or hypolipoproteinemia
Mucolipidoses (I-cell disease)
Lipid storage diseases
  Niemann-Pick disease
  Gaucher disease
  GM_1 and GM_2 gangliosidosis
Mucopolysaccharidoses
Hurler syndrome
Hunter syndrome

Toxic Causes

Drugs
Hypervitaminosis A

Autoimmune Causes

Autoimmune hepatitis
Primary sclerosing cholangitis

Juvenile rheumatoid arthritis

Systemic lupus erythematosus

Miscellaneous Causes

Obesity

Diabetes mellitus

Protein-calorie malnutrition

Chronic intravenous alimentation

Reye syndrome

Chronic granulomatous disease

Histiocytic disorders

    Langerhans cell histiocytosis

Hemophagocytic lymphohistiocytosis

Malignant histiocytic disorders

Amyloidosis

Sarcoidosis

Nonalcoholic steatohepatitis

Focal nodular hyperplasia of the liver

Idiopathic neonatal giant cell hepatitis

DIFFERENTIAL DIAGNOSIS DISCUSSION

Benign Viral Infection

It is not uncommon for children with viral syndromes to have **mild hepatomegaly.** The liver is nontender, and serum transaminase levels are occasionally slightly high. Only **observation** for resolution of the infection is required.

Liver Abscess

Etiology

Bacterial agents are the usual culprits; occasionally, a **parasitic agent** can cause a liver abscess. The following are risk factors for liver abscess:

- Bacteremia
- Intra-abdominal infection
- Anti-inflammatory drug therapy
- Antineoplastic drug therapy
- Immunodeficiency
- Umbilical vein catheterization

Clinical Features

Patients present with **right upper quadrant pain, fever, anorexia, weight loss,** and, occasionally, **jaundice.**

Evaluation

The patient's liver enzyme levels, white blood cell count, and erythrocyte sedimentation rate are usually increased. Blood culture results may be positive. **Ultrasound, computed tomography (CT),** and **magnetic resonance imaging (MRI)** are useful diagnostic modalities.

Treatment

Therapy includes the use of **antibiotic agents** in concert with CT- or ultra-sound-guided **aspiration or surgical drainage.** Appropriate empirical antibiotic therapy includes a penicillinase-resistant penicillin (e.g., naf-cillin, oxacillin) and an aminoglycoside (e.g., gentamicin). Anaerobic coverage is sometimes added as well. Common antimicrobial choices for anaerobic abscesses include clindamycin, cefoxitin, or metronidazole.

Viral Hepatitis

Viral hepatitis is discussed in Chapter 45, "Jaundice."

Infectious Mononucleosis

Infectious mononucleosis is discussed in Chapter 50, "Lymphadenopathy."

Cytomegalovirus Infection

CMV infection is discussed in Chapter 73, "Splenomegaly."

AIDS

AIDS is discussed in Chapter 70, "Sexually Transmitted Diseases."

Sepsis

Sepsis is discussed in Chapter 56, "Neonatal Infections."

Neuroblastoma

Neuroblastoma is discussed in Chapter 8, "Abdominal Mass."

Biliary Atresia

Biliary atresia is discussed in Chapter 46, "Jaundice, Newborn."

Wilson Disease (Hepatolenticular Degeneration)

Etiology

Wilson disease is an autosomal recessive disease of **copper metabolism.** Decreased biliary excretion of copper causes copper accumulation in hepatocytes and other organs.

Clinical Features

The onset of symptoms, which are usually the result of **hepatic or neurologic involvement,** usually occurs during **late childhood or adolescence.** There may be a family history of undiagnosed hepatic, neurologic, or psychiatric disease.

- **Hepatic involvement** is characterized by a variety of different manifestations. Patients may present with increased transaminase levels, hepatomegaly, or cirrhosis with complications of portal hypertension.

Some patients have an acute fulminant presentation of Wilson disease, with liver failure and a brisk hemolysis that can cause unconjugated hyperbilirubinemia.

- **Psychiatric and neurologic manifestations** include subtle problems (e.g., a decline in school performance or behavioral changes) that progress if a diagnosis is not made and therapy initiated. Late symptoms include tremors, slurring of speech, and severe dystonia.

Evaluation

Urine copper levels are increased, and the **serum ceruloplasmin level is decreased.** Slit-lamp examination to detect the presence of Kayser-Fleischer rings should be performed, but a negative examination does not rule out the diagnosis. **Cranial CT and MRI scans** may show central nervous system (CNS) lesions caused by copper deposition. Definitive diagnosis is by liver biopsy with quantitative copper measurement. Genetic testing for mutations in ATP7B is also available.

Treatment

Dietary intake of copper should be minimized, and **copper chelation therapy** with d-penicillamine or trientine is initiated. Patients with advanced chronic liver disease or fulminant presentation require **liver transplantation.**

α₁-Antitrypsin Deficiency

α_1-AT deficiency is discussed in Chapter 45, "Jaundice."

Tyrosinemia

Etiology

Tyrosinemia is an aminoacidopathy characterized by an increased level of **plasma tyrosine and elevated urine and plasma succinylacetone.** This autosomal recessive disorder is caused by mutations in the FAH gene, encoding fumarylacetoacetate hydrolase, in the tyrosine degradation pathway. The liver, the kidneys, and the CNS are primarily affected.

Clinical Features

Symptoms, which include **vomiting and irritability,** develop early in the first year of life. Other manifestations include acute liver failure, jaundice, hypoglycemia, failure to thrive, rickets, and developmental delay. Patients with untreated tyrosinemia are at high risk of developing hepatocellular carcinoma.

Evaluation

Laboratory test results may show **anemia, hyperbilirubinemia,** and an **increase in liver enzyme values.** Typically these infants present with a severe coagulopathy out of proportion to the elevations in liver enzymes. Signs of a renal Fanconi syndrome, including hypouricemia, hypophosphatemia, and aminoaciduria, may also be present. The α-fetoprotein level is usually highly elevated.

Treatment

Treatment includes **dietary management** and **liver transplantation.** NTBC is a novel compound that blocks the tyrosine metabolic pathway above FAH and thereby prevents the accumulation of toxic metabolites. This medication is now used as standard therapy in tyrosinemia and has allowed affected infants to survive without liver transplantation.

Urea Cycle Disorders

Etiology

Urea cycle disorders involve **defects or deficiencies** in the **enzymes** that detoxify ammonia to urea.

Clinical Features

After a few days of dietary protein intake, neonates develop **vomiting, seizures, lethargy,** and even **coma.** Infants and older children present with vomiting and neurologic symptoms.

Evaluation

Increased levels of ammonia, a **decreased blood urea nitrogen** (BUN) level, and **metabolic acidemia** are present.

Treatment

Treatment entails **dietary protein restriction** and the oral administration of **ammonia-removing compounds** (e.g., sodium benzoate, sodium phenylacetate, arginine, lactulose). Liver transplantation is indicated in some patients with urea cycle defects.

Galactosemia

Etiology

Classic galactosemia is caused by galactose-1-phosphate uridylyltransferase deficiency, which leads to the inability to metabolize **galactose-1-phosphate** and the **accumulation** of this substance in the liver, kidney, and brain.

Clinical Features

Infants and children may present for examination with **irritability, lethargy, vomiting, jaundice, hepatosplenomegaly, failure to thrive, cataracts,** and **hypoglycemia.** It is important to make the diagnosis at birth to prevent permanent brain damage.

TABLE 42-1 Comparison of Glycogen Storage Diseases

	Von Gierke disease	Pompe disease
Etiology	Hepatorenal glycogenosis	Cardiac glycogenosis
Clinical features	"Doll face" appearance; failure to thrive; hydronephrosis; gout; normal mental status; hypoglycemia with an increase in the amount of lactic acid, lipids, and uric acid; no muscle involvement	Cardiomegaly, hypotonia, normal mental status, muscle involvement
Treatment	Dietary control	No effective therapy
Prognosis	Near-normal life	Death, usually from respiratory muscle failure

Treatment

Treatment entails reduction or **exclusion of dietary galactose.**

Glycogen Storage Diseases

Table 42-1 compares von Gierke disease and Pompe disease.

Niemann-Pick Disease

Etiology

Classic Niemann-Pick disease is an autosomal recessive disease caused by a sphingomyelinase deficiency, which results in **excess storage of sphingomyelin and cholesterol** in the liver, spleen, brain, and bone marrow ("foam" cells). Classic Niemann-Pick disease ultimately **progresses to mental retardation, neurologic deterioration, and death.**

Clinical Features and Evaluation

Infants present for evaluation with **developmental delay, hearing and vision abnormalities, hypotonia, feeding difficulties,** and **failure to thrive.** Other findings on physical examination include a "wasted" appearance, hepatosplenomegaly, and, in some, a "cherry-red" spot on the macula. The diagnosis is made by means of **enzyme analysis.**

> **HINT:** Patients with Tay-Sachs disease, another devastating lipid storage disorder, classically have the "cherry-red" spot on the macula of the eye, but notably they do not have associated hepatosplenomegaly.

Mucopolysaccharidoses

Table 42-2 compares Hunter syndrome and Hurler syndrome.

TABLE 42-2 Comparison of Mucopolysaccharidoses

	Hunter Syndrome	Hurler Syndrome
Etiology	X-linked recessive disorder caused by iduronate-2-sulfatase deficiency	Autosomal recessive disorder caused by α-l-iduronidase deficiency
Clinical features	Coarse facial features, short stature, hearing abnormalities, cardiac abnormalities, hepatosplenomegaly, hernias, joint stiffness, skin problems, mental retardation	Developmental delay, macrocephaly, coarse facial features, clouded corneas, nasal discharge, hepatosplenomegaly, hernias, kyphosis
Prognosis	More mild course than that of Hurler syndrome	Joint immobility, skeletal disturbances, developmental regression, and neurologic deterioration progress to death by early adolescence

Drug Toxicity

Drugs that can cause hepatitis and cholestasis through direct hepatotoxicity or fatty infiltration are summarized in Chapter 45, "Jaundice," Table 45-1.

Protein-Calorie Malnutrition

Etiology

Starvation states are commonly associated with **hepatomegaly. Kwashiorkor,** which is characterized by **severe protein deficiency,** is the most prevalent form of malnutrition in the world.

Clinical Features

Children with kwashiorkor have a **severely wasted appearance, growth retardation, apathy, lethargy, dermatitis,** and **edema. Susceptibility to infection** is increased. Severely ill patients may develop stupor and coma.

Evaluation

Laboratory test abnormalities include **anemia, hypoglycemia, hypoalbuminemia,** and **hypoproteinemia. Vitamin and mineral deficiencies are universal.** Urinalysis is notable for the presence of **ketones.** Bone age, measured by radiographic study of the left hand and wrist, shows a **delay in skeletal maturation** with respect to chronologic age.

Treatment

Enteral "refeeding" (with careful monitoring of laboratory nutritional indexes and electrolytes) is usually curative.

Chronic Intravenous Alimentation

Etiology

Hyperalimentation hepatitis, or total parenteral nutrition hepatitis, is a common complication when parenteral nutrition using crystalline amino acid solutions is provided long term.

Clinical Features

Elevated liver enzymes and jaundice usually mark the onset of this complication. Chronic liver disease may ensue.

Evaluation

Liver enzymes, bilirubin, and nutritional indicators (e.g., albumin, protein) should be monitored.

Treatment

When possible, attempts should be made to use enteral nutrition.

Autoimmune Hepatitis

Etiology

Autoimmune hepatitis, which is characterized by the presence of circulating autoantibodies, may be caused by an abnormality of suppressor T cells.

Clinical Features

Like most autoimmune diseases, autoimmune hepatitis is most common in girls. Symptoms include fever, fatigue, weakness, abdominal pain, and joint pain. Symptoms of other autoimmune manifestations may also be present (e.g., thyroiditis, autoimmune hemolytic anemia).

Evaluation

Physical examination signs include hepatosplenomegaly, jaundice, palmar erythema, and spider angiomata. Laboratory results may show hypergammaglobulinemia; the presence of specific anti-smooth muscle, anti-liver kidney microsomal antibodies; and hemolytic anemia.

Treatment

Patients often respond to immunosuppressive therapy with corticosteroids (e.g., prednisone) or azathioprine, but relapse often occurs when the patient is weaned from the steroids. Liver transplantation may be necessary.

Reye Syndrome

Etiology

Reye syndrome is a rare, reversible, noninflammatory encephalopathy of unknown etiology, characterized by fatty degeneration of the liver.

There is an **association between Reye syndrome and aspirin use** during varicella infection or an influenza-like illness.

Clinical Features

The initial presentation is the **abrupt onset of vomiting** following prodromal viral (or varicella) symptoms. **Neurologic changes** rapidly develop. The ensuing **progressive encephalopathy** is characterized by quietness, irritability, combativeness, confusion, delirium, stupor, and coma.

Evaluation

Laboratory test abnormalities include increases in liver enzyme levels, ammonia level, BUN value, and prothrombin time. Decreases in the serum glucose level, bicarbonate level, and arterial carbon dioxide tension ($Paco_2$) may also be present. **Liver biopsy** is usually confirmatory.

Treatment

Fluid restriction, hyperventilation, and **mannitol therapy** are commonly used to combat the lethal effects of cerebral edema.

Histiocytic Disorders

Etiology

Reactive disorders associated with the proliferation of the mononuclear phagocytic system are classified into three groups:

- Langerhans cell histiocytosis (LCH)
- Hemophagocytic lymphohistiocytosis (HPLH)
- Malignant histiocytic disorders

> **HINT:** Langerhans cell histiocytosis (dendritic cell-related disorders) was previously classified as a "histiocytosis X syndrome" and referred to as Hand-Schüller-Christian syndrome, Letterer-Siwe disease, and eosinophilic granuloma.

- LCH is characterized by cells similar to the Langerhans cells of the skin, causing organ damage to multiple body systems through the production of cytokines and prostaglandins.
- HPLH is a macrophage-related disorder characterized by a proliferation of erythrophagocytic histiocytes in the bone marrow, spleen, lymph nodes, skin, or CNS. The underlying pathophysiology is related to impaired natural killer cells and cytotoxic T-cell activity.

Both LCH and HPLH are **linked to underlying immunodeficiencies and viruses.**

Clinical Features

- LCH may present as a **single-system disease,** with isolated bony lesions, or as a **multisystem disease involving the skin, teeth, liver, bone marrow, lungs, liver, spleen, gastrointestinal tract, or CNS.** Complications include pulmonary and hepatic fibrosis, liver and bone marrow failure, and neurologic abnormalities.
- HPLH patients commonly present with **fever, fatigue, jaundice,** and **hepatosplenomegaly.** Complications include overwhelming infection, bleeding, and progressive CNS disease.

Evaluation

Complete blood count (CBC), coagulation studies, liver enzymes, and **chest radiograph** are important initial studies in all the histiocytic disorders. A **skeletal survey** is used in LCH to search for bony lesions. HPLH is usually associated with pancytopenia, hypertriglyceridemia, hepatitis, and hyperferritinemia. **Bone marrow evaluation** is usually confirmatory.

Treatment

Chemotherapy, radiotherapy, immunotherapy (cyclosporin A, antithymocyte globulin), and **bone marrow transplantation** have been used in the histiocytic disorders with variable success.

EVALUATION OF HEPATOMEGALY

Patient History

The following questions may lead to a diagnosis:

- **Is there a history of a minor preceding viral illness?** Mild hepatomegaly may be apparent with even benign viral illnesses.
- **Did a prodromal illness lead to jaundice?** Hepatitis A infection is a common diagnosis in the setting of a jaundiced child after a mild prodromal illness.
- **Is there a history of poor feeding with respiratory distress?** Hepatomegaly in the setting of poor feeding and respiratory distress is a classic clinical triad for congestive heart failure in infants. Pneumonia may also present with these findings.
- **Is there a history of trauma?** Abdominal trauma may result in a liver laceration or hematoma.
- **Is the patient lethargic or irritable?** Sepsis and metabolic disorders may present with a history of lethargy or irritability.
- **Is there a history of vomiting with developmental delay or behavioral abnormalities?** Metabolic disorders may present with vomiting and nonspecific neurodevelopmental abnormalities.

- **Is there a family history of early death or neurologic disease?** Metabolic disorders should be considered with vague family histories of infantile deaths of unknown etiology.
- **What is the patient's medication history?** Many drugs can cause liver abnormalities and hepatomegaly. Aspirin use is associated with Reye syndrome.
- **Is there a maternal history of perinatal illness or poor prenatal care?** Infectious etiologies such as AIDS, hepatitis, CMV, and syphilis should be considered with perinatal illness or when prenatal care was absent or incomplete.
- **Is there a history of umbilical catheterization?** Hepatic abscess is a known complication of umbilical catheterization.
- **Is there a history of foreign travel?** Malaria, as well as other infectious etiologies, should be considered if the patient has recently traveled abroad.
- **Is there a history of a tick bite?** Rocky Mountain spotted fever, ehrlichiosis, and babesiosis are all concerns after tick bites.
- **Is there a history of animal contact?** Cats or kittens are the main culprits in cat-scratch disease (via scratches) and toxoplasmosis (commonly from the litter box); contact with cat or dog feces is also a risk factor for toxocariasis; dogs are also occasional carriers of echinococcus, as are coyotes, wolves, and other canines; leptospirosis is usually caused by contact with the urine or waters contaminated by rats, dogs, or cattle; brucellosis should also be considered if there has been contact with cattle (or unpasteurized milk), goats, sheep, or swine; exposure to infected dogs may also lead to brucellosis; inhalation of spores containing the fecal droppings of birds or bats might lead to histoplasmosis.

Physical Examination

- **Jaundice** is often the presenting sign in patients with viral hepatitis, hemolytic anemia, anatomic pathologies, and drug hepatotoxicity.
- **Fever** supports an infectious or inflammatory diagnosis.
- **Exudative pharyngitis** suggests EBV or CMV infection.
- **Adenopathy** raises suspicion for an infectious or oncologic process.
- **An abdominal mass** raises concern for neuroblastoma or other neoplastic process.
- **Splenomegaly** occurs with metabolic, infectious, oncologic, and anatomic (obstructive) disorders, as well as with any process that causes hepatic fibrosis and portal hypertension.
- **Eye findings** may be seen in metabolic (e.g., Wilson disease) or infectious (e.g., CMV) disorders.
- **Facial dysmorphism** suggests a metabolic disorder or Alagille syndrome.

Laboratory Studies

Appropriate laboratory studies may include the following:

- **Liver enzymes.** Hepatocellular injury is marked initially by rises in liver enzymes. Alanine aminotransferase (ALT) and aspartate aminotransferase (AST) are the two most common markers. The ALT level is more specific for liver disease because the AST level also rises with muscle disorders. Alkaline phosphatase (which is also nonspecific) and gamma-glutamyltransferase levels rise—especially with cholestatic disorders. Lactate dehydrogenase is another nonspecific marker of liver injury.
- **Bilirubin.** Elevations in conjugated (direct) bilirubin are found in cholestatic disorders; rises in unconjugated (indirect) bilirubin are seen in hemolytic processes and congenital disorders of bilirubin metabolism.
- **Prothrombin time (PT), albumin, and glucose.** The true "liver function tests" are PT, albumin, and glucose. These studies reflect the synthetic function of the liver.
- **CBC.** The white blood count and platelet counts are useful when certain infections are suspected. The hemoglobin should be closely monitored in hemolytic processes, as well as traumatic hepatic injuries. The CBC is important when oncologic processes are suspected.
- **Reticulocyte count.** The reticulocyte count is diagnostic in hemolytic anemias.
- **Routine blood smear.** Evidence of hemolysis can be also seen on the blood smear. Parasitic diseases like malaria and babesiosis often can be identified on blood smears.
- **Ammonia.** The ammonia level is important in many metabolic disorders as well as in Reye syndrome.
- **Viral serologies.** Serologic studies are confirmatory in cases of many viral infections (e.g., hepatitis A to E, EBV, CMV).
- **Blood cultures.** Blood cultures should be obtained in cases of sepsis or suspected liver abscess.
- **Urinalysis (UA).** Hemoglobinuria is a common finding in hemolytic anemias. Metabolic disorders are sometimes associated with abnormalities on the UA.
- **Plasma amino acids and urine organic acids.** Metabolic studies of the plasma and urine are warranted when metabolic disorders are suspected.

Appropriate ancillary studies may include the following:

- **Ultrasound.** Ultrasound is useful to visualize the anatomy of the liver and surrounding structures noninvasively. Intrahepatic and extrahepatic masses are readily identified, and the anatomy of the biliary tree can be evaluated. Doppler studies add important information about hepatic blood flow.

- **CT scan and MRI scan.** CT and MRI are useful to detect smaller masses and may better delineate among tumors, cysts, and abscesses. CT is the most useful study when liver trauma is a possibility.
- **Radionuclide scan.** Nuclear scintography is excellent in distinguishing hepatitis (impaired liver uptake) from biliary atresia (impaired intestinal excretion).
- **Cholangiography.** Direct visualization of the intrahepatic and extrahepatic biliary tree is possible through cholangiography.
- **Liver biopsy.** Biopsy of the liver is indicated in cases of suspected autoimmune or oncologic processes, metabolic disorders, and anatomic pathologies (e.g., atresia).
- **Bone marrow biopsy.** Bone marrow biopsy is confirmatory in many oncologic and metabolic (e.g., storage) disorders.

TREATMENT OF HEPATOMEGALY

Most patients with hepatomegaly require **supportive care** only. Most importantly, however, it must be ensured that the **synthetic function of the liver is adequate.** Prolongation of the PT, which is seen earlier than decreases in albumin, is treated with vitamin K and, sometimes, fresh-frozen plasma. Albumin infusions are sometimes used for hypoalbuminemia. A "burned-out" liver also loses its ability to maintain satisfactory glucose levels, and these patients must be vigorously supported with glucose infusions.

Additionally, the **cause of the hepatomegaly should be treated** if possible (e.g., antibiotics for infections, antineoplastics for oncologic disorders, surgical management for anatomic disorders). Traumatic liver injuries are usually managed conservatively with **observation,** but surgical intervention is occasionally necessary. **Surgical intervention** is also used in cases of biliary atresia, choledochal cysts, and sometimes liver abscesses.

APPROACH TO THE PATIENT (FIGURES 42-1 AND 42-2)

The approach to hepatomegaly is guided by the patient's acuity and age; neonatal management differs from older infants and children.

- **Acutely ill neonate. Infection** must be considered first and foremost. If infection is likely, broad-spectrum antibiotics are initiated, and then the distinction of bacterial versus viral should be investigated. **Noninfectious causes** that should be considered in an acutely ill neonate include hemolytic, metabolic, congestive, and anatomic abnormalities.

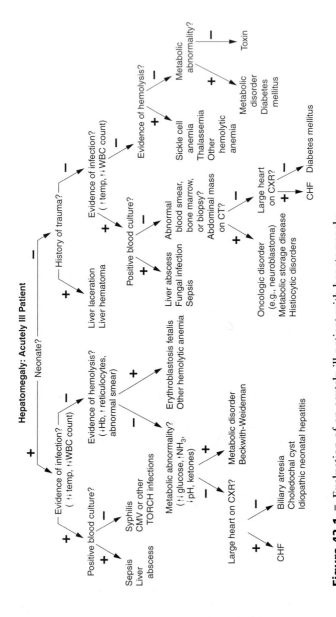

Figure 42-1 ■ Evaluation of an acutely ill patient with hepatomegaly

CHF = congestive heart failure; CMV = cytomegalovirus; CT = computed tomography; CXR = chest radiograph; Hb = hemoglobin; NH₃ = ammonia; TORCH = toxoplasmosis, other infections (congenital syphilis and viruses), rubella, cytomegalovirus, herpes simplex; WBC = white blood cell

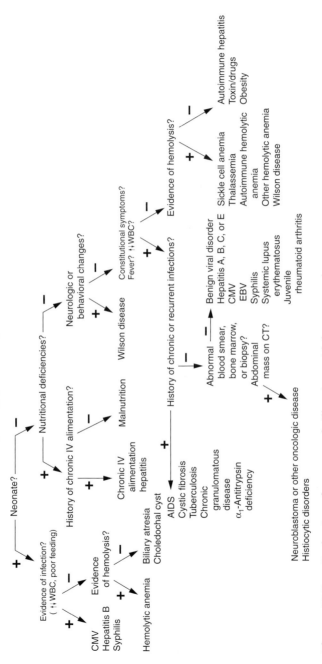

Figure 42-2 ■ Evaluation of a nonacutely ill patient with hepatomegaly

CMV = cytomegalovirus; CT = computed tomography; EBV = Epstein-Barr virus; IV = intravenous; WBC = white blood cell

- **Acutely ill older infant or child.** Beyond the neonatal age groups, oncologic, metabolic and toxic causes must also be considered.
- **Nonacutely ill neonate.** Bacterial sepsis is unlikely, whereas **viral causes** and **syphilis** are more common. Hemolytic anemias and anatomic causes are likely considerations in a nonacutely ill neonate with hepatosplenomegaly but no evidence of infection. Importantly, **biliary atresia** is a serious diagnosis that should be made swiftly because surgical correction is most likely to be successful in the first few months of life. Clues to this diagnosis include a conjugated hyperbilirubinemia, elevated liver enzymes, and acholic stools in a relatively well-appearing infant.
- **Nonacutely ill older infant or child.** Viral hepatitis is one of the most common diagnoses, but many other possibilities need to be eliminated first. Toxic, hemolytic, and oncologic causes are not uncommon, and nutritional, rheumatologic, and metabolic disorders are also possible.

Suggested Readings

De Kerguenec C, Hillaire S, Molinie V, et al.: Hepatic manifestations of hemophagocytic syndrome. *Am J Gastroenterol* 96:852–857, 2001.

Elisofon SA, Jonas MM: Hepatitis B and C in children: current treatment and future strategies. *Clin Liver Dis* 10(1):133–148, 2006.

Emerick KM, Whitington PF: Neonatal liver disease. *Pediatr Ann* 35(4):280–286, 2006.

Lee CK, Jonas MM: Pediatric hepatobiliary disease. *Curr Opin Gastroenterol* 23(3):306–309, 2007.

Lipton JM, Westra S, Haverty CE, et al.: Case records of the Massachusetts General Hospital. Weekly clinicopathological exercises. Case 28-2004. Newborn twins with thrombocytopenia, coagulation defects, and hepatosplenomegaly. *N Engl J Med* 351(11): 1120–1130, 2004.

Misra S, Ament ME, Vargas JH, et al.: Chronic liver disease in children on long-term parenteral nutrition. *J Gastroenterol Hepatol* 11:S4–S6, 1996.

Smith K: Hepatomegaly. *Clin Pediatr* 44(9):813–814, 2005.

Troy SB, Rickman LS, Davis CE: Brucellosis in San Diego: epidemiology and species-related differences in acute clinical presentations. *Medicine* 84(3):174–187, 2005.

Wolf AD, Lavine JE: Hepatomegaly in neonates and children. *Pediatr Rev* 21:303–310, 2000.

chapter 43

Hypertension

Christine B. Sethna and Kevin E. C. Meyers

INTRODUCTION

- **Normotension** is defined as blood pressure (BP) (systolic, diastolic, or both) that is ≤90th percentile for the patient's age, height percentile, and sex.
- **Prehypertension** is defined as BP levels ≥90th percentile but <95th percentile.
- **Hypertension** is defined as average systolic and/or diastolic BP ≥95th percentile for gender, age, and height on three or more separate occasions.
  - **Stage 1 hypertension** is the designation for BP levels that range from the 95th percentile to 5 mm Hg >99th percentile.
  - **Stage 2 hypertension** is the designation for BP levels >5 mm Hg above the 99th percentile.
  - **Labile blood pressure** refers to BP (systolic, diastolic, or both) that is sometimes above and sometimes below the 95th percentile and **does not result in hypertensive damage to organs.** Labile blood pressure is frequently found in teenagers.
  - **White coat hypertension** is present when elevated BP readings are found in a medical setting with normal BPs measured elsewhere.
  - **Hypertensive urgency** is severely elevated BP with no evidence of secondary end-organ damage.
  - **Hypertensive emergency** is severely elevated BP with clinical evidence for **end-organ damage** (retinopathy, papilledema, encephalopathy, seizures, cardiac failure, or renal insufficiency).
- Hypertension in the pediatric population is estimated to be between 1% and 5%.
- Younger children are more likely to have an underlying cause for hypertension than adolescents and adults. However, primary (essential) hypertension is now seen in children and adolescents and is associated with obesity, metabolic syndrome, and a family history of hypertension.

> **HINT:** The younger the patient and the higher the blood pressure, the more likely a secondary cause for hypertension will be found.

DIFFERENTIAL DIAGNOSIS LIST 🔒

Primary Hypertension (Essential Hypertension)

Monogenetic Causes
Gordon syndrome
Liddle syndrome
Syndrome of apparent mineralocorticoid excess (AME)
Glucocorticoid remediable aldosteronism (GRA)

Renoparenchymal Causes
Glomerulonephritis—acute and chronic
Hemolytic uremic syndrome
Focal segmental glomerulosclerosis
Lupus nephritis
Pyelonephritis (acute or chronic) or reflux nephropathy
Polycystic kidney disease— autosomal recessive, autosomal dominant
Wilms tumor
Obstructive uropathy
Trauma

Vascular Causes
Coarctation of the aorta
Large arteriovenous fistula
Midaortic syndrome (idiopathic, Williams syndrome, NF-1, Takayasu arteritis)
Renal artery stenosis (fibromuscular dysplasia)
Renal artery thrombosis
Renal venous thrombosis

Endocrine Causes
Cushing syndrome
Hyperthyroidism or hypothyroidism
Hyperparathyroidism
Pheochromocytoma
Neuroblastoma
Congenital adrenal hyperplasia
Conn syndrome (hyperaldosteronism)

Neurologic Causes
Traumatic brain injury
Intracranial hemorrhage (epidural, subdural, subarachnoid)
Increased intracranial pressure
Familial dysautonomia
Guillain-Barré syndrome
Pain

Drug-Related Causes
Corticosteroids
Calcineurin inhibitors
Epinephrine
Cocaine
Amphetamines
Sympathomimetics
Oral contraceptives
Caffeine
Cyclosporin

Miscellaneous Causes
Stress
Orthopedic traction
Burns
"White coat" hypertension
Malignant hyperthermia
Acute intermittent porphyria

APPROACH TO THE PATIENT

History

- Hypertension is **often asymptomatic.** If symptoms are present they may include headache, blurry vision, epistaxis, chest pain, flushing, fatigue, and difficulty sleeping.
- **Neonatal history**—history of umbilical artery catheter placement, neonatal asphyxia, bronchopulmonary dysplasia.
- **Renal disease**—history of renoparenchymal disease or symptoms of gross hematuria or edema.
- **Urinary tract infections** can be associated with reflux nephropathy or renal scars.
- **Family history**—hypertension, obesity, familial endocrinopathies, renal disease.
- Assess for history of **obesity** or **metabolic syndrome.**
- **Medications.**
- **Pheochromocytoma** and **neuroblastoma** may present with sweating, flushing, palpitations, or abdominal pain.

Physical Examination

- Systolic, diastolic, and mean BP should be obtained in the upper extremity at the level of the heart while calm.

> **HINT:** Falsely high readings stem from using a cuff that is too small. The cuff should cover two thirds of the upper arm from the tip of the acromion to the elbow, and the bladder width should cover 80% to 100% of the circumference of the arm.

- BP should be checked in all four extremities and femoral pulses should be palpated to rule out coarctation of the aorta.
- **Stigmata for syndromes**—café au lait, neurofibromas, malar rash, acanthosis, moon facies, short stature, obesity, virilization, ambiguous genitalia, proptosis, thyromegaly.
- **Other**—retinal changes seen on funduscopic examination, abdominal bruit, heart murmur, gallop, Bell palsy.

Evaluation

- A **24 hour ambulatory blood pressure** monitoring may be helpful to diagnose white coat hypertension, masked hypertension, or labile hypertension.
- Laboratory studies should include complete blood count, urinalysis, urine culture, serum electrolytes, blood urea nitrogen, serum creatinine, and fasting lipid profile.

TABLE 43-1 Commonly Used Antihypertensive Agents in Children

Category	Agent	Common Side Effects
Diuretics	Chlorothiazides	Hypokalemia, hypochloremic alkalosis, volume depletion, hyperuricemia, hyperlipidemia, hyperglycemia,
	Furosemide	Volume depletion, hypokalemia, alkalosis, nephrocalcinosis
	Spironolactone	Hyperkalemia, mild acidosis, gynecomastia
	Eplerenone	Hyperkalemia, mild acidosis
Vasodilators	Hydralazine	Flushing, tachycardia, headaches
	Minoxidil	Hypotension, hirsutism
β blockers	Atenolol	Bronchospasm, hypoglycemia
	Labetalol	Bronchospasm, hypotension, tingling in skin or scalp, headache
Calcium channel blockers	Nifedipine	Hypotension, peripheral edema, elevated liver enzymes
	Amlodipine	Peripheral edema, flushing, palpitations
	Diltiazem	Flushing
ACE inhibitors	Captopril, Enalapril, Lisinopril, Benazepril	Hyperkalemia, dry cough, increase in serum creatinine, angioedema
ATIIR blockers	Losartan, Valsartan, Candesartan, Irbesartan	Hyperkalemia, increase in serum creatinine
Renin inhibitors	Aliskiren	Hyperkalemia

ACE = angiotensin-converting enzyme; ATIIR = angiotensin II receptor

- Ultrasound studies include renal ultrasound and echocardiogram.
- Further evaluation is based on history, physical examination, and/or to prove secondary causes: **voiding cystourethrogram, nuclear renal scan, 3D computed tomography angiography** or **magnetic resonance angiography,** serum metanephrines, plasma renin activity, and aldosterone level.
- More extensive studies include renal angiogram, metaiodobenzyl-guanidine scan, renal biopsy, and genetic studies for monogenetic causes of hypertension.

Treatment

- **Hypertensive emergencies** should be treated with intravenous blood pressure medications, aiming to decrease the blood pressure by 25% over the first 8 hours and gradually normalizing blood pressure over 24 to 48 hours.
- **Hypertensive urgencies** can be treated by either intravenous or oral antihypertensives depending on symptomatology.
- **Mild primary hypertension** may be managed with nonpharmacologic treatment: weight reduction, exercise, and sodium restriction.

■ **Pharmacologic therapy** should be directed to the cause of secondary hypertension when this is known or for severe, sustained primary or secondary hypertension. Chronic oral antihypertensive pharmacologic therapy is generally required for sustained primary or secondary hypertension. Medications may be needed in children with mild-to-moderate hypertension if nonpharmacologic therapy has failed or if end-organ changes are present.

■ The physician should be familiar with potential medication interactions and side effects (Table 43-1). Drug doses should be maximized prior to adding a second agent.

Suggested Readings

Feld L, Corey H: Hypertension in childhood. *Pediatr Rev* 28(8):283–298, 2007.

National Heart, Lung, and Blood Institute: The fourth report on the diagnosis, evaluation and treatment of high blood pressure in children and adolescents. *Pediatrics* 114(2):S555–576, 2004.

Portman R, McNiece K, Swinford R, et al.: Pediatric hypertension: diagnosis, evaluation, management, and treatment for the primary care physician. *Curr Probl Pediatr Adolesc Health Care* 35(7):262–294, 2005.

Portman R, Sorof J, Ingelfinger J (eds): *Pediatric Hypertension*. Totowa, NJ, Humana Press, 2004.

44

Hypotonia

Courtney J. Wusthoff
Douglas J. Hyder (Third Edition)

INTRODUCTION

Hypotonia is defined as **abnormally low resting muscle tone.** It primarily manifests as **decreased resistance to passive movement and abnormalities in resting posture.** Hypotonia most commonly presents in infancy (often called **"floppy babies"**), although low tone may present acutely with a variety of illnesses at any age.

The first task when confronted with a patient with possible hypotonia is to **differentiate decreased tone from weakness or lethargy.** Likewise, hyporeflexia is a separate finding with a distinct differential diagnosis.

A careful history and physical examination, including a thorough neurological examination, frequently narrows the differential diagnosis enough to necessitate only confirmatory diagnostic tests, sparing the patient a shotgun approach including unnecessary and often painful, costly, or invasive procedures.

DIFFERENTIAL DIAGNOSIS LIST

In Infants

Central Hypotonia

Infection (e.g., sepsis, meningitis, encephalitis)

Genetic abnormalities (e.g., Down syndrome, Prader-Willi syndrome, fragile X)

Metabolic disease (e.g., leukodystrophy, glycogen storage disease)

Trauma (e.g., birth trauma, nonaccidental trauma)

Hypoxic ischemic encephalopathy (e.g., decreased perinatal perfusion)

Vascular (e.g., stroke, intracranial hemorrhage)

Anatomic (e.g., congenital brain malformations)

Drug/toxin (e.g., narcotics)

Other causes (e.g., benign congenital hypotonia, hypothyroidism)

Peripheral Hypotonia

Spinal muscular atrophy

Nerve injury (e.g., brachial plexus injury)

Myasthenia gravis

Medications/toxins (e.g., botulinum toxin, hypermagnesemia)

Congenital myopathies

Congenital myotonic dystrophy

In Children

Central Hypotonia

Infection (e.g., sepsis, encephalitis)

Metabolic disease (e.g., adrenoleukodystrophy, glycogen storage disease)

Neoplasm (e.g., brain tumor, infiltrative neoplasm)
Vascular (e.g., stroke)
Toxins/electrolyte abnormalities (e.g., ingestion)
Peripheral Hypotonia
Spinal muscular atrophy
Infection (e.g., myositis)

Trauma (e.g., nerve injury)
Neuropathy (e.g., Charcot-Marie-Tooth disease)
Guillain-Barré syndrome
Myasthenia gravis
Muscular dystrophy
Dermatomyositis
Tick paralysis

DIFFERENTIAL DIAGNOSIS DISCUSSION

Most "floppy babies" do not have hypotonia of a neurological etiology but are weak and/or lethargic from other causes, such as infection or dehydration. Likewise, older children with focal "decreased tone" can actually be manifesting orthopedic problems or joint laxity. The first step in considering the differential diagnosis of hypotonia for any patient, therefore, is to consider the possibility of nonneurological illness.

> **HINT:** The two most common pitfalls in diagnosing hypotonia are confusing weakness or lethargy for hypotonia and assuming a neurological etiology, without consideration for nonneurological causes.

Once careful history and physical examination confirm that the problem is truly hypotonia, the next step is to determine localization in the neuraxis (see later). Central hypotonia is caused by problems in the central nervous system; peripheral hypotonia is related to disturbance somewhere at the level of the spinal cord, nerve, neuromuscular junction, or muscle. There are myriad causes of hypotonia, and a full differential is often beyond the scope of the general pediatrician. Distinguishing central from peripheral hypotonia, however, is easily accomplished during the initial evaluation and can help guide appropriate evaluation and referral (see Table 44-1).

TABLE 44-1 Features of Central Versus Peripheral Hypotonia

	Central Hypotonia	Peripheral Hypotonia
History	Encephalopathy	Joint contractures
	Hypoxic ischemic injury	Normal mental status
	Seizures	No seizures
Examination	No weakness	Muscle weakness
	Dysmorphic features	Sensory deficits
	Normal or brisk reflexes	Diminished or absent reflexes

The differential diagnosis differs extensively between infants and children >1 year of age; therefore, they are divided accordingly here. Selected diagnoses are described here, but the full differential is extensive and beyond the scope of this book.

INFANTS

Central Hypotonia

Etiology and Clinical Features

Central hypotonia is caused by problems in the **central nervous system** (i.e., the brain or upper motor neurons in spinal cord). Tone abnormalities are **global,** involving the whole body, and often accompanied by **encephalopathy,** or altered mental status. Seizures and sleep/wake cycle disturbances also may suggest a central problem. Babies with central hypotonia have low resting tone but usually have **preserved strength** when they do make effort with their limbs. The numerous causes of central hypotonia may be grouped into larger categories.

- **Infection.** Consider sepsis, meningitis, encephalitis, and (toxoplasmosis, other, rubella, cytomegalovirus, herpes simplex (TORCH) infections.
- **Genetic abnormalities.** A number of genetic syndromes include hypotonia as a presenting feature in the neonatal period, even before dysmorphic features or other affected organs might be apparent. Important and common syndromes include:
  - **Trisomy 21** (Down syndrome) is the most commonly observed chromosomal abnormality, occurring in approximately 1 in 1,000 births. Children with Down syndrome have characteristic facial features, dermatoglyphic and hand abnormalities, and are at higher risk for cardiac and gastrointestinal (GI) defects.
  - **Prader-Willi syndrome** is usually the result of a paternally inherited deletion in chromosome 15. Affected neonates have severe hypotonia, feeding difficulties, and failure to thrive. Mental retardation, hypogonadism, and hyperphagia with obesity become prominent features later in childhood.
  - **Turner syndrome** is caused by the 45 X0 genotype, occurring in 1 in 5,000 infants. It only occurs in females, who also may have short stature, broad chest, webbed neck, hearing loss, and coarctation of the aorta.
  - **Fragile X syndrome** is caused by increased triplet nucleotide repeat in the region of the FMR1 gene. Although girls may present with a milder phenotype, the profound symptoms seen in infancy are usually only seen in boys. Mental retardation and autism are prominent features.
- **Metabolic disease.** A host of inborn errors of metabolism can cause hypotonia. This category should be suspected particularly in patients who are initially asymptomatic but fall ill after initiation of feeding

or during intercurrent illness. Developmental regression raises special concern for metabolic disease. If metabolic disorders are suspected, a neurologist or geneticist with expertise in metabolic disorders should be consulted because effective dietary or gene replacement therapy is available for some conditions.

- **Trauma.** Birth trauma and the possibility of subsequent nonaccidental trauma must always be considered and evaluated by appropriate imaging. Spinal cord trauma, as in complicated delivery, may cause spinal shock, signaled by autonomic changes and acute deficits in bladder and bowel function; immediate neurological consultation is indicated.
- **Hypoxic ischemic encephalopathy** can result from any impairment in oxygenation and blood flow to the brain. This may include difficult delivery or be secondary to other disease, such as respiratory or cardiac failure.
- **Vascular insults.** Neonatal stroke may include arterial ischemic stroke, venous sinus thrombosis, and intracranial hemorrhage. Each of these may include focal symptoms that are mild and much less obvious than global hypotonia.
- **Anatomic abnormalities.** Neuroimaging may reveal congenital anomalies in brain and/or cord development causing hypotonia.
- **Drugs/Toxins.** Medications given to the mother prior to delivery, particularly **narcotics, sedatives, and magnesium (to prevent preterm labor),** may lead to congenital hypotonia.
- **Other causes.** Benign congenital hypotonia is a diagnosis of exclusion. These children initially present with hypotonia in the newborn period or first months of life. Because motor milestones are so important in infancy, they may present with developmental delay but catch up by early childhood. Hypotonia usually resolves in the first years of life but can persist into adulthood. **Hypothyroidism** is treatable if identified early so must always enter the differential.

Peripheral Hypotonia

Etiology and Clinical Features

Peripheral hypotonia is caused by problems at the level of the lower motor neuron, nerve, muscle, or neuromuscular junction. The characteristic findings are preserved mental status, accompanying weakness, and decreased or absent deep tendon reflexes.

- **Spinal muscular atrophy (SMA)** is the result of a mutation in the SMN1 gene on chromosome 5p. Affected patients have progressive degeneration of anterior horn cells. SMA type I (Werdnig-Hoffmann disease) may present as early as the newborn period with hypotonia and weakness, and it progresses in the first year of life to include weakness of facial muscles. Tongue fasciculation may be present.

The disease is universally fatal; although treatment trials show promise, supportive care is the current standard.

- **Nerve injuries** can lead to focal hypotonia and weakness. The most common type in neonates is brachial plexus injury (**Erb palsy**). It is caused by stretching of the nerves of the brachial plexus. This may occur with difficult deliveries of macrosomic neonates, especially if traction on the head or arm is required. The affected arm is adducted and internally rotated, with the forearm extended and the wrist flexed. The diagnosis is made clinically and may be confirmed with nerve conduction studies (NCS) and electromyography (EMG).

- **Myasthenia gravis** occurs when **antibodies against the acetylcholine** receptor cause blockade of signal transmission at the **neuromuscular junction.** Antibodies are transferred from the affected mother in 10% of neonates born to mothers with myasthenia gravis. Other forms of **congenital myasthenia** also result from impaired neuromuscular junction signaling and can be caused by a genetic defect in receptor, synaptic vesicle, or enzyme production. The diagnosis may be made via Tensilon test, nerve conduction studies with electromyography, and serum testing for specific antibodies.

- **Medications/toxins** may act on the nerves, muscles, or neuromuscular junction to cause hypotonia. A well-known example is **botulinum toxin.** In infants, disease is produced by an enteric-toxin mechanism (as opposed to ingestion of preformed toxin in tainted food seen in older children and adults). Spores of *Clostridium botulinum* may be ingested in contaminated honey, but they are also often ingested during contact with contaminated soil, as in homes near construction, or when parents have been involved in labor in contaminated soil. Germination leads to toxin production in the immature GI tract, which produces constipation. Absorption of toxin leads to disease, often beginning with diplopia and followed by progressive bulbar and extremity weakness. Pupils do not constrict in response to light, a characteristic finding that helps distinguish botulism from other causes of hypotonia. Diagnosis is made with NCS/EMG and detection of organism or toxin in stool sample. Treatment includes aggressive supportive care in the intensive care unit, avoidance of aminoglycoside antibiotics, and use of botulinal antitoxin.

- **Congenital myopathies** include central core and nemaline rod myopathy. Decreased muscle bulk and abnormal creatine kinase (CK) are suggestive of these diseases.

- **Congenital myotonic dystrophy.** Myotonic dystrophy is an inherited condition demonstrating anticipation. Affected mothers may only demonstrate weak handshake, mild facial diplegia, or prolonged labor, but their children may be much more severely affected, with arthrogryposis and profound weakness, including the need for mechanical ventilation.

IN CHILDREN

Although some of the disease categories in children are similar to infants, important differences are highlighted here.

Central Hypotonia

- **Infection.** Encephalitis should be considered if encephalopathy is a feature.
- **Metabolic disease.** Although many metabolic diseases present in infancy, several storage diseases do not become apparent until later in life. History of developmental regression, or repeated encephalopathy or profound weakness in times of illness, suggest this category.
- **Neoplasm.** In addition to brain tumor, infiltrative neoplasms of the spinal cord may cause hypotonia.
- **Vascular insults.** These include spinal cord infarction.
- **Toxin/electrolyte abnormalities.** Ingestions of medications, recreational drugs, and toxins can cause subacute onset of hypotonia. Inhalants should also be considered if encephalopathy occurs. Lead poisoning, although decreased in recent decades, remains of concern.

Peripheral Hypotonia

- **Spinal muscular atrophy,** types II and III, present later in life than Werdnig-Hoffmann disease (type I). Type II presents in toddlers; type III has a mean onset of 9 years of age. Each may present with weakness, most notably in the proximal muscles, as well as difficulty with motor skills. NCS and EMG or genetic testing can make the diagnosis.
- **Infection.** Although rare in infants, myositis in children can cause myalgias, weakness, and hypotonia.
- **Trauma.** A careful history can reveal recent trauma causing focal nerve injury in the area affected by hypotonia.
- **Neuropathy.** Hereditary neuropathy, such as Charcot-Marie-Tooth disease, can cause mild, diffuse hypotonia. Acquired neuropathy caused by toxins or infection (such as HIV) is also considered when sensory or motor deficits are present.
- **Guillain-Barré syndrome** is an parainfectious, autoimmune disease that causes demyelination of the peripheral nerves. Ascending, progressive weakness typically develops approximately 2 weeks following mild flu-like or GI illness. Paresthesias are also common. Cerebrospinal fluid (CSF) abnormalities with elevated protein and no leukocytosis may aid the diagnosis, but findings may not be seen until the second week of symptoms or later. NCS/EMG testing can also be helpful. Supportive treatment is essential, and the disease course may be modified with intravenous immunoglobulin.

- Myasthenia gravis is caused by **acetylcholine receptor antibodies** as described earlier. In children, myasthenia gravis is an acquired illness caused by the production of **autoantibodies.** Children have both hypotonia and fluctuating weakness, usually **worsened by activity** or at the end of the day.
- Muscular dystrophy is of many types and can present in childhood. Progressive weakness and decreased muscle bulk are clues toward this diagnosis.
- Dermatomyositis is an autoimmune illness with characteristic rash, myalgias, and weakness. The weakness comes in flares; diagnosis is aided by skin findings, elevation of CK, and abnormal erythrocyte sedimentation rate.
- Tick paralysis occurs when the patient has a tick attached to the affected limb. Careful inspection of skin reveals the causative insect, and removal results in quick recovery.

APPROACH TO THE PATIENT

Conditions that are amenable to rapid treatment (e.g., electrolyte imbalance, infection) must be excluded and treated first. Correction removes complicating factors from further evaluation and may even relieve symptoms alone.

Stabilization of the patient is the highest priority. A number of central and peripheral causes of hypotonia have the potential for rapid progression and life-threatening consequences. Constant attention must be paid to airway stabilization and respiratory function because these are commonly impaired in diseases causing hypotonia.

After the patient is stable, the evaluation may proceed as described next. Because the differential diagnosis of hypotonia is broad, care should be taken to ascertain all of the historical facts and to perform a complete examination. A neurology consult is generally necessary to help narrow the differential diagnosis after the preliminary categorization is performed.

EVALUATION OF HYPOTONIA

Patient History

- When did the symptoms first appear?
- Are the symptoms worsening or staying the same?
- Was the onset acute or gradual? Paroxysmal onset suggests an acute event, such as stroke or trauma. Ingestion or infection is more likely to be subacute; metabolic and degenerative diseases have more chronic progressions.
- Where are the symptoms? Clarify if the problem is global or affects only one limb.

- Are there any associated symptoms? Multisystem disease should raise the suspicion for a genetic syndrome. Encephalopathy points toward central hypotonia. Sensory deficits suggest nerve disease.
- What is the birth history? Decreased fetal movements prior to birth suggest problems existing before delivery. Prematurity should adjust the examiner's expectations for normal tone and strength. Traumatic delivery can point toward brachial plexus injury. Acidotic cord blood gas, neonatal seizures, and other evidence of birth depression may support hypoxic-ischemic encephalopathy.
- Is there a family history of hypotonia, nerve, or muscle problems? Affected parents may have a milder phenotype, so hereditary neuropathies or muscle disease may have never been diagnosed.

Physical Examination

In addition to a general physical examination, special care should be taken with the following points:

- Mental status—altered mental status strongly supports a central cause of hypotonia.
- Posture of trunk and extremities—the most accurate examination is performed with the child awake, relaxed, and (in infants) the head at midline. In older children, low truncal tone may manifest as slumped posture or poor head control.
- A "frog-leg" position (i.e., hips abducted, flexed, and externally rotated) is seen in hypotonic infants.
- Head lag when the infant is pulled from a supine to sitting position supports the diagnosis of hypotonia.
- Vertical suspension should be performed in all infants; in the hypotonic infant, there is a tendency to slip through the examiner's hands when held under the axillae.
- Horizontal suspension results in a hypotonic infant draping over the examiner's hands, rather than holding the head and extremities up in the air ("inverted comma sign").
- Muscle bulk, when decreased, is concerning for primary muscle disease.
- Fasciculations are concerning for SMA.
- Deep tendon reflexes are more likely to be normal or brisk in central hypotonia, diminished or absent in peripheral hypotonia.

Laboratory Studies

Care should be taken to gather as much information as possible with the history and physical examination before proceeding with laboratory assessment. **Complete blood count and urinalysis** can be helpful in evaluating for infection. **Metabolic panel, bilirubin level** (in infants), and **thyroid function** testing can be helpful screening tests. If metabolic disease is suspected, serum amino acids, urine organic acids, and ammonia levels can be helpful screens. Newborn screen results should be obtained. Creatine phosphokinase can indicate muscle disease. CSF analysis can indicate infection or an autoimmune disease, such as Guillain-Barré syndrome. Chromosome analysis is helpful if genetic disease is suspected.

Diagnostic Modalities

- NCS and EMG are helpful in peripheral hypotonia and may even be diagnostic.
- Magnetic resonance imaging of the brain can identify structural abnormalities, vascular lesions, and evidence of genetic or metabolic disease in central hypotonia.
- Muscle ultrasound can help identify myopathic changes and identify those patients who might benefit from muscle biopsy.

Suggested Readings

Chen C, Visootsak J, Dills S, et al.: Prader-Willi syndrome: an update and review for the primary pediatrician. *Clin Pediatr* 46:580–591, 2007.

Cherington M: Clinical spectrum of botulism. *Muscle Nerve* 21:701–710, 1998.

Dubowitz V: Evaluation and differential diagnosis of the hypotonic infant. *Pediatr Rev* 6:237–243, 1985.

McNeely PD, Drake JM: A systematic review of brachial plexus surgery for birth-related injury. *Pediatr Neurosurg* 38:57–62, 2003.

Paro-Panjan D, Neubauer D: Congenital hypotonia: is there an algorithm? *J Child Neurol* 19:439–442, 2004.

Petersen MC, Palmer FB: Advances in prevention and treatment of cerebral palsy. *Ment Retard Dev Disabil Res Rev* 7:30–37, 2001.

Stiefel L: Hypotonia in infants. *Pediatr Rev* 17:104–105, 1996.

Thompson CE: Benign congenital hypotonia is not a diagnosis. *Dev Med Child Neurol* 44:283–284, 2002.

Thompson JA, Filloux FM, Van Orman CB, et al.: Infant botulism in the age of botulism immune globulin. *Neurology* 64: 2029–2032, 2005.

Jaundice *

James M. Callahan

INTRODUCTION

Jaundice (icterus) is a **yellow discoloration** of the skin, mucous membranes, and sclerae caused by **increased levels of circulating bilirubin.** Jaundice signals either increased production or decreased elimination of bilirubin.

The major source of bilirubin is the breakdown of heme pigment released from degraded red blood cells (RBCs). Normally, the liver clears bilirubin from the circulation via conjugation, and then the bilirubin is excreted in bile and eliminated in the feces. **Hemolytic processes and diseases affecting the liver** are the major causes of jaundice.

DIFFERENTIAL DIAGNOSIS LIST

Unconjugated Hyperbilirubinemia
Hemolytic Causes
Hemoglobinopathies
RBC defects
Autoimmune hemolytic anemia
Wilson disease (mixed conjugated and unconjugated)
Hepatic Disorders
Gilbert syndrome
Crigler-Najjar syndrome (types 1 and 2)

Conjugated Hyperbilirubinemia
Infectious Causes
Viral infections—hepatitis A to E, cytomegalovirus infection, Epstein-Barr virus (EBV) infection

Bacterial infections—sepsis, liver abscess, pneumonia, peritonitis
Toxic Causes
Amanita mushrooms
Carbon tetrachloride and other solvents
Medications
Total parenteral nutrition
Metabolic or Genetic Causes
α_1-Antitrypsin (α_1-AT) deficiency
Wilson disease
Cystic fibrosis
Hemochromatosis (primary or secondary)
Inflammatory Causes
Autoimmune hepatitis
Primary sclerosing cholangitis

---

*The most common causes of jaundice in infants <3 months of age are described in Chapter 46, "Jaundice, Newborn." Jaundice in children >3 months is always pathologic.

Vascular Causes
 Budd-Chiari syndrome
 Veno-occlusive disease
Miscellaneous Causes
 Biliary tract disorders—
  cholangitis, cholecystitis,

choledochal cyst,
 cholelithiasis
Pancreatic disease
Kawasaki syndrome
Rare hepatic disorders

> **HINT:** If a toddler or an older child presents with yellowish discoloration of the skin, one must first determine whether jaundice actually exists. Children who eat a large amount of yellow, orange, or red vegetables or fruits can develop keratodermia (owing to ingestion of carotene-containing vegetables) or lycopenemia (owing to ingestion of certain red foods, such as tomatoes). In both conditions, the child is healthy, active, and without other significant findings. In these conditions, the sclerae remain white and the serum bilirubin levels are within normal limits.

DIFFERENTIAL DIAGNOSIS DISCUSSION

Hemolytic Processes

A complete discussion of hemoglobinopathies, RBC defects, and autoimmune hemolytic anemia can be found in Chapter 40, "Hemolysis."

Gilbert Disease and Crigler-Najjar Syndrome

In the absence of hemolysis, **unconjugated hyperbilirubinemia in older children is usually attributable to a relative deficiency in glucuronyl transferase** and the resulting decrease in conjugation of bilirubin seen in Gilbert and Crigler-Najjar syndromes. Gilbert syndrome is diagnosed much more often in older children and adults than it is in infants. Patients with Gilbert syndrome present with a benign increase in unconjugated bilirubin, caused by a mild decrease in uridine diphosphate-glucuronosyltransferase (UDPGT) activity. Crigler-Najjar syndrome is an autosomal recessive disorder caused by mutations in the UDPGT gene. Patients with the most severe form of Crigler-Najjar syndrome require either lifelong phototherapy or liver transplantation to prevent kernicterus. Table 45-1 compares Gilbert and Crigler-Najjar syndromes.

Hepatitis

Etiology

The **most common cause of conjugated hyperbilirubinemia in older infants and children is an acute viral infection that causes hepatitis.** Hepatitis A, B, C, D, and E viruses are agents that specifically attack

TABLE 45-1 Defects in Hepatic Bilirubin Conjugation

Disease	Degree of Hyperbilirubinemia	Defect	Genetics
Gilbert disease	Mild (usually <5 mg/dL; may increase with intercurrent viral illnesses)	Underactivity of UDPGT, defective uptake of albumin-bound bilirubin from the plasma	Autosomal recessive
Crigler-Najjar syndrome			
Type I	Marked (usually 25–35 mg/dL; patients at risk of kernicterus)	Complete absence of UDPGT activity	Autosomal recessive
Type II	Moderate (usually <20 mg/dL; usually decreases rapidly with phenobarbital therapy)	Partial absence of the UDPGT activity (less severe than type I)	Autosomal recessive

UDPGT = uridine diphosphate-glucuronosyltransferase

the liver. **Hepatitis A virus (HAV)** and **hepatitis E virus (HEV,** mainly found in developing countries) are usually passed by the fecal-oral route; child-care center outbreaks of hepatitis A are not unusual.

Clinical Features

HAV is the most common cause of foodborne hepatitis in the United States. It usually has a **2- to 6-week incubation period.** A preicteric phase characterized by **fever, headache, malaise, and abdominal complaints** (e.g., abdominal pain, nausea, vomiting, anorexia) may last up to 5 days. This phase is followed by the appearance of **dark urine and frank icterus,** usually as the fever begins to resolve (although children <3 years may never develop jaundice). There is usually **hepatomegaly and right upper quadrant tenderness.** Other symptoms tend to lessen as the jaundice resolves (which may take as long as 1 month). **Complete resolution** without the development of chronic liver disease or a chronic carrier state **is characteristic.** However, **occasional patients** may **progress to liver failure and even death.**

Hepatitis B is usually **transmitted parenterally via contaminated blood products or by sexual contact with an infected person.** Hepatitis B may also be transmitted **vertically in the perinatal period.** The incubation period is longer than for hepatitis A **(2 to 6 months).** There is a preicteric and an icteric phase in this illness, as with hepatitis A. The **preicteric phase** may be accompanied by **rash, arthritis, arthralgia, and even urticaria.** Late sequelae include **fulminant hepatitis, hepatic necrosis, cirrhosis, and hepatocellular carcinoma. Chronic carrier states** and **chronic active hepatitis** are occasionally seen after infection with hepatitis B virus (HBV). The **younger the patient** is at the time of infection, the **higher the likelihood of development of chronic infection**—infants infected at the time of delivery have a 60% to 90% risk of developing a chronic infection.

Hepatitis C constitutes most of what was previously called non-A, non-B hepatitis. It is **transmitted parenterally or through sexual contact.** Previously most pediatric hepatitis C infections occurred in children who had received blood products prior to 1992 when universal screening for this virus in the blood supply was introduced. These children would now be in late adolescence. **Hepatitis C may also be transmitted vertically, which is now the most common mode of acquisition in pediatric patients.** Cases of hepatitis C are documented in teenage patients who have received **tattoos** and who use **intranasal crack cocaine** (because of sharing of glass paraphernalia). Intranasal crack cocaine use may also be associated with HBV infection. The **incubation period is 1 to 5 months,** and the disease usually has an insidious onset and produces a **mild clinical illness.** Jaundice occurs in only 25% of patients. Infection with hepatitis C virus (HCV) is associated with **chronic liver disease and a chronic carrier state,** and it may lead to **cirrhosis or hepatocellular carcinoma.**

Hepatitis D occurs only as a **coinfection or superinfection** in patients with **acute or chronic disease secondary to HBV infection. Except for perinatal transmission,** hepatitis D virus is **acquired similarly to HBV.** The **incubation period is 3 weeks to 3 months.** The **onset is usually acute,** and the symptoms are usually more severe than with hepatitis B. A **chronic carrier state, chronic hepatitis, or cirrhosis** may develop, and the **mortality rate is higher than with hepatitis B** alone.

Hepatitis E is usually benign, although there has been a **high fatality rate in pregnant women** infected with HEV. HEV is mainly seen in **developing countries with poor sanitation.**

Evaluation

When viral hepatitis is suspected, **evaluation to determine the causative agent** is appropriate. A **history of exposures** (e.g., shellfish [hepatitis A], blood transfusions [hepatitis B] or sexual activity or parenteral drug use) may guide testing.

Testing for **IgM antibody to hepatitis A, hepatitis B surface antigen (HBsAg),** and **IgM antibody to hepatitis B core antigen (IgM-HBcAg),** as well as for **EBV** and possible **noninfectious causes,** is indicated. **Hepatic transaminases** (alanine aminotransferase, aspartate aminotransferase), **gamma-glutamyltransferase,** and the **prothrombin time** should be obtained and monitored.

- During infection with HAV, hepatic transaminase levels peak at about the time that jaundice appears. Hepatitis A antibody is present at the onset of disease. IgM antibody predominates initially, but within several months, it is completely replaced by IgG.

- With HBV infection, hepatic transaminase and bilirubin levels increase rapidly after the onset of symptoms. HBsAg is detectable one to several weeks before the onset of symptoms and the rapid increase in hepatic transaminase and bilirubin levels. HBcAb appears about 1 week after the onset of increased transaminase levels, and is initially predominantly of the IgM class. If the infection is cleared, HBsAg usually disappears about 2 months after the onset of symptoms. Some time after this, antibody to HBsAg becomes detectable. The intervening period is known as the "window phase." Positive results on IgM-HBcAb testing during this phase confirm the diagnosis of hepatitis B. Patients who develop chronic hepatitis B infection remain positive for HBsAg, HBeAg, and HBV DNA, indicating active viral replication.

- Diagnosis of HCV infection is accomplished by detection of anti-HCV antibodies. A positive polymerase chain reaction for HCV RNA is a confirmatory test.

Treatment

Treatment for acute hepatitis A, B, and C is **mainly supportive. Intravenous fluids** may be required to ensure adequate hydration. Hepatic function should be monitored closely until the acute infection resolves. Any patient with acute hepatitis B or C should have a gastrointestinal (GI) consult; in some cases treatment of acute HCV can be beneficial. Patients with chronic or **progressive cases of hepatitis B and hepatitis** C should be referred to a pediatric gastroenterologist for consideration of treatment. Hepatitis B can be treated with α-interferon or with oral antiviral agents. The standard of care for HCV treatment is combination therapy with pegylated interferon and ribavirin.

Epstein-Barr Virus Infection

Clinical Features

EBV, the agent that **causes infectious mononucleosis,** can be associated with hepatic involvement and jaundice. Children with this disease often have a **high fever,** and the illness is usually associated with **splenomegaly** as well as **hepatomegaly, pharyngitis, and lymphadenopathy.** The course of this disease is usually **benign;** often, jaundice does not develop at all.

Treatment

Treatment is **supportive. Steroids** may be administered if **tonsilloadenoidal hypertrophy or lymphadenopathy threaten airway patency.**

TABLE 45-2 Commonly Used Pediatric Medications That May Cause Cholestasis and Hepatotoxicity

Anticonvulsants	Immunosuppressants
Phenobarbital	Cyclosporine
Diphenylhydantoin	Azathioprine
Carbamazepine	Methotrexate
Valproic acid	
Antimicrobials	**Steroids**
Tetracycline	Corticosteroids
Erythromycin (estolate preparations)	Androgens
Sulfonamides	Oral contraceptives
Ketoconazole	
Isoniazid	
Rifampin	
Griseofulvin	
	Miscellaneous Drugs
	Acetaminophen
	Salicylates
	Chlorpromazine
	Cimetidine
	Iron preparations (with overdosage)

Note: A large number of less commonly encountered agents, including antineoplastic agents, antidepressants, antipsychotics, and tranquilizers, can also cause cholestasis and hepatotoxicity.

Hepatotoxicity

Etiology

Many drugs (Table 45-2) **and environmental toxins** can produce hepatic injury, elevated transaminases, and cholestasis. **Acetaminophen overdose,** either accidental or intentional, is probably the **most common drug-induced cause** of hepatic toxicity in children and adolescents.

Clinical Features

The clinical picture in a patient with drug- or toxin-induced hepatotoxicity **is similar to** that seen in patients with **infectious hepatitis;** however, there is **no prodrome** before the onset of hepatitis. **Liver failure usually occurs late** in the clinical course unless there is an overwhelming drug or toxin exposure or a continued exposure that is unrecognized. **Occasionally,** a toxic exposure can lead to **fulminant hepatic failure,** including coagulopathy and encephalopathy. **Acetaminophen overdose rarely causes acute symptoms;** liver injury becomes evident 2 to 4 days after ingestion. In **iron toxicity, GI symptoms** (e.g., vomiting, diarrhea, hematochezia) **predominate early,** and hepatotoxicity and cholestasis occur during the late stages.

Evaluation

The patient's **medication, social, and psychiatric histories** should be obtained. The **absence of prodromal symptoms and the acute onset of symptoms** can be clues to a possible toxic exposure.

Transaminase levels, the bilirubin level, and coagulation studies should be followed. An **acetaminophen level** (or a qualitative toxicology screen for acetaminophen) should be obtained **for any adolescent who has attempted suicide by ingestion with any substance** because acetaminophen is often an unrecognized coingestant.

Treatment

Acetaminophen and iron are the only agents in Table 45-2 for which **specific antidotes are available. n-Acetylcysteine** is a specific **antidote for acetaminophen poisoning,** which, if used early, can **prevent hepatic failure and death.** Of interest are recent reports of the use of n-acetylcysteine in the treatment of hepatic failure due to a variety of causes. Similarly, prompt recognition of the symptoms of **iron ingestion** and appropriate **treatment with deferoxamine** prevent most late complications, including hepatotoxicity and cholestasis. When there is **no available antidote** for the toxin, **withholding the toxic agent and supportive care** are the only available treatments. **Liver transplantation** has been successfully used for patients who have developed frank liver failure.

α_1-Antitrypsin Deficiency

Etiology

α_1-AT deficiency is a **genetic disorder** characterized by decreased serum concentrations of α_1-AT, an **important protease inhibitor.** There are **many phenotypic variants** denoted by "Pi-typing." Individuals with a homozygous Pi ZZ phenotype are at risk for developing hepatic dysfunction because of an accumulation of abnormally folded α_1-AT proteins in hepatocytes. Patients with heterozygous phenotypes have intermediate serum levels of α_1-AT.

Clinical Features

Patients may develop **premature pulmonary emphysema, chronic liver disease, and nephritis in infancy;** however, if the disease is not detected at that time, some or all of these **manifestations may appear in later life. Progressive liver disease,** characterized by jaundice, hepatomegaly, and acholic stools, occurs in 10% to 20% of patients. **Cirrhosis and hepatic failure** may develop by late childhood.

Evaluation

Diagnosis is established by finding **decreased serum levels of α_1-AT along with performing protein electrophoresis for protease inhibitor typing.**

Phenotype determination and characteristic findings on **liver biopsy** confirm the diagnosis.

Treatment

There is **no specific treatment** for individuals who have this disorder and progressive liver disease. **Infusions of the deficient serum protein have slowed the progression of lung disease in adult patients,** but are not helpful in pediatric patients with hepatic dysfunction. There is hope that gene therapy will be available in the future. Presently, **hepatic transplantation** is the only hope for children who develop hepatic failure as a result of α_1-AT deficiency.

Wilson Disease

Wilson disease is discussed in detail in Chapter 42, "Hepatomegaly." Patients presenting with fulminant liver dysfunction may demonstrate Coombs-negative hemolysis and unconjugated hyperbilirubinemia. More often, Wilson disease presents with signs of **hepatic involvement** (including conjugated hyperbilirubinemia, liver enzyme elevation, signs of chronic liver disease) **and neurologic involvement.**

Autoimmune Hepatitis

Autoimmune chronic active hepatitis is discussed in Chapter 42, "Hepatomegaly."

Hepatobiliary Tract Disorders

Etiology

Hepatobiliary tract disease is **rare in most pediatric patients;** however, **patients with variants of hemolytic anemia** (especially sickle cell disease) **often develop cholelithiasis (gallstones).** Although rare, **choledochal cysts** may present in late childhood.

Clinical Features

The **acute onset of right upper quadrant pain or recurring episodes** of right upper quadrant pain in a patient with a **history of ongoing hemolysis** should prompt consideration of the possibility of cholelithiasis. If **fever** is present, **acute cholecystitis** may be complicating the picture. A **palpable right upper quadrant mass** may be felt.

Usually, patients with **choledochal cysts** complain of **right upper quadrant pain or diffuse abdominal pain and vomiting.**

Evaluation

Abdominal ultrasonography demonstrates the presence of gallstones or anatomic abnormalities.

HINT: Cholestasis can also be associated with hydrops of the gallbladder in patients with Kawasaki syndrome. Other manifestations of this multisystem disease should be evident. Hydrops can be demonstrated on an abdominal ultrasound.

HINT: Patients with pancreatic disease and abdominal tumors can have hepatobiliary obstruction and cholestasis. Patients with vascular disease (e.g., Budd-Chiari syndrome in patients with hypercoagulable states or vaso-occlusive disease in patients following bone marrow transplantation) may have hepatic vein obstruction and resultant jaundice, ascites, and hepatomegaly. An ultrasound or computed tomography scan of the abdomen demonstrates these obstructions.

EVALUATION OF JAUNDICE

Patient History

Important questions to ask when evaluating a patient with jaundice include the following:

- Has the child eaten a large amount of yellow, red, or orange vegetables (suggestive of keratodermia or lycopenemia)?
- Is there a past history or a family history of a blood disorder (suggestive of hemolysis)?
- Is the jaundice acute in onset and associated with right upper quadrant pain (suggestive of cholelithiasis or cholecystitis, especially in patients with a history of a hemolytic disorder)?
- Were there prodromal symptoms before the onset of jaundice (suggestive of an infectious cause)?
- Was the onset acute in the absence of prodromal symptoms (suggestive of toxic injury)?
- What is the patient's medication history?
- Is there a history of psychiatric illness or social stress (suggestive of intentional ingestion)?
- Is there a history of behavioral changes, diminished school performance, or other subtle neurologic changes (suggestive of Wilson disease)?
- Is there a family history of unexplained psychiatric, neurologic, or hepatic disease (suggestive of Wilson disease or another genetic cause)?
- Has the patient had symptoms of chronic illness, such as weight loss or pruritus (suggestive of an inflammatory or metabolic process)?
- Has the patient complained of unusual bleeding or a marked change in mental status (suggestive of hepatic failure)?

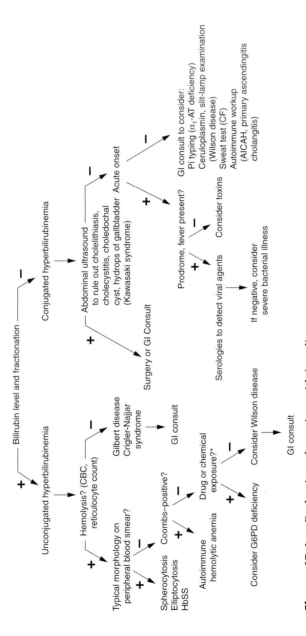

Figure 45-1 ■ Evaluation of a patient with jaundice

In patients with a negative Coombs test, a history of drug ingestion (e.g., salicylates, sulfonamides) or chemical exposure (e.g., naphthalene moth balls, fava beans) should be sought because glucose-6-phosphate dehydrogenase (G6PD) deficiency can lead to hemolysis on exposure to these agents. G6PD deficiency is especially common in African American boys. AICAH = autoimmune-type chronic active hepatitis; α₁-AT = α₁-antitrypsin; CBC = complete blood cell count; CF = cystic fibrosis; GI = gastrointestinal; HbSS = hemoglobin SS; RUQ = right upper quadrant

Physical Examination

- **Hepatomegaly and splenomegaly** are common associated findings in patients with viral hepatitides or inflammatory liver disease.
- **Tenderness over the liver,** but not marked hepatomegaly, is often seen in patients with hepatotoxicity.
- **Right upper quadrant tenderness or a mass** can be seen with biliary tract disease. A mass may not be distinguishable from a finding of hepatomegaly.
- **Signs of systemic or chronic disease** may be present if hepatic involvement is a component of a more protean disorder. Rash, fever, adenopathy, oral lesions, and changes in the hands and feet are seen with Kawasaki disease. Cachexia, edema, palmar erythema, pruritus, and spider angiomata may be detected in patients with autoimmune chronic active hepatitis. Digital clubbing and pulmonary symptoms may be found in patients with cystic fibrosis and hepatic involvement.
- **Abnormal bleeding and a decreased level of consciousness** are worrisome findings in jaundiced patients because these findings may herald the onset of hepatic failure.

TREATMENT OF JAUNDICE

Until the cause of the jaundice is determined, treatment is supportive and may entail:

- Administration of intravenous fluids
- Administration of vitamin K, clotting factors, or both
- Intubation (for patients with a decreased level of consciousness)
- Administration of lactulose and neomycin for treatment of hepatic encephalopathy in patients with hepatic failure
- N-acetylcysteine may be useful as an adjunctive therapy in children with hepatic failure due to a variety of causes.

APPROACH TO THE PATIENT (FIGURE 45-1)

Suggested Readings

Elisofon SA, Jonas MM: Hepatitis B and C in children: current treatment and future strategies. *Clin Liver Dis* 10(1):133–148, 2006.

Gubernick JA, Rosenberg HK, Ilaslan H, et al.: US approach to jaundice in infants and children. *RadioGraphics* 20:173–195, 2000.

Köhnlein T, Welte T: Alpha-1 antitrypsin deficiency: pathogenesis, clinical presentation, diagnosis, and treatment. *Am J Med* 121(1):3–9, 2008.

Lee CK, Jonas MM: Pediatric hepatobiliary disease. *Curr Opin Gastroenterol* 23(3):306–309, 2007.

Nizar NZ: Hepatitis C in children: recent advances. *Curr Opin Pediatr* 19:570–574, 2007.

Pashankar D, Schreiber RA: Jaundice in older children and adolescents. *Pediatr Rev* 22:219–226, 2001.

Shah U, Habib Z, Kleinman RE: Liver failure attributable to hepatitis A virus infection in a developing country. *Pediatrics* 105:436–438, 2000.

Walker WA, Mathis RK: Hepatomegaly: an approach to differential diagnosis. *Pediatr Clin North Am* 22:929–942, 1975.

Jaundice, Newborn

Clyde J. Wright and Michael A. Posencheg

INTRODUCTION

"Jaundice" is a term used to describe the visible manifestation of elevated serum concentrations of bilirubin. The breakdown of heme proteins, the most abundant of which is hemoglobin, is the major source of bilirubin. The heme moiety is broken down to biliverdin by heme oxygenase and reduced to unconjugated bilirubin via the action of biliverdin reductase. Unconjugated bilirubin travels to the liver through the bloodstream, mostly bound to albumin, where it is transformed into the conjugated form. Conjugated bilirubin enters the small intestine and is excreted in the stool. Enzymes in the small intestine convert a portion of this conjugated bilirubin back into unconjugated bilirubin, which can return to the bloodstream. Here, it can reenter the hepatic circulation and add to the bilirubin load. This process is called the *enterohepatic circulation of bilirubin*. Note that elevations of either conjugated or unconjugated bilirubin can cause jaundice, and each etiology has a distinct laboratory evaluation and treatment. For unconjugated hyperbilirubinemia, elevations may be caused by increased production, decreased conjugation or excretion, or increased enterohepatic circulation of bilirubin. Alterations in conjugated bilirubin are mostly caused by bile duct/excretion abnormalities or hepatic dysfunction. Figure 46-1 represents a basic schematic for the consideration of the broad differential diagnosis of hyperbilirubinemia.

DIFFERENTIAL DIAGNOSIS LIST

Unconjugated Hyperbilirubinemia: Physiologic

Increased Bilirubin Production

Blood group incompatibility— Rh, ABO, minor blood group

Red blood cell enzyme abnormalities— glucose-6-phosphate dehydrogenase (G6PD), pyruvate kinase, hexokinase deficiency

RBC membrane defects— hereditary spherocytosis, elliptocytosis, pyknocytosis.

Hemoglobinopathies— α-thalassemia, sickle cell disease

Increased RBC load— cephalohematoma, polycythemia, ecchymosis

Infants of diabetic mothers

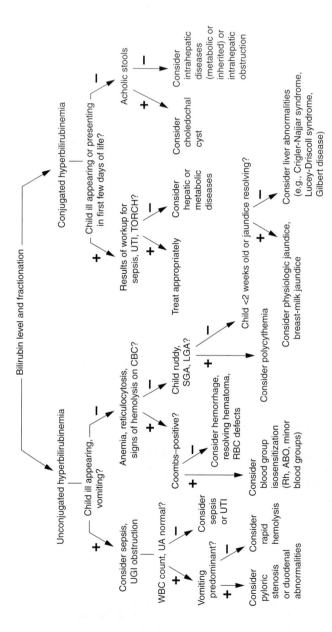

Figure 46-1 ■ Evaluation of a newborn with jaundice

CBC = complete blood count; LGA = large for gestational age; SGA = small for gestational age; TORCH = toxoplasmosis, other infections, rubella, cytomegalovirus, herpes simplex; UA = urinalysis; UTI = urinary tract infection; WBC = white blood cell

Decreased Bilirubin
Conjugation or Excretion
  Hormonal deficiency—
  hypothyroidism,
  hypopituitarism
  Bilirubin metabolism
  disorders—Gilbert
  syndrome, Crigler-Najjar
  (types 1 and 2),
  Lucey-Driscoll syndrome
  Sepsis—bacterial, viral, fungal
Increased Enterohepatic
Circulation
  Breast-feeding failure
  jaundice
  Breast-milk jaundice
  Bowel obstruction or ileus
  Pyloric stenosis

Conjugated Hyperbilirubinemia

The differential diagnosis of conjugated hyperbilirubinemia is an extensive list, encompassing more than a hundred distinct disease entities. The majority of the disorders causing conjugated hyperbilirubinemia in the neonate can be organized into obstructive, infectious, metabolic, and miscellaneous categories. Some of the most important etiologies are listed here.

Bile Duct Abnormalities
  Biliary atresia
  Choledochal cyst
Infection
  Hepatic—toxoplasmosis, other, rubella, cytomegalovirus, herpes simplex (TORCH) infections, herpes simplex virus, enterovirus, and so on
  Systemic—bacterial sepsis, urinary tract infection
Metabolic/Genetic Disorders
  Galactosemia
  Tyrosinemia.
  α_1-Antitrypsin deficiency
  Alagille syndrome
Miscellaneous
  Total parenteral nutrition (TPN)–related cholestasis
  Neonatal hemochromatosis
  Idiopathic neonatal hepatitis

SELECTED DIFFERENTIAL DIAGNOSIS DISCUSSION

Unconjugated Hyperbilirubinemia

Physiologic Jaundice

 HINT: Over 50% of infants have clinical jaundice in the first few days of life, but visible jaundice in the first 24 hours of life is pathologic until proven otherwise.

In utero, fetal unconjugated bilirubin easily crosses the placenta and is conjugated and excreted by the mother. Following birth, the neonate is solely responsible and somewhat ill prepared for bilirubin metabolism. Because of this, jaundice develops in >50% of infants in the first few days of life.

Physiologic jaundice never appears in the first 24 hours, but peaks at 4 days in term infants. Many physiologic factors contribute to this "physiologic hyperbilirubinemia," including a larger RBC mass, decreased RBC life span (70 to 90 days in neonates versus 120 days in adults), reduced bilirubin uridine diphosphate-glucuronosyltransferase (UDPGT) activity (<1% that of adults in the first 10 days of life), and delayed meconium passage leading to increased enterohepatic circulation.

It is important to note that breast-fed infants have higher bilirubin levels, and with more neonates breast-feeding, clinicians have to reassess what "normal" levels of total serum bilirubin (TSB) are in these otherwise healthy neonates. Historically, 95% of term infants had bilirubin levels that did not exceed 12.9 mg/dL. However, recent studies have shown that in breast-fed infants, the normal mean peak TSB level is 8 to 9 mg/dL, with an upper limit of 17 to 18 mg/dL.

Increased Bilirubin Production

Blood Group Incompatibility

If a blood group incompatibility exists between the fetus and the mother, maternal IgG against fetal red cells can cross the placenta, resulting in hemolysis and increased bilirubin production in the fetus and newborn. An incompatibility can exist in the Rh, ABO, or minor blood group antigens.

> **HINT:** Rh incompatibility requires prior sensitization and therefore does not happen in a first pregnancy, whereas ABO incompatibility can occur in a first-born infant.

Rh Incompatibility

Rh incompatibility occurs when an Rh-negative mother carries an Rh-positive fetus. The mother must have had previous sensitization to the Rh antigen, usually via a prior pregnancy. Rh-positive infants born to Rh-negative mothers display a wide spectrum of disease, ranging from unaffected (15% to 20%) to severe disease, including erythroblastosis fetalis and fetal death (25%). The administration of blocking antibodies (RhoGAM) to pregnant Rh-negative mothers prevents Rh sensitization and has reduced the incidence of erythroblastosis fetalis caused by Rh sensitization to 1 per 1,000 live births in the United States.

ABO Incompatibility

ABO incompatibility occurs when a mother with type O blood carries a fetus with type A or B blood. This condition is confined to mothers with type O blood because these women carry anti-A and anti-B IgG antibodies that cross the placenta. Mothers with type A or type B blood produce mostly IgM antibodies against their respective antigens, and these IgM antibodies fail to cross the placenta. Because A and B antigens are common in nature, group O mothers are previously sensitized to these antigens and hemolysis may occur in a first pregnancy. Although ABO incompatibility occurs in 15% of all pregnancies, ABO hemolytic disease occurs in only 5% of ABO-incompatible mother-infant pairs. Hemolysis tends to be less severe than with Rh incompatibility. The classic presentation is anemia, reticulocytosis, and hyperbilirubinemia occurring in the first 24 to 72 hours of life.

RBC Enzyme Abnormalities

Glucose is the primary metabolic substrate for the red cell, and because the mature red cell lacks organelles including mitochondria, glucose can only be metabolized via anaerobic pathways. Defects in glucose metabolism or pathways that protect against red cell oxidation can result in hemolysis and hyperbilirubinemia.

Glucose-6-Phosphate Dehydrogenase Deficiency

> **HINT:** Consider the diagnosis of G6PD in infants from the appropriate ethnic backgrounds with severe hyperbilirubinemia or who are poor responders to phototherapy.

G6PD is the most common red cell enzyme deficiency, occurring most commonly in infants of Mediterranean, Middle Eastern, African, and Southeast Asian descent. This disorder occurs in up to 15% of African American newborns. The mode of inheritance is X-linked recessive. Presence of this deficiency confers resistance against *Plasmodium falciparum*, the infectious agent causing malaria. G6PD generates substrates that protect the red cell against oxidative stress. Erythrocytes lacking these substrates undergo hemolysis with oxidative stress. Important triggers in the neonate include sepsis or exposure to other stressors (naphthalene, sulfa drugs, acetaminophen, breast milk of a mother who has eaten fava beans, etc.). However, the pathogenesis of hyperbilirubinemia appears to be more complicated than simple hemolysis. Often, the offending agent is not identified, and infants with significant hyperbilirubinemia have no evidence of hemolysis, leading some authorities to postulate a concurrent impairment in bilirubin conjugation or clearance. Classically, hyperbilirubinemia appears between 24 and 96 hours postpartum, and it can be severe, even in the absence of significant anemia. Up to 50% of patients also have Gilbert syndrome (see later), and this combination increases the risk of hyperbilirubinemia and kernicterus. Many states include G6PD in the routine newborn screen. In the 2004 American Academy of Pediatrics

(AAP) guidelines for hyperbilirubinemia, the committee emphasized the possibility for the underdiagnosis of G6PD deficiency in the newborn period, and encouraged practitioners to consider this diagnosis in infants with the appropriate ethnic backgrounds who are poor responders to phototherapy.

Pyruvate Kinase Deficiency

Deficiency in pyruvate kinase causes ineffective adenosine triphosphate generation from glucose, resulting in shortened red cell survival. This disorder is inherited in an autosomal recessive pattern and is most common in whites of northern European descent. Clinical expression ranges from severe neonatal jaundice to compensated hemolytic anemia.

RBC Membrane Defects

Defects that affect the red cell membrane and cytoskeletal structure alter the shape and deformability of the cell and result in hemolysis and hyperbilirubinemia. Conditions include hereditary spherocytosis, elliptocytosis, and pyknocytosis.

Hereditary Spherocytosis

With an incidence of 1 in 5,000, hereditary spherocytosis is the most common congenital RBC membrane disorder. This disease is inherited in an autosomal dominant manner, with 25% of cases arising from new mutations. Family history can be significant for splenectomy, gallstones, and anemia.

Increased Red Blood Cell Load

Any condition that results in increased red blood cell load can result in hyperbilirubinemia secondary to breakdown of extravascular or sequestered erythrocytes. Common conditions include cephalohematoma, extensive bruising after traumatic delivery, and polycythemia.

Infants of Diabetic Mothers

Macrosomic infants of insulin-dependent diabetic mothers represent a unique group of patients at risk for hyperbilirubinemia. These infants have high levels of erythropoietin and increased erythropoiesis; thus ineffective red cell production and polycythemia are probably responsible for the resulting hyperbilirubinemia.

Decreased Bilirubin Conjugation or Excretion

Hormone Deficiency

The pathogenesis of hyperbilirubinemia in infants with hypothyroidism and hypopituitarism is poorly understood. Hypothyroidism results in unconjugated hyperbilirubinemia, whereas hypopituitarism can result in either unconjugated or conjugated hyperbilirubinemia.

Bilirubin Metabolism Disorder

Bilirubin uridine diphosphate-glucuronosyltransferase (UDPGT) is responsible for converting unconjugated bilirubin into the conjugated form. Defects in this enzyme can result in unconjugated hyperbilirubinemia.

Crigler-Najjar Syndromes, Types I and II

> **HINT:** Crigler-Najjar syndrome type II is less severe than type I disease and is uniquely responsive to phenobarbital, which induces enzymatic activity.

Type I is a rare disease that results from an autosomal recessive inheritance of a deficiency in UDPGT activity. These patients develop severe hyperbilirubinemia in the first 2 to 3 days of life and often require exchange transfusion. Patients with type II disease (also known as Arias syndrome) retain some UDPGT activity, and infants typically have less severe hyperbilirubinemia. Furthermore, infants with type II disease are also partially responsive to phenobarbital, which induces enzyme activity.

Gilbert Syndrome

Gilbert syndrome affects from 5% to 10% of the general population, and both autosomal dominant and recessive patterns of inheritance are described. Infants may have mildly elevated levels of unconjugated bilirubin when compared to controls because of decreased UGT1 activity. Presentation with pathologic hyperbilirubinemia in the newborn period is rare, unless a concurrent condition such as G6PD deficiency or hereditary spherocytosis exists.

Lucey-Driscoll Syndrome

Lucey-Driscoll syndrome can be associated with significant hyperbilirubinemia and is thought to be related to a hormone or antibody from the maternal serum that inhibits the action of UDPGT. This is a self-limited process and should be considered in unexplained familial severe hyperbilirubinemia.

Sepsis

Sepsis results in hyperbilirubinemia secondary to hemolysis and impaired conjugation. Patients with sepsis may have both elevated unconjugated and conjugated bilirubin levels.

Increased Enterohepatic Circulation of Bilirubin
Breast-Feeding Failure Jaundice and Breast-Milk Jaundice

> **HINT:** Breast-feeding failure jaundice is early onset, occurring in the first 2 to 4 days of life, whereas breast-milk jaundice is responsible for later-onset or persistence of jaundice from the end of the first week through the first few weeks of life.

Multiple studies have indicated a link between breast-feeding and an increased incidence and severity of neonatal hyperbilirubinemia. Breast-fed infants are three times more likely to develop bilirubin levels of >12 mg/dL within the first week of life, and levels commonly peak at 10 to 30 mg/dL. Additionally, up to 10% to 30% of breast-fed infants continue to have elevated serum bilirubin levels into the second to sixth weeks of life. Jaundice that occurs in the first 2 to 4 days is called "breast-feeding failure jaundice" and that occurring later, from 4 to 7 days and continuing to cause prolonged jaundice, is termed "breast-milk jaundice." There is considerable overlap with these two conditions. Both maternal and newborn factors that lead to inefficient nutritional intake by the infant are thought to contribute to the etiology of breast-feeding failure jaundice. These include lack of proper technique, engorgement, cracked nipples, and ineffective suck or latch. Delayed meconium passage and increased enterohepatic circulation are thought to cause the indirect hyperbilirubinemia that appears under these conditions. Multiple factors found in breast milk are implicated in causing the prolonged unconjugated hyperbilirubinemia known as breast milk jaundice, including the presence of a glucuronidase enzyme that deconjugates bilirubin in the intestinal lumen allowing for increased enterohepatic circulation. However, the absolute etiology remains unclear.

CONJUGATED HYPERBILIRUBINEMIA

Conjugated hyperbilirubinemia is defined as a level ≥ 1 mg/dL if the total bilirubin is <5 mg/dL or a conjugated fraction that accounts for >20% of the total bilirubin if the total bilirubin is >5 mg/dL. The differential diagnosis of conjugated hyperbilirubinemia, or cholestasis, is long, with both hepatocellular and ductal disturbances of bilirubin excretion playing a role. However, after a full diagnostic workup is performed, between 70% and 80% of cases can be attributed to either biliary atresia or idiopathic neonatal hepatitis in term infants. In preterm infants, the most likely cause is TPN-related cholestasis.

Bile Duct Abnormalities

Biliary Atresia

> HINT: For biliary atresia, the Kasai portoenterostomy procedure is more successful if performed in the first 8 weeks of life. For this reason, infants with persistent jaundice into the second or third week of life require a fractionated bilirubin to ensure the conjugated fraction is not elevated.

Biliary atresia is one of the most common diagnoses responsible for cholestasis, occurring in 1 per 10,000 births and accounting for one-third of all cases of conjugated hyperbilirubinemia. A progressive, inflammatory sclerotic process results in extrahepatic obstruction of the bile ducts and ongoing inflammation of the intrahepatic bile ducts that can lead to biliary cirrhosis. Although multiple etiologies are proposed, the causative agent remains obscure. Infants often appear well at birth, but persistent jaundice develops in the first few weeks of life. Early diagnosis is critical because the definitive treatment to reestablish bile flow, the Kasai portoenterostomy, is most successful when done at <8 weeks of age. Despite treatment, most patients eventually require liver transplantation.

Infection

Several congenital infections can manifest as conjugated hyperbilirubinemia. These include the TORCH infections. Viral infections of the neonate, including hepatitis A and B, and enterovirus can cause liver failure and hyperbilirubinemia. Additionally, bacterial sepsis and urinary tract infections can cause conjugated hyperbilirubinemia.

Metabolic/Genetic Disorders

Multiple metabolic disorders, including tyrosinemia and galactosemia, may have conjugated hyperbilirubinemia and fulminant liver disease as part of their clinical presentation. α_1-Antitrypsin deficiency, inherited in an autosomal recessive fashion, affects 1 in 2,000 live births. Only 5% of these patients develop rapidly progressive liver disease requiring transplant within the first 4 years of life, with the remaining 95% manifesting variable symptoms extending into adult life. Alagille syndrome (arteriohepatic dysplasia) consists of dysmorphic facies and cholestasis associated with paucity of intrahepatic bile ducts. This disorder occurs in 1 in 70,000 live births.

Miscellaneous

Cholestasis Related to Total Parenteral Nutrition

TPN is essential in many conditions that require withholding feeds from neonates. Prolonged administration of TPN results in liver injury, resulting in elevated transaminases, elevated gamma-glutamyltransferase, and jaundice. The longer the duration of TPN administration, the higher the risk of cholestasis tends to be. The onset of cholestasis usually occurs following 2 weeks of TPN administration. In most patients, cholestasis slowly resolves with initiation of feeds and discontinuation of parenteral nutrition. This condition most commonly affects preterm infants because of their greater exposure to TPN.

Idiopathic Neonatal Hepatitis

Idiopathic neonatal hepatitis is defined as conjugated hyperbilirubinemia without general viral illness or an etiology specific to a metabolic abnormality. Liver biopsy shows transformation of hepatocytes into multinucleated giant cells. Distinguishing this from biliary atresia is difficult but essential for proper clinical management. Jaundice frequently occurs in the first week of life, but can manifest as late as 4 months. Familial cases have poor prognosis, with <30% recovery. Sporadic cases resolve in 60% to 80% of patients.

CLINICAL FINDINGS

History

Family History

- Family history of hematological disorders, splenectomy, gallstones, and previously affected children: inherited causes of hyperbilirubinemia

Pregnancy, Labor, and Delivery

- Maternal blood type and Rh status: Rh and ABO incompatibility
- TORCH titers
- Maternal diabetes
- Maternal medications: sulfonamides, nitrofurantoins, antimalarials, oxytocin
- Abnormal fetal anatomy ultrasound: gastrointestinal (GI) obstruction, choledochal cyst
- Traumatic delivery: hemorrhage, hematoma

Infant History

- Gestational age, postnatal age, and ethnicity of the infant
- Intrauterine growth restriction/small for gestational age—may be associated with inherited, metabolic, or infectious causes as well as polycythemia

- Newborn screen results, if available
- Infant blood type and direct Coombs test results, often sent on cord specimen
- Nutrition—breast-feeding versus formula feeding; TPN exposure
- Voiding and stooling pattern

Physical Examination

Level of Jaundice

> **HINT:** Jaundice becomes clinically apparent at levels ≥5 mg/dL and progresses cephalocaudally. Studies show, however, that prediction of bilirubin levels by evaluating the progression of jaundice from head to toe is unreliable.

It has long been noticed that jaundice progresses in a cephalocaudal manner. Clinical jaundice appears at total serum bilirubin (TSB) >5 mg/dL and can be elicited by blanching the skin with slight pressure and evaluating the color of the underlying skin and subcutaneous tissue. It is best to evaluate for the presence of jaundice in natural light. The clinical use of cephalocaudal progression of jaundice to gauge TSB levels appears less reliable in darkly pigmented neonates and when TSB levels exceed 12 mg/dL.

General Physical Examination

- **Signs of extravascular blood**—cephalohematoma, ecchymosis
- **Plethoric infant**—polycythemia
- **Ascites, pleural effusion, hepatomegaly**—Rh isoimmunization, α-thalassemia
- **Pallor, hepatosplenomegaly**—hemolysis
- **Fever, temperature instability, lethargy, respiratory distress, vomiting, seizures**—sepsis or acute bilirubin encephalopathy
- **Microcephaly, petechiae, hepatosplenomegaly, chorioretinitis**—TORCH infections
- **Abdominal mass**—choledochal cyst, intestinal obstruction
- **Dark urine and acholic stool**—cholestasis

Acute Bilirubin Encephalopathy and Kernicterus

> **HINT:** "Acute bilirubin encephalopathy" is the preferred term for the initial symptoms of neurological dysfunction associated with elevated levels of bilirubin. Kernicterus is reserved for the chronic manifestations.

The prevention of acute bilirubin encephalopathy that may progress to kernicterus is the main reason for timely diagnosis and appropriate treatment of hyperbilirubinemia in the newborn period. Unconjugated bilirubin, in the free or unbound form, that crosses the blood-brain barrier is toxic to neurons of the basal ganglia and various brainstem nuclei. Clinical manifestations of acute bilirubin encephalopathy are often mistaken for sepsis, asphyxia, or hypoglycemia. In term babies, several phases of acute bilirubin encephalopathy are described. The early phase consists of lethargy, poor feeding, and hypotonia. The intermediate phase follows with stupor, irritability, and hypertonia and occasionally fever and high-pitched cry. The hypertonia may consist of backward arching of the neck (retrocollis) and trunk (opisthotonos). The advanced phase consists of opisthotonos, shrill cry, no feeding, apnea, coma, and occasionally seizures and death. "Kernicterus" is the term reserved for describing the chronic form of bilirubin encephalopathy. With survival, the infant may develop choreoathetosis, sensorineural deafness, dental enamel dysplasia, and paralysis of upward gaze.

The level of hyperbilirubinemia at which kernicterus occurs is unclear. In patients with Rh hemolytic disease, treatment of levels >20 mg/dL prevent long-term sequelae. Recent studies suggest that with hemolysis, both the level and duration of hyperbilirubinemia contribute to the development of kernicterus. It has been shown that otherwise healthy infants without hemolysis may develop marked hyperbilirubinemia (20 to 25 mg/dL), and this does not appear to lead to adverse neurologic outcomes; however, contradictory reports exist. Conditions that increase bilirubin deposition in the brain include low albumin, acidosis, hypercarbia, hypoxemia-ischemia, and systemic illness (shock, sepsis, respiratory distress syndrome). Relatively little is known about bilirubin levels and kernicterus in the preterm infant, although most experts recommend treatment at lower levels than those recommended for term infants. Only careful attention by the clinician to individual risk factors can ensure that neonates with hyperbilirubinemia are treated appropriately.

Data from the Kernicterus Registry suggest an increasing incidence of kernicterus, with 1 case per 624,000 live births in the United States. Some have postulated that early discharge with delayed follow-up, failure to check bilirubin levels in newborns with jaundice that presents in the first 24 hours of life, and an insufficient response to jaundice by clinicians may play a role in this phenomenon.

Laboratory Evaluation

Unconjugated Versus Conjugated Versus Indirect Versus Direct Hyperbilirubinemia

When ordering bilirubin levels, clinicians often have to choose between unconjugated, conjugated, indirect, and direct levels. These levels are determined via different laboratory methods and deserve mention here. Traditional methods of bilirubin measurement took advantage of the reaction between bilirubin and a diazo reagent. Direct bilirubin reflects the conjugated component that reacts directly with the diazo reagent. This includes delta bilirubin, which is the fraction of conjugated bilirubin covalently bound to albumin that appears after prolonged hyperbilirubinemia. Total bilirubin levels can be determined by adding an accelerant to the reaction, and the indirect component is calculated by taking the difference between total and direct bilirubin. Various nontraditional methods have been developed to assess conjugated and unconjugated bilirubin directly. Conjugated levels do not include delta bilirubin. Thus direct bilirubin and conjugated bilirubin are slightly different, as are indirect and unconjugated levels. Often, conjugated and unconjugated levels are more quickly obtained and the tests of choice for evaluating newborn hyperbilirubinemia.

Transcutaneous Bilirubin Measurement

Transcutaneous bilirubinometry (TcB) is a noninvasive method of measuring total bilirubin levels. Some concerns have been raised regarding the accuracy of these readings at levels >15 mg/dL and in African American and Hispanic populations. Further studies must be done to evaluate the utility of TcB at high levels of bilirubin and during phototherapy. However, this technique has gained widespread use as a screening tool to help detect early hyperbilirubinemia in the newborn nursery.

Unconjugated Hyperbilirubinemia

Any infant with clinically visible jaundice should have a TSB with unconjugated and conjugated levels determined. Serial TSB levels are helpful because special attention should be paid to the neonate whose bilirubin rises ≥0.5 mg/dL per hour over 4 to 8 hours or >5 mg/dL per day. Levels increasing this quickly may indicate active hemolysis. Further laboratory studies include checking a blood type and direct Coombs test (can be done on cord blood) in neonates born to mothers with type O blood. Of these patients, one third have positive Coombs, and of those, only 15% to 20% have bilirubin ≥12.8 mg/dL. The result of this test alone should not be used to rule in or rule out ABO incompatibility as a cause of hyperbilirubinemia. A complete blood count, peripheral smear, and reticulocyte count can lead to the diagnosis of anemia secondary to hemolysis. If sepsis is suspected, blood culture, urine culture, and cerebrospinal fluid analysis may also be indicated. A serum albumin can be useful in assessing the risk of acute bilirubin encephalopathy (see later). Newborn screen results should be checked (hypothyroidism), and G6PD enzyme activity should be determined in the correct clinical scenario. G6PD levels in the setting of hemolysis may be normal in a G6PD-deficient infant. If clinical suspicion remains, a repeat level should be drawn when the hemolysis has resolved.

The frequency of laboratory evaluation is based on the severity of hyperbilirubinemia and the pathologic process involved. TSB levels should be checked every 2 to 3 hours when levels are >25 mg/dL, every 3 to 4 hours when TSB is 20 to 25 mg/dL, every 4-6 hours when TSB is <20 mg/dl, and every 8 to 12 hours when TSB is decreasing on phototherapy.

Conjugated Hyperbilirubinemia

The North American Society for Pediatric Gastroenterology, Hepatology and Nutrition (see web address in Suggested Readings section) has developed clinical practice guidelines. Conjugated hyperbilirubinemia is never physiologic and requires immediate evaluation. Any infant with clinical jaundice at 2 weeks of age should be evaluated for cholestasis by checking TSB and conjugated or direct bilirubin levels. Multiple studies can lead to the correct diagnosis. These include blood/urine cultures, viral titers, ophthalmologic exam, α_1-antitrypsin genotyping, liver function tests including coagulation studies, and newborn screen results (galactosemia, tyrosinemia). For the diagnosis of biliary atresia and neonatal hepatitis, abdominal ultrasound, radionucleotide scans, and percutaneous liver biopsy may need to be done. Close follow-up of these infants is essential because the diagnosis of biliary atresia must be made early to optimize the chances for success of surgical therapy.

TREATMENT

Unconjugated Hyperbilirubinemia

Preventive Measures and Nomograms

The AAP has developed an algorithm for the systematic evaluation of all infants for the development of hyperbilirubinemia (see web address in Suggested Readings section). Every newborn should be assessed clinically every 8 to 12 hours for the development of jaundice. Special attention should be paid to those infants at high risk for developing marked hyperbilirubinemia (see Table 46-1). Any jaundice occurring in the first 24 hours requires further workup. Additionally, if the clinical assessment suggests significant jaundice, TSB should be checked. Once a TSB is obtained, multiple nomograms exist to assist the clinician with management. The hour-specific bilirubin nomogram developed by Bhutani (see AAP guideline reference) is helpful in determining a neonate's risk of developing hyperbilirubinemia with the next measurement, and it is used mostly as a tool for determining the appropriate time for follow-up. The AAP has developed treatment nomograms for neonates born at 35 or greater weeks of gestation that are stratified by gestational age and the presence or absence of risk factors associated with the development of acute bilirubin encephalopathy. These nomograms

TABLE 46-1 Risk Factors for Developmental Disabilities

Major Risk Factors

Predischarge TSB or TcB level in the high-risk zone
Jaundice observed in the first 24 hr
Blood group incompatibility with positive direct antiglobulin test, other known hemolytic disease (e.g., G6PD deficiency), elevated ETCO$_c$
Gestational age 35–36 wk
Previous sibling received phototherapy
Cephalohematoma or significant bruising
Exclusive breast-feeding, particularly if nursing is not going well and weight loss is excessive
East Asian race*

Minor Risk Factors

Predischarge TSB or TcB level in the high intermediate-risk zone
Gestational age 37–38 wk
Jaundice observed before discharge
Previous sibling with jaundice
Macrosomic infant of a diabetic mother
Maternal age ≥25 yr
Male gender

Decreased Risk (these factors are associated with decreased risk of significant jaundice, listed in order of decreasing importance)

TSB or TcB level in the low-risk zone
Gestational age ≥41 wk
Exclusive bottle-feeding
Black race*
Discharge from hospital after 72 hr

*Race as defined by mother's description.
Adapted from *Pediatrics* 114(1):297–316, 2004. Used with permission.
ETCO$_c$ = end-tidal carbon monoxide concentration; *G6PD* = glucose-6-phosphate dehydrogenase; *TcB* = transcutaneous bilirubin; *TSB* = total serum bilirubin;

help the clinician decide whether a neonate should receive phototherapy (see Figure 46-2) or exchange transfusion (see Figure 46-3).

Measurement of serum albumin can assist the clinician in determining which infants may benefit from exchange transfusion. An albumin <3.0 g/dL is considered a risk factor for developing acute bilirubin encephalopathy, and an elevated bilirubin-to-albumin ratio may be considered when making treatment decisions regarding exchange transfusion.

Early hospital discharge increases the risk of missing neonates who may go on to develop significant hyperbilirubinemia. The AAP recommends follow-up of these infants at the following intervals:

Age at Discharge	Age at Follow-Up
Before age 24 hours	72 hours
Between 24 and 48 hours	96 hours
Between 48 and 72 hours	120 hours

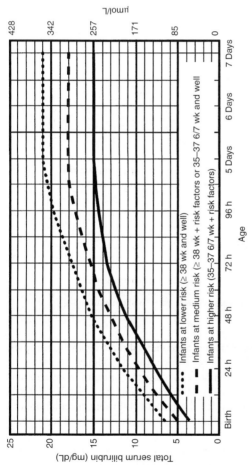

• Use total bilirubin. Do not subtract direct reacting or conjugated bilirubin.
• Risk factors = isoimmune hemolytic disease, G6PD deficiency, asphyxia, significant lethargy, temperature instability, sepsis, acidosis, or albumin < 3.0 g/dL (if measured)
• For well infants 35–37 6/7 wk can adjust TSB levels for intervention around the medium risk line. It is an option to intervene at lower TSB levels for infants closer to 35 wks and at higher TSB levels for those closer to 37 6/7 wk.
• It is an option to provide conventional phototherapy in hospital or at home at TSB levels 2–3 mg/dL (35–50 mmol/L) below those shown but home phototherapy should not be used in any infant with risk factors.

Figure 46-2 ■ Guidelines for phototherapy

Used with Reprinted with permission from Pediatrics 114(1):297–316, 2004

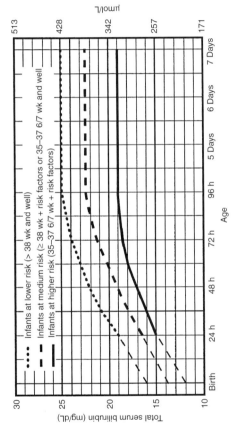

Figure 46-3 ■ Guidelines for exchange transfusion
Reprinted with permission from Pediatrics 114(1):297–316, 2004

- The dashed lines for the first 24 hours indicate uncertainty due to a wide range of clinical circumstances and a range of responses to phototherapy.
- Immediate exchange transfusion is recommended if infant shows signs of acute bilirubin encephalopathy (hypertonia, arching, retrocollis, opisthotonos, fever, high pitched cry) or if TSB is ≥5 mg/dL (85 µmol/L) above these lines.
- Risk factors—isoimmune hemolytic disease, G6PD deficiency, asphyxia, significant lethargy, temperature instability, sepsis, acidosis.
- Measure serum albumin and calculate B/A ratio (See legend).
- Use total bilirubin. Do not subtract direct reacting or conjugated bilirubin.
- If infant is well and 35–37 6/7 wk (median risk) can individualize TSB levels for exchange based on actual gestational age.

Infants at high risk for developing hyperbilirubinemia may require follow-up at earlier intervals; infants with minimal risk factors may be seen at longer intervals.

Phototherapy

> **HINT:** Phototherapy is the mainstay of therapy for hyperbilirubinemia and works by converting unconjugated bilirubin, in a nonenzymatic fashion, into a polar, water-soluble, and therefore more-readily excretable form.

Phototherapy should be instituted as dictated by the AAP guidelines, which contain specific postnatal age and gestational age nomograms guiding therapy. Unconjugated bilirubin absorbs light maximally in the blue portion of the visible spectrum (450 nm). The use of phototherapy results in the photoisomerization of bilirubin into a polar, water-soluble, and more readily excretable form. Both configurational and structural isomers are formed as a result, and the most common structural isomer is lumirubin. Multiple factors affect the efficacy of phototherapy, including spectrum of light, irradiance (dosage of light) of the phototherapy unit, exposed surface area of the infant, and the distance of the infant from the light source. Fiberoptic pads placed under the infant increase surface area exposure. The current AAP guidelines call for the use of intensive phototherapy, with an irradiance of at least 30 μW/cm^2 per nanometer for all infants with gestational age ≥ 35 weeks requiring phototherapy. Phototherapy should be discontinued when TSB reaches <13 to 14 mg/dL or when values reach <40th percentile on the Bhutani nomogram. The utility of checking "rebound bilirubin" levels remains unclear but can be helpful when phototherapy was stopped before the peak bilirubin was suspected to occur (i.e., 4 days of life) or in the setting of possible ongoing hemolysis.

Side effects of phototherapy include disruption of the mother-baby unit, increased insensible water loss, retinal injury from ultraviolet light, and, in the setting of an elevated conjugated fraction, a brown discoloration of the skin called "bronze-baby syndrome." The presence of an elevated conjugated fraction or bronzing of the skin is not a contraindication to the use of phototherapy. The conjugated fraction should not be subtracted from the TSB in determining when to use phototherapy or perform exchange transfusion. However, if an infant's bilirubin increases during phototherapy and is associated with purpura or bullous eruptions on the skin, the diagnosis of congenital erythropoietic porphyria should be entertained (resulting from photosensitivity and induced hemolysis).

Intravenous Fluids

Administration of intravenous fluids does not lower TSB levels, although an infant receiving phototherapy has increased insensible water losses that may be compounded by poor feeding and thus may benefit from parenteral fluid therapy.

Exchange Transfusion

HINT: The bilirubin-to-albumin ratio can be used as an adjunct in determining the need for exchange transfusion because it emphasizes the risk factor of a low serum albumin.

Exchange transfusion should be performed based on the age-specific nomograms published in the AAP guidelines. Replacing twice the infant's circulating blood volume can rapidly correct hyperbilirubinemia and remove offending antibodies in the setting of isoimmune hemolytic disease. Typically, type O blood and AB+ plasma are used to reconstitute whole blood because time does not allow cross-matching infant blood. Presence of skilled personnel and close monitoring of the patient in an intensive care setting are required. Secure intravascular access is essential, and if umbilical lines are to be used, their position must be confirmed before starting the procedure. Slow withdrawal from umbilical catheters at a rate of approximately 1 to 2 mL/kg per minute is recommended with concomitant infusion of the reconstituted whole blood. Peripheral lines are preferred to minimize the risk of GI complications, but their use may be complicated by the limitations of their small caliber. An effective double-volume exchange transfusion (160 mL/kg) reduces serum bilirubin by nearly 85%; a single-volume exchange transfusion reduces the level by 63%. A posttransfusion rebound to 60% to 80% of pretransfusion levels is common, likely representing reequilibration between vascular and extravascular compartments. Complications include transfusion reaction, infection, ischemic bowel/necrotizing enterocolitis, hypocalcemia (especially with packed red blood cells stored in sodium citrate), thrombocytopenia, and hemodynamic instability. Risk of death is 1% in healthy infants and may be as high as 12% in sick neonates.

Intravenous Immune Globulin for Isoimmune Hemolytic Hyperbilirubinemia

In the setting of an isoimmune hemolytic disease causing hyperbilirubinemia (Rh, ABO, or minor blood group antigens), intravenous immunoglobulin (IVIG) attenuates hemolysis and, therefore, hyperbilirubinemia. Use of IVIG for this condition is recommended by the AAP for hyperbilirubinemia unresponsive to phototherapy or levels approaching exchange transfusion criteria, based on studies demonstrating reduced need for exchange transfusion with fewer side effects. The current recommendation is for the administration of IVIG (0.5 to 1 g/kg over 2 hours) if the TSB is rising despite intensive phototherapy or is within 2 to 3 mg/dL of the exchange level. This dose can be repeated in 12 hours if necessary.

Phenobarbital

Phenobarbital is used in certain populations to increase the conjugation and excretion of bilirubin by inducing the expression of the glucuronyl transferase enzyme. It has been studied for the treatment of both conjugated and unconjugated hyperbilirubinemia. Currently, phenobarbital is not a mainstay of therapy.

Synthetic Metalloporphyrins (Tin-Mesoporphyrin)

These compounds limit the production of bilirubin because they act as a competitive inhibitor of the heme oxygenase enzyme responsible for the first step in bilirubin production. Tin-mesoporphyrin is the best studied of these compounds and has been used with some success to avoid the need for exchange transfusion in certain populations (e.g., Jehovah's Witnesses), whose beliefs do not allow exposure to blood products. Currently, these products are not approved by the Food and Drug administration.

Conjugated Hyperbilirubinemia

Treatment of conjugated hyperbilirubinemia depends on the ultimate diagnosis and should be coordinated with a pediatric gastroenterologist. Care should be made to optimize nutrition, with attention paid to fat-soluble vitamins (A, D, E, and K). Medical management is limited and believed to be purely supportive. Phenobarbital increases conjugation and excretion of bilirubin, but it is not routinely recommended because of sedative effects. Ursodeoxycholic acid may increase bile flow, but efficacy is not confirmed. For patients with biliary atresia, outcomes after Kasai portoenterostomy are improved if the surgery is performed in the first 8 weeks of life.

Suggested Readings

American Academy of Pediatrics: Management of hyperbilirubinemia in the newborn infant 35 or more weeks of gestation. *Pediatrics* 114(1): 297–316, 2004. Available at: http://aappolicy.aapublications.org/cgi/content/abstract/pediatrics;114/1/297.

Bhutani VK, Johnson L, Sivieri EM: Predictive ability of a predischarge hour-specific serum bilirubin for subsequent significant hyperbilirubinemia in healthy term and near-term neonates. *Pediatrics* 103:6–14, 1999.

Dennery PA, Seidman DS, Stevenson DK: Neonatal hyperbilirubinemia. *N Engl J Med* 344(8):581–590, 2001.

Moyer V, Freese DK, Whittington PF, et al.: Guideline for the evaluation of cholestatic jaundice in infants: recommendations of the North American Society for Pediatric Gastroenterology, Hepatology, and Nutrition. *J Pediatr Gastroenterol Nutr* 39(2):115–128, 2004. Available at: http://www.naspghan.org.

Wong RJ, Stevenson DK, Ahlfors CE, et al.: Neonatal jaundice: bilirubin physiology and clinical chemistry. *NeoReviews* 8(2):e58–67, 2007.

47 *Joint Pain*

Jeffrey A. Seiden and Joel A. Fein

INTRODUCTION

Arthritis is defined as limitation of motion of a joint with associated **swelling, pain with motion, tenderness, or warmth. Arthralgia** is joint pain in which there is **no limitation of range of motion and** in which **none of the other associated findings** are present. Arthritis or arthralgia may present as **polyarticular** (multiple joint), **pauciarticular** (few joints), or **monoarticular** (one joint).

DIFFERENTIAL DIAGNOSIS LIST 🔒

Traumatic/Structural Causes

Recent trauma—fracture, sprain
Foreign body synovitis
Overuse syndromes—stress fracture, apophysitis (tendonitis), Osgood-Schlatter disease
Degenerative—Legg-Calvé-Perthes disease, slipped capital femoral epiphysis (SCFE), patellofemoral pain syndrome, osteochondritis dissecans, chondromalacia patella

Infectious Causes

Septic arthritis
Osteomyelitis
Viral arthritis
Postinfectious arthritis—acute rheumatic fever (ARF), poststreptococcal arthritis, Lyme disease, postdysenteric arthritis (Reiter syndrome)

Inflammatory Causes

Transient (toxic) synovitis
Reactive arthritis

Kawasaki disease
Systemic lupus erythematosus
Dermatomyositis
Polyarteritis nodosa
Henoch-Schönlein purpura
Behçet syndrome
Psoriatic arthropathy

Immunologic Causes

Serum sickness
Erythema multiforme
Inflammatory bowel disease
Juvenile idiopathic arthritis (JIA)

Congenital Causes

Hemophilia
Sickle cell disease (SCD)
Hypermobility syndromes
Multiple epiphyseal dysplasias

Neoplastic Causes

Bone tumors
Leukemia, lymphoma
Neuroblastoma

Miscellaneous Causes

Functional (growing pains)

DIFFERENTIAL DIAGNOSIS DISCUSSION

Traumatic/Structural Causes of Joint Pain

Recent Trauma: Fractures and Sprains

Etiology

Fractures located **near the growth plate** are a common cause of posttraumatic joint pain.

Clinical Features and Evaluation

The growth plate is often the **weakest portion of the joint** in children. For this reason, it is difficult to diagnose anything but the most minor joint injuries as "sprains" in patients whose growth plates have not yet fused. Fractures near the growth plate can be classified by their radiographic appearance and severity.

Treatment

Injuries that reveal **localized or "point" tenderness** at a child's joint require **immobilization and orthopedic follow-up, even if radiographs fail to reveal an obvious fracture site** (Salter I fracture classification).

Foreign Body Synovitis

Etiology

Splinters, glass, or other **foreign material located near a joint space** can induce an **inflammatory response,** causing **synovitis or tendonitis.** This process can occur over a period of months, or it can develop earlier if it is complicated by infection.

Clinical Features and Evaluation

Diagnosis is based on a **high index of suspicion** and a **review of the history. Plain radiographs** are helpful **only with radiopaque foreign materials,** such as glass.

Treatment

Treatment consists of **surgical exploration and removal** of the foreign material.

Overuse Injury

Overuse injuries occur when a **small amount of stress** is placed on the joint **for a long period of time.** Although these injuries are **most common in the knee joint,** overuse injuries of other joints can occur secondary to exercise of inappropriate rate, intensity, or both (e.g., "Little Leaguer's elbow").

Stress Fractures

Stress fractures occur most commonly in the **lower extremity** and may be difficult to diagnose without a **bone scan.**

Apophysitis

Apophysitis is **inflammation of a tendon or ligament at its insertion site near the joint.** It occurs more commonly in children than pure tendonitis. In apophysitis, the tenderness is usually **localized to the area just above or below the joint,** and radiographs are generally normal.

Osgood-Schlatter Disease

Osgood-Schlatter disease is thought to be either **apophysitis or an avulsion of the tibial tubercle secondary to recurrent traction of the patellar tendon.** The patient, usually an **active preadolescent or adolescent,** complains of **tenderness below the patella** and has **pain on extension of the knee against force.** Radiographs may be normal but can reveal **irregularity** and, possibly, **fragmentation** of the tibial tubercle. Treatment consists of **limiting activity until the natural fusion of the tubercle** occurs during midadolescence.

Degenerative Disease
Legg-Calvé-Perthes Disease

Legg-Calvé-Perthes disease is an avascular necrosis of the femoral head that can produce **hip or thigh pain.** The diagnosis should be considered in **5- to 10-year-old boys** with an **indolent presentation of limp** and with **painful abduction and internal rotation of the affected hip.** Plain **radiographs** might reveal changes in the femoral head on the affected side; a **bone scan** allows earlier detection of the disease. Other causes of avascular necrosis include SCD and **chronic steroid use.**

Slipped Capital Femoral Epiphysis

SCFE, **displacement of the femoral head from the femoral neck,** is commonly seen in **obese adolescents.** These children complain of **hip or thigh pain** and walk with the **affected leg externally rotated.** Hip radiographs **(both anteroposterior and frog-leg projections)** are diagnostic. Orthopedic referral is mandatory.

Patellofemoral Pain Syndrome

Patellofemoral pain syndrome results from **recurrent transmission of force onto a malaligned patella.** The common scenario is an adolescent girl who complains of pain on flexion of a previously rested knee joint, pain when traveling down an incline, or **weakness,** causing the knee to "give out from under her." **Damage to the articular cartilage** (i.e., idiopathic adolescent anterior knee pain syndrome) can occur. Radiographs are frequently normal. **Exercise that strengthens the medial quadriceps muscles** may help realign the patella. **Surgical realignment** may be necessary.

Osteochondritis Dissecans

Osteochondritis dissecans is a **degenerative** process in which **cartilage replaces bone at an articular surface**, usually the **lateral epicondyle of the distal femur, the radial capitellum, or the talus.** It can develop as a result of **acute trauma** or as a result of the **repeated application of smaller forces,** which cause a **small subchondral fracture.** Osteochondritis dissecans is most common in children undergoing a **growth spurt.** Radiographs may be normal early in the course of the disease. **Immobilization in a non-weight-bearing cast** frequently alleviates the problem. However, **surgical removal of the avulsed fragment** occasionally is necessary.

Infectious Causes of Joint Pain

Septic Arthritis
Etiology

The cause is predominantly **bacterial,** occurring by **hematogenous delivery, direct extension from osteomyelitis, or from a penetrating injury** to the joint. *Staphylococcus aureus* and *Streptococcus pyogenes* are the most commonly involved organisms. Other bacterial causes include group B streptococcus and Gram-negative organisms in neonates, *Neisseria gonorrhoeae* in adolescents, *Salmonella* in patients with SCD, and *Haemophilus influenzae* in unimmunized children. **Pyogenic infection** in the joint space causes increased pressure within the joint capsule, resulting in **derangements of the vascular and lymphatic supply. Bacterial and leukocyte proliferation** may also occur, causing the release of proteolytic enzymes. These changes can rapidly **damage cartilage and bone tissue.**

Clinical Features

Most patients with septic arthritis develop **fever** within the first few days of infection. If the **hip or shoulder joints** are involved, the patient holds the extremity **slightly flexed, abducted, and externally rotated** to relieve the pressure within the joint. The **knee and elbow,** if affected, are **slightly flexed,** and the **ankle is plantar flexed.** The **application of pressure** to the joint **or movement of the joint** through almost **any range of motion produces pain.** This finding contrasts with that found in purely traumatic injuries, which may be asymptomatic through a limited range of motion. **Erythema, heat, and swelling** may be present but are difficult to detect in the hip and shoulder joints because these joints are relatively deep beneath the skin surface.

Neisseria infections can produce either **monoarticular or polyarticular** disease. Gonococcal arthritis may begin as polyarthralgia, with a progression to monoarticular arthritis within a few days. These **symptoms** begin within 2 to 4 weeks of the initial urethritis and commonly **increase in severity 1 week following the menstrual period** in girls. Acute cases

TABLE 47-1 Characteristics of Synovial Fluid

	Appearance	WBC/mm^3	% Neutrophils	Glucose Synovial Fluid to Blood
Normal	Clear	<2,000	<40	>0.5
Infectious	Turbid	>75,000	>75	<0.5
Inflammatory (JIA, SLE)	Clear or turbid	5,000–75,000	50	>0.5
Traumatic	Bloody or clear	<5,000	<50	>0.5

JIA = juvenile idiopathic arthritis; SLE = systemic lupus erythematosus; WBC = white blood cell.

may be associated with **fever, malaise, or dermatitis.** Tenosynovitis (painful tendon sheaths) may also be present.

Evaluation

Plain radiographs may not be helpful early in the course of illness, but they may reveal distortion of the normal fat pads and dislocation of the bone from the joint.

Although the peripheral leukocyte count alone is not often helpful, laboratory data including an elevated C-reactive protein (CRP) and erythrocyte sedimentation rate (ESR) can be helpful in diagnosing septic arthritis. The joint fluid may appear turbid and reveals a large number of leukocytes and a low fluid-to-serum glucose ratio, as described in Table 47-1.

Joint fluid cultures identify the causative organism in about 60% of patients. In contrast, blood culture results are positive in only 30% of all patients. Joint fluid culture results are more likely to reveal the organism **within the first week of infection. Chronic meningococcemia** presents a **similar clinical picture** to gonococcal joint disease; however, **joint fluid cultures** are usually **sterile.**

Treatment

Septic arthritis is a **medical and surgical emergency.** Management of septic arthritis involves **evacuation of the purulent material** from the joint space **as soon as possible. Open surgical drainage** is preferred for the hip joint and remains an option for other joints that contain thick purulent material as well. Empirical **parenteral antibiotic therapy** directed at the presumed causative organisms should be initiated immediately after the diagnosis is made. A combination of **intravenous therapy and oral therapy** is given for **2 to 4 weeks** after diagnosis.

Osteomyelitis
Etiology

Osteomyelitis in children can present with symptoms **similar** to those of septic arthritis: **fever, limp, or refusal to use an extremity in younger** children, or discrete localized pain in older children. Although the patho-physiology of osteomyelitis differs from that of septic arthritis, the **pre-dominant causative bacteria** remain the same. Occasionally, **viral, fungal, and mycobacterial causes** are reported.

Clinical Features

Because osteomyelitis tends to affect the metaphyseal portion of the bone, symptoms can often be confused with joint pain. However, in contrast to septic arthritis, **isolated movement of the affected joint** in an older child with osteomyelitis **does not cause as much pain as does pal-pation of the affected portion of the bone.** The **CRP and the ESR are usually increased** and are helpful in monitoring the response to therapy.

Evaluation

- **The triple-phase bone scan** is a sensitive and specific test of osteo-myelitis, except in neonates.
- **Plain radiographs** may reveal periosteal elevation or bone destruction 10 to 21 days after the onset of illness.
- **Magnetic resonance imaging** can be used to detail the extent and degree of bone and soft tissue injury and to define the presence of a bone abscess ("Brodie abscess"). It is the study of choice for suspected pelvic or vertebral body osteomyelitis and provides better spatial res-olution, which is helpful in cases for which a surgical procedure is warranted (e.g., abscess drainage). However, it is more expensive than bone scan, and for younger children, sedation is often necessary to complete the study. Bone scan is the study of choice in suspected cases of multifocal infection.
- **Blood culture results** identify the causative organism in approxi-mately 50% of patients with osteomyelitis.
- Needle aspiration of metaphyseal bone, in combination with a blood culture, can increase the yield of a microbiologic diagnosis to 80%.

Treatment

High-dose antibiotic therapy is required to ensure adequate penetration of the bone and complete eradication of the bacterial nidus. A **combi-nation of intravenous and oral antibiotics** may be required for a longer total course than in patients with septic arthritis. However, recent evidence suggests that **shorter courses of intravenous antibiotics, fol-lowed by oral antibiotics** can be administered successfully to treat osteomyelitis caused by *S. aureus*. The decision to switch from par-enteral to oral antibiotic therapy is based on the absence of signs and symptoms of inflammation, improvement in serum inflammatory markers, and the child's ability to comply with and appropriately absorb the oral regimen. The total duration of therapy should be no less than 3 weeks because the rates of chronic infection are highest in those receiving shorter courses of antibiotic therapy.

Viral Arthritis

Young children <5 years of age can often present with pain caused by infection of the joint by viruses. Parvovirus and adenovirus are two of the more common culprits, and the fever, rash, and polyarthritis are frequently preceded by an upper respiratory infection.

Postinfectious Arthritis
Acute Rheumatic Fever

The arthritis of ARF is migratory and involves several large joints in quick succession. Commonly, each joint is affected for <1 week, and the entire polyarthritis rarely lasts >1 month. The arthralgia is also migratory but is differentiated from the arthritis by the absence of swelling, redness, and decreased range of motion in an otherwise painful joint. One cannot use both the arthritis and arthralgia as criteria for diagnosis.

Because the joint manifestations of ARF occur within 5 weeks of the initial streptococcal infection, antistreptococcal antibody levels are almost always increased during this period. Children with poststreptococcal reactive arthritis do not fulfill the Jones criteria for ARF (Table 47-2) but may still complain of prolonged polyarthritis after group A hemolytic streptococcal infection. These children may still develop recurrent arthritis and are thought to carry a greater risk of development of a subsequent "second attack" of rheumatic fever. Some physicians therefore treat these patients similarly to those with acute rheumatic fever. Treatment consists of antistreptococcal and anti-inflammatory medications. The arthritis associated with ARF responds dramatically to treatment with aspirin.

TABLE 47-2 Revised Jones Criteria (1992) for Diagnosis of Acute Rheumatic Fever

Major Criteria	Minor Criteria
Carditis	Fever
Polyarthritis	Arthralgia
Erythema Marginatum	Elevated ESR, CRP
Sydenham Chorea	Prolonged PR interval on ECG
Subcutaneous nodules	

Diagnosis of acute rheumatic fever requires both of the following:

1) Evidence of a preceding group A streptococcal infection, defined as either an elevated or rising antistreptolysin O (ASO) titer, a positive throat culture, or a positive rapid antigen test.

   AND

2) Either **two major** or **one major and two minor** criteria listed above

Adapted from Dajani AS, Ayoub E, Bierman FZ, et al. Guidelines for the diagnosis of rheumatic fever: Jones criteria, updated 1992. Circulation. 1993; 87: 302–307.
CRP = C-reactive protein; ECG = electrocardiogram; ESR = erythrocyte sedimentation rate.

Lyme Disease

Approximately 60% of patients with documented Lyme disease complain of **painful joints** at some point during their illness. The knee is the most frequently affected joint. Initially, many patients suffer from **polyarthralgias** within the first few weeks of illness. **Frank arthritis** of one or more large joints can occur **2 weeks to 2 years after the onset** of disease, and episodes of **arthritis and arthralgia** can recur over **subsequent years in untreated patients.** Each episode usually lasts a few weeks but can last as long as 1 year.

Many patients **do not report a history of deer tick bite** and **do not exhibit the pathognomonic rash** of erythema migrans. The diagnosis, albeit difficult to confirm, is supported by the finding of **concurrent clinical manifestations and serologic evidence** of recent infection. Examination of **synovial fluid** for polymerase chain reaction to the *Borrelia* **antigens** can be diagnostic but is less sensitive than the blood test for Lyme exposure.

Intravenous therapy is warranted only for cases of arthritis that do not respond to treatment with **amoxicillin (or doxycycline in children >8 years of age)** for 1 month.

Postdysenteric Arthritis

Occasionally, patients who have recently suffered **acute gastroenteritis** experience **subsequent aseptic arthritis** affecting the large joints. This may occur days to weeks after the infection. It is most common after *Yersinia, Campylobacter,* and *Shigella* infections. In some patients, the **arthritis lasts for years** and may produce **destructive changes** in the joint. **Reiter syndrome,** which consists of **arthritis, urethritis, and uveitis,** may present similarly after gastrointestinal or chlamydial infections in HLA-B27–positive patients.

Inflammatory Causes of Joint Pain

Transient (Toxic) Synovitis

Etiology

The cause of transient synovitis is **unknown,** but it is associated with **upper respiratory infections.**

Clinical Features

The child with transient synovitis is most commonly a boy **3 to 9 years** of age who has a **preceding or concurrent upper respiratory infection.** The **hip** is the most commonly affected joint, causing a **limp** as well as **hip, thigh, or knee pain.**

Evaluation

Differentiation from septic arthritis and osteomyelitis is based on the child's **nontoxic appearance** and his **ability to move the hip through some range of motion without pain.**

Treatment

Treatment of transient synovitis includes **rest** of the affected extremity, **administration of oral analgesic medications**, and **follow-up** to assure resolution within 1 week.

Reactive Arthritis

Reactive arthritis is a sterile inflammatory condition that occurs in response to an infection at a distant site in the body. This is often very difficult to distinguish from infectious causes of arthritis. Nonsteroidal anti-inflammatory medications may be beneficial in treating reactive arthritis.

Other Inflammatory Causes

Joint pain can be a minor manifestation of other known conditions, such as Kawasaki disease, systemic lupus erythematosus, dermatomyositis, polyarteritis nodosa, Henoch-Schönlein purpura, Behçet syndrome, and psoriatic arthropathy. The nonmusculoskeletal symptoms and signs of these conditions often overshadow the joint or bone involvement, and the musculoskeletal findings rarely contribute in a unique manner to the diagnosis.

Immunologic Causes

Serum Sickness

Serum sickness is an antigen-antibody mediated disease of **immune complex** deposition. It commonly occurs 1 to 2 weeks after **exposure to viral antigens or to certain medications**, such as cephalosporin or sulfa drugs. However, many **other infectious or medicinal agents** have been implicated. Symptoms consist of an **urticarial rash, arthralgias in the large joints, and constitutional symptoms, such as fever**. The **rash may turn purple** within a few days. **Steroid treatment** is reserved for the most severe cases.

Erythema Multiforme

Erythema multiforme is an illness with causes similar to those of serum sickness, **in which erythematous target lesions found over the entire** body are accompanied by **pauciarticular arthritis**.

Inflammatory Bowel Disease

Inflammatory bowel disease can present **initially as a form of arthritis**. There are multiple forms of arthritic manifestations of inflammatory bowel disease. The most common is the **pauciarticular enteropathic arthritis of large joints associated with erythema nodosum**. The attacks can last up to 6 weeks and coincide with the acute exacerbations of inflammatory bowel disease.

TABLE 47-3 Main Subsets of Juvenile Idiopathic Arthritis and Their Characteristics

Subset Frequency	Number of Joints	Gender	Age	+ANA	+RF	Uveitis	Outcome
Pauciarticular	1–4	F	2 yr	++	−	Yes	Good
Polyarticular	≥5	F	3–9 yr	+	−	Yes	Poor
Polyarticular RF+	≥5	F	Teens	+	+	No	Very poor
Systemic	Any	Either	0–16 yr	−	−	No	Very poor*

*Intriguingly, it is excellent in some patients.
(Reprinted with permission from Polin A, Ditmar M: Pediatric Secrets, 3rd ed. Philadelphia, Hanley & Belfus, 2001, 681.)
ANA = antinuclear antibody testing; F = female; RF = rheumatic fever.

Ankylosing Spondylitis

Ankylosing spondylitis is a less common form of arthritis associated with inflammatory bowel disease in HLA-B27–positive children.

Juvenile Idiopathic Arthritis

JIA is a systemic illness with arthritis as one of its manifestations. It carries an incidence of approximately 3 in 100,000 children, with a female predominance of 2:1.

The clinical presentation of JIA may be divided into three types: pauciarticular, polyarticular, and systemic. Within these types, the age of onset and the presentation of illness may vary, as delineated in Table 47-3.

The key to the diagnosis of JIA is the presence of symptoms for at least 6 weeks, with a fluctuating clinical course. The diagnosis is made primarily from historical and physical examination findings. Laboratory analysis should be guided toward the evaluation of other illnesses that may be causing the joint pain, but antinuclear antibody testing can be included. Rheumatoid factor testing is usually not helpful, and it is positive only in older girls with polyarticular manifestations. The ESR is often normal in all patients except those with systemic JIA. A thorough search for other illnesses with similar manifestations should ensue before diagnosing this condition. Anti-inflammatory drugs are the mainstay of treatment for the arthritis of JIA. Intra-articular corticosteroid injections, low-dose methotrexate, and biologic agents that act as tumor necrosis factor blockers are successful in alleviating symptoms in children with JIA.

Neoplastic

Primary Bone Tumors
Etiology

Primary bone tumors are uncommon in children; however, they can cause joint pain if they are localized to the proximal or distal portions of the bone.

- Osteogenic sarcoma (osteosarcoma) is the most common primary bone tumor in children and can spread to the joint space by direct extension or as a "skip" lesion.
- Ewing sarcoma, another malignant bone tumor in children, involves the joint space less often than does osteogenic sarcoma.
- Eosinophilic granuloma, a benign bone lesion that can cause joint pain, often mimics the more malignant tumors.
- Osteoid osteoma, another benign bone lesion that can cause joint pain, has a predilection for the femur or tibia and may present as nighttime bone pain that awakens the child from sleep and responds dramatically to anti-inflammatory drugs.

Clinical Features

Frequently, the symptoms are **subtle,** with **progressive development of bone or joint pain,** a **soft tissue mass,** and possibly **recurrent fevers.** The patient or parents may relate the symptoms to a **single episode of trauma,** and **pathologic fractures** may occur when minor trauma causes a break in a bone that is weakened by the presence of tumor.

Evaluation

The diagnosis is usually made after review of the **plain radiographs,** which reveal the tumor and corresponding bony changes.

Leukemia and Lymphoma

Leukemia and lymphoma can cause either **bone or joint pain** in children. Most often, the patient presents with **arthralgias** in conjunction with **other systemic problems.** The concomitant findings include **hepatomegaly or splenomegaly, petechiae, lymphadenopathy, anemia, and fever.** The joint pain is usually **chronic and remitting. Peripheral blood smear** and **bone marrow aspiration or lymph node biopsy** are diagnostic.

Miscellaneous

Limb Pain of Childhood

"Growing pains" result from **muscle overuse.** The pain lasts **less than a few hours,** frequently **awakens the child at night,** and is usually **local-ized to the muscles of the lower extremities.** The pain is **rarely (if ever)** localized to the joint.

EVALUATION OF JOINT PAIN

Patient History

The medical history should include questions regarding the presence of **rash, fever, or recent illness.** In addition, the **time course** of the joint

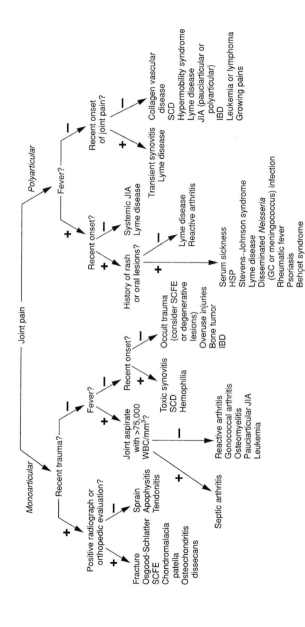

Figure 47-1 ■ Approach to the child with joint pain

GC = gonococcus; HSP = Henoch-Schönlein purpura; IBD = inflammatory bowel disease; JIA = juvenile idiopathic arthritis; SCD = sickle cell disease; SCFE = slipped capital femoral epiphysis; WBC = white blood cell pain should be elicited. A **history of trauma** can account for any acute event or be the disclosing event in a more chronic problem, such as SCFE, chondromalacia patella, stress fractures, bone tumors, and hemophilia.

Physical Examination

Physical examination should concentrate on the **range of motion** of each joint in comparison with the corresponding contralateral joint. A thorough **neurologic examination** should be performed, with attention to **muscle strength and tone** as well as careful observation of the **child's gait.** The remainder of the physical examination may reveal specific rashes, mucosal lesions, lymphadenopathy, or fever.

Laboratory Studies

- ESR
- CRP
- Joint fluid analysis
- Plain radiographs
- Bone scans
- Electrocardiogram
- White blood count

APPROACH TO THE PATIENT (FIGURE 47-1)

Although many of the illnesses that cause joint pain can be diagnosed and treated by the pediatrician or family physician, **referral to an orthopedist, a rheumatologist, or an oncologist** may be necessary.

Suggested Readings

Adebajo AO: Rheumatic manifestations of infectious diseases in children. *Curr Opin Rheumatol* 9:68–74, 1997.

Ansell BM: Rheumatic disease mimics in childhood. *Curr Opin Rheumatol* 12:445–447, 2000.

Caird MS, Flynn JM, Leung YL, et al.: Factors distinguishing septic arthritis from transient synovitis of the hip in children. *J Bone Joint Surg Am* 88(6):1251–1257, 2005.

Carek PJ, Dickerson LM, Sack JL: Diagnosis and management of osteomyelitis. *Am Fam Physician* 63:2413–2420, 2001.

Oudjhane K, Azouz EM: Imaging of osteomyelitis in children. *Radiol Clin North Am* 39:251–266, 2001.

Peltola H, Unkila-Kallio L, Kallio MJT, and the Finnish Study Group: Simplified treatment of acute staphylococcal osteomyelitis of childhood. *Pediatrics* 99:846–850, 1997.

Sherry DD: What's new in the diagnosis and treatment of juvenile rheumatoid arthritis. *J Pediatr Orthop* 20:419–420, 2000.

Sorokin R, Ward SB: Joint pain. *Med Clin North Am* 79:247–260, 1995.

48

Leukocytosis

Leslie J. Raffini
Cynthia Norris (Third Edition)

INTRODUCTION

Leukocytosis is defined as an increase in the total number of white blood cells (WBCs). The normal WBC count varies by age, with infants having the highest total leukocyte count. Leukocytosis may result from an increase in any of the types of WBCs found in the bone marrow. Neutrophilia is most common, but lymphocytosis, monocytosis, basophilia, eosinophilia, and atypical lymphocytosis can also occur. Lymphoblasts or myeloblasts can be seen in abundance in the peripheral blood in leukemia, causing leukocytosis. Leukemoid reactions, which consist of benign but excessive leukocytosis (WBC counts of >50,000/mm³) associated with an increase in the number of immature myeloid cells (blasts, promyelocytes, myelocytes, and metamyelocytes) in the peripheral blood, can also occur.

DIFFERENTIAL DIAGNOSIS LIST

Neutrophilia
Infectious Causes
  Bacterial Infection
    Staphylococcus
    Streptococcus
    Gonococcus
    Meningococcus
    Escherichia coli
    Pseudomonas
    Corynebacterium diphtheriae
    Pasteurella
  Viral Infection
    Herpes zoster
    Varicella
    Rabies
    Poliomyelitis
    Epstein-Barr virus (infectious mononucleosis)
  Fungal Infection
    Actinomyces
    Coccidioides

Mycobacterial Infection
  Tuberculosis
Rickettsial Infection
Spirochetal Infection
  Leptospira
  Lyme disease
  Syphilis
Other Infection
  Kawasaki disease
Toxic/Drug/Hormonal Causes
  Corticosteroids, adrenocorticotrophic hormone
  Mercury, lead, kerosene, camphor
  Epinephrine, norepinephrine, serotonin, histamine, acetylcholine
Neoplastic Causes
  Eclampsia
  Uremia
  Anorexia

Inflammatory Causes
Collagen vascular diseases
(e.g., rheumatoid arthritis)
Acute rheumatic fever
Hematologic Causes
Hemolysis—associated
with both acute hemolysis,
as in autoimmune
hemolytic anemia, and
chronic hemolysis, as in
sickle cell anemia
Acute blood loss
Myeloproliferative
disorders
Surgical or functional
asplenia
Leukemoid reaction
Miscellaneous Causes
Physical Stimuli
Burns
Pain
Electric shock
Trauma/surgery
Physiologic
Pregnancy/labor
Ovulation/menstruation
Vigorous exercise
Emotional stress

Eosinophilia (>4% of Total WBC Count)

Infectious Causes (Especially Parasites)
Ascaris infestation
Hookworm infestation
Strongyloides infestation
Trichinosis
Visceral larva migrans
Filariasis
Malaria
Toxoplasmosis
Pneumocystis carinii

Schistosomiasis
Scabies
Scarlet fever
Aspergillosis
Coccidioidomycosis
Toxic Causes
Drug hypersensitivity
reaction
Postirradiation
Neoplastic Causes
Leukemia
Hodgkin and non-Hodgkin
lymphoma
Brain tumors
Myeloproliferative
disorders
**Inflammatory/Allergic/
Immune Conditions**
Polyarteritis nodosa
Sarcoidosis
Goodpasture syndrome
Milk precipitin disease
Enteritis/ulcerative colitis
Environmental allergies
Asthma
Hay fever
Urticaria
Miscellaneous Causes
Hereditary eosinophilia
Tropical eosinophilia
(syndrome of pulmonary
infiltrates, asthmalike
symptoms, lymphadenopa-
thy, and eosinophilia
thought to be secondary
to an unidentified filarial
parasite)
Peritoneal dialysis
Chronic renal or liver
disease
Immune deficiency
syndromes

Monocytosis (>8% to 10% of Total WBC Count in Childhood; >2% of Total WBC Count in Newborn Period)

Infectious Causes
Tuberculosis
Syphilis
Brucellosis
Malaria
Bacterial endocarditis
Rocky Mountain
  spotted fever
Typhoid fever
Neoplastic Causes
Preleukemia
Acute myelogenous
  leukemia—
  myelomonocytic and
  monocytic forms
Juvenile myelomonocytic
  leukemia
Chronic myelogenous
  leukemia
Hodgkin
  and non-Hodgkin
  lymphoma
Inflammatory Causes
Systemic lupus
  erythematosus
Rheumatoid arthritis
Ulcerative colitis/Crohn
  disease
Sarcoidosis
Miscellaneous Causes
Chronic neutropenia
  syndromes (e.g., Kostmann
  syndrome)
Postsplenectomy

Basophilia (>1% of Total WBC Count)

Infectious Causes
Varicella
Tuberculosis
Influenza
Neoplastic Causes
Chronic myelogenous
  leukemia
Hodgkin disease
Inflammatory Causes
Ulcerative colitis
Rheumatoid arthritis
Miscellaneous Causes
Asthma
Drug hypersensitivity
  reaction
Chronic hemolytic anemia
Postsplenectomy or
  postradiation

Lymphocytosis

Infectious Causes (Associated with an Increased Number of Atypical Lymphocytes)
Bacterial Infection
Pertussis*
Tuberculosis
Brucellosis
Typhoid fever
Viral Infection
Infectious mononucleosis
  (Epstein-Barr virus)†
Cytomegalovirus†
Acute viral lymphocytosis
  (with common viral
  infections)*
Infectious hepatitis
  (A, B, or C)†

---

*Frequently associated with very *high* lymphocyte counts.
†Frequently associated with high *atypical* lymphocyte counts.

Rubeola
Rubella
Mumps
Varicella
Other Infection
Syphilis
Toxoplasmosis
Miscellaneous Causes
Physiologic lymphocytosis
(percentage of lymphocytes
is greater than percentage
of polymorphonuclear

leukocytes from 2 to
5 years of age)
Relative lymphocytosis
(secondary to neutropenia)
Endocrine—thyrotoxicosis,
Addison disease
Drug hypersensitivity
reaction
Crohn disease/ulcerative
colitis
Leukemia

DIFFERENTIAL DIAGNOSIS DISCUSSION

Neutrophilia

 HINT: Healthy newborn infants normally experience a period of neutrophilia associated with a "left-shifted" differential (an increase in the
percentage of early myeloid forms in the peripheral blood). The peak
WBC count occurs during the first few days of life and decreases to
adult levels within the first few weeks.

Neutrophilia is the **most common type of leukocytosis.** The cause of
neutrophilia is **most frequently an infection,** although drugs, inflammation, and other conditions listed in the differential diagnosis can be
responsible. Neutrophilia is a result of one or more of the following
mechanisms:

- Increased neutrophil production by the bone marrow
- Increased release of neutrophils from bone marrow storage
- A shift of neutrophils from the marginating to the circulating pool
- Prolonged neutrophil survival owing to decreased neutrophil entry
  into tissue or decreased removal by the spleen

Some forms of neutrophilia develop within minutes of exposure to the
stimulus. For example, the neutrophilia that follows exposure to epinephrine is a result of neutrophils shifting from the marginating to the
circulating pool. Other forms of neutrophilia take longer to develop
because they occur by a combination of these mechanisms. The **duration
of neutrophilia is usually days to weeks,** although in some instances it
may persist for months.

Eosinophilia

> **HINT:** Allergy is the most common cause of eosinophilia in children in the United States. Outside of the United States, parasites are the most common cause.

Normal eosinophil counts vary with age, reaching the adult value by 6 to 8 years of age. **Boys have slightly higher counts than girls,** and most individuals experience a **diurnal variation** in eosinophil count, with the **peak at night.** Most eosinophils reside in the tissues (especially in areas exposed to the external environment, such as the gastrointestinal and respiratory tracts), and their **release into the bloodstream is the primary cause** of eosinophilia. Histamine release in allergic conditions or chronic inflammation tends to make blood vessel walls permeable, resulting in a release of eosinophils into the peripheral blood. Although allergy is the most common cause, skin diseases, parasitic infections, and conditions associated with chronic inflammation can also be factors. The **hypereosinophilic syndromes** are a poorly understood grouping of disorders characterized by persistent profound, chronic neutropenia ($>1,500/mm^3$ for at least 6 months) of unclear cause.

Acute Lymphoblastic Leukemia

Incidence

Acute lymphoblastic leukemia (ALL) is the **most common malignancy** seen in the pediatric population. The peak age for development of acute lymphoblastic leukemia is approximately 4 years, although all ages can be affected. Certain individuals, such as those with **Down syndrome** are at **increased risk** of development of this disorder.

Etiology

The **cause is unknown,** although genetic, environmental, infectious, and immune-mediated factors are all implicated.

Clinical Features

Symptoms at presentation may include **pallor, fatigue, fever, bleeding, or bruising.** Bone pain is common, and young children may present for evaluation with a **limp or refusal to walk.** Physical findings include **bruises, petechiae, lymphadenopathy, and hepatosplenomegaly.**

Evaluation

Laboratory evaluation may reveal **leukocytosis, anemia, and thrombocytopenia.** In approximately 50% of patients, the WBC count is $>10,000/mm^3$ at the time of diagnosis, and in 20% of patients, it is $>50,000/mm^3$. **Neutropenia** (absolute neutrophil count of $<500/mm^3$) is also frequently seen. **Lymphoblasts** can be found **in the peripheral blood,** but the inexperienced observer may report them as atypical lymphocytes. Definitive diagnosis of leukemia is made by a **bone marrow aspiration** that demonstrates >25% lymphoblasts. Immunologic, cytogenetic, and biochemical characterization of the cells should also be performed. The **spinal fluid** also needs to be examined because the central nervous system is a sanctuary site of extramedullary disease.

Treatment

Prognostic factors such as the initial WBC count and the patient's age dictate the treatment indicated. High-risk patients require more intensive therapy. Most treatment plans last **2 to 3 years** and begin with a **remission induction phase intended to decrease the detectable leukemic burden to <5%.** The following phases of therapy aim to decrease and eventually eliminate all leukemic cells from the body:

- **Central nervous system preventive therapy** is incorporated into all protocols.
- **Multiagent chemotherapy** is the mainstay of treatment, although irradiation to the central nervous system is used for some high-risk patients.
- **Bone marrow transplantation** is another treatment approach used for the child who has experienced a relapse in the bone marrow.

Other sites of relapse include the central nervous system and the testes. The prognosis for long-term disease-free survival with current therapy is approximately 75% for all risk groups.

> **HINT:** Tumor lysis syndrome (a metabolic triad of hyperuricemia, hyperkalemia, and hyperphosphatemia) is a complication of therapy that occurs when leukemic cells lyse in response to cytotoxic chemotherapy and release their intracellular contents into the bloodstream. This occurs commonly in cells with a high-growth fraction (T-cell leukemia/lymphoma and Burkitt lymphoma). Aggressive hydration, alkalinization, and allopurinol administration before initiating chemotherapy may alleviate serious renal dysfunction. The first two maneuvers promote uric acid and phosphate excretion, and allopurinol reduces uric acid formation. Potassium should not be added to hydration fluids. By monitoring the electrolyte concentrations and renal function closely, one can often avoid the development of renal failure.

Acute Myelogenous Leukemia

Incidence

Acute myelogenous leukemia (AML) represents approximately 15% to 20% of all cases of leukemia seen in the pediatric population. It is slightly more common in older children but affects all ages.. It affects both sexes equally. The **incidence is increased in** individuals with **Down syndrome and Fanconi anemia.** It is also a **common "secondary malignancy"** resulting from **prior exposure to chemotherapy** (especially regimens that included alkylating agents).

Etiology

The **cause is unknown.** Predisposing factors include the earlier mentioned syndromes, exposure to large doses of **ionizing radiation,** and exposure to certain **chemicals.**

Clinical Features

Symptoms at presentation are similar to those of ALL and include **pallor, fatigue, fever, infection, bruising, and bleeding.** The physical examination may reveal **hepatosplenomegaly, lymphadenopathy, bruises, or petechiae. Leukemic infiltration of the skin** (leukemia cutis) may occur; it appears as colorless or slightly purple lesions. **Localized tumors or chloromas** can also be seen.

Evaluation

Laboratory evaluation typically reveals **neutropenia, anemia, and thrombocytopenia.** The WBC count is variable, although approximately 25% of children have a WBC count of >100,000/mm^3 at the time of diagnosis. Blasts may be seen in the peripheral blood. The definitive diagnosis is made by examination of the **bone marrow aspirate,** which demonstrates **>25% blasts.** As in ALL, the **spinal fluid** must also be examined for evidence of leukemia. Up to 15% of patients have evidence of blasts in the spinal fluid at the time of diagnosis.

Based on morphologic characterization and the result of histochemical staining, AML is divided into **seven subgroups.** The FAB (French-American-British system) subclasses are as follows:

- **M1, acute myeloblastic leukemia without differentiation**
- **M2, acute myeloblastic leukemia with differentiation**
- **M3, acute promyelocytic leukemia**
- **M4, acute myelomonocytic leukemia**
- **M5, acute monocytic leukemia**
- **M6, erythroleukemia**
- **M7, acute megakaryoblastic leukemia**

The subclasses differ from each other in their method of presentation, associated chromosome abnormalities, and prognosis. **Poor prognostic variables** include having a **high WBC count at the time of diagnosis** and the M5 subtype.

Treatment

Standard treatment consists of **multiagent chemotherapy** that includes central nervous system preventive therapy. **Allogeneic bone marrow** transplanted **from a matched sibling donor during first remission** is the **treatment of choice.** Despite advances in AML therapy, the **prognosis remains poor,** with long-term disease-free survival rates of approximately 50%. In addition, AML therapy is generally more toxic than the therapy for ALL. **Serious infection rates** are higher during therapy, and the **late effects of treatment** can be problematic.

Complications

Three complications of AML deserve mention:

- Disseminated intravascular coagulation (DIC)
- Leukostasis
- Tumor lysis syndrome (mentioned previously)

> **HINT:** DIC can occur with any subtype of AML but is especially common in the M3 and M5 subtypes. Aggressive treatment with platelet and fresh-frozen plasma transfusions is often indicated. The initiation of chemotherapy frequently causes the coagulopathy to worsen before it improves.

> **HINT:** Leukostasis (intravascular WBC clumping) rarely occurs unless the WBC count is >200,000/mm^3. Because myeloblasts are larger and more "sticky" than lymphoblasts, leukostasis occurs more frequently in AML than in ALL. The most commonly involved organs are the brain and the lungs. Central nervous system hemorrhage or stroke can occur. The pulmonary involvement is manifested by tachypnea and development of a need for supplemental oxygen. Treatment consists of leukapheresis and prompt initiation of cytotoxic therapy. Red blood cell transfusion should be used with caution because it can increase whole blood viscosity. (Hemoglobin level should not exceed 10 g/dL.)

> **HINT:** Children with Down syndrome deserve special mention. Neonates with Down syndrome may develop a transient myeloproliferative syndrome that mimics congenital leukemia in every way except that it regresses spontaneously without therapy. For older children with Down syndrome and AML, there is also a better prognosis than for the average child with AML. The reasons are unclear.

Chronic Myelocytic Leukemia

Incidence and Etiology

Chronic myelocytic leukemia accounts for approximately 3% of all pediatric cases of leukemia. Individuals of any age can be affected, but most cases occur in late childhood. The disease is relatively **indolent** as compared with the acute leukemias. The **cause is unknown.**

Clinical Features

The patient is often **asymptomatic** and presents with a **high WBC count or splenomegaly** that was discovered at a routine well-child visit. However, symptoms such as **fever, night sweats, abdominal pain, or bone pain** can occur. Physical examination reveals impressive splenomegaly. **Hepatomegaly** can also be present.

Evaluation

Laboratory evaluation typically reveals impressive **leukocytosis, thrombocytosis, and mild anemia.** The bone marrow is hypercellular but with normal myeloid maturation. An abundance of blasts is not seen. In approximately 90% of cases, the characteristic cytogenetic hallmark of chronic myelocytic leukemia is seen: the **Philadelphia chromosome.** This is associated with the classic t(9;22).

Treatment

There are **three phases** of chronic myelocytic leukemia: **chronic phase, accelerated phase, and blast crisis.** The **chronic phase** may last for years and represents **hyperproliferation of mature myeloid elements.** Treatment during this phase is aimed at **cytoreduction** to decrease the risk of development of leukocytosis and massive splenomegaly. Administration of **hydroxyurea** is the mainstay of cytoreductive treatment. With time, **all patients enter the accelerated and blast phases,** developing frank leukemia. In most instances, **myeloblasts** are seen morphologically, but **lymphoblast transformation** can also occur. **Once the blast phase has begun, the prognosis is poor.** Bone marrow transplantation is the only curative therapy and should be undertaken while the patient is still **in the chronic phase.**

General Therapy Guidelines for Leukemia

- **Prevent bleeding.** Aim to keep the platelet count $>20,000/mm^3$ by means of platelet transfusions. Watch for signs of DIC, which is especially common in the M3 and M5 subtypes of AML.
- **Treat anemia.** Most oncologists aim to keep the hemoglobin level >8 g/dL (but not more than 10 g/dL if hyperleukocytosis is present). Some oncologists treat anemia only if the patient is symptomatic.

- **Identify and treat infection.** Because all neutropenic patients are at increased risk for development of an infection, fever should be treated aggressively. Blood should be drawn for culture, and use of broad-spectrum antibiotics (to cover both Gram-positive and Gram-negative organisms) should be instituted. Prolonged fever in the neutropenic host raises the question of the existence of fungal disease.
- **Watch for tumor lysis.** This was described in the discussion of ALL.
- **Watch for complications of hyperleukocytosis.** This was described in the discussion of AML.
- **Begin definitive chemotherapy promptly** once the diagnosis has been established.

Leukemoid Reactions

Etiology

Leukocytosis that develops in **response to an infection** or other stimuli can occasionally become **exaggerated,** often with WBC counts of >50,000/mm^3. If the **white cells are not malignant blasts,** this syndrome is termed a leukemoid reaction (Table 48-1). Frequently, there is an associated **increase in the number of immature myeloid or lymphoid precursors** in the peripheral blood. Examination of the bone marrow typically reveals **myeloid hyperplasia** with normal maturation. Myeloid leukemoid reactions (comprising two thirds of all cases) most often occur in association with **bacterial infection.** The etiologic agents most frequently involved are *Staphylococcus, Haemophilus, Neisseria meningitidis, Meningococcus,* and *Salmonella.* Lymphoid leukemoid reactions (which comprise a third of all cases) occur most commonly in individuals infected with *Bordetella pertussis* or in common acute viral infections. **Other causes** of a leukemoid reaction include **granulomatous**

TABLE 48-1 Features of Leukemoid Reactions, ALL, and CML (Chronic Phase)

	Leukemoid Reaction	ALL	CML
Common physical examination findings	Evidence of infection	Hepatospleno-megaly or lym-phadenopathy	Splenomegaly
Predominant WBC morphologic characteristics	Myelocytes or lymphocytes	Lymphoblasts	Myelocytes
WBC count	>50,000/mm^3	Wide range	>100,000/mm^3
Other cell lines	Normal hemo-globin and platelet counts	Anemia and thrombocyto-penia	Mild anemia and thrombocytosis

ALL = acute lymphoblastic leukemia; CML = chronic myelocytic leukemia; WBC = white blood cell.

disease, severe hemolysis, vasculitis, drugs, and the presence of a tumor that metastasizes to the bone marrow.

Evaluation

Distinguishing a leukemoid reaction from chronic myelogenous leukemia in the chronic phase may be difficult. The acute leukemias may also exhibit excessive leukocytosis, usually composed of predominantly blast forms.

Suggested Readings

Ebb DH, Weinstein HJ: Diagnosis and treatment of childhood acute myelogenous leukemia. *Pediatr Clin North Am* 44:847–862, 1997.

Kelly KM, Lange B: Oncologic emergencies. *Pediatr Clin North Am* 44:809–830, 1997.

Pui CH: Acute lymphoblastic leukemia. *Pediatr Clin North Am* 44:831–846, 1997.

Webb D, Roberts I, Vyas P: Haematology of Down syndrome. *Arch Dis Child Neonatal Ed* 92:F503–507, 2007.

49 *Leukopenia*

Leslie J. Raffini
Cynthia Norris (Third Edition)

INTRODUCTION

Leukopenia is defined as a **decrease in the total white blood cell (WBC) count, usually to <4,000/mm³**. Neutropenia is defined as a **decrease in the number of circulating neutrophils** (both segmented and band forms). An absolute neutrophil count (ANC) of <1,500/mm³ is considered neutropenia. **Severe neutropenia is defined as an ANC <500/mm³.** The absolute neutrophil count is calculated by multiplying the total WBC count by the sum of the percentage of segmented neutrophils plus the percentage of band forms in the differential count. For example, if the WBC count is 4,000, with 12% segmented neutrophils/polymorphonuclear leukocytes, 10% bands, 60% lymphocytes, and 18% monocytes, the ANC will be 880 [4,000 × (0.12 + 0.10)]. The differential diagnoses of isolated leukopenia and neutropenia are similar; the two conditions are therefore considered as one entity for the purpose of this chapter.

> **HINT:** In 3% to 5% of African American children, the total WBC count normally may be as low as 3,600/mm³, and the ANC may be as low as 1,000/mm³.

DIFFERENTIAL DIAGNOSIS LIST

Infectious Causes

Bacterial Infection
  Sepsis syndrome, bacteremia
    (especially group B streptococcal disease in neonates)
  Tuberculosis
  Brucellosis
  Tularemia
  Typhoid
  Paratyphoid
Viral Infection
  Hepatitis A or B
  Parvovirus B19
  Respiratory syncytial virus
  Influenza A or B
  Rubeola
  Varicella
  Rubella
  Infectious mononucleosis
    (Epstein-Barr virus)
  HIV
  Cytomegalovirus
Protozoal Infection
  Malaria
  Kala azar (visceral
    leishmaniasis)
Rickettsial Infection
  Scrub typhus
  Sandfly fever

Toxic Causes
  Ionizing radiation
  Heavy metals (gold, arsenic,
    mercury)

TABLE 49-1 Drugs that Can Induce Neutropenia or Leukopenia

Cytotoxic Chemotherapeutics

Alkylating agents (e.g., cyclophosphamide), antimetabolites (e.g., methotrexate), anthracyclines (e.g., doxorubicin)

Antimicrobials

Sulfonamides, penicillin, cephalosporins, macrolides, ciprofloxacin, acyclovir, isoniazid, imipenem

Analgesics

Aspirin, ibuprofen, indomethacin, acetaminophen

Anticonvulsants

Valproic acid, Dilantin, carbamazepine

Antithyroid Drugs

Thiouracil, thiocyanate

Antirheumatic Agents

Gold, penicillamine, phenylbutazone

Antihistamines

Cimetidine, ranitidine

Cardiovascular Drugs

Procainamide, captopril, nifedipine, hydralazine, propanolol

Antipsychotics, Antidepressants, and Neuropharmacologic Agents

Phenothiazines, risperidone, barbiturates, benzodiazepines

Miscellaneous

Allopurinol, retinoic acid, metoclopramide, spironolactone, intravenous immunoglobulin

Medications

See Table 49-1

Congenital Causes

Kostmann syndrome

Cyclic neutropenia

Shwachman-Diamond syndrome (neutropenia and exocrine pancreatic insufficiency)

Reticular dysgenesis

Barth syndrome (neutropenia, cardiomyopathy, myopathy)

Neutropenia associated with X-linked agammaglobulinemia

Neutropenia associated with dysgammaglobulinemia type I (neutropenia, absent immunoglobulin A [IgA] and IgG, and increase in IgM)

Neutropenia associated with metabolic disease (hyperglycemia, isovaleric acidemia, propionic acidemia, methylmalonic acidemia)

Neutropenia as part of bone marrow failure syndrome (Fanconi anemia, dyskeratosis congenital, Blackfan-Diamond syndrome)

(SLE) (lymphopenic common in SLE)

Neonatal alloimmune neutropenia (antibody derived from mother)

Immune-Mediated Causes

Autoimmune neutropenia (owing to IgG-mediated destruction of neutrophils)

Felty syndrome (triad of neutropenia, splenomegaly, and rheumatoid arthritis)

Secondary to collagen vascular disease—juvenile rheumatoid arthritis or systemic lupus erythematosus

Miscellaneous Causes

Aplastic anemia

Splenic sequestration

Nutritional deficiency (B_{12} or folate deficiency)

Copper deficiency)

Familial benign neutropenia

Leukemia

Bone marrow infiltration (with tumor, osteopetrosis, Gaucher disease)

Chronic idiopathic neutropenia

DIFFERENTIAL DIAGNOSIS DISCUSSION

Neutropenia Associated with Infection

Infection, usually viral, is the most common cause of neutropenia in childhood. Typically, neutropenia develops during the first few days of infection and persists for 3 to 8 days. Neonates are at especially high risk for developing neutropenia because they have only a small neutrophil reserve in their bone marrow, and they release neutrophils too quickly into the circulation when stressed. The mechanism by which an infection causes neutropenia is most often caused by direct marrow suppression or viral-induced immune neutropenia. Leukopenia is common in patients with AIDS. Management of neutropenia in patients with infections consists of treating the underlying infection.

Drug-Induced Neutropenia

Etiology

Drug-induced neutropenia may be caused by a cytotoxic effect, immunologic effect, or may be an idiosyncratic reaction. Neutropenia can be a result of the following:

- Increased sensitivity of myeloid precursors to appropriate drug concentrations.
- Altered drug metabolism resulting in toxic levels of the drug in the bone marrow.

- An **immunologic response** that occurs after exposure to the drug, resulting in neutrophil destruction. In some cases, the drug serves as a hapten in promoting antibodies that can destroy neutrophils. In other cases, the drug causes the formation of circulating immune complexes that attach to the surface of the neutrophil and lead to its destruction.

Clinical Features

Fever, chills, and fatigue may occur patients with **immune-mediated drug-induced neutropenia.** These symptoms typically develop **7 to 14 days after exposure** to the drug. The duration of the neutropenia is usually brief (1 to 2 weeks) after cessation of the drug.

Drug-induced neutropenia that is **not immune mediated is less predictable.** It may present several days to more than a month after exposure to the drug. The duration may be brief, or it may last months or years.

Table 49-1 shows a partial list of drugs that may cause neutropenia.

Treatment

Treatment consists of **prompt discontinuation** of the offending drug.

Kostmann Syndrome

Etiology

Kostmann syndrome, or **severe congenital neutropenia,** is a rare disorder that most commonly arises as a result of new autosomal dominant mutations in the gene ELA2, which encodes the neutrophil elastase. The gene responsible for many cases of autosomal recessive forms is HAX1.

Clinical Features

Children with this disorder frequently present for medical care in the **first few months of life. Fever, cellulitis, stomatitis, and perirectal abscesses** are the most common findings. These children are **at risk for** developing severe bacterial infections, which may be **life threatening.**

Evaluation

Laboratory test results reveal **profound neutropenia** (absolute neutrophil count of $<200/mm^3$) with or without leukopenia. The differential count may reveal **monocytosis and eosinophilia.**

Bone marrow biopsy findings are variable. Usually, there is normal myeloid maturation up to the promyelocyte or myelocyte stage but **no evidence of mature neutrophils** (maturational arrest). Erythroid precursors and megakaryocytes are present in normal numbers, with a normal maturational sequence noted.

Treatment

The natural course of this disease is **death at an early age secondary to overwhelming infection.** Prophylactic antibiotics are not beneficial.

Therapeutic use of the **cytokine granulocyte colony-stimulating factor (G-CSF)** has resulted in an improvement in the neutrophil count, decreased risk of development of serious infections, and improved survival in many patients with Kostmann syndrome.

Autoimmune Neutropenia

> **HINT:** Autoimmune neutropenia is the most common cause of chronic neutropenia in children.

Etiology

Autoimmune neutropenia is a **benign and self-limited condition in the majority of patients.** Children with this disorder develop **antibodies against their own neutrophils, often after a recent viral infection.** This disorder affects individuals of all ages, but the highest incidence occurs in infants and young children.

Clinical Features

The majority of patients are asymptomatic. A small percentage of patients develop **skin infections, oral ulcerations, and pharyngitis.** Serious infections are uncommon. Some children have mild to moderate **splenomegaly** on physical examination.

Evaluation

Laboratory testing results reveal neutrophil counts that are often <250/mm^3. Monocytosis is common. Bone marrow examination typically reveals normal cellularity with **myeloid hyperplasia** and a **paucity of mature neutrophils.** Diagnosis is made by demonstrating **antineutrophil antibodies** in the serum or on the surface of the neutrophil, although this is not necessary for the diagnosis in patients with the typical clinical features.

Treatment

In most children with this disorder, the neutrophil count usually increases in response to infection. Although the prognosis is good, **aggressive treatment of bacterial infections** is important. In many children, the WBC count completely normalizes within 1 to 3 years.

Cyclic Neutropenia
Etiology

Cyclic neutropenia, a **rare** diagnosis, is characterized by regular **oscillation in the number of circulating neutrophils** in the peripheral blood. The periodicity is usually every 21 days, with the period of neutropenia spanning 3 to 6 days. Cyclic neutropenia is the result of dominantly inherited mutations in the neutrophil elastase gene (ELA2).

Clinical Features

Symptoms usually appear before 10 years of age. Diagnosis is made from analysis of **serial complete blood counts (CBCs)** and **differential counts** (two to three times a week for 4 to 6 weeks). Clinical findings include **stomatitis, oral ulcers, pharyngitis with lymph node enlargement, and skin infection.** Laboratory test results reveal **severe neutropenia. Monocytosis and eosinophilia** occur in some patients. The **platelet and reticulocyte counts may also fluctuate,** although not consistently in the same direction. The **morphological characteristics of the bone marrow change** according to the time in the cycle, varying from normal to hypocellular, with maturational arrest of the myeloid line. The **ANC is low for 3 to 10 days and then begins to increase.**

Symptoms disappear as the ANC returns to normal. The **severity of infection varies** with each child and with the ANC. Some children do not have infections despite profound neutropenia, although there are reports of death in up to 10% of patients.

Treatment

Therapeutic use of G-CSF has been demonstrated to decrease the risk of infection.

Shwachman-Diamond Syndrome

Etiology

Shwachman-Diamond syndrome is a **rare congenital form of neutropenia** inherited as an autosomal recessive trait. The syndrome consists of neutropenia with **exocrine pancreatic insufficiency.** Some children also have metaphyseal **chondrodysplasia and dwarfism.**

Clinical Features

The symptoms of **weight loss, diarrhea, steatorrhea, and failure to thrive** usually develop in infancy, resembling the **clinical presentation of cystic fibrosis.** Patients experience **recurrent infections;** the mortality rate from infection or bone marrow failure is 15% to 25%.

Evaluation

The sweat electrolyte values are normal in this syndrome. The neutrophil count is usually 200 to 400/mL.

Chronic Idiopathic Neutropenia

Chronic idiopathic neutropenia of childhood is a **poorly understood** disorder. Symptoms of **skin infections** may appear in early childhood and vary with the degree of neutropenia. Laboratory test results reveal **neutropenia and associated monocytosis**. The diagnosis is essentially one of **exclusion** and should be considered in any child with **persistent chronic neutropenia, a benign clinical course, and no evidence of another neutropenic disorder**. The prognosis is good.

EVALUATION OF LEUKOPENIA

Patient History

- **Does the child have a fever?** This raises the question of infection, especially in a neutropenic patient. It may also give a clue to the cause because some infections can cause neutropenia.
- Does the child have any skin infections? Abscesses and cellulitis require prompt treatment in the setting of neutropenia.
- Has the child previously had a normal CBC? If so, this will exclude congenital causes of neutropenia, such as Kostmann syndrome.
- Has the child recently taken any medication (e.g., sulfonamides, penicillin, phenothiazines)?
- Does the child have any symptoms of a systemic infection, such as fever, rash, and upper respiratory symptoms? This could indicate infectious mononucleosis, rubeola, rubella, or varicella.
- Does the child have any symptoms of the following infections: tuberculosis, brucellosis, tularemia, or malaria?
- Is there a history of jaundice (seen in hepatitis A and B)?
- Is the child a sick neonate? This could indicate group B streptococcal infection or isoimmune neonatal neutropenia.
- Does the child have a history of recurrent skin infections or oral ulcerations? This suggests a more chronic, perhaps congenital neutropenia such as cyclic neutropenia or Kostmann syndrome.
- Does the child have an unusual diet or look malnourished? This could indicate malnutrition or an isolated B_{12}, folate, or copper deficiency.
- Is there a family history of neutropenia, recurrent infection, or death at an early age from infection? This would be seen in any of the congenital neutropenia syndromes—Kostmann syndrome, chronic benign neutropenia, or familial aplastic anemia.
- Is there any bruising or bleeding? Is the child pale or fatigued? If the answer is yes, this suggests that other cell lines are involved, such as in aplastic anemia, leukemia, or megaloblastic anemia.

Physical Examination

- **Is the child ill appearing?** Infection, either as the cause or the result of neutropenia, is likely and should be treated promptly.

- Is there evidence of cellulitis, perirectal abscesses, labial abscesses, or pharyngitis? All are seen in neutropenic patients and require prompt treatment.
- Are there oral ulcerations or swollen red gums common in many neutropenic disorders?
- Are there bruises, petechiae, or pallor suggesting leukemia or aplastic anemia?
- Is there splenomegaly (found in hypersplenism, Felty syndrome, and leukemia?)
- Is there hepatomegaly (occurring in hepatitis, leukemia, and infectious mononucleosis)?
- Are there phenotypic abnormalities, such as thumb anomalies (Fanconi anemia), dwarfism (Shwachman-Diamond syndrome or cartilage-hair hypoplasia), or skin hyperpigmentation (Fanconi anemia, dyskeratosis congenita)?
- Are there joint findings suggesting arthritis (seen in juvenile rheumatoid arthritis, SLE, or Felty syndrome)?
- Is there fever or rash? See corresponding list in "Patient History."

Laboratory Studies

HINT: In infants, the total WBC count is higher than in later childhood. Lymphocytes are the predominant WBC form in children 2 to 5 years of age. Neutrophils are the predominant WBC form in infants and in children >5 years of age.

- CBC, differential count (sometimes serially)
- Bone marrow aspirate with or without biopsy
- Antineutrophil antibodies

Factitious Causes of Leukopenia (False-Positive Test Result)

- Delay in testing blood sample drawn from the patient
- Excessive leukocyte clumping (in the presence of cold agglutinins, increased immunoglobulin levels, or certain paraproteins)
- Leukocyte fragility (owing to certain drugs or leukemia)
  Note: Results of a WBC count determined manually should identify the last two conditions.

TREATMENT OF LEUKOPENIA

Antibiotics
Prompt treatment of infection with antibiotics is indicated.

Cytokines

Cytokine Granulocyte Colony-Stimulating Factor

G-CSF is a **hematopoietic growth factor** produced by recombinant DNA technology that stimulates the growth of committed neutrophil progenitors. G-CSF is approved for use in treating the neutropenia that results from **cancer chemotherapy.**

Granulocyte Transfusions

Granulocyte concentrates are usually prepared by **leukapheresis of a single donor.** The indications for a granulocyte transfusion are few and include the following:

- Gram-negative sepsis not responding to antibiotics in a neutropenic host
- Life-threatening infections in a neutropenic patient who shows no sign of bone marrow recovery

Complications are many and include the **risks of infection, allergic or febrile transfusion reactions, and graft-versus-host disease.** A hematologist or blood bank physician should be involved in this decision.

HINT: WBC concentrates should not be run through a leukoreduction filter.

APPROACH TO THE PATIENT

- If the child is ill appearing, the workup should be delayed while administration of appropriate antibiotics is started. If the cause of the fever is not evident, broad-spectrum antibiotics should be chosen.
- If a recent infection or drug exposure is noted in the history and the child is clinically well with isolated neutropenia, close follow-up with performance of several repeat CBCs and differentials may be all that is indicated.
- If the neutropenia is chronic or if there is a history of recurrent infection, a more extensive workup should be initiated that includes (a) antineutrophil antibody testing; (b) serial CBCs and differential counts two to three times a week for 3 to 4 weeks; and (c) bone marrow aspirate and biopsy. More specific testing (i.e., gene mutation analyses for congenital syndromes) is dictated by the history and physical examination findings.

Suggested Readings

Bernini JC: Diagnosis and management of chronic neutropenia during childhood. *Pediatr Clin North Am* 43:773–792, 1996.

Calhoun DA, Christensen RD: Recent advances in the pathogenesis and treatment of nonimmune neutropenias in the neonate. *Curr Opin Hematol* 5:37–41, 1998.

Segel GB, Halterman S: Neutropenia in pediatric practice. *Pediatr Rev* 29:12–24, 2008.

Shastri KA, Logue GL: Autoimmune neutropenia. *Blood* 81:1984–1995, 1993.

Zeidler C, Boxer L, Dale DC: Management of Kostmann syndrome in the G-CSF era. *Br J Haematology* 109:490–495, 2000.

Chapter 50

Lymphadenopathy

Leslie J. Raffini
Cynthia Norris (Third Edition)

INTRODUCTION

Healthy children frequently have **palpable lymph nodes,** most commonly in the cervical, axillary, and inguinal areas. Palpable nodes are present in a third of neonates and over half of children 1 to 12 months of age. In general, palpable lymph nodes normally become more prominent as the child approaches puberty and then tend to regress as the child approaches adulthood. **Benign lymph nodes should be small, soft, and freely mobile. Cervical or axillary nodes >1 cm** diameter or **inguinal nodes >1.5 cm,** or nodes that are **firm, hard, erythematous, tender, warm, fluctuant, or fixed** in position **require further attention.** Occipital, preauricular, popliteal, and epitrochlear nodes may be palpable but are typically enlarged in the presence of local inflammation or infection. **Hilar adenopathy** is the nonspecific enlargement of lymph nodes at the pulmonary hilum often detected on a chest radiograph. A thorough physical examination will determine whether the enlarged node is isolated to one region or is part of a generalized adenopathy. This will help narrow the differential diagnosis.

> **HINT:** Supraclavicular nodes are normally not palpable and should be considered pathologic because of their association with mediastinal malignancy.

DIFFERENTIAL DIAGNOSIS LIST

Generalized Lymphadenopathy

Infectious Causes
  Bacterial Infection
  Bacteremia, sepsis
  Scarlet fever
  Syphilis
  Tuberculosis (TB)
  Subacute bacterial
    endocarditis
  Brucellosis
  Leptospirosis
  Typhoid fever

Plague
Lyme disease
Tularemia
Viral Infection
Epstein-Barr virus (EBV)
HIV
Varicella
Cytomegalovirus (CMV)
Rubeola
Rubella
Infectious hepatitis
Influenza
Fungal Infection

Histoplasmosis
Coccidioidomycosis
Parasitic Infection
Toxoplasmosis
Malaria
Neoplastic Causes
Primary Lymphoid
Neoplasm
Hodgkin disease
Non-Hodgkin lymphoma
Metastatic Neoplasm
Acute lymphocytic leukemia
Acute myelogenous
leukemia
Neuroblastoma
Rhabdomyosarcoma
Metabolic Causes
Gaucher disease
Niemann-Pick disease
Immunologic Causes
Systemic lupus erythematosus
Juvenile rheumatoid arthritis
Vasculitis syndromes
Serum sickness
Autoimmune hemolytic
anemia
Medications
Dilantin
Isoniazid
Endocrine Causes
Hyperthyroidism
Miscellaneous Causes
Skin disorders
Atopic dermatitis
Sinus histiocytosis with
massive lymphadenopathy
(Rosai-Dorfman disease)
Chronic granulomatous
disease
Chédiak-Higashi syndrome
Sarcoidosis
Nonspecific reactive
hyperplasia

Castleman disease (benign
giant lymph node
hyperplasia)

Regional Lymphadenopathy

Cervical
Infectious Causes
Viral Infection
Upper respiratory tract
infections
Systemic viral infections
(rubeola, rubella, varicella,
CMV, EBV)
Bacterial Infection
Pharyngitis (streptococcal,
diphtheria)
Primary adenitis (staphylo-
coccal, streptococcal)
Infections of head/neck
Systemic bacterial infections
(tularemia, brucellosis,
leptospirosis)
TB
Atypical mycobacterium
Cat-scratch disease
(*Bartonella henselae*)
Fungal Infection
Histoplasmosis
Parasitic Infection
Toxoplasmosis
Other Infection
Kawasaki syndrome
Neoplastic Causes
Hodgkin disease
Non-Hodgkin lymphoma
Carcinoma of thyroid
Rhabdomyosarcoma
Neuroblastoma
Other Causes
Sinus histiocytosis
(benign)
Sarcoidosis

Occipital
  Tinea capitis
  Seborrheic dermatitis
Preauricular
  Conjunctivitis (viral,
    bacterial, chlamydial)
  External ear infections
  Cat-scratch disease
    (*B. henselae*)
  Tularemia
Submaxillary/Submental
  Herpetic gingivostomatitis
  Dental infections
Epitrochlear
  Local infection of
    hand/forearm
  Rheumatologic disease of
    fingers/wrist
  Tularemia
  Cat-scratch disease
    (*B. henselae*)
Axillary
  Infectious Causes
  Local infection of upper
    extremity, chest wall, or
    breast
  Cat-scratch disease
    (*B. henselae*)
  Neoplastic Causes
  Rhabdomyosarcoma of
    extremity
  Other Causes
  Postvaccination (when
    administered in arm)
  Chronic inflammation of
    skin (rash) or joints
    (juvenile rheumatoid
    arthritis) of upper extremity
Mediastinal/Hilar
  Infectious Causes

TB
EBV
Histoplasmosis
Coccidioidomycosis
Blastomycosis
Inflammatory Causes
Sarcoidosis
Neoplastic Causes
Hodgkin disease
Non-Hodgkin lymphoma
Supraclavicular
  Hodgkin disease
  Lung, mediastinal, or
    abdominal malignancy
  TB
  Sarcoid
Inguinal
  Infectious
  Genital herpes
  Syphilis
  Chancroid
  Chlamydia
  Lymphogranuloma
    venereum
  Staphylococcal or strepto-
    coccal cellulitis
**Chronic Inflammation of
  Lower Extremity**
  Skin—diaper dermatitis,
    insect bites
  Joints—juvenile rheumatoid
    arthritis
  Neoplastic Causes
  Rhabdomyosarcoma of
    extremity
  Neuroblastoma
Popliteal
  Local infection of lower
    leg/foot

HINT: Are your physical examination or radiographic findings truly consistent with lymphadenopathy? For a list of possible entities confused with adenopathy, see Table 50-1.

TABLE 50-1 Possible Entities Confused with Adenopathy

Cervical Area

Thyroglossal cyst
Branchial cleft cyst
Epidermal cyst
Cystic hygroma
Ectopic thyroid tissue

Anterior Mediastinum

Thymic neoplasm/thymoma
Teratoma/dermoid cyst
Cystic hygroma
Rhabdomyosarcoma
Lymphangioma/hemangioma
Bronchogenic cyst
Foreign body

Middle Mediastinum

Neuroblastoma
Bronchogenic cyst
Teratoma
Pericardial cyst
Foreign body

Posterior Mediastinum

Neurogenic tumor
Bronchogenic cyst
Ewing sarcoma
Rhabdomyosarcoma
Thoracic meningocele

DIFFERENTIAL DIAGNOSIS DISCUSSION

Acute Infective Lymphadenitis

Etiology

Acute infective lymphadenitis is a problem frequently encountered in the pediatric population. It represents a **primary infection of the lymph node**. The causative organism frequently gains entry to the body via the **pharynx, nares, dentition, or a break in the skin**. The cause is most often **bacterial**, with *Staphylococcus aureus* the organism most frequently isolated. Other pathogens that may be found include group A streptococci, *Mycobacterium tuberculosis*, atypical mycobacteria, Gram-negative bacilli (thought to be etiologic agents in cat-scratch disease), *Haemophilus influenzae*, anaerobic bacteria, *Francisella tularensis*, and *Yersinia pestis*.

Clinical Features

Physical examination usually reveals a **unilateral, tender, warm, often fluctuant lymph node with erythema** of the overriding skin. Fever and elevated white blood cell (WBC) count occur occasionally, most often in the younger child.

Evaluation and Treatment

Aspiration often reveals the cause and may provide symptomatic relief if the lymph node is large or in an awkward position. In uncomplicated cases, treatment with an **oral antibiotic** is frequently all that is needed. Recent increases in antibiotic resistance such as methicillin-resistant *Staphylococcus aureus* may impact the choice of antibiotics. Infants as well as children who appear clinically ill or have an underlying immunodeficiency should be admitted to the hospital for **intravenous antibiotics.**

Reactive Lymphadenopathy

Etiology

Reactive hyperplasia of lymph nodes represents the body's **response to antigenic stimuli** (foreign material, cellular debris, or infectious organisms and their toxic products).

Clinical Features

The resulting lymphadenopathy can be **acute or chronic.** The cervical, axillary, and inguinal nodes are most commonly involved and can sometimes grow to be quite large. The nodes clinically enlarge secondary to infiltration with histiocytes or plasma cells. Acute cellular infiltration and edema causes distention of the capsule, producing **tenderness when the lymph node is palpated.**

Evaluation

- **In the acute setting:** Careful history and physical examination, with attention to symptoms of upper respiratory infections (influenza or adenovirus are commonly associated with cervical lymphadenopathy), symptoms of EBV or CMV, local infections of the ear, nose, teeth, or skin, or Kawasaki disease.
- **In chronic situations:** Chronic lymph node hyperplasia can pose a diagnostic dilemma (see "Evaluation of Lymphadenopathy"). Lymph node biopsy may be helpful. Reactive hyperplasia is the most common histologic diagnosis seen in children undergoing lymph node biopsy.

Treatment

Because reactive hyperplasia represents the body's normal response to stimuli, treatment is not indicated in most cases. The nodes usually **regress** with time.

Infectious Mononucleosis

Etiology

EBV, a member of the herpesvirus group, is the causative agent in infectious mononucleosis. EBV is also **associated with nasopharyngeal carcinoma** and some cases of **Burkitt lymphoma.** The virus, **transmitted by saliva,** gains entry through the pharynx and spreads throughout the lymphatic system.

Clinical Features

The **primary infection** is frequently **asymptomatic.** Individuals who experience primary infection in adolescence or young adulthood are more likely to develop the clinical syndrome of infectious mononucleosis. After an **incubation period of 4 to 8 weeks,** the patient begins to experience **fatigue, anorexia, headache, and malaise. Fever and sore throat** usually develop within 1 week, bringing the patient to medical attention.

Physical findings at presentation include **pharyngitis, lymphadenopathy, and hepatosplenomegaly.** Not uncommonly, the patient is **misdiagnosed with streptococcal pharyngitis** and treated with ampicillin. For reasons that are unclear, **80% to 100% of patients** with infectious mononucleosis **treated with ampicillin develop a pruritic maculopapular rash,** which can prove very helpful in making the diagnosis. Symptoms usually persist for **several weeks,** although **fatigue and malaise may persist for months.** Central nervous system (CNS) complications include aseptic meningitis, encephalitis, Bell palsy, and Guillain-Barré syndrome. Other complications include splenic rupture, autoimmune hemolytic anemia, thrombocytopenia, granulocytopenia, myocarditis, interstitial pneumonitis, and airway obstruction.

Evaluation

Diagnosis is suggested by the **clinical triad of fever, lymphadenopathy, and pharyngitis combined** with the laboratory finding of **atypical lymphocytosis.** If the clinical presentation is unclear, **serologic testing** is available. **Heterophile antibodies** (e.g., **Monospot**) are usually positive in patients >4 years. **EBV titers** are a quantitative measure and more useful in younger children.

Treatment

Treatment is **supportive** because the disease is **self-limiting.** Patients should be advised to **avoid contact sports for 6 to 8 weeks** to decrease the risk of splenic rupture. The lymphadenopathy may persist for as long as 6 months after diagnosis.

Cat-Scratch Disease

Etiology

Cat-scratch disease is a benign **self-limited regional adenitis** that develops 1 to 2 weeks after a cat scratch or bite. Cervical, axillary, or epitrochlear nodes are most commonly involved. The etiologic agent is a Gram-negative bacillus (*B. henselae*).

Clinical Features

The presenting symptom is usually a **large swollen, erythematous, painful solitary lymph node.** History and examination may reveal an erythematous papule that appeared approximately **2 weeks earlier** in the area drained by the lymph node. Most patients recall a cat scratch or bite approximately 10 days before papule formation. **Suppuration of the involved node** occurs in 30% of cases. Atypical presentations of the disease include encephalitis, Parinaud oculoglandular syndrome (granulomatous conjunctivitis and unilateral preauricular node enlargement), erythema nodosum, osteolytic lesions, and thrombocytopenic and nonthrombocytopenic purpura.

Evaluation

Diagnosis is established by serologic detection of antibodies to *B. henselae.*

Treatment

In most instances, the nodes **regress within 8 weeks without intervention.** Occasionally drainage is required. Antibiotic treatment may be considered for acutely ill patients who are immunocompromised.

Non-Hodgkin Lymphoma

Incidence

Non-Hodgkin lymphoma, the third most common pediatric cancer, is a **heterogeneous group of lymphomas** whose incidence increases with age. The incidence of non-Hodgkin lymphoma varies with geographic area. **Africa and the Middle East** have the highest rates of non-Hodgkin lymphoma, with Burkitt lymphoma especially prevalent in Africa.

Etiology

EBV has been recovered from many of these tumors, raising the question of its role in the etiology of the tumor. Risk factors for development of non-Hodgkin lymphoma include **genetically determined immunodeficiency syndromes** (ataxia-telangiectasia, Wiskott-Aldrich syndrome, severe combined immunodeficiency disease, and X-linked lymphoproliferative disease) and **acquired immunodeficiency syndromes** (AIDS and postrenal/cardiac/bone marrow transplant).

Clinical Features

Childhood non-Hodgkin lymphoma is divided into **three main histo-logic patterns: lymphoblastic** (40%), **small noncleaved cell** (including Burkitt and non-Burkitt lymphoma) (40%), **and large cell** (20%).

- **Lymphoblastic.** Most lymphoblastic lymphomas are of T-cell origin. The patient may present with **cervical adenopathy and respiratory distress.** A chest radiograph frequently reveals a **mediastinal mass** and **pleural effusions. Superior vena cava syndrome is a life-threatening emergency** that may arise in this setting. The mediastinal mass compresses the superior vena cava and/or trachea, impeding blood return and air flow. Symptoms include **cough, dyspnea, and difficulty lying down secondary to respiratory distress.** Physical findings include **edema and cyanosis of the face, neck, and upper extremities and wheeze or stridor. Immediate therapy with radiation or chemotherapy** may obscure the diagnosis but may be lifesaving.
- **Small noncleaved cell.** Most patients with small noncleaved cell lymphomas present with abdominal findings. **Abdominal pain and swelling** are common complaints. Physical findings include a **rapidly enlarging abdominal mass and inguinal adenopathy.** Signs of **intestinal obstruction** may be present.
- **Large cell lymphomas.** Large cell lymphomas have various clinical presentations.

Evaluation

Workup should include a **complete blood cell count (CBC) with WBC differential, serum lactate dehydrogenase, serum uric acid, and examination of the bone marrow and spinal fluid. Chest radiography or computed tomography (CT)** of the chest should be performed to evaluate supradiaphragmatic disease; **abdominal ultrasonography or CT** should be performed to evaluate subdiaphragmatic disease. Ascites, pleural, or pericardial fluid can also be used to establish the diagnosis.

Treatment

Because this tumor grows rapidly, prompt diagnosis is vital so treatment can be initiated. **Combination chemotherapy** is the mainstay of treatment. These patients are at increased **risk for tumor lysis syndrome** (see discussion of leukemia in Chapter 48, "Leukocytosis"), as a result of the tumor's high growth rate and sensitivity to chemotherapy. **Prognosis is good,** except in patients with advanced disease (bone marrow or CNS involvement).

Hodgkin Disease

Etiology

Hodgkin disease is a form of lymphoma most frequently seen in **late adolescence.** Although it can occur at other ages, it is especially rare in those <5 years. The etiology is unknown.

Clinical Features

The patient usually presents with **painless cervical or supraclavicular adenopathy,** although other nodes may be involved. Systemic symptoms include **fever, weight loss, night sweats, anorexia, and fatigue.**

Evaluation

Physical examination reveals **firm, nontender lymph nodes** in the areas just mentioned. **Hepatosplenomegaly** is a common finding and may indicate advanced disease.

If Hodgkin disease is suspected, a **chest radiograph should be obtained promptly** because two thirds of patients have some degree of **mediastinal involvement.** The **airway should be assessed** for evidence of tracheal compression before any procedures are performed. **Lymph node biopsy** establishes the definitive diagnosis, revealing the **characteristic Reed-Sternberg cell and one of four histologic patterns** (nodular sclerosing, lymphocytic predominance, lymphocytic depletion, and mixed cellularity). Further workup is necessary for staging purposes and to establish a baseline for following response to treatment. Studies should include a **complete blood count (CBC) with differential, erythrocyte sedimentation rate, chest and abdominal CT scans, bone scan, and bone marrow aspirate/biopsy. Gallium scans and staging laparotomies** are helpful in some instances.

Treatment

Treatment consists of **combination chemotherapy and/or radiation therapy,** based on the patient's age, pubertal status, and stage of disease. Long-term survival continues to improve but still varies greatly with stage of disease.

Tuberculosis

Incidence

The incidence of TB has risen in recent years. **Early detection and prompt treatment** are becoming increasingly important to prevent spread of the disease. The highest rates of infection are currently seen in minority populations, in urban settings, and in association with crowded living conditions. **Patients with HIV infection** are especially likely to present with active disease. Transmission of the etiologic agent

Mycobacterium tuberculosis is by inhalation of infected droplets. The **incubation period** from time of infection to the development of a positive skin test is 2 to 10 weeks. Clinical disease develops in a minority of infected patients. When disease does develop, it is usually within the first 2 years after infection.

Clinical Features

Patients most commonly present with either an **asymptomatic infection or pulmonary disease.** Those with a positive skin test and no evidence of clinical disease should have a **screening chest radiograph.** Individuals with pulmonary disease may have symptoms that include **fever, weight loss, and cough,** and physical examination may reveal **lymphadenopathy. A chest radiograph** reveals an **infiltrate or hilar adenopathy. Extrapulmonary disease** (miliary, meningeal, lymph node, bone/joint disease, etc.) can also occur in a minority of patients.

Evaluation

An infection is diagnosed by a **positive skin test or by culture** (which takes months to grow) from infected **body fluids** (sputum, gastric washings). The tuberculin preparation recommended for skin testing is the purified protein derivative (PPD). The standard dose is 5 tuberculin units in 0.1 mL of solution, which should be injected intradermally on the forearm. A positive reaction is defined as >10 mm of induration after 48 to 72 hours. Tine tests should not be used for definitive diagnosis and are of questionable value for screening.

Treatment

Treatment of patients with asymptomatic infection consists of **isoniazid for 9 months.** Patients with clinical disease should be treated with **multiple-drug regimens.**

EVALUATION OF LYMPHADENOPATHY

Patient History

> **HINT:** Because infections are the most common cause of acute and chronic lymphadenopathy, the history should focus on the presence of or exposure to infections.

- When were the swollen glands first noted?
- Are they getting larger? (in general, the larger the node, the more worrisome)
- Is the node red, tender, or painful? (lymphadenitis)
- Has there been fever, weight loss, night sweats? (lymphoma, TB)

- Is there any bruising or bleeding? Is the child fatigued or pale? (leukemia)
- Is there fever, rash, systemic symptoms? (scarlet fever, rubeola, rubella, infectious mononucleosis, Kawasaki disease)
- Are there joint complaints? (juvenile rheumatoid arthritis, systemic lupus erythematosus)
- Is there a history of a cat scratch (cat-scratch disease), tick bite (Lyme disease), or other animal exposure (tularemia)?
- Has there been exposure to an individual with TB?
- Is there a history of high-risk sexual behavior, substance abuse, or transfusion? Does a parent have any of these risk factors? (HIV)
- Is there a history of travel? (malaria)

Physical Examination

Are the nodes generalized or regional? (see "Differential Diagnosis" section earlier in this chapter)

- What size are the nodes? (baseline measurement important to ensure proper follow-up)
- Are the nodes erythematous, tender, warm, fluctuant? (lymphadenitis)
- Are the nodes firm/hard and fixed in position? (malignancy)
- Is there fever, rash? (scarlet fever, rubeola, rubella, infectious mononucleosis, Kawasaki disease)
- Is there pharyngitis? (streptococcal disease)
- Is there hepatosplenomegaly? (infectious mononucleosis, leukemia)
- Are there bruises, petechiae, pallor? (leukemia)
- Are there joint findings? (juvenile rheumatoid arthritis, systemic lupus erythematosus)
- Is there a palpable abdominal mass? (neuroblastoma)
- Is there any skin infection and/or inflammation? (tinea, atopic dermatitis)

Laboratory Studies

- CBC, differential count
- Peripheral blood smear (atypical lymphocytes)
- Lactate dehydrogenase, uric acid (for suspected lymphoma, leukemia)
- Screening for specific infectious diseases
  - *B. henselae*
  - EBV
  - CMV
  - HIV
  - Toxoplasmosis
- PPD skin test
- Chest radiograph

- Ultrasound (distinguish suppurative from nonsuppurative lymphadenitis)
- Needle aspiration (may identify organism in suppurative lymphadenitis)
- Lymph node biopsy

APPROACH TO THE PATIENT

- Do you have a probable diagnosis (e.g., fever, sore throat, cervical lymphadenopathy, exudative pharyngitis, probable streptococcal pharyngitis) after completing the history and physical examination? If so, perform appropriate diagnostic tests (throat culture) and begin treatment with antibiotics if indicated.
- Are you unsure of the diagnosis in a patient who looks ill or is febrile without a clear cause? Consider admission to the hospital and a more extensive laboratory screen for infectious or malignant causes.
- Does the patient exhibit any particularly worrisome symptoms or physical findings, such as the following?
  - Supraclavicular adenopathy
  - Hard, rubbery, or matted adenopathy
  - Fever, constitutional symptoms >1 week without infectious cause identified
  - Cervical nodes that continue to increase in size despite adequate antibiotic therapy
  - A node that continues to increase in size after 1 to 2 weeks
  - An enlarging node that does not regress in size after 4 weeks
- If the answer to one or more of these questions is yes, these children should all have a CBC with differential, PPD skin test, and a chest radiograph. Lymph node biopsy should be considered in the absence of a diagnosis.
- Are you unsure of the diagnosis in a patient who looks well and does not have any high-risk symptoms or physical findings? Consider empirical antibiotics to cover common staphylococcal and streptococcal infections and close follow-up with serial examinations.

Suggested Readings

Kelly CS, Kelly RE Jr: Lymphadenopathy in children. *Pediatr Clin North Am* 45:875–888, 1998.

Nield LS, Kamat D: Lymphadenopathy in children: when and how to evaluate. *Clin Pediatr* 43:25–33, 2004.

chapter 51

Macrocephaly

Cynthia Campen
Mitchell Roberts (Third Edition)

INTRODUCTION

The skull provides a fixed space for the brain, blood vessels, and cerebrospinal fluid (CSF) (thereby causing symptoms of increased intracranial pressure in the case of a space-occupying lesion) in adults and older children, but in **infants** it has the capability of growth that can accommodate expansion of any intracranial compartment. Macrocephaly is defined by **head circumference greater than two standard deviations from the mean for gender** (i.e., 98th percentile). It arises from the enlargement of any of the four major constituents of the head: **ventricles** (hydrocephalus), **brain parenchyma** (megalencephaly), **skull** (osteodysplasia), or **extracerebral fluid collections** (subdural, subgaleal, or subperiosteal).

Hydrocephalus is typically described as **communicating** (with free flow of CSF between the ventricles and subarachnoid space) or **noncommunicating** (obstructive). Either type can be congenital or acquired. Communicating hydrocephalus is usually caused by **overproduction of CSF** or **blockage of CSF reabsorption** at the arachnoid villi. Common causes include intraventricular hemorrhage, infection, or inflammation (e.g., bacterial, tuberculous or cryptococcal meningitis, viral encephalitis), meningeal infiltration by tumor, and metabolic conditions (e.g., Hurler syndrome with associated mucopolysaccharidosis deposition at the leptomeninges).

Congenital hydrocephalus is increasingly being diagnosed in utero by routine ultrasonography. It usually presents during the newborn period or in early infancy with lethargy or irritability, vomiting, poor feeding, or poor weight gain. Signs of increased intracranial pressure (ICP) include apnea, bradycardia, a tense and bulging fontanelle, split sutures, the "setting sun sign" (i.e., downward deviation of the eyes showing sclera superiorly), vomiting, sixth nerve palsies, and increased blood pressure with bradycardia. Scalp veins may be prominent and tortuous.

- Diagnosis is made by serial head measurements (see Table 51-1) and neuroimaging.
- In patients with progressive hydrocephalus, treatment includes ventriculoperitoneal (VP) shunting.

DIFFERENTIAL DIAGNOSIS LIST 🔓

Congenital

Infectious—cytomegalovirus, toxoplasmosis, mumps, rubella

Anatomic—Chiari malformation, hydranencephaly, aqueductal stenosis

TABLE 51-1 Head Growth Velocity

Full Term		Preterm	
Age	Rate of Growth	Age	Rate of Growth
0–3 months	2 cm/month	0–2 months	1 cm/week
3–6 months	1 cm/month	2–4 months	0.5 cm/week
7–12 months	0.5 cm/month	>4 months	1cm/month

Neoplasm—medulloblastoma, choroid plexus papilloma, meningioma

Acquired

Neoplasm—posterior fossa tumor: medulloblastoma, ependymoma, cerebellar astrocytoma

Intraventricular tumor—ependymoma, choroids

plexus papilloma, giant cell astrocytoma, meningioma

Intraparenchymal mass—cyst, abscess, tumor

Trauma—cephalohematoma, subdural or subgaleal fluid collections

Vascular—aneurysm of the vein of Galen, intraparenchymal bleed, intraventricular hemorrhage

> **HINT:** Papilledema is uncommon in infancy because open fontanelles and unfused sutures allow skull expansion, thus relieving pressure.

DIFFERENTIAL DIAGNOSIS DISCUSSION

Congenital Infection

Congenital infections are discussed in detail in Chapter 56, "Neonatal Infections." Calcification seen on a computed tomography (CT) scan of the head increases the suspicion for congenital infection.

Chiari Malformations

There are four types of Chiari malformations. The most common is **type II** (Arnold-Chiari malformation), often associated with **spina bifida.** In this variant, the cervical canals of both the brainstem and cerebellum are displaced downward, the fourth ventricle is elongated, and hydrocephalus results from obstruction of the flow of CSF through the foramina of Magendie and Luschka. At birth, some patients already have advanced hydrocephalus; others show rapid head enlargement during the first weeks of life. Patients with Chiari malformations may exhibit signs and symptoms related to brainstem dysfunction (lower cranial nerve findings, breathing difficulty, apnea, poor feeding, swallowing problems, poor gag, and tongue fasciculations) as well as symptoms of increased ICP.

- Serial head circumference measurements need to be performed.
- Ultrasonography (US), CT, or magnetic resonance imaging (MRI) of the head can confirm the diagnosis. MRI is recommended to evaluate brain anatomy.
- Brainstem auditory evoked responses complement the MRI assessment.

> **HINT:** A child who presents with headache that worsens with cough or other Valsalva maneuvers should be evaluated for Chiari malformation.

Genetic Syndromes

Hydrocephalus is seen in many genetic disorders. Fifty percent of patients with trisomy 13 syndrome have meningomyelocele with hydrocephalus. **Warburg syndrome,** an autosomal recessive disorder, includes findings of hydrocephalus, retinal lesions, Dandy-Walker cyst, occipital encephalocele, agyria, and pachygyria. **Klippel-Feil syndrome,** with many modes of inheritance, causes malformation of the skull and cervical vertebrae that can be associated with Chiari malformation and hydrocephalus.

Hydranencephaly

Hydranencephaly is caused by the replacement of cortex by enlarged ventricles, presumably secondary to ex vacuo dilation following massive intrauterine infarctions. The infant may initially appear normal, with a normal head circumference and intact primitive reflexes, but developmental arrest and long tract signs make the absence of cortex evident as the child grows. Many patients die in early infancy, but prolonged survival is possible. Positive transillumination and percussion of the skull strongly support the diagnosis, which is made by prenatal ultrasound or neuroimaging after birth.

Congenital Aqueductal Stenosis

Cerebral aqueductal atresia or stenosis can occur following intrauterine hemorrhage, infection, brain tumor, venous malformation, or as an isolated developmental anomaly. Diagnosis is made by prenatal US or postnatal neuroimaging. Management includes placement of a VP shunt.

Acquired Hydrocephalus

Neoplasm

The most common tumors in children <2 years are choroid plexus papilloma, ependymoma, and medulloblastoma. Children with posterior fossa masses (e.g., medulloblastoma, ependymoma, cerebellar astrocytoma) present to medical care with signs of increased ICP, ataxia, papilledema, and meningismus. Persistent torticollis in a child should raise the suspicion of tumor. Intraventricular tumors (e.g., choroid plexus papilloma) can lead to hydrocephalus by increased CSF production or blockage of CSF pathways. Diagnosis is made by CT or MRI scans. Treatment of hydrocephalus is by surgical resection of the tumor with or without VP shunt.

Intraventricular Hemorrhage

Intraventricular hemorrhage is common in low birthweight infants because of immaturity of the germinal matrix vessels. Perinatal and neonatal stresses (e.g., sepsis, respiratory distress syndrome, hyperglycemia and hypoglycemia, hypoxemia, and shock) trigger hemorrhage. Low-grade intraventricular hemorrhage is usually asymptomatic. Grade III or IV hemorrhages (significant subependymal involvement, intraparenchymal extension) may result in obstructive hydrocephalus by compression of critical pathways or communicating hydrocephalus by blocking the CSF reabsorption in the arachnoid villi.

Infection and Inflammation

Inflammation and meningeal seeding (from tumor cells) may result in communicating hydrocephalus. In addition, irritation or entrapment of the nerves throughout their course in the brain may cause patchy cranial nerve abnormalities. Massive subdural effusion or empyema complicating bacterial meningitis may contribute to head enlargement. Diagnosis is made by MRI with gadolinium enhancement.

Trauma

Cephalohematoma and subdural collections may result from traumatic delivery, either spontaneously or as a result of a forceps or vacuum delivery. Patients with a large subdural collection may experience rapid head enlargement associated with an acute **encephalopathy** characterized by lethargy, poor feeding, vomiting, and seizures.

- CT of the head should be performed immediately in all symptomatic infants with a history of traumatic birth injury because diagnostic delay can be fatal.
- Large symptomatic subdural collections may require neurosurgical intervention.

Megaloencephaly or parenchymal enlargement is caused by anatomic or metabolic abnormalities including the following:

- **Benign familial macrocephaly,** in which there is a family history of large head, with normal intelligence and normal neurologic examination. Although the head circumference is greater than two standard deviations above the mean, it remains parallel to the expected percentile with serial measurements. No workup is necessary, although if neuroimaging is performed, one finds top normal size of the ventricles and subarachnoid spaces.

> **HINT:** Even if head growth velocity is crossing percentiles, measuring the head circumference of the parents can be helpful in diagnosing benign familial macrocephaly and quickly reducing anxiety.

- **Sotos syndrome** (megalencephaly with gigantism) is characterized by cerebral gigantism with excessive somatic growth, advanced bone age, megalencephaly, and mild mental retardation.
- **Symptomatic megalencephaly** is a description for a group of diseases associated with megalencephaly, for example, degenerative diseases (e.g., Tay-Sachs disease, Canavan disease, Alexander disease) and neurocutaneous syndromes (e.g., neurofibromatosis, tuberous sclerosis).
- **Osteodysplasia** presents with increased skull thickness caused by anemia, osteochondrodysplasia, or rickets, and can also lead to macrocephaly.
- **Idiopathic megalocephaly** is a diagnosis of exclusion when there are no identifiable causes, associated syndromes, or a family history of macrocephaly. MRI shows normal or mildly dilated ventricles.

Suggested Readings

Alper G, Ekinci G, Yilmaz Y, et al.: Magnetic resonance imaging characteristics of benign macrocephaly in children. *J Child Neurol* 12(10):678–682, 1999.

Archibald SL, Fennema-Notestine C, Gamst A, et al.: Brain dysmorphology in individuals with severe prenatal alcohol exposure. *Dev Med Child Neurol* 43(3):148–154, 2001.

Charney E: Management of Chiari II complications. *J Pediatr* 3(3):364–371, 1989.

Mercuri E, Ricci D, Cowan FM, et al.: Head growth in infants with hypoxic-ischemic encephalopathy: correlation with neonatal magnetic resonance imaging. *Pediatrics* 105(2 Pt 1):235–243, 2000.

Sher PK, Brown SB: A longitudinal study of head growth in preterm infants. I: Normal rates of head growth. *Dev Med Child Neurol* 17:705–710, 1975.

Sher PK, Brown SB: A longitudinal study of head growth in preterm infants. II: Differentiation between "catch up" head growth and early infantile hydrocephalus. *Dev Med Child Neurol* 17:711–718, 1975.

52 *Mediastinal Mass*
Jonathan D. Fish

INTRODUCTION

The mediastinum is a potential space within the thoracic cavity, between the two pleura. It is divided into anterior, middle, and posterior regions. The etiology of a mediastinal mass is often suggested by its regional location because it likely formed from the normal structures within that region.

■ Anterior mediastinum.
Anatomy: The anterior mediastinum is bounded by the first rib superiorly, the posterior surface of the sternum anteriorly, the anterior border of the upper dorsal vertebra posteriorly, and by an imaginary curved line that follows the cardiac border and extends backward until it reaches the border of the dorsal vertebra.
Structures: This area contains the thymus, lymph nodes, and, rarely, extensions of the thyroid gland. The superior vena cava is an easily compressible, thin-walled vessel with a low intraluminal pressure that is surrounded by the lymph nodes and thymus.

> **HINT:** Superior vena cava syndrome is generally associated with anterior mediastinal masses.

■ Posterior mediastinum.
Anatomy: The posterior mediastinum is bounded posteriorly by the anterior surface of the curve of the ribs, anteriorly by the posterior border of the pericardium, and inferiorly by the diaphragm.
Structures: The primary structures in this area are the sympathetic ganglia and esophagus.
■ Middle mediastinum.
Anatomy: The middle mediastinum is the area between the anterior and posterior regions with the diaphragm as its base.
Structures: This region contains the trachea, bronchi, heart, great vessels, and lymph nodes.

DIFFERENTIAL DIAGNOSIS LIST

Anterior Mediastinum
Lymphoma—non-Hodgkin lymphoma (NHL), Hodgkin lymphoma
Germ cell tumor

Thymic hyperplasia or cyst
Lymphangioma (cystic hygroma)
Hemangioma
Histiocytosis

Lipoma

Thymoma

Substernal thyroid

Middle Mediastinum

Histoplasmosis

Tuberculosis (TB)

Sarcoidosis

Bronchogenic cyst

Pericardial cyst

Fibromatosis

Posterior Mediastinum

Tumors of neurogenic origin—
neuroblastoma, ganglioneuroblastoma, ganglioneuroma

Thoracic meningocele

Esophageal duplication cyst

Note: **Ewing sarcoma** and **rhabdomyosarcoma** can form masses in **any** of the mediastinal regions.

DIFFERENTIAL DIAGNOSIS DISCUSSION

Anterior Mediastinum

> **HINT:** Most, but not all, symptomatic anterior mediastinal masses in children are malignant.

Superior Vena Cava Syndrome/Superior Mediastinal Syndrome

Superior vena cava and superior mediastinal syndromes are **life-threatening complications of anterior mediastinal masses. Superior vena cava syndrome** implies **venous obstruction** from compression or thrombosis. When **coupled with tracheal compression**, the syndrome is called **superior mediastinal syndrome.** Tracheal compression without signs of venous obstruction is more common than the full-blown syndrome but is equally worrisome. The mediastinal mass compresses the superior vena cava, the trachea, or both, impeding blood return and air flow and producing the signs and symptoms summarized in Table 52-1.

TABLE 52-1 Signs and Symptoms of Superior Vena Cava Syndrome or Superior Mediastinal Syndrome

History	Physical Examination
Cough, especially when supine	Retractions
Dyspnea or orthopnea	Wheezing or stridor
Headache	Papilledema
Dizziness or syncope, especially when symptoms are exacerbated with Valsalva maneuver	Prominence of neck or chest veins
	Suffusion or edema of conjunctiva
	Cyanosis or plethora
Facial swelling	Anxiety or confusion
Visual changes	
Sense of fullness in ears	

These are rare syndromes; only 10% to 15% of pediatric patients with malignant anterior mediastinal tumors have superior vena cava syndrome or superior mediastinal syndrome. However, it is **critical to recognize these patients** because their condition can **deteriorate dramatically** with disastrous consequences. **Immediate consultation with an oncologist** is always appropriate.

Lymphoma

> **HINT:** Lymphoma is the most common cause of superior vena cava syndrome and superior mediastinal syndrome in children.

Non-Hodgkin Lymphoma

Mediastinal masses in patients with NHL are almost exclusively caused by lymphoblastic lymphoma (see Chapter 50, "Lymphadenopathy"). Approximately 60% of patients with lymphoblastic lymphoma present with a mediastinal mass, and they often have pleural effusions.

Hodgkin Lymphoma

Although NHL has a slightly higher incidence than Hodgkin lymphoma, the mediastinum is more often the primary site of involvement in Hodgkin disease. **Cervical adenopathy** is the most common clinical presentation, but approximately 52% to 65% of patients with Hodgkin lymphoma also present with a mass consisting of **anterior mediastinal, paratracheal, and tracheobronchial lymph nodes. Tracheobronchial compression** has been observed on chest radiographs in 50% of children with newly diagnosed Hodgkin lymphoma. Half of these patients also have systemic symptoms of Hodgkin disease, including **fever, night sweats, and weight loss** of >10% in the previous 6 months. (Hodgkin lymphoma is discussed in detail in Chapter 50, "Lymphadenopathy.")

Germ Cell Tumors

The **anterior mediastinum** is the second most common site of extragonadal germ cell tumors.

> **HINT:** Up to 20% of boys with mediastinal germ cell tumors have Klinefelter syndrome.

Teratomas

Teratomas are classified histologically as follows:

- **Mature teratoma.** The tumor is composed of well-differentiated tissues derived from the three germinal layers of the embryo (i.e., endoderm, mesoderm, and ectoderm).

- **Immature teratoma.** In addition to mature elements, the mass contains embryonic-appearing elements. In infants, immature teratomas behave as mass lesions, but in adolescents, they behave as highly malignant tumors.
- **Teratoma with malignant germ cell tumor components.** These teratomas contain one or more of the components of germinomas, embryonal carcinomas, endodermal sinus tumors, or choriocarcinoma, in addition to characteristics of either a mature or immature teratoma.

Germinoma

Germinomas histologically **resemble primordial germ cells.** Previously, germinomas were designated "seminomas" when they occurred in the testes and "dysgerminomas" when they occurred in the ovaries.

Embryonal Carcinoma

Embryonal carcinomas histologically **resemble a poorly differentiated or anaplastic carcinoma with extensive necrosis.** These tumors are most commonly found in the **testes of young adults.**

Endodermal Sinus (Yolk Sac) Tumor

Endodermal sinus tumors are **the most common malignant germ cell tumors in children.** They are most commonly found in the **sacrococcygeal area.** Patients test **positive for** α-fetoprotein (the principal serum protein of the fetus, with a structure and function similar to that of albumin).

Choriocarcinoma

Choriocarcinoma is rare in children, but two forms have been described: **gestational** (arising from the placenta) and **nongestational.** β-Human chorionic gonadotropin (hCG) is invariably produced.

Thymic Hyperplasia

An enlarged thymus is the most common cause of a widened anterior mediastinum in neonates. This is a **benign incidental finding** that does not cause symptoms unless the hyperplastic thymus is located in an abnormal position. Thymic enlargement is sometimes the result of a **thymic cyst,** which can be delineated by computed tomography (CT), although this would rarely be indicated clinically.

Lymphangioma (Cystic Hygroma)

Lymphangiomas are **rarely localized to the mediastinum** but can extend into the mediastinum from a neck lesion and cause symptoms. Lymphangiomas are almost always noted by the time the patient reaches 3 years of age. **Surgical resection** is necessary.

Hemangioma

Like lymphangiomas, hemangiomas are reported in all portions of the mediastinum, but approximately **75% of mediastinal hemangiomas occur in the anterior region.** Many are **asymptomatic,** but they may cause **airway compression** or, rarely, **bleeding into the pleural cavity.** Mediastinal hemangiomas are associated with hemangiomas at other sites in the body. Generally, hemangiomas **grow during the first and second year of life and then slowly regress.**

Histiocytosis

Histiocytosis is an increase in the number of mononuclear phagocytic cells (histiocytes). Rarely, patients with Langerhans cell histiocytosis (which is caused by immunologic stimulation of the normal antigen-processing Langerhans cell in an uncontrolled manner) present with a mediastinal mass.

Lipoma

Lipomas are benign tumors composed of aberrant fat cells. They grow very slowly and generally do not undergo malignant transformation.

Thymoma

A neoplasm of the thymus is not considered a thymoma unless it contains **neoplastic epithelial components.** Such tumors are rare in adults and even rarer in children. Thymomas are slow-growing tumors that extend locally and rarely metastasize. Rarely, **autoimmune disorders** (e.g., myasthenia gravis, systemic lupus erythematosus, rheumatoid arthritis, cytopenias, thyroiditis) are reported in **association with thymomas.**

Middle Mediastinum

> **HINT:** Mediastinal lymph node granulomas, usually from histoplasmosis, are the second most common cause of mediastinal masses.

Histoplasmosis

This disease is caused by the fungus *Histoplasma capsulatum.* It is endemic in the Mississippi, Ohio, and Missouri River valleys, where up to 80% of the population has a positive histoplasmin skin test by 20 years of age. The diagnosis is best made by either noting a fourfold increase in the complement fixation titer between acute and convalescent sera (using *Histoplasma* yeast and mycelial antigens) or by performing a tissue diagnosis.

Tuberculosis

TB, a mycobacterial disease, commonly affects **mediastinal lymph nodes** in children. Infection of nodes without significant pulmonary involvement is more common in primary pulmonary TB than in reactivation of the disease. Of note, as many as 20% of patients with culture-proven TB have negative Mantoux skin test reactions during the early phase of their illness (even when the skin testing is performed with 250 tuberculin units). A definitive diagnosis requires **histologic and bacteriologic confirmation.**

Sarcoidosis

This **chronic, multisystemic disease** of obscure origin is uncommon in patients <10 years and is more common in **African American children.** The pathologic lesion is a noncaseating granuloma; the **lung** is the most frequently affected organ. **Hilar and paratracheal adenopathy** is often found in association with parenchymal infiltrates and may be far more dramatic than the parenchymal lesions. **Biopsy** of the affected tissue is the most valuable diagnostic tool.

Bronchogenic Cysts

These cysts, which are lined with ciliated epithelium, can be found in any portion of the mediastinum but most often are found **near the carina in the middle mediastinum.** Cysts can become **symptomatic** either **by becoming infected or by enlarging in size,** thereby compromising the function of an adjacent airway. **Surgical excision is curative.**

Pericardial Cysts

Pericardial cysts are benign mediastinal lesions. They are usually unilocular cystic lesions with a thin connective tissue wall and clear fluid contents. Although they are considered developmental anomalies, they can be acquired. They are very rare in children.

Posterior Mediastinum

> **HINT:** Most posterior mediastinal masses in children are neurogenic in origin.

Tumors of Neurogenic Origin

Neuroblastoma, a malignant tumor, may arise **anywhere along the sympathetic nervous system chain.** Approximately 15% of neuroblastomas arise in the paraspinal ganglion of the thorax. **Thoracic neuroblastomas** are almost always attached to the **intervertebral foramina** and thus can cause **spinal cord compression.** Interestingly, **less than gross total resection of such lesions can provide a cure.**

Differentiation of neuroblasts into benign ganglion cells occurs both spontaneously and after therapy. The term **ganglioneuroma** refers to such differentiated lesions. **Ganglioneuroblastoma** refers to **lesions containing malignant cells and benign ganglion cells.**

Thoracic Meningocele

Anterior spinal meningoceles are rare and associated with neurofibromatosis type 1 or Marfan syndrome.

Esophageal Duplication Cysts

Approximately 10% of alimentary tract duplications are esophageal, and two thirds are **right-sided.** The **duplication does not communicate with the esophagus** unless there is ulceration of the gastric mucosa within the cyst. Neurenteric cysts are esophageal duplication cysts that **contain glial elements;** vertebral anomalies usually accompany these cysts.

Ewing Sarcoma

This **small, round, blue-cell tumor** rarely occurs in children <5 years and has a very low incidence in African American children. Ewing sarcoma most frequently involves the **axial skeleton,** and some "mediastinal" masses actually originate from the chest wall (or a rib). True mediastinal involvement rarely occurs at diagnosis but is not infrequent in advanced cases.

Ewing sarcoma must be **differentiated from** other small, round, blue-cell tumors, including **neuroblastoma, lymphoma, and rhabdomyosarcoma.** Previously a diagnosis of exclusion, Ewing sarcoma can now be **diagnosed by demonstrating the characteristic t(11;22) chromosomal abnormality.**

Rhabdomyosarcoma

This sarcoma, which arises from **primitive mesenchymal cells,** is the **most common soft tissue sarcoma in children.** However, in large series, only 1% of these tumors arise in the mediastinum, and these series do not stratify masses into the anterior, posterior, or middle mediastinum. Most patients with mediastinal rhabdomyosarcomas are **boys (65%)** with a mean age of 10 years. Metastatic disease may be seen in the **lungs (including pleura), bone, and bone marrow** of these patients.

EVALUATION OF MEDIASTINAL MASS

> **HINT:** As many as a third of masses in the mediastinum are found acciden-
> tally when radiographs are performed to evaluate fever or other
> complaints.

History and Physical Examination

Table 52-1 lists the important features of the history and physical
examination that should be specifically addressed to **rule out an emergency.** The **presence or absence of hepatosplenomegaly, adenopathy,
systemic signs of a malignant tumor** (e.g., fever, weight loss), **or neurologic signs** (e.g., Horner syndrome, signs of cord compression) are
equally important.

Laboratory Studies

Laboratory tests are tailored to the individual, but the following may
be appropriate:

- **Complete blood count with differential.** The presence of lymphoblasts
  on smear or cytopenias from marrow infiltration may allow the physician to establish the diagnosis without biopsying tissue from the mediastinal mass.
- **Chemistry panel, including uric acid.** A high uric acid level, lactate dehydrogenase level, or both are often seen in patients with lymphoblastic
  lymphomas.
- **α-Fetoprotein and β-hCG levels** are helpful in suggesting the diagnosis of germ cell tumor, and useful in following the response to therapy.
- **Quantitative vanillylmandelic and homovanillic acid analysis.**
  Elevations of these substances in the urine are suggestive of neuroblastoma.
- **Histoplasma complement fixation titers** should be obtained in endemic
  areas.

Other Diagnostic Modalities

- **CT and magnetic resonance imaging (MRI).** A CT scan can delineate
  the cystic nature of a lesion and reveals calcifications in 95% of patients
  with neuroblastomas and 35% of patients with germ cell tumors.
  Visualization of a tooth is pathognomonic of a teratoma. CT is more
  sensitive for bony erosion than MRI, but MRI is more helpful for
  detecting intraspinous extension and should be considered for patients
  with posterior mediastinal masses.

HINT: Before performing CT or MRI, a careful history should be taken for orthopnea because having a patient with superior mediastinal syndrome lie supine can lead to decreased blood return to the heart and arrest, or airway compromise.

- **Bone marrow aspirate.** Performed while the patient is sitting, bone marrow aspirate is indicated for ill patients in whom the diagnosis of lymphoma or another disease involving the marrow is suspected.
- **Pleurocentesis or pericardiocentesis.** It is usually possible to make a definitive diagnosis of lymphoblastic lymphoma by assessing cells collected during these procedures.
- **Biopsy** may be necessary to make a definitive tissue diagnosis and requires general anesthesia.

 HINT: Before considering a biopsy to make a tissue diagnosis definitively, an echocardiogram (preferably upright and supine) and a (pulmonary) flow-volume loop should be obtained. Patients who do not tolerate these procedures are not candidates for general anesthesia. Cardiopulmonary changes associated with general anesthesia can aggravate superior vena cava syndrome and superior mediastinal syndrome, leading to total airway obstruction, cardiac arrest, or both. Particularly worrisome is the fact that these complications can develop in patients with mild or no preoperative symptoms.

TREATMENT OF MEDIASTINAL MASS

Thirty years ago it was stated "early, vigorous treatment, designed to cause rapid shrinkage of the tumor, should not be delayed by an overly diligent pursuit of the diagnosis." This is equally true today. **If a patient is critically ill and cannot tolerate a definitive diagnostic procedure, empirical chemotherapy, emergency radiation therapy, or both are indicated.** One must be aware, however, that **steroids or even low-dose radiotherapy** (200 cGy) **may render definitive diagnosis impossible—** even if a biopsy is done only 24 hours later. Biopsy of a node that is out of the field or intentionally shielded is, of course, still possible after the patient is stabilized.

Some authors recommend **concurrent treatment with steroids** during radiotherapy because patients can transiently worsen, presumably as a result of edema. A significant percentage of patients improve within 12 hours of the first dose of radiation. **Chemotherapy with steroids,** cyclophosphamide, or both in combination with vincristine or an anthracycline is a reasonable **alternative empirical approach,** although this too can render the subsequent histologic picture uninterpretable. Even when the histologic diagnosis is lost, **continued treatment of the diagnosis that best fits the clinical picture** usually results in long-term disease-free survival.

Suggested Readings

Filler RM, Simpson JS, Ein SH: Mediastinal masses in infants and children. *Pediatr Clin North Am* 14:677–690, 1979.

Franco A, Mody NS, Meza MP: Imaging evaluation of pediatric mediastinal masses. *Radiol Clin North Am* 43:325–353, 2005.

Issa PY, Brihi ER, Janin Y, et al.: Superior vena cava syndrome in childhood: report of ten cases and review of the literature. *Pediatrics* 71:337–341, 1983.

53 | *Murmurs*
Jack Rychik

INTRODUCTION

A murmur is an **auditory vibration produced by turbulent flow within the cardiac structures.** A murmur may be **physiologic** (i.e., a normal finding) or **pathologic.**

Heart Sounds

Variations in the normal heart sounds, as well as **adventitious** heart sounds, may be associated with murmurs and are essential clues to diagnostic interpretation of the murmur.

First Heart Sound (S₁)

The S_1 is produced by **closure of the mitral and tricuspid valves,** in that order. The mitral component and tricuspid component are **best heard at the apex and the lower sternal border region,** respectively.

- The intensity of the S_1 is accentuated in conditions characterized by increased cardiac output and a short PR interval because in these circumstances maximal excursion of the leaflets occurs during closure.
- Wide splitting of the S_1 with a delayed tricuspid component may be noted in patients with tricuspid stenosis, Ebstein anomaly, right bundle branch block, or when there is pacing of the left ventricle.

Second Heart Sound (S₂)

The S_2 is produced by **closure of the aortic valve (A_2) immediately followed by closure of the pulmonic valve (P_2)** and is best heard at the base of the heart. The P_2 is normally softer than the A_2 and is less widely transmitted. **Splitting of the S_2** is normally appreciated during quiet respiration. Inspiration results in two physiologic phenomena: an **increased capacitance of the lung vasculature,** with a greater period of systole for the right ventricle relative to the left ventricle, and **increased venous return to the right-sided structures.** Both of these phenomena result in **delayed closure of the pulmonic valve.**

- In mild forms of aortic or pulmonic stenosis, the A_2 or the P_2 may be soft.
- The S_2 is single and loud in the following circumstances: when there is fusion of the two components, such as in severe pulmonary hypertension; when there is only one semilunar valve, such as in atresia of either the aortic or pulmonic valves or truncus arteriosus; and when the P_2 is inaudible because of an anteriorly positioned aorta, such as in tetralogy of Fallot or transposition of the great arteries.

TABLE 53-1 Common Causes of Abnormally Wide Splitting of the Second Heart Sound (S$_2$)
Atrial septal defect
Mild pulmonic stenosis
Complete right bundle branch block
Left ventricular paced beats
Massive pulmonary embolus

■ Abnormally wide splitting of the S$_2$ is noted in the conditions listed in Table 53-1.

Third Heart Sound (S$_3$) and Fourth Heart Sound (S$_4$)

Heart sounds are occasionally heard during ventricular diastole. **Early rapid filling of the ventricle,** which follows the opening of the atrioventricular valve, **may produce the third heart sound (S$_3$); ventricular filling related to the forceful expulsion of blood from the atrium into the ventricle** with atrial contraction **may produce the fourth heart sound (S$_4$).** These sounds are **best heard at the apex with the bell of the stethoscope.** An **audible S$_3$ may be normal in infants and young children,** whereas an **audible S$_4$ is distinctly abnormal.**

■ Conditions that cause ventricular volume overload produce an abnormally prominent S$_3$ and are summarized in Table 53-2.
■ Conditions that result in ventricular hypertrophy produce an S$_4$ and are summarized in Table 53-3.

Characteristics of a Murmur

■ **Phase.** Murmurs are described as being **systolic** (occurring during systole following S$_1$, corresponding with ventricular contraction), **diastolic** (occurring during diastole following S$_2$, corresponding with ventricular relaxation), or **continuous** (occurring throughout the cardiac cycle).
■ **Length and timing.** Murmurs are described as having a short, medium, or long duration and occurring in the early, mid-, or late part of the cardiac cycle. The terms "holosystolic" and "pansystolic" refer to a murmur that begins with S$_1$ and ends with S$_2$.

TABLE 53-2 Conditions Causing a Prominent Third Heart Sound (S$_3$)
Physiologic (infants and children)
Congestive heart failure
Ventricular septal defect, with large pulmonary to systemic flow (Qp-to-Qs) ratio
Mitral insufficiency
Tricuspid insufficiency
Hyperdynamic ventricle with high output (e.g., anemia, thyrotoxicosis, arteriovenous fistula)

TABLE 53-3 Conditions Causing a Prominent Fourth Heart Sound (S₄)

Left ventricular outflow tract obstruction (e.g., aortic stenosis)
Right ventricular outflow tract obstruction (e.g., pulmonic stenosis)
Hypertrophic cardiomyopathy
Heart block (atrium contracting against a closed valve)

- **Peak intensity (grade)** is summarized in Table 53-4.
- **Variation in intensity.** The term "crescendo" implies that the murmur starts low and builds to a peak; "decrescendo" implies that the murmur starts at its greatest intensity and subsequently diminishes. The term "crescendo-decrescendo" is used to describe a murmur that starts low, builds to a peak, and then diminishes over the course of the murmur (i.e., a "diamond-shaped" murmur).
- **Location and radiation.** The location of the murmur is described in relation to a chest wall landmark such as the sternum or intercostal spaces (e.g., the left upper sternal border second intercostal space). The direction of projection (i.e., the radiation) is also noted (e.g., originating at the apex of the heart and radiating toward the left axilla).

Physical Maneuvers

The following maneuvers can alter the characteristics of a murmur:

- **Supine position.** Having the patient lie supine increases venous return to the heart and augments murmurs that are volume dependent (e.g., those associated with aortic stenosis or pulmonic stenosis; functional murmurs). Pericardial rubs are diminished when the patient is supine because the visceral and parietal membranes move away from each other when the heart shifts posteriorly in the chest.
- **Valsalva maneuver.** Forced exhalation against a closed glottis or straining with the mouth and nose closed increases the intrathoracic pressure and reduces venous return to the heart. During the Valsalva maneuver, the two components of S₂ become single, and volume-dependent murmurs are attenuated.

TABLE 53-4 Grading of Murmurs

Grade	Description
I	Very soft, no thrill
II	Easily audible, of moderate intensity, no thrill
III	Prominent intensity but no thrill
IV	Loud murmur accompanied by a thrill
V	Very loud murmur accompanied by a thrill; heard with the stethoscope partially off the chest wall
VI	Very loud murmur accompanied by a thrill; heard with the stethoscope completely off the chest wall

DIFFERENTIAL DIAGNOSIS LIST 🔓

Heart murmurs can be categorized into three groups: **functional or inno-cent** murmurs, which are **normal**; **physiologic** murmurs, which are caused by an **abnormality of flow not of primary cardiac origin**; and **pathologic** murmurs, which are caused by an **abnormality of primary cardiac origin**.

Functional or Innocent Murmurs
Still murmur
Cervical venous hum
Peripheral pulmonic stenosis

Physiologic Murmurs
High cardiac output
  states
Arteriovenous fistula

Pathologic Murmurs
Ventricular septal defect
  (VSD)—nonrestrictive
  and restrictive
Atrial septal defect (ASD)
Patent ductus arteriosus (PDA)
Pulmonic stenosis
Aortic stenosis
Coarctation of the aorta

DIFFERENTIAL DIAGNOSIS DISCUSSION

Still Murmur (Innocent "Flow" Murmur)

Etiology

This sound, described in the early 20th century by Dr. George Frederick Still of Great Ormond Street Children's Hospital, London, is **one of the most common findings in the physical examination of a normal child.** It is heard in children **between 2 years of age and early adolescence** and may even persist into adulthood. Although its **cause is uncertain,** some evidence points to turbulent flow across the left ventricular outflow tract as the source.

Clinical Features and Evaluation

The Still murmur is a **systolic murmur, grade II to III** (never associated with a thrill), and **heard best at the left lower sternal border.** It is described as **vibratory, scratchy, or musical,** and it is **accentuated when the patient is supine** (i.e., with increased venous return to the heart). The **intensity and splitting of the S_2 are always normal.** Additional test-ing is usually not indicated if the murmur fits this description.

Cervical Venous Hum

Turbulent flow may occur **at the junction of the subclavian vein and head vessels as they join to form the superior vena cava,** resulting in a **contin-uous murmur** called a venous hum. It is **low-pitched** and **heard best just beneath the right clavicle** while the child is **sitting up. Turning the patient's head to either the extreme right or left,** placing the patient in a **supine position,** or **applying gentle pressure in the supraclavicular fossa** may dramatically **eliminate the murmur** and is **pathognomonic.** This murmur **may be confused with a PDA,** although the latter does not change with position and is best heard in the left clavicular region. Venous hums **usually disappear during adolescence** but may persist in thin adults.

Murmurs Associated with a High Cardiac Output State

Etiology

Murmurs secondary to a high cardiac output state (e.g., **fever, anemia, thyrotoxicosis**) are usually caused by a **relative stenosis of normal-size structures** in relation to increased blood flow.

Clinical Features

These murmurs are usually located at the **left mid- to upper sternal border, are grade II to III,** and of **medium pitch.** These are typically called ejection murmurs because the timing and intensity of the murmur follow the upstroke and downstroke of the systolic pressure curve. An S_3 **may be audible,** creating a gallop sound.

Evaluation

A **chest radiograph** may show **cardiac enlargement secondary to an increased end-diastolic volume,** but the **ECG** (electrocardiogram) **should be normal.** In patients with **chronic anemia** (e.g., those with sickle cell disease), high-output physiology may lead to **compensatory left ventricular hypertrophy,** which will be evident on ECG.

Treatment

Because the murmur is caused by an increased volume of flow, **treatment of the primary problem** (e.g., with **antipyretics** or **blood transfusion**) diminishes the intensity of the murmur.

Arteriovenous Fistula

Etiology

Congenital anomalous connections between arteries and veins may occur in the **lung, head, or liver.** Because of the constant pressure differential between the artery and vein, the **potential exists for a torrential amount of shunting** to occur, leading to **increased venous return to the right chambers** of the heart.

Clinical Features

A **continuous murmur** is heard over the site of the anomalous arteriovenous connection. In addition, increased flow across the pulmonic and aortic outflow tracts results in a **systolic murmur,** usually of **grade II to III,** along the **left mid- or upper sternal border.**

Evaluation

Auscultation over the liver and the head should be a routine part of the evaluation of all newborn infants with a heart murmur. Chest radiographs may reveal a **giant heart with increased pulmonary arterial markings.**

Peripheral Pulmonic Stenosis

Etiology

This murmur is **heard only in newborn infants,** primarily **premature** ones, and involves a **relative stenosis of the branch pulmonary arteries** in relation to the amount of pulmonary blood flowing across them.

Clinical Features

The murmur of peripheral pulmonic stenosis is a **low-pitched systolic** murmur with **occasional decrescendo run-off into diastole,** and it is heard **loudest in the back over both the right and left lung** fields. At times the murmur is heard **equally in both the right and left axillae. No thrill** is present and the S_2 is normal.

Evaluation

Most infants **outgrow this murmur by 12 to 18 months of age,** but if it persists, an ECG may be indicated **to rule out a fixed anatomic steno-sis of the branch pulmonary arteries.**

Nonrestrictive (Large) Ventricular Septal Defect

Etiology

In a **nonrestrictive VSD,** a **large communication between the lower pumping chambers** exists and allows blood to flow from the left to the right ventricle, resulting in **increased blood flow to the lungs** and increased pulmonary venous return to the left atrium and the left ven-tricle. Hence, in a large VSD, the left ventricle pumps a significantly larger volume of blood than normal.

> **HINT:** In a large nonrestrictive VSD, the right and left ventricular pressures are equal. As a result, a murmur related to a large VSD is not heard until there is a significant difference in the pulmonary and systemic vascular resistances. As pulmonary vascular resistance decreases, increasing amounts of blood shunts across the VSD from left to right. A murmur related to a large VSD may not become evident until pul-monary vascular resistance falls at 1 month of age.

Clinical Features

The murmur of a large VSD is **holosystolic**, reflecting the movement of blood between the right and left ventricles throughout systole. It is **heard best at the left lower sternal border**, frequently **radiating to the right lower sternal border**. A thrill is not palpable because the defect is large and nonrestrictive, producing little turbulence. **As the pulmonary vascular resistance continues to drop during the first 3 months of life, a greater amount of blood flow ("shunt") across the defect occurs,** so that **two to three times the amount of blood exiting the aorta** may end up **circulating through the lungs.**

A **low-pitched diastolic rumble murmur** may be **heard at the apex.** This rumble murmur is caused by a **relative mitral stenosis secondary to the increased blood volume returning to the left atrium** via the normal-size mitral valve.

Evaluation

In patients with a large VSD, the **ECG reveals left ventricular hypertrophy initially** and **biventricular hypertrophy over time.** A **chest radiograph** reveals a **large heart with increased pulmonary vascular markings.** If a large VSD is suspected, an **echocardiogram** to assess the location and anatomy of the defect is indicated. **Cardiac catheterization** may be necessary if complete anatomic detail is not satisfactorily delineated on the echocardiogram or if hemodynamic information is needed to aid in the decision making.

Treatment

A large VSD does not undergo spontaneous closure; therefore, **surgery is required.** A VSD with a **pulmonary to systemic flow (Qp-to-Qs) ratio >2:1** (as calculated by cardiac catheterization) is considered physiologically large and **requires closure.**

Restrictive (Small) Ventricular Septal Defect

By definition, small defects are **not hemodynamically significant** but **may produce a very prominent murmur.**

Clinical Features

Small defects in the muscular portion of the ventricular septum produce a **short, high-pitched, systolic murmur heard best along the left lower sternal border or apex** of the heart. The murmur may be **truncated—** not extending to the end of systole—and may even **abruptly stop at midsystole.** This occurs when the defect is closed off by its muscular borders at the peak of ventricular contraction. Because of the potential for tremendous turbulence across a restrictive narrow orifice in small muscular defects, a **thrill** may be appreciated, and the murmur **may be** as loud as grade VI. The natural tendency is for **muscular defects to become smaller with time,** and hence it is not uncommon for the **murmur to get louder with subsequent examinations.**

A small defect may also be noted in the **inlet portion of the ventricular septum adjacent to the septal leaflet of the tricuspid valve;** this is called a **perimembranous or conoventricular VSD.** A small conoventricular VSD produces a **high-pitched holosystolic murmur, heard best at the left lower sternal border and radiating to the right lower sternal border.** The septal leaflet of the tricuspid valve may fill in the defect, and **aneurysmal tissue may develop,** surrounding the VSD. This may produce an **early systolic click** that precedes the onset of the murmur. Additional **growth of aneurysmal tissue** adjacent to a perimembranous VSD **may result in its spontaneous closure.**

Evaluation

In a small VSD, the S_2 is normal, as are the ECG and chest radiographs. More than 50% of small VSDs undergo **spontaneous closure** by the time the patient reaches **2 years of age.**

Atrial Septal Defect

Etiology

ASD allows for **passive low-pressure flow of blood from the left atrium to the right atrium,** resulting in a volume load on the right ventricle and causing a **relative pulmonic stenosis** (i.e., normal-size pulmonic structures but increased flow) and a **murmur similar to that heard in** patients with **pulmonic stenosis.** The murmur in an ASD is therefore not caused by flow at the defect site; rather, it is a **physiologic consequence of increased flow at the pulmonic valve level.**

Clinical Features

The murmur is **systolic, ejection type, usually grade II to III,** and **low to medium pitched.** It is **heard best at the left upper sternal border and second intercostal space,** with **occasional radiation to the lung fields in the back.**

A widely split S_2 caused by the large right ventricular ejection volume is frequently found in patients with an ASD. The S_2 **does not vary with respiration** because the usual effect of inspiration on right-sided volume is not as great in the presence of a large atrial communication.

In the presence of a **large shunt,** a **diastolic rumble murmur** may be heard at the **right lower sternal border** relating to **increased flow across the tricuspid valve** (normal flow returning via the superior and inferior vena cavae plus flow across the ASD).

Evaluation

Typically, the ECG shows a mild right ventricular conduction delay (i.e., a regular sinus rhythm prime [rSR'] pattern in the anterior precordial leads—V_{3R}, V_{4R}, V_1). A **chest radiograph** reveals a **normal to slightly enlarged heart** with a **prominent pulmonary artery shadow** along the left heart border. Pulmonary vascular markings are normal or slightly increased. An echocardiogram is sufficient to confirm the diagnosis; cardiac catheterization is rarely indicated.

Patent Ductus Arteriosus

Etiology

Persistence in patency of the ductus arteriosus is a common cause of murmurs within the **first year of life**. In utero, the ductus arteriosus functions as the **conduit through which blood from the right ventricle is shunted away from the lungs to the descending aorta**. This structure is **highly sensitive to oxygen** and **usually undergoes spontaneous closure within 24 hours of birth**. In some infants, a stimulus (e.g., **prematurity, sepsis, volume overload**) may be identified as the **cause of the PDA**.

Clinical Features

Classically, the murmur heard in a PDA is a **continuous rumbling murmur**, at times even **harsh and machinelike**. It is **best heard in the left upper sternal border area and under the left clavicle**. The continuity of the murmur is caused by the **persistent pressure differential** that exists **between the aorta and pulmonary artery,** both in systole and diastole, leading to **continuous left-to-right shunting** throughout the cardiac cycle. The S_2 is **normal** and may be **masked by the murmur.**

When **patients present** at the nadir of the pulmonary vascular resistance decrement (**at approximately 3 months,** earlier in premature infants), the **amount of shunting from aorta to pulmonary artery may lead to left ventricular volume overload and congestive heart failure** (CHF). In these patients, a **diastolic rumble** may be apparent at the **apex** as a result of increased flow across the mitral valve, and the **ECG** may show left **ventricular hypertrophy**. The diagnosis is confirmed on echocardiogram.

Treatment

Treatment consists of **close observation during the first 6 months** because **spontaneous closure** in this period is **still possible.** In patients who are >6 months, or in whom **CHF is present** and is **poorly controlled** with anticongestive medication (e.g., digoxin, diuretics), **surgical ligation** is recommended. In **premature infants, indomethacin treatment** is reported as extremely successful, although it is less effective after 2 weeks of age.

Pulmonic Stenosis

Etiology

Dysplasia of the pulmonary valve leaflets or a bicuspid pulmonary valve may cause pulmonic stenosis.

Clinical Features

When stenosis is severe, the infant may present with cyanosis from impedance of flow out of the right ventricle and right-to-left shunting at the level of the foramen ovale. Emergent intervention in this circumstance is necessary.

In patients with mild to moderate pulmonary stenosis, the typical presentation is a murmur noted on physical examination in a child without symptoms. The murmur is systolic, low pitched, crescendo-decrescendo, and best heard at the second intercostal space at the left upper sternal border. An early, dull-sounding systolic ejection click may be appreciated at the left upper sternal border. Frequently, the murmur radiates along the course of the branch pulmonary arteries and may be heard over the lungs in the right and left back. The S_2 may split widely, with normal respiratory variation, but the P_2 component is soft.

Evaluation

The ECG and chest radiograph may be normal in patients with mild to moderate pulmonic stenosis.

Treatment

In cases of mild stenosis, treatment is not necessary; however, in moderate or severe stenosis, cardiac catheterization with balloon valvuloplasty is required. Although pulmonic insufficiency is always created at the time of balloon valvuloplasty, the insufficiency is well tolerated as long as the tricuspid valve remains competent.

Aortic Stenosis

Etiology

Dysplasia, or more commonly, fusion, of the aortic leaflets may cause aortic stenosis. A bicuspid aortic valve is the most common form of congenital heart "disease" in the older child and adult and often results in very mild or no obstruction.

Clinical Features

> **HINT:** Severe aortic stenosis seen in infancy may not cause a murmur if obstruction to aortic outflow is of such a degree that a PDA is present to supply the systemic circulation.

In an **older child** aortic stenosis **always produces a murmur.** The murmur is typically **systolic crescendo-decrescendo,** at times **harsh,** and **heard best at the right upper sternal border at the second intercostal space** radiating along the course of the aortic arch up into the carotid vessels.

A **thrill** may be palpable in the **suprasternal notch.** The S_2 is **softer than normal** and may be **single.** In patients with **mild to moderate cases** of aortic stenosis, a **high-pitched ejection click** may be heard in **early systole,** just preceding the onset of the murmur. Of note is that the click is best appreciated at the **apex of the heart,** not at the base, and its cause may relate more to inertial forces in the left ventricular outflow tract than to the opening of the aortic valve.

> **HINT:** Aortic stenosis may be a progressive disease. Increased harshness of the murmur as well as disappearance of the click may indicate an increased gradient across the aortic valve.

Evaluation

ECG findings of left ventricular hypertrophy and cardiac enlargement on the chest radiograph are present when the aortic stenosis is hemodynamically significant.

Coarctation of the Aorta

Etiology

Coarctation of the aorta is a **narrowing or shelf-like protuberance in the aortic arch distal to the left subclavian artery.** In **infancy,** coarctation is usually a **diffuse narrowing** of the area just **proximal to the insertion of the ductus arteriosus** (isthmus of the aortic arch). In **older children,** a **discrete shelf** is more commonly found and is thought to relate to remnants of ductal tissue within the aorta.

Clinical Features

A **long systolic** murmur **heard best along the left upper sternal border** is most commonly noted in patients with coarctation of the aorta. It is **loudest in the interscapular region in the back.** Bicuspid aortic valve is found in 80% of patients with coarctation of the aorta. As a result, an **early systolic ejection click may be heard at the base of the heart** in patients with coarctation of the aorta because of the presence of a bicuspid aortic valve.

In **older patients** with long-standing coarctation, **continuous murmurs** may be appreciated along the **lateral chest wall.** These are caused by intercostal collateral flow to the portion of the aorta distal to the narrowing.

Evaluation

On physical examination, a blood pressure gradient is noted between the right upper and lower extremities. Diminished femoral pulses may also be present. An ECG may show **left ventricular hypertrophy.** A chest **radiograph** is either **normal or reveals mild cardiomegaly.** Occasionally, **poststenotic dilation of the descending aorta distal to the coarctation** can be seen.

Suggested Readings

Allen HD, Phillips JR, Chan DP: History and physical examination. In *Moss and Adams' Heart Disease in Infants, Children, and Adolescents,* 6th ed. Edited by Allen HD, Gutgesell HP, Clark EB, et al. Philadelphia, Lippincott Williams & Wilkins, 2001, 143–152.

Menashe V: Heart murmurs. *Pediatr Rev* 28(4):e19–e22, 2007.

Park MK: Routine cardiac evaluation in children. In *The Pediatric Cardiology Handbook Third Edition.* Philadelphia, Mosby, 2003, 1–51.

Sivarajan VB, Vetter VL, Gleason MM: Pediatric evaluation of the cardiac patient. In *Pediatric Cardiology: The Requisites in Pediatrics.* Edited by Vetter VL. Philadelphia, Mosby Elsevier, 2006, 1–30.

INTRODUCTION

Neck masses are a common clinical problem in children. Although the list of potential causes is extensive, most are caused by **benign processes** that can be readily diagnosed after a complete history and physical examination. **Close follow-up** is important to ensure that less common causes in children such as malignancy are not overlooked.

DIFFERENTIAL DIAGNOSIS LIST

Infectious Causes
Cervical Adenitis
 Bacterial infection—
  Streptococcus pyogenes,
  Staphylococcus aureus,
  Group B *Streptococcus*,
  oral anaerobes, *Pasteurella*
  multocida
 Cat-scratch disease
 Tularemia
 Nocardia
 Mycobacterium tuberculosis
 Atypical mycobacterium
Reactive Adenopathy
 Viral infection—upper
  respiratory viruses, mumps,
  measles, Epstein-Barr virus,
  cytomegalovirus, HIV
 Bacterial infection—syphilis,
  brucellosis
 Fungal infection—
  histoplasmosis, coccid-
  ioidomycosis,
 Parasitic infection—
  toxoplasmosis
 Other infections—head and
  neck infections (tonsillitis,
  otitis media, tinea capitis)
 Lemierre's syndrome

Congenital or Vascular Causes
 Thyroglossal duct cyst
 Branchial cleft cyst
 Cystic hygroma
 Laryngocele
 Dermoid
 Cervical thymic cyst
 Arteriovenous fistula

Neoplastic Causes
 Malignant neoplasms—
  Hodgkin lymphoma, non-
  Hodgkin lymphoma, rhab-
  domyosarcoma, fibrosarcoma,
  thyroid carcinoma, neuroblastoma, metastatic deposits
 Benign neoplasms—lipoma,
  fibroma, neurofibroma,
  teratoma, osteochondroma,
  hemangioma

Metabolic or Genetic Causes
 Goiter
 Thyroid nodule

Traumatic Causes
 Hematoma
 Congenital muscular torticollis

Subcutaneous emphysema
Cervical spine fracture

**Inflammatory Causes
(Cervical Adenopathy)**

Kawasaki syndrome
Systemic lupus erythematosus

Sinus histiocytosis
Sarcoidosis
Lemierre's syndrome

Toxic Causes

Drug-related adenopathy
(e.g., phenytoin)

DIFFERENTIAL DIAGNOSIS DISCUSSION

Reactive Adenopathy

Familiarity with regional anatomy helps narrow the differential diagnosis in a child who presents with a neck mass. Because **most neck masses in infants and children are enlarged lymph nodes,** it is important to be familiar with areas of lymphatic drainage. In addition, certain masses present in typical locations that help identify the cause. The neck is divided into the anterior and posterior triangles, with the sternocleidomastoid muscle (SCM) forming the posterior border of the anterior triangle (Figure 54-1).

It is **important to distinguish adenopathy from adenitis.** Adenopathy is defined by nodal enlargement. **In adenitis, the swelling is usually accompanied by signs of inflammation** such as warmth, tenderness, and erythema. The vast **majority of children with adenopathy** have a **benign viral or easily treatable bacterial cause.** However, **follow-up is important** to assess resolution of symptoms and progressive reduction in size so as not to miss unusual infectious, inflammatory, or oncologic processes. Moreover, any node >2 cm warrants further attention because it falls outside the range of benign hyperplasia. A more detailed review of this topic is covered in Chapter 50, "Lymphadenopathy."

> **HINT:** Epitrochlear, popliteal, supraclavicular, or occipital nodes in children <2 years are rarely caused by benign lymph node hyperplasia. These nodes, as well as any palpable nodes in the newborn infant, deserve further investigation.

Lemierre Syndrome

Lemierre syndrome (also known as necrobacillosis or postanginal sepsis) is a rare disease characterized by sepsis secondary to an anaerobic infection of the tonsillar or peritonsillar region and **superficial thrombophlebitis of the internal jugular vein.** It typically presents with prolonged pharyngitis or tonsillitis followed by lateral neck pain, swelling, and subsequent pulmonary symptoms. The most common bacteria isolated are *Fusobacterium necrophorum.* The key to diagnosis is having an appropriate index of suspicion based on clinical findings. Confirmation is by ultrasound,

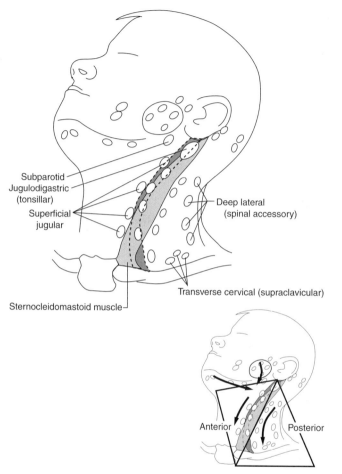

Subparotid
Jugulodigastric
(tonsillar)

Superficial
jugular

Deep lateral
(spinal accessory)

Transverse cervical (supraclavicular)

Sternocleidomastoid muscle

Anterior   Posterior

Figure 54-1 ■ Division of the neck into anterior and posterior triangles

computed tomography (CT), or magnetic resonance imaging (MRI) demonstrating phlebitis of the internal jugular vein. Management consists of appropriate antibiotics and possible anticoagulation.

Congenital Malformations

Thyroglossal Duct Cyst
Etiology

Thyroglossal duct cyst (TGDC) results from the cellular proliferation of embryonic remnants of the thyroglossal duct.

Clinical Features and Evaluation

TGDC is the **most common congenital neck mass** and usually presents in the **first decade of life**. TGDC may become apparent during an upper respiratory infection that causes cyst inflammation. Physical examination is best done with the **neck fully extended** and reveals a **midline or paramedian swelling of the anterior neck.** The location can be anywhere along the embryonic pathway from the base of the tongue to the thyroid cartilage. The **mass is round and changes position when the child swallows or sticks out his tongue.** Children with TGDC should be **referred to an otorhinolaryngologist** for further evaluation. When suspected, it is important to differentiate TGDC from ectopic thyroid. The surgeon may consider further testing to confirm normal thyroid function and location.

Treatment

Almost all TGDC require **surgical excision** for definitive diagnosis and to prevent recurrent infections of the cyst.

Branchial Cleft Cyst/Fistula/Sinus
Etiology

The embryological branchial clefts give rise to the structures of the face and neck. Cysts result from the **proliferation of the remnants of these clefts, usually involving the second cleft.**

Clinical Evaluation

Branchial cleft remnants are the **second most common congenital neck mass.** A fistula or sinus is obvious in the newborn; however, a cyst often does not become clinically apparent until early school age. Second branchial cleft cysts are found **anterior to the lower third of the sternocleidomastoid muscle as a small, round, nontender, soft mass.** An upper respiratory infection or infection of the cyst itself may lead to an **inflammatory appearance.** Diagnosis should be suspected if a **mass lateral to the SCM persists or recurs despite antibiotic treatment** for an adenitis and can be further delineated by CT or MRI.

Treatment

If there is evidence of cyst infection, an **antibiotic** that covers skin flora should be initiated. Definitive treatment requires **surgical excision,** which can be done electively.

Cystic Hygroma
Etiology

Cystic hygromas arise from the **nonmalignant proliferation of lymphatic tissue that does not connect with normal lymphatic drainage.** These sacs become **filled with lymphatic fluid** secreted by the endothelial lining. They can compress or stretch surrounding tissues.

Clinical Evaluation

Cystic hygromas are the **third most common congenital neck mass.** The vast majority of hygromas are found in the **posterior cervical triangle,** and most are diagnosed within the first year of life. The mass is **soft, easily compressible, and, if not secondarily infected, transilluminates.** Upper respiratory infections or trauma may cause a rapid increase in size. **Encroachment on the airway may lead to respiratory symptoms such as stridor.** Diagnosis is usually clinical, but **ultrasound or CT imaging** may be necessary to delineate the extent of the lesion.

Treatment

Spontaneous regression is rare. Currently, **staged surgical excision** is the mainstay of therapy. **Sclerosing agents** and other therapies may have an adjunctive role. Timing of surgery depends on the location of the lesion, age of the child, and involvement of vital structures. **Tracheostomy and gastric tube feedings** are sometimes required.

Dermoid

Dermoids consist of ectoderm and mesoderm and are considered **true developmental neoplasms.** This rare midline mass is often **doughy, non-tender, mobile,** and is found **above the level of the hyoid bone.** It may initially be confused with a TGDC; however, it **does not change position with tongue protrusion.** Signs of **inflammation** may occur with cyst infection. **Ultrasound and CT imaging** help delineate the nature and extent of the lesion. **Surgical excision** is required.

Laryngocele

Laryngocele is an **extremely rare** congenital anomaly. It is an **air-filled mass that arises from the larynx.** External extension through the thyrohyoid membrane results in a **compressible mass,** lateral to midline, that **increases in size with a Valsalva maneuver.** Hoarseness, cough, dyspnea, or dysphagia may be suggestive of a laryngocele. Lateral radiographs may demonstrate the air-filled sac. **Surgical excision** is required.

Oncologic Masses

See Chapter 50, "Lymphadenopathy," and Chapter 36, "Goiter," for more details on this topic.

> **HINT:** Fortunately, neck masses in children are rarely caused by an oncologic process. A mass that is rapidly growing, found in a neonate, adherent to underlying tissues, ulcerated, >3 cm, or located in the posterior triangle is more of a concern for malignancy.

Lymphoma

Hodgkin lymphoma is the **most frequent malignant neck mass** in children. Hodgkin lymphoma often presents with a **unilateral slowly enlarging mass of the neck**, whereas non-Hodgkin lymphoma is more often bilateral. Systemic symptoms of **fatigue, fever, weight loss, night sweats ("B symptoms"), and respiratory distress** may be present. Findings related to **bone marrow dysfunction, mediastinal involvement, and spinal cord impingement** may also be found. **Node biopsy** is necessary for diagnosis. **Immediate referral to a pediatric oncologist** is indicated to plan the diagnostic and therapeutic evaluation.

Neuroblastoma

Neuroblastoma of the cervical region may present in a child ≤5 years **with a neck mass and Horner syndrome** (miosis, ptosis, and anhidrosis). Neuroblastoma may also **metastasize** from other regions to the neck, but neurologic symptoms will be absent until the mass causes nerve compression.

Thyroid Masses

See Chapter 36, "Goiter."

Traumatic Causes

Congenital Muscular Torticollis (Fibromatosis of Infancy)
Etiology

Although the exact etiologic mechanism of this condition is unclear, **birth trauma causing injury and bleeding into the SCM** with subsequent fibrosis and contracture is implicated. An **intrauterine position that obstructs SCM venous outflow** may also cause muscle injury and contracture.

Clinical Evaluation

Parents usually notice a neck mass or torticollis in the baby's **first month of life**. Physical examination reveals a **nontender, firm, mobile mass within the SCM.** The **head is in lateral flexion** and the **chin is pointed away from the mass.** Diagnosis can usually be made clinically. **Cervical spine radiographs** and **ultrasound** may assist in ruling out other less common causes.

Treatment

Delayed diagnosis and treatment may lead to irreversible asymmetric development of facial features. The vast majority of children improve with **passive stretching exercises.** If the torticollis persists past 6 to 12 months, a **surgical release of the muscle** may be necessary.

Inflammatory Causes

Inflammatory disease processes may have **associated cervical adenopathy.** It is rare that cervical adenopathy is the first or only presenting finding.

Kawasaki Disease (Mucocutaneous Lymph Node Syndrome)

In Kawasaki disease, the lymph node must be ≥1.5 cm. When present, it is usually found in the cervical chain. However, it is the least common finding of the five criteria (discussed in more detail in Chapter 64, "Rashes").

Sinus Histiocytosis (Rosai-Dorfman Syndrome)

This is an **extremely rare disorder** of unknown etiology. The typical patient is a young **African American child** who presents with **prolonged fever** and **massive, nontender, bilateral cervical adenopathy.** Diagnosis depends on characteristic findings on **lymph node biopsy.** Treatment may include **chemotherapeutic agents,** and these patients should be **referred to an oncologist.**

APPROACH TO THE PATIENT

Most neck masses in children are benign. A thorough history and physical examination coupled with a follow-up visit is sufficient to diagnose most masses. **Systemic symptoms, persistence or recurrence of a mass, or a history of exposure to an infectious agent** such as tuberculosis should prompt **further evaluation.** Further evaluation may include a **complete blood count, purified protein derivative tuberculin test, other pathogen-specific assays, or imaging with ultrasound or CT. Biopsy** should be considered in a patient whose mass has increased in size at 2 weeks, unchanged in size in 4 to 6 weeks, or not returned to normal at 8 to 12 weeks. **Inpatient evaluation and treatment** is often necessary for neonates or for patients who are ill appearing, have signs of impending airway compromise, are immunocompromised, or have failed outpatient oral antibiotic treatment.

Suggested Readings

Chesney PJ: Cervical adenopathy. *Pediatr Rev* 15:276–283, 1994.

May M: Neck masses in children: diagnosis and treatment. *Pediatr Ann* 5:518–535, 1976.

Nagy M, Backstrom J: Comparison of the sensitivity of lateral neck radiographs and computed tomography scanning in pediatric deep-neck infections. *Laryngoscope* 109(5):775–779, 1999.

Pounds LA: Neck masses of congenital origin. *Pediatr Clin North Am* 28:841–844, 1981.

Turkington JRA, Paterson A, Sweenery LE, et al.: Neck masses in children. *Br J Radiol* 78(10):75–85, 2005.

Wetmore RF, Mahboubi S, Soyupak SK: Computed tomography in the evaluation of pediatric neck infections. *Otolaryngol Head Neck Surg* 119(6):624–627, 1998.

Neck Pain/Stiffness

Jill C. Posner

INTRODUCTION

In children, the chief complaint of neck pain often may represent neck stiffness or torticollis. **Torticollis** describes a **characteristic malpositioning of the head and chin** in which the head is tilted to one direction and the chin points oppositely. It is a sign of an underlying disease process and does not imply a specific diagnosis. The head and neck regions are highly complex anatomically, and many structures within these areas can give rise to symptoms. **Pain or stiffness can arise from structures within the neck** such as the cervical musculature, the vertebral bones, or lymph nodes. Alternatively, **pain from the scalp, ear, oropharynx, or mandible** can refer and be perceived in the neck region. **Pressure** originating from the head either external to the dura or from within the brain or spinal cord can cause neck pain or stiffness. Finally, processes involving the upper thorax (e.g., clavicular fracture or upper lobe pneumonia) can also cause pain that might radiate to the neck region.

DIFFERENTIAL DIAGNOSIS LIST

Trauma

Fracture of cervical spine
Subluxation of cervical spine
Spinal cord injury without radiographic abnormality (SCIWORA) syndrome
Atlantoaxial rotary subluxation
Muscular contusions/spasm
Subarachnoid hemorrhage
Epidural hematoma of cervical spine
Clavicular fracture

Infectious

Meningitis
Retropharyngeal abscess
Peritonsillar abscess
Epiglottitis
Osteomyelitis
Diskitis

Epidural abscess
Cervical adenitis
Pharyngitis
Upper respiratory tract infection
Upper lobe pneumonia
Viral myositis
Otitis media/mastoiditis

Inflammatory

Atlantoaxial rotary subluxation
Grisel syndrome
Collagen vascular diseases
Juvenile intervertebral disk calcification

Congenital

Congenital muscular torticollis
Skeletal malformations
Klippel-Feil syndrome
Atlantoaxial instability

Toxic Metabolic

Dystonic reaction
Tetanus

Neurologic

Space-occupying lesions
Brain tumor
Spinal cord tumor
Arnold-Chiari malformation
Syringomyelia
Arteriovenous malformation

Strabismus
Cranial nerve palsies
Myasthenia gravis
Migraine headaches

Miscellaneous

Benign paroxysmal torticollis
Gastroesophageal reflux
 (Sandifer syndrome)
Psychogenic

DIFFERENTIAL DIAGNOSIS DISCUSSION

Major Trauma

Etiology

Cervical spine fracture, subluxation of the vertebral bodies, or spinal cord injury without radiographic abnormality (SCIWORA) syndrome may result from high-risk mechanisms of injury (e.g., motor vehicle collision, pedestrian struck by motor vehicle, falls from heights, high-impact sports activities). The larger head size, weaker neck muscles, and increased ligamentous laxity render children more likely to sustain injury in the upper cervical area as compared with adults, who are more likely to sustain lower cervical injuries.

Clinical Features

Cervical spine injury should be suspected in the patient with a high-risk mechanism of injury or suggestive signs or symptoms: pain on neck palpation, neck muscle spasm, limited range of motion, torticollis, transient or persistent sensory changes, hyporeflexia, muscle weakness or flaccidity, priapism, bladder or bowel dysfunction, or hypotension with bradycardia (spinal shock). In addition, in the nonverbal or uncooperative child or the child who has an altered mental status or an associated severe head injury, the physical examination may be difficult or unreliable. In these children, the possibility of cervical spine injury should be considered at the outset of the evaluation and spinal immobilization and precautions maintained until proved otherwise.

Evaluation

Suspected cervical spine injury generally requires emergent evaluation. The child should be immobilized with a rigid cervical collar and pediatric spine board.

- The evaluation should begin by assessing the patient's respiratory and hemodynamic status. In some alert, verbal, and cooperative children, an attempt to "clinically clear" the cervical spine may be made through a careful physical examination.
- A complete sensory and motor neurologic exam should be performed and must be without deficits.
- A careful examination of the cervical spine with the collar removed, but with manual immobilization maintained, should yield no tenderness or deformity.

At this point, the patient may be allowed to attempt **active** (not passive) **neck flexion, extension,** and **lateral rotation.** Any limitation or complaint of pain with range of motion should prompt the immediate reinstitution of cervical spine immobilization and cervical radiography.

- The **radiographic evaluation** should include a minimum of three views: the lateral, anteroposterior, and open-mouth (odontoid) radiographs. Flexion and extension views are used to assess for ligamentous injury in a child with persistent neck pain after a normal three-view series.
- **Computed tomography (CT) scan** provides excellent bone detail, whereas magnetic resonance imaging (**MRI) scan** is used to evaluate the soft tissues and spinal cord.

Treatment

In addition to **supportive care,** a treatment adjunct for spinal cord injury with associated neurologic abnormality is the administration of **methylprednisolone,** 30 mg/kg over 15 minutes, followed by 5.4 mg/kg per hour for 23 hours. Based on studies in adults, this treatment is most effective if given within 8 hours of the injury.

Atlantoaxial Rotary Subluxation

Etiology

The odontoid process of the second cervical vertebrae is normally positioned squarely within the ring of C1, and the two vertebrae are secured by the transverse and alar ligaments. The increased laxity and longer lengths of the ligaments renders **children more susceptible** to traumatic cervical spine injury than their adult counterparts.

As the name implies, in patients with rotary subluxation, **C1 and C2** are **rotationally malpositioned.** This commonly results from a **minor traumatic mechanism,** as might occur during light wrestling or gymnastics. Some conditions such as **tonsillectomy** (Grisel syndrome), **upper respiratory infections,** or **juvenile rheumatoid arthritis** may cause inflammation and laxity of the transverse ligament, resulting in C1-C2 instability with rotary subluxation. Additionally, certain conditions such as **Down syndrome** or **congenital odontoid dysplasias** may predispose to rotary subluxation.

Clinical Features

Patients commonly present with **neck pain** or **stiffness.** Physical examination reveals **torticollis, tender paracervical muscles,** and **decreased range of motion** of the neck. The torticollis results as the ipsilateral sternocleidomastoid muscle attempts to reestablish normal positioning. Rotary subluxation is a **stable cervical spine injury,** rarely causing spinal cord impingement, and neurologic signs are infrequently encountered.

The lateral radiograph may be normal or show distorted anatomy. Particular attention should be paid to check the **predental space** that may be widened. The diagnostic modality of choice, however, is the **static and dynamic neck CT scan.** A static CT scan usually shows the asymmetric location of the dens within the anterior arch of C1. In the dynamic CT, the rotation of C2 on C1 is fixed, persisting despite lateral rotation of the head to both directions.

Treatment

Most patients have resolution of symptoms with **supportive care with a soft collar** and the administration of nonsteroidal **anti-inflammatory drugs.** Orthopedic referral is suggested for the patients with persistent symptoms who may require reduction and stabilization with traction.

Meningitis

Meningitis is discussed in Chapter 21, "Coma."

Retropharyngeal Abscess, Peritonsillar Abscess, Epiglottitis, Cervical Adenitis, and Pharyngitis

Retropharyngeal abscess, peritonsillar abscess, epiglottitis, cervical adenitis, and pharyngitis are discussed in Chapter 72, "Sore Throat."

Diskitis

Etiology

Infectious diskitis is a **rare illness** with an unclear etiology. In approximately 50% of patients with diskitis, an aspirated culture of the affected area yields a bacterial pathogen (*Staphylococcus aureus* in most, also coagulase-negative *Staphylococcus, Kingella, Salmonella*), which has led some to believe the process is **infectious** in etiology. Yet the outcome in patients is the same with or without antimicrobial treatment. Others suggest a **traumatic or inflammatory** etiology, theorizing that a preceding traumatic event induces the release of tissue enzymes from the disk, resulting in inflammation. Diskitis more commonly affects the **lumbar area** but can occur in the cervical region.

Clinical Features

The clinical presentation is **gradual in onset** with few constitutional symptoms. The patient may present with mild irritability or more obvious pain. The physical examination is often near normal except that the child may refuse to move his neck.

The peripheral white blood count and differential are usually normal. **Nonspecific indicators of inflammation (erythrocyte sedimentation rate [ESR], C-reactive protein [CRP]) are almost always elevated.** Blood cultures are rarely positive. Radiographs are usually normal early in the course of the illness but may demonstrate erosion of the adjacent vertebral plates by 4 to 8 weeks after the onset. **Repair and residual sclerosis** is the typical progression. **Bone scan** may detect disease earlier, showing increased uptake in the disk and vertebral bodies.

Treatment

The management of diskitis is **controversial.** Supportive treatment with immobilization and analgesia generally renders patients free of discomfort in about 48 hours. The role of parenteral antibiotics remains unclear.

Epidural Abscess

Epidural abscess is discussed in Chapter 58, "Paraplegia."

Congenital Muscular Torticollis

Etiology

Congenital muscular torticollis (CMT) is a relatively common entity, occurring with a prevalence of 3 to 19 per 1,000 newborns. The **etiology is unknown,** although several theories exist. The **intrauterine theory** suggests that abnormal fetal positioning results in a shortened sternocleidomastoid muscle. Another theory contends that **birth trauma** during difficult deliveries leads to bleeding into the sternocleidomastoid muscle with subsequent compartment syndrome, fibrosis, and contracture. There is no genetic predisposition.

Clinical Features

CMT is **often undetected** in the **immediate newborn period.** The head tilt becomes more obvious, however, as the infant develops head control. The **head tilts** toward the shorted muscle and the chin points away. A **mass** can be palpated in the inferior portion of the sternocleidomastoid muscle in about a third of cases. Rarely, other musculoskeletal anomalies are associated, including hip dysplasia, metatarsus adductus, and talipes equinovarus.

Evaluation

A thorough **physical examination** to eliminate other causes of torticollis should be performed. **Radiographic evaluation** of the cervical spine can identify rare congenital vertebral anomalies such as Klippel-Feil syndrome (congenital fusion of any number of cervical vertebrae).

Treatment

Treatment is usually **nonsurgical** with **strengthening and stretching exercises.** Early **physical therapy** referral correlates with improved outcome. **Recurrence** of torticollis may occur in 11% of patients and can happen years later.

Paroxysmal Torticollis

Etiology

The etiology is unclear but felt to be either a **migraine** variant or related to **vestibular dysfunction.**

Clinical Features

The syndrome, generally presenting in the **first few months of life,** is characterized by **recurrent episodes of head tilt,** often alternating in sides. Torticollis is rarely the only finding. Other **associated symptoms** may include **vomiting, pallor, irritability,** and **ataxia.** Although frightening for the parents to witness, paroxysmal torticollis is a **benign, self-limited process.** The frequency of attacks progressively decreases and ultimately it resolves in 1 to 5 years.

Evaluation and Treatment

Evaluation of the initial episode consists of a careful history and physical examination to **rule out other causes of vomiting** and **ataxia** such as central nervous system (CNS) processes or intoxication. Subsequent attacks are managed by **supportive therapy** including intravenous fluid hydration if necessary. Pharmacologic treatment has not been well studied.

Dystonic Reactions

Etiology

Antiemetics, neuroleptics, and **other medications** with dopamine receptor antagonism can cause dystonia when taken either in overdose or in therapeutic doses.

Clinical Features

Patients with dystonic reactions experience a **severe, uncomfortable contraction of the sternocleidomastoid muscle.** Often the **facial muscles,** and sometimes the muscles of the **extremities and trunk,** are also involved.

Evaluation and Treatment

The administration of **diphenhydramine** (1.25 mg/kg) can be both diagnostic and therapeutic. The response is **rapid and dramatic**. The offending agent should be discontinued and diphenhydramine continued every 6 to 8 hours for several days to avoid recurrence.

Neurologic Causes

CNS processes can induce torticollis via a variety of mechanisms. **Space-occupying lesions** exerting pressure on the dura can cause irritation that can cause neck stiffness. Alternatively, **tonsillar herniation** may cause stretching or irritation of the accessory nerve, which then induces sternocleidomastoid spasm. In addition, a child with diplopia secondary to **cranial nerve dysfunction or strabismus** may attempt compensation through tilting his head to realign the visual axis. This head tilt may be perceived by the examiner as torticollis. The evaluation of the child with neck stiffness or torticollis must include a **careful neurologic examination** to assess for the presence of a neurologic cause.

Atlantoaxial Rotary Subluxation

Inflammatory conditions involving the transverse ligament of C1 and C2 can result in torticollis as described earlier.

Juvenile Rheumatoid Arthritis

The **cervical spine** is involved in 50% of patients with juvenile rheumatoid arthritis. It is rarely an early complication of the disease and is usually found in patients with >6 months of illness.

Juvenile Intervertebral Disk Calcification

Etiology

The uncommon disease entity of juvenile intervertebral disk calcification (JIDC) has an **unknown etiology** but has been postulated to arise from developmental changes in the water content, blood supply, and cellular matrix of the nucleus of the disk. There are several distinguishing features of JIDC, and therefore it is believed to be a **different** entity **than adult intervertebral disk calcification.**

- **The location of involvement in children is distinct from that in adults.** In JIDC, the cervical region is most commonly involved and the calcification occurs within the nucleus. In adults, the annulus of the disks in the thoracic or lumbar regions is affected.
- Childhood disease may be either asymptomatic or transiently symptomatic. Adults generally have asymptomatic, permanent calcification.

Clinical Features

Patients with JIDC may be divided into **symptomatic** and **asymptomatic** groups, depending on clinical features. It is unknown what triggers the development of symptoms. Many asymptomatic patients never develop symptoms, but resolution does not occur without a symptomatic period. In most symptomatic patients, symptoms develop over 24 to 48 hours and most commonly consist of **neck pain, torticollis,** and **fever.** Neurologic symptoms and signs are rare.

Evaluation and Treatment

In the symptomatic patient, **nonspecific laboratory evidence of inflammation** is apparent in one-third to one-half of patients (leukocytosis, elevated ESR). Blood cultures are negative. Radiographs of the spine demonstrate **intervertebral disk calcification** of the nucleus pulposus. During the acute episode, the involved **interspace may widen** and then normalize as the symptoms resolve. **Extruded calcified disk material** may be seen posteriorly within the spinal canal or within the prevertebral soft tissues. There is no destruction of the adjacent vertebral bodies and the retropharyngeal space is not enlarged. MRI can be used to evaluate for canal compromise that is secondary to disk herniation.

Given that the disease is usually benign and self-limited, treatment is generally **supportive** with bed rest, analgesics, heat, and muscle relaxants. Operative removal of the disk is usually not indicated. Symptoms resolve in 3 weeks (67%) to 6 months (95%). **Complete radiographic resolution** is the rule.

EVALUATION OF NECK PAIN

A child who presents with neck pain may have a **potentially life-threatening illness.** The immediate priority is to ensure the adequacy of the **airway, breathing,** and **circulation.** The possibility of **cervical spine injury** is **considered early,** and spinal immobilization and precautions are instituted if warranted. Most diagnoses are made based on the history and physical examination findings alone. Further evaluation with laboratory and radiographic tests are based on these findings.

History

In the history, it is important to characterize the nature of the chief complaint, **distinguishing neck pain from stiffness or torticollis.** Is the pain acute or chronic in nature? Is it constant or intermittent? Has there been any response to any home therapies? It is particularly important to elucidate any evidence of acute or chronic **CNS pathology** such as weakness, paresthesias, loss of bowel or bladder continence, or loss of developmental milestones. There should be a careful probing for any symptoms of increased intracranial pressure such as headaches, vomiting, or changes in school performance. Preceding **major trauma** is usually evident, but the possibility of **minor trauma** should be explored. Has the patient had fever, sore throat, cough, upper respiratory symptoms, or ear or mouth pain? Is the patient, or are any household contacts, taking any medications, either prescription or over the counter?

Physical Examination

A **general review of all systems** should occur. The diagnosis of meningitis usually can be excluded by physical examination. When in doubt, a **lumbar puncture** should be performed. The examination of the neck begins with **observation of positioning.** If **palpation** of the cervical spinous processes yields **localized tenderness or deformity,** a **cervical collar** should be placed and no further manipulation done until a **radiographic evaluation** shows the absence of fracture, subluxation, or ligamentous injury. Barring this, the rest of the neck should be carefully palpated for masses and muscle spasm. At this point, the child should be allowed to attempt **active (not passive) neck flexion, extension, and lateral rotation.**

Diagnostic Evaluation

The diagnostic evaluation is selective and based on history and physical examination clues to the diagnosis. **Laboratory studies** such as a complete blood count, ESR, CRP, and blood culture may provide nonspecific evidence for an infectious or inflammatory etiology. **Radiographic studies** such as plain films, CT, MRI, and nuclear medicine scans can be useful in selected circumstances.

TREATMENT OF NECK PAIN

Until the cause of the neck pain is established, treatment is **supportive** and may entail the following:

- Administration of analgesics, usually in the form of nonsteroidal anti-inflammatory drugs
- Application of warm compresses
- Administration of antipyretic agents

Suggested Readings

Ballock RT, Song KM: The prevalence of nonmuscular causes of torticollis in children. *J Pediatr Orthop* 16(4):500–504, 1996.

Bredenkamp JK, Maceri DR: Inflammatory torticollis in children. *Arch Otolaryngol Head Neck Surg* 116:310–313, 1990.

Dias MS, Pang D: Juvenile intervertebral disc calcification: recognition, management, and pathogenesis. *Neurosurgery* 28(1):130–135, 1991.

Do TT: Congenital muscular torticollis: current concepts and review of treatment. *Curr Opin Pediatr* 18(1):26–29, 2006.

Fernandez M, Carrol CL, Baker CJ: Discitis and vertebral osteomyelitis in children: an 18 year review. *Pediatrics* 105(6):1299–1304, 2000.

Galer C, Holbrook E, Treves T, et al.: Grisel's syndrome: a case report and review of the literature. *Int J Pediatr Otorhinolaryngol* 69(12): 1689–1692, 2005.

Gupta AK, Roy DR, Conlan ES, et al.: Torticollis secondary to posterior fossa tumors. *J Pediatr Orthop* 16(4):505–507, 1996.

Hadjipavlou, AG, Mader, JT, Necessary JT, et al.: Hematogenous pyogenic spinal infections and their surgical management. *Spine* 25(13): 1668–1679, 2000.

Hall DE, Boydston W: Pediatric neck injuries. *Pediatr Rev* 20(1):13–19, 1999.

Khanna G, El-Khoury GY: Imaging of cervical spine injuries of childhood. *Skeletal Radiol* 36(6):477–494, 2007.

Lewis D, Pearlman E: The migraine variants. *Pediatr Ann* 34(6):486–488, 490–492, 494–497, 2005.

Pang D: Spinal cord injury without radiographic abnormality in children, 2 decades later. *Neurosurgery* 55(6):1325–1342; 2004.

Parker C: Complicated migraine syndromes and migraine variants. *Pediatr Ann* 26:417–421, 1997.

Robin NH: In brief: congenital muscular torticollis. *Pediatr Rev* 17(10): 374–375, 1996.

Singer JI: Evaluation of the patient with neck complaints following tonsillectomy or adenoidectomy. *Pediatr Emerg Care* 8(5):276–279, 1992.

Neonatal Infections

Samir S. Shah

NEONATAL SEPSIS

Overview

The most common classification of neonatal sepsis is by age at onset.

- **Early-onset infection.** Clinical manifestations of early-onset infection occur **within the first 7 days of life** (95% present within the first 72 hours). Frequently, **maternal complications of labor or delivery** lead to these infections. Organisms from the maternal genital tract during the intrapartum period colonize the infant's skin and gastrointestinal and respiratory tracts. The reasons for progression from colonization to infection are not well understood. The most common organisms causing early-onset infection are group B streptococci (GBS), *Escherichia coli,* and, occasionally, *Listeria monocytogenes.*

- **Late-onset infection.** Clinical manifestations of late-onset infection occur **between 7 and 30 days of life.** Infection may be the result of **colonization during birth or during hospitalization** in the intensive care unit. Although most infants do not become ill as a result of this colonization, necessary invasive procedures put them at increased risk for infection. The most common organisms causing late-onset infection are coagulase-negative staphylococci, *Staphylococcus aureus, Enterococcus* spp., GBS, *Escherichia coli, Klebsiella pneumoniae,* and *Candida* spp.

- **Late, late-onset infection.** The improved survival rate of **very low birthweight infants** (<1,500 g) has prompted the addition of this third category: late, late-onset infection. Although these infants are no longer neonates, their "corrected" gestational age (usually 28 to 34 weeks) and continued need for hospitalization because of complications of prematurity accord them "newborn" status. A quarter of all very low birthweight infants who survive beyond 3 days of life have at least one episode of late-onset or late, late-onset sepsis. These infants usually have **central venous catheters or endotracheal tubes** in place. Infection in this group is **nosocomially acquired** and often caused by coagulase-negative staphylococci, *Pseudomonas aeruginosa, Enterobacter cloacae, Serratia marcescens,* and *Candida* spp.

Common Pathogens

Group B *Streptococcus* Infection

The maternal colonization rate for GBS is 15% to 30%, and 50% of these women deliver infants who are **colonized at birth;** 1% of colonized

TABLE 56-1 Select Risk Factors for Group B Streptococcal Infection

Maternal Risk Factors

Prior infant with group B streptococcal sepsis
Group B streptococcal bacteriuria
Prolonged rupture of membranes (≥18 hr)
Premature rupture of membranes (<37 wk of gestation)
Preterm labor (<37 wk of gestation)
Intrapartum fever >100.4°F (37.9°C)

infants develop invasive GBS infection. Women with prenatal colonization are 25 times more likely to deliver an infant with early-onset GBS disease. Table 56-1 shows other risk factors for infection. The most common clinical manifestations for **early-onset infection are sepsis, pneumonia, and, less often, meningitis** (5% to 10% of early-onset GBS cases). Early-onset GBS infection has a fulminant presentation; 50% of infected infants are symptomatic at birth. Initial manifestations include **respiratory distress, hypoxia, and shock.** The mortality rate of early-onset GBS infection is 5% to 10%. Late-onset infections typically occur within the first month of life, but a small subset of infants develops GBS infection 3 to 6 months after birth. **Late-onset infections** include **sepsis, meningitis** (30% to 40% of late-onset GBS cases), and, occasionally, **skin or soft tissue infections, osteomyelitis, or septic arthritis.** The mortality rate of late-onset GBS infection is 2% to 6%. **Permanent neurologic sequelae** occur in approximately 50% of patients with meningitis caused by GBS infection.

The use of **intrapartum antibiotics** to treat GBS colonized women has decreased the incidence of early-onset GBS infection in neonates by about 30%; the incidence of late-onset disease remains unchanged because intrapartum antibiotic administration does not effectively eradicate neonatal colonization. Currently, half of all cases of invasive GBS disease are late onset. American Academy of Pediatrics (AAP) and American College of Obstetrics and Gynecology (ACOG) recommendations include vaginal and rectal GBS screening of all pregnant women at 35 to 37 weeks of gestation. **Intrapartum penicillin is administered** in the following situations: previous infant with GBS; GBS bacteriuria; positive GBS screening culture; and unknown GBS status if there is preterm labor, membrane rupture ≥18 hours, or intrapartum temperature ≥100.4°F (38°C). Cefazolin, clindamycin, erythromycin, or vancomycin may be given to penicillin-allergic women based on results of GBS isolate susceptibility testing. Other **factors that increase the risk** of neonatal sepsis include a **multiple gestation pregnancy and maternal chorioamnionitis.**

E. coli Infection

E. coli, like GBS, is passed from **mother to infant,** and the ratio of infected to colonized babies is similar. **Early-onset and late-onset infections** occur.

Organisms that have the K1 surface antigen are more apt to cause infection, especially meningitis.

Coagulase-negative Staphylococcal Infection

Coagulase-negative staphylococci (primarily *S. epidermidis*) are most commonly associated with nosocomial infection. Risk factors include **prematurity** and the use of **indwelling catheters.** The organism produces a slime coating that allows it to adhere to the surfaces of synthetic polymers used to make central venous catheters and also enables it to evade the immune system. **Clinical manifestations** of staphylococcal sepsis are **often subtle,** and a **high index of suspicion** is needed to diagnose the infection early.

Fungal Infection

Candida albicans has been the most common cause of neonatal fungal infection; however, *C. parapsilosis* and other non-*albicans Candida* species (*C. tropicalis, C. glabrata*) are becoming more prevalent. Risk factors for fungal infection include gestational age <32 weeks, indwelling intravascular catheter, endotracheal intubation >7 days, receipt of intralipids or parenteral nutrition, and broad-spectrum antibiotic use, especially third-generation cephalosporins. Systemic infection occurs after hematogenous dissemination. Infants with persistently positive blood cultures for *Candida* spp. (>3 days) with a central venous catheter in place are three times more likely to have disseminated disease. The most commonly involved sites are the **heart** (15%), **retina** (6%), **kidneys** (5%), and **liver** (3%). *Malassezia furfur* **bloodstream infection** is associated with intralipid infusion.

Differential Diagnosis

Neonatal sepsis may present with a variety of clinical presentations. These same presentations can have a variety of other causes simulating or accompanying sepsis. Table 56-2 summarizes the differential diagnosis for sepsis.

Evaluation of Sepsis

All infants with suspected sepsis should receive antibiotics while awaiting blood culture results. The remainder of the evaluation, including lumbar puncture (LP), can be completed once the infant is stabilized.

Patient History

- Are there maternal factors that place the infant at risk for sepsis (see Table 56-1)?
- Is there a family history of infection or other diseases in newborns?
- Does the infant have poor feeding, feeding intolerance (e.g., vomiting, abdominal distention), decreased activity, lethargy, or irritability?

TABLE 56-2 Differential Diagnosis of Sepsis

Category	Disorder	Associated Symptoms and Signs	Differentiating Features
Metabolic	Hypoglycemia	Respiratory distress, jitteriness, lethargy, seizures	Hypoglycemia can occur with sepsis; check blood glucose in sick infants; especially common in infants of diabetic mothers and small for gestational age infants.
	Hypocalcemia	Respiratory distress, jitteriness, seizures	Check calcium; especially common in infants of diabetic mothers and preterm infants.
	Inborn error of metabolism	Lethargy, vomiting, seizures, tachypnea	Urea cycle defects and organic acidemias often present after the first few feedings.
Pulmonary	Respiratory distress syndrome	Respiratory distress in preterm infant	CXR shows hazy, "ground-glass" appearance; often indistinguishable from bacterial pneumonia.
	Meconium aspiration	Respiratory distress in term infant	Classic CXR shows diffuse, patchy interstitial infiltrates with hyperinflation; may have severe cyanosis from pulmonary hypertension and right-to-left shunting.
	Transient tachypnea of the newborn	Tachypnea without significant respiratory distress	CXR clear or with fluid in fissures; usually minimal supplemental oxygen requirement; usually seen after cesarean section delivery.
Cardiac	Cyanotic congenital heart disease: tetralogy of Fallot, TGA, tricuspid atresia, truncus arteriosus, TAPVR	Tachypnea, cyanosis unresponsive to oxygen, cardiac murmur, extra heart sounds, or abnormal S_2	CXR without infiltrates but with abnormal pulmonary vasculature or cardiac silhouette; difference in pre- and postductal pulse oximetry; lack of response to hyperoxia test (Pao_2 <100 mm Hg breathing 100% O_2).
	Congestive heart failure (VSD, patent ductus arteriosus, myocarditis, AVM—especially hepatic or cerebral)	Poor feeding, tachypnea, poor perfusion, hepatomegaly, S_2	Congestive heart failure from a left-to-right shunt is unusual in the immediate newborn period when the pulmonary vascular resistance is high; onset is gradual.
	Ductal-dependent lesions (aortic coarctation, hypoplastic left heart, critical pulmonic stenosis)	Poor perfusion, tachypnea, metabolic acidosis, cyanosis	Often sudden in onset, from hours to weeks after birth; check arterial blood gas, four-extremity blood pressures, and preductal and postductal pulse oximetry.

Neurologic	Hemorrhage	Pallor, hypotonia, tachycardia, hypotension	Especially common in preterm infants and following traumatic vaginal delivery.
	Cerebral infarct	Seizures	May be associated with polycythemia or cocaine exposure; often idiopathic.
Gastrointestinal	Necrotizing enterocolitis	Feeding intolerance, abdominal distention, bloody stools	Usually associated with prematurity; abdominal radiograph may show pneumatosis, portal venous air, or free air; associated laboratory findings may include metabolic acidosis and thrombocytopenia.
	Malrotation, volvulus	Bilious emesis, abdominal distention, bloody stools, and shock	All newborns with bilious emesis should be evaluated for GI obstruction; **volvulus is a surgical emergency.**
Hematologic	Profound anemia	Pallor, tachycardia, jaundice (if caused by hemolysis)	Hemolysis, perinatal bleeding (vasa previa, placental abruption), or postnatal hemorrhage.

AVM = arteriovenous malformation; CXR = chest radiograph; GI = gastrointestinal; Pao_2 = arterial oxygen tension; S_2 = second heart sound; S_3 = third heart sound; $TAPVR$ = total anomalous pulmonary venous return; TGA = transposition of the great arteries; VSD = ventricular septal defect.

TABLE 56-3 Standard Sepsis Workup

Complete blood count with differential
Blood culture
Lumbar puncture (LP) and cerebrospinal fluid (CSF) analysis*
Urinalysis and urine culture†
Chest radiograph‡

*If the infant is clinically stable and has a platelet count >50,000/mm³, an LP can be per-
formed to obtain CSF for analysis of cell count, protein level, and glucose level, and for
Gram stain and culture.
†If infant is >72 hours of life.
‡If respiratory symptoms are present.

Physical Examination

Signs of infection in the newborn infant are nonspecific and include the
following disturbances:

■ **Temperature**—fever (>100.2°F [37.9°C]) or hypothermia (<96.8°F
  [36.0°C])
■ **Neurologic**—bulging fontanel, lethargy, irritability, weak suck or cry,
  hypotonia, hypertonia
■ **Respiratory**—tachypnea (respiratory rate >60/minute), grunting,
  nasal flaring, retractions, hypoxemia, apnea
■ **Cardiovascular**—tachycardia, bradycardia, hypotension (systolic blood pres-
  sure <60 mm Hg in term infants), delayed capillary refill (>2 seconds)
■ **Cutaneous**—jaundice, mottled skin, cyanosis, or petechiae
■ **Skeletal**—focal bone tenderness

Laboratory Studies

Table 56-3 lists the studies included in a standard sepsis workup.

■ **Complete blood count (CBC).** The range of normal values for the white
  blood cell (WBC) count and differential changes with the gestational and
  chronological age of the baby. The normal WBC count is 10,000 to
  30,000/mm³ at birth and decreases to 5,000 to 15,000/mm³ by the second week of life. Although elevated total WBC and absolute neutrophil
  counts (ANCs) are not helpful as single indicators of sepsis, neutropenia
  (ANC <1,500/mm³) and an elevated immature-to-total WBC ratio >0.2
  are more often associated with infection. Positive and negative predictive
  values in large enough studies have not been established to use these values for treatment decisions. The initial WBC count may be normal in an
  infected newborn, with abnormalities developing 24 to 48 hours later.

> **HINT:** Remember that several noninfectious conditions can cause neu-
> tropenia in newborns, including pregnancy-induced hypertension,
> asphyxia, intraventricular hemorrhage, hemolytic disease, and alloim-
> mune neutropenia.

- **Cerebrospinal fluid (CSF) analysis.** The CSF sample should be evaluated for the cell count and differential and protein and glucose levels. Newborns have higher CSF cell counts and protein levels than older children and adults. The average CSF WBC count in an uninfected newborn is 6 WBCs/mm^3, and several studies have determined the normal range to be up to 20 WBCs/mm^3. The average value for protein in the CSF is 90 mg/dL in full-term infants and 120 mg/dL in preterm infants. Normal babies may have CSF protein of 150 to 200 mg/dL. Traumatic ("bloody") LPs can give results that are difficult to interpret. The correction factor applied to a traumatic LP is based on the WBC-to-RBC (red blood cell) ratio in the CSF and in the peripheral blood. Unfortunately, it is often inaccurate in determining the true WBC and protein counts of the CSF.
- **Other studies.** Additional tests to consider include C-reactive protein, prothrombin time, partial thromboplastin time, hepatic function panel, serum electrolytes, glucose, CSF enteroviral and herpes simplex virus detection by polymerase chain reaction (PCR), and viral cultures of nasopharyngeal secretions, rectal swabs, or CSF.
- **C-reactive protein.** The level of C-reactive protein, an acute phase reactant, is often increased in response to infection. The negative predictive value of two C-reactive protein measurements <1 mg/dL measured 24 hours apart and within 48 hours of birth was >97% in one study. Routine use of C-reactive protein to guide initiation of antibiotic therapy in the asymptomatic newborn infant is not advocated because of insufficient data.

Treatment of Sepsis

Stabilization and Monitoring

One must always remember the ABCs: **airway, breathing, and circulation.** Close monitoring of the **respiratory status, perfusion, and urine output** is necessary in all newborns with sepsis.

Initial Empirical Antibiotic Therapy

Empirical antimicrobial therapy for suspected bacterial infections is guided by knowledge of pathogens suspected, associated focus of infection, and the antimicrobial susceptibility patterns in a particular intensive care unit. The standard therapy for suspected early-onset sepsis is **ampicillin** (which is effective against GBS, *L. monocytogenes*, most enterococci, and 50% of *E. coli* strains) plus **gentamicin** (provides good Gram-negative coverage and is synergistic with ampicillin against many organisms). **Cefotaxime** may be used in place of gentamicin for treatment of meningitis or when resistance to aminoglycosides is suspected. **Vancomycin plus an aminoglycoside** (gentamicin, tobramycin, or amikacin) can be used as empirical therapy for nosocomial infections in the intensive care nursery. Obviously, the therapy should be altered appropriately when an organism is isolated and susceptibilities are available.

Specific Antibiotic Therapy

- **Group B _Streptococcus_.** Bacteremia or pneumonia can be treated with administration of ampicillin alone. If meningitis is present, aminoglycoside administration should be continued.
- **_L. monocytogenes_.** Ampicillin plus an aminoglycoside is recommended.
- **_E. coli_ and _K. pneumoniae_.** Combination therapy with an aminoglycoside and a third-generation cephalosporin is generally recommended. A single agent may be used for an uncomplicated urinary tract infection.
- **Other Gram-negative organisms.** Therapy is more complicated because of development of strains resistant to gentamicin and cephalosporins. Administration of a carbapenem and amikacin (or tobramycin) should be considered. This decision should be made in conjunction with a specialist in pediatric infectious diseases. Cephalosporins should not be used as monotherapy to treat Gram-negative rod bloodstream infections because of the risk of inducing resistant strains.
- **Coagulase-negative staphylococci.** Oxacillin can be used if sensitivity to this agent is demonstrated in vitro. Otherwise, vancomycin should be continued. Meningitis should be treated with a combination of vancomycin and an aminoglycoside.
- **_Candida albicans_.** Treat with amphotericin B. For meningitis, add oral flucytosine. For severe amphotericin B-associated toxicity (e.g., renal insufficiency), consider lipid amphotericin B or fluconazole. Caspofungin is being studied for use in neonates. Removal of the infected catheter is an important part of treatment of candidemia. Failure to remove the catheter as soon as candidemia is detected results in prolonged duration of candidemia and increased mortality rates.

Duration of Antibiotic Therapy

Expected duration of therapy depends on many variables, including **virulence of pathogen, rapidity of clinical response, removal of infected catheter, and adequacy of drainage of purulent foci,** if present. Table 56-4 presents the approximate duration of therapy for selected infections.

In cases of **bacterial meningitis,** a LP should be repeated several days into therapy to document sterilization of the CSF for Gram-negative meningitis and meningitis caused by highly resistant bacteria. Therapy should continue **2 weeks after obtaining a negative culture result for Gram-positive meningitis** and **3 weeks after obtaining a negative culture result for Gram-negative meningitis.**

Other Treatment Modalities

- **Blood products.** Some centers treat coagulation disorders with administration of fresh-frozen plasma (15 mL/kg) to replenish clotting factors. Platelets should be given to maintain a count of $>20,000/mm^3$ (or $>50,000/mm^3$ if there is evidence of bleeding).

TABLE 56-4 Approximate Duration of Therapy for Selected Infections in the Newborn Infant

Site of Infection	Duration of Therapy (days)
Skin/soft tissue	7–10
Bacteremia	10
Bacteremia with CVC	10–14
Necrotizing enterocolitis	10–14
Pneumonia	10–14
Meningitis (Gram positive)	14
Meningitis (Gram negative)	21
Osteomyelitis/septic arthritis	28–42
Endocarditis	28–42
Fungemia (CVC removed)	14
Fungemia (disseminated)	>28

CVC = central venous catheter.

- **Alternative therapies.** Various strategies for prophylaxis or treatment of sepsis in the newborn have been studied, including exchange transfusion, neutrophil transfusion, administration of intravenous immunoglobulin, and cytokine therapy. Unfortunately, none has consistently proven effective for routine use. Hemopoietic colony-stimulating factors in recent trials increased ANC and decreased mortality rates in critically ill neutropenic neonates.

Approach to the Asymptomatic Patient with Risk Factors for Sepsis

The decision on whether to evaluate an asymptomatic newborn for infection should be based on **maternal and fetal risk factors,** such as those listed in Table 56-1. In asymptomatic infants with gestational age >35 weeks, the duration of intrapartum prophylaxis before delivery determines subsequent management. If **two or more doses of maternal prophylaxis** were given before delivery, **no laboratory evaluation or antimicrobial treatment** is required. These infants should be **observed in the hospital for at least 48 hours.** If fewer than two doses were given, the AAP and ACOG recommend a **limited evaluation** (CBC with differential and blood culture) and **at least 48 hours of observation** before discharge from the hospital.

Premature neonates have at least a **10-fold higher risk for early-onset GBS sepsis** compared with term neonates. Furthermore, as the degree of prematurity increases, clinical evaluation for signs and symptoms of sepsis are less reliable. Therefore, asymptomatic infants <35 weeks of gestation should receive **limited evaluation** (CBC with differential and blood culture) and **at least 48 hours of observation** prior to hospital discharge. Empirical antibiotic therapy is not required. If, during the period of observation, the clinical course **suggests systemic infection, complete**

TABLE 56-5 Clinical Features Suggesting Infection with TORCH Agents

Intrauterine growth retardation
Hydrops
Microcephaly, hydrocephalus, intracranial calcifications
Eye abnormalities (chorioretinitis, cataracts, glaucoma)
Cardiac malformations, myocarditis
Pneumonitis
Hepatosplenomegaly
Anemia, thrombocytopenia, petechiae
Jaundice (especially conjugated hyperbilirubinemia)
Bone abnormalities (osteochondritis, periostitis)

TORCH = toxoplasmosis, other (congenital syphilis and viruses), rubella, cytomegalovirus, and herpes simplex virus.

diagnostic evaluation and administration of empiric antibiotic therapy are indicated. This degree of surveillance and treatment is justified by the high morbidity and mortality rates associated with neonatal infection.

CONGENITAL (TORCH) AND PERINATAL INFECTIONS

Overview

A congenital infection is acquired by the infant transplacentally during the first, second, or early third trimester. Table 56-5 lists the clinical features associated with these infections. The classic acronym for the agents that cause these congenital infections is TORCH. Infections that are acquired in the perinatal period are frequently included in this group:

Toxoplasmosis
Other (includes HIV, syphilis, enterovirus, parvovirus, hepatitis
 B virus, varicella-zoster virus)
Rubella
Cytomegalovirus (CMV)
Herpes simplex virus (HSV)

Common Infections

Cytomegalovirus Infection

CMV is the **most common viral cause** of congenital infection. Approximately 50% to 80% of women of childbearing age are seropositive for CMV, but the risk of reactivation during pregnancy causing fetal infection is small (<1%). Primary CMV infection occurs in 1% to 4% of pregnancies and the fetus is infected in 40% of these cases. Most affected infants are **asymptomatic at birth** and develop normally. Approximately

10% to 15% of infected infants have symptoms at birth, and 90% of these infants develop sequelae (e.g., mental retardation, hearing loss, seizures).

Congenital CMV infection is diagnosed by detection of the virus from the urine (PCR rather than culture is used at some hospitals) within 2 weeks of birth; after this time, a detection of the virus could indicate intrapartum or postnatal infection, which is usually not clinically significant unless the baby is premature.

Treatment of congenital CMV infection usually involves supportive care and close follow-up. Ganciclovir treatment for 6 weeks reduces the progression of hearing loss in affected infants. Criteria for ganciclovir use include evidence of neurologic involvement such as intracranial calcifications, microcephaly, or CSF pleocytosis.

Syphilis

Congenital syphilis results from transplacental passage of the spirochete *Treponema pallidum;* rarely, infant contact with a maternal chancre results in perinatal transmission. Maternal syphilis in any stage can lead to fetal infection.

Fetal or perinatal death occurs in 40% of congenital syphilis infections. The surviving infants are asymptomatic at birth but, if not treated, develop symptoms within the first few weeks of life. The most common manifestations of early congenital syphilis are hepatosplenomegaly, bone abnormalities, hemolytic anemia, and jaundice. Less common findings include ocular involvement, bloody nasal discharge (snuffles), mucocutaneous rash, and pneumonia alba.

Maternal testing for syphilis involves nontreponemal serology using either the Venereal Disease Research Laboratory (VDRL) or the rapid plasma reagent (RPR) test. Treponemal test (i.e., the microhemagglutination-*Treponema pallidum* [MHA-TP] test or the fluorescent treponemal antibody absorbed [FTA-ABS] test) are positive for life; therefore, they indicate disease history, not activity at the time of the blood study. In many cities, the health department keeps records of previous infection and treatments.

Indications for treatment of the infant vary; consult the latest AAP Committee on Infectious Disease report, the *Red Book,* for recommendations. Maternal history of treatment and response to treatment by a fourfold drop in titers are major factors to consider in management plans. Testing of the newborn infant includes the following:

- **Serum RPR.** Umbilical cord testing can show false-positive results.
- **LP.** Send CSF for VDRL; CSF analysis reveals pleocytosis and elevated protein.
- **Radiographs of the long bones.**

In the newborn period, the normally high CSF protein and infrequency of abnormal bone findings make the criteria just listed less absolute. Pregnancy can slightly elevate the RPR. Infants should be treated for congenital syphilis if

- They were born to a mother with untreated syphilis.
- There is evidence of maternal relapse or reinfection.
- There is physical, radiologic, or laboratory evidence of syphilis.
- Their CSF VDRL is reactive.
- Their serum quantitative nontreponemal titer is at least fourfold greater than the mother's titer.

Treatment of early asymptomatic infection prevents long-term clinical sequelae. **Penicillin G** (50,000 U/kg given intravenously every 12 hours for 10 to 14 days) is the treatment of choice. **Infants born to mothers treated in the last month of pregnancy** should be evaluated; if the workup is normal, they may receive a single dose of **intramuscular benzathine penicillin G.** Detailed recommendations for the treatment of syphilis in pregnancy and infancy can be found in the *2006 Red Book: Report of the Committee on Infectious Diseases,* published by the AAP.

> **HINT:** False-positive VDRL tests occur in patients with lupus. Patients with Lyme disease have positive treponemal tests (MHA-TP or FTA-ABS) and negative VDRL.

Hepatitis B

In utero infection with the hepatitis B virus rarely occurs; **perinatal transmission** is more common. Overall, there is a 60% to 70% chance of perinatal transmission if the mother has acute symptomatic infection. If the mother is seropositive for hepatitis B e antigen (HBeAg), the perinatal transmission rate is 90%, as opposed to only 10% if the mother is HBeAg negative.

Infected infants are asymptomatic at birth but may develop antigenemia and an increased level of transaminases by 2 to 6 months of age.

Hepatitis B can be **prevented by either active or passive immunization.** Current recommendations include treating all infants born to mothers who are hepatitis B surface antigen positive with hepatitis B immune globulin and hepatitis B vaccine.

> **HINT:** Mothers with hepatitis B may breast-feed their infants.

Herpes Simplex

Approximately 75% of neonatal HSV infections are caused by HSV type 2. Congenital infection with this organism is extremely rare; usually, the baby is infected via the maternal genital tract shortly **before or during delivery.** Primary maternal infection results in neonatal HSV infection in approximately 50% of cases, whereas recurrent infection poses a risk of approximately 5%. Transmission of HSV may be **prevented by cesarean delivery** when the mother has active genital lesions and the membranes have been ruptured for <4 hours.

Neonates with HSV infection manifest in three distinct clinical groups:

- Disease localized to the skin, eye, and/or mouth (SEM disease)
- Encephalitis with or without skin involvement (central nervous system [CNS] disease)
- Disseminated disease that involves multiple organ systems, including the CNS, lung, liver, adrenals, skin, eye, and mouth

Disease onset occurs at <24 hours of life in 9%, at days 1 to 5 in 30%, and at >5 days in 60% of infants.

Skin lesions are seen in 60% of infants **with CNS or disseminated disease. Seizures** occur in 50% with CNS disease and in 20% with disseminated disease. **Pneumonia** occurs in 35% to 40% of infants with disseminated disease. **Disseminated infection** appears **clinically similar to bacterial sepsis** (e.g., lethargy, poor feeding, temperature instability). As the disease progresses, **jaundice, disseminated intravascular coagulation, hepatosplenomegaly, and shock** develop. Common CSF findings include **pleocytosis** (with a lymphocyte predominance), an **increased RBC count,** and an **increased protein level.** A positive CSF HSV PCR test confirms the diagnosis of meningitis. The CSF HSV PCR test has a high sensitivity (>98%) and specificity. Skin or conjunctival cultures are positive in >90% of neonates with any type of HSV infection. HSV is difficult to isolate from CSF culture.

Neonatal HSV infection is treated with **high-dose acyclovir** (60 mg/kg per day, divided, every 8 hours). Duration of treatment is **14 days for SEM disease** and **at least 21 days for CNS or disseminated disease.**

HIV

The risk of transmission of HIV from a seropositive mother to her fetus is approximately 20% to 30%, although **treatment of the infected mother during pregnancy and delivery reduces the transmission** dramatically. The **risk increases** to approximately 50% **if the mother has AIDS or if she previously had a child who was infected.** It is not known whether cesarean section delivery reduces the probability of transmission. Because the virus can also be **transmitted through breast milk,** the current recommendation in the United States is to counsel HIV-positive mothers not to breast-feed.

For babies of mothers with **unknown HIV status,** antibody level is the initial screening. **If the mother is HIV positive, HIV DNA PCR of the infants' blood should be performed at birth, 1 month, and 4 months** of age, and **blood for HIV culture** should be sent at **1 month** of age. HIV DNA PCR is positive in 30% of HIV-infected infants on the first day of life (the false-positive rate of HIV DNA PCR is 2%). The false-negative rate of HIV culture is approximately 0.5%. The combination of HIV culture and HIV DNA PCR detects 98% of all positive infants by 1 month of age and >99% by 4 months of age. **Infants with negative HIV DNA PCR** (at birth, 1 month, and 4 months of age) and HIV culture (at 1 month of age) should undergo **HIV antibody testing at 12, 15, and 18 months** of age to confirm that maternal HIV antibody is no longer present.

Opportunistic infections are reported in young infants; therefore, **Bactrim prophylaxis** is usually **started at 6 weeks of age and discontinued at 4 months of age** if testing reveals that the infant does not have HIV. Clinical trials have shown that **treatment of HIV-positive women** with **zidovudine** during the **second and third trimesters** of pregnancy and **intrapartum,** followed by **treatment of the newborn** for the first 6 weeks of life, **decreases the rate of transmission** of infection from mother to infant to approximately 8%.

Evaluation of Congenital Infection

Patient History

Confirm the results of maternal serologic screening for rubella, hepatitis B, syphilis, and HIV.

Physical Examination

Examine the baby for organ system involvement, including funduscopic examination. Table 56-6 lists the findings suggestive of particular infections.

TABLE 56-6   Clinical Findings in Specific TORCH Infections
Toxoplasmosis
Hydrocephalus with generalized calcifications Chorioretinitis, microphthalmia Deafness
Rubella
Cataracts, glaucoma, pigmented retinopathy, microphthalmia Deafness Cardiac malformation (PDA, pulmonary artery stenosis) "Blueberry muffin" appearance (extramedullary hematopoiesis)

(Continued)

TABLE 56-6 Clinical Findings in Specific TORCH Infections *(Continued)*

CMV

Microcephaly with periventricular calcifications
Chorioretinitis
Inguinal hernias (boys)
Petechiae with thrombocytopenia

Herpes

Acute CNS findings
Keratoconjunctivitis
Skin, eye, mucous membrane vesicles

Syphilis

Interstitial keratitis, pigmentary retinopathy
Snuffles (persistent and often bloody nasal discharge)
Fissures (lips, nares) and mucous patches (mouth, genitalia)
Eczematoid skin rash
Osteochondritis and periostitis

Modified with permission from Stagno S, Pass   Alford CA: Perinatal infections and maldevelopment. In *The Fetus and the Newborn,* Volume 17, Series 1. Edited by Bloom AD, James LS. New York, Wiley-Liss, 1981.
CMV = cytomegalovirus; *CNS* = central nervous system; *PDA* = patent ductus arteriosus.

Laboratory Studies

It is not necessary to perform a complete TORCH evaluation for every baby with suspected congenital infection. A **thorough history and physical examination** of the baby and **knowledge of maternal prenatal laboratory studies** (rubella, syphilis, hepatitis, and HIV serologies) can narrow the differential diagnosis. Table 56-7 lists the studies to consider in the evaluation of an infant with a suspected TORCH infection.

- **Serology.** Maternal IgG antibody crosses the placenta; therefore, the absence of rubella- or *Toxoplasma*-specific IgG in the infant excludes congenital infection. However, positive IgG titers in the infant for rubella or *Toxoplasma* are not diagnostic of congenital infection. If the serology is positive, check specific IgM titers. In suspected congenital syphilis, serum RPR and CSF VDRL should be tested.

- **Viral culture.** All infants with suspected HSV should have surface viral cultures performed. Urine viral culture can be used to diagnose congenital CMV infection, but many centers use PCR. Testing for CMV must be sent within 2 weeks of birth, otherwise postnatal acquisition cannot be excluded. Enteroviral culture of nasopharyngeal and rectal swabs and CSF may be indicated for a baby with myocarditis, hepatitis, or aseptic meningitis.

TABLE 56-7 Evaluation of the Infant with a Suspected TORCH Infection

Cerebrospinal Fluid

CSF cell count, protein, glucose (enterovirus, rubella, syphilis)
CSF PCR (enterovirus, HSV)
CSF VDRL (syphilis)

Blood

IgG (specify *Toxoplasma* or rubella—if positive, send IgM)
RPR (syphilis)
Hepatitis B surface antigen
PCR (enteroviruses, HIV)

Skin Lesions

Darkfield examination (syphilis)
Direct fluorescent antibody (HSV, varicella)
PCR (HSV, varicella)
Tzanck smear (HSV)*
Culture (HSV)

Urine

PCR (CMV, enteroviruses)
Culture (CMV)

Mucosa

Conjunctiva culture (HSV)
Mouth or nasopharynx culture (HSV, enterovirus)[†]
Rectum culture (enterovirus, HSV)[†]

Other Studies

Audiologic evaluation (CMV, rubella, toxoplasmosis)
Head CT (CMV, toxoplasmosis)
Ophthalmologic examination (toxoplasmosis, rubella, CMV, HSV, varicella, syphilis)
Radiograph of long bones (rubella, syphilis)

See text for evaluation of an infant for HIV.
*Tzanck smear rarely used. PCR and direct fluorescent antibody testing more common.
[†]Enteroviral cultures rarely performed given the high sensitivity of enteroviral PCR for detection of enterovirus in blood, urine, and stool specimens.
CMV = cytomegalovirus; *CSF* = cerebrospinal fluid; *CT* = computed tomography; *HSV* = herpes simplex virus; *IgM* = immunoglobulin M; *PCR* = polymerase chain reaction; *RPR* = rapid plasma reagent; *VDRL* = Venereal Disease Research Laboratory.

■ **Other laboratory studies** include a CBC, bilirubin (conjugated and unconjugated), and transaminases. Darkfield examination of nasal discharge in patients with "snuffles" may reveal syphilis.

Suggested Readings

American Academy of Pediatrics: Revised guidelines for prevention of early-onset group B streptococcal (GBS) infection. *Pediatrics* 99: 489–496, 1997.

Centers for Disease Control and Prevention: Prevention of perinatal group B streptococcal disease. Revised guidelines from CDC. *MMWR* 51(R-11):1–22, 2002.

Freeman J, Goldmann DA, Smith NE, et al.: Association of intravenous lipid emulsion and coagulase-negative staphylococcal bacteremia in neonatal intensive care units. *N Engl J Med* 323:301–308, 1990.

Kimberlin DW, Lin CY, Jacobs RF, et al.: Natural history of neonatal herpes simplex virus infections in the acyclovir era. *Pediatrics* 108:223–229, 2001.

Kimberlin DW, Lin CY, Sanchez PJ, et al.: Effect of ganciclovir therapy on hearing in symptomatic congenital cytomegalovirus disease involving the central nervous system: a randomized, controlled trial. *J Pediatr* 143:16–25, 2003.

Nielsen K, Bryson YJ: Diagnosis of HIV infection in children. *Pediatr Clin North Am* 47:39–62, 2000.

Remington JS, Klein JO (eds): *Infectious Diseases of the Fetus and Newborn Infant,* 6th ed. Philadelphia, Elsevier, 2006.

Rowley AH, Stumos JK: Timely diagnosis of congenital infections. *Pediatr Clin North Am* 41:1017–1034, 1994.

Schrag SJ, Stoll BJ: Early-onset neonatal sepsis in the era of widespread intrapartum chemoprophylaxis. *Pediatr Infect Dis J* 25(10):939–940, 2006.

Stoll BJ, Gordon T, Korones SB, et al.: Late-onset sepsis in very low birth weight neonates: a report from the National Institute of Child Health and Human Development Neonatal Research Network. *J Pediatr* 129:63–71, 1996.

57 *Pallor (Paleness)*

Kim Smith-Whitley

INTRODUCTION

Pallor (paleness) results from a **decreased amount of circulating hemoglobin or vasoconstriction of dermal blood vessels.** Causes can be classified as hematologic or nonhematologic.

DIFFERENTIAL DIAGNOSIS LIST

Hematologic Causes

Increased red blood cell (RBC) destruction —see Chapter 40, "Hemolysis"
  Isoimmune or alloimmune hemolytic anemia (hemolytic disease of the newborn)
  Autoimmune hemolytic anemia
  RBC membrane defects
  RBC enzyme defects
  Qualitative hemoglobin disorders
  Quantitative hemoglobin disorders
  Microangiopathic hemolytic anemia
  Drugs
  Toxins
  Infections
Bone Marrow Failure
  Transient erythroblastopenia of childhood
  Aplastic crisis with underlying congenital hemolytic anemia
  Diamond-Blackfan anemia
  Anemia associated with systemic illness
  Drug-related anemia

Infection
Aplastic anemia—idiopathic or secondary to drugs, chemicals, viruses, radiation, pregnancy
Transient bone marrow suppression—caused by viral or bacterial infection, drugs, pregnancy, radiation
Fanconi anemia
Dyskeratosis congenita
Pure red cell aplasia
Congenital dyserythropoietic anemia
Pregnancy
Bone Marrow Infiltration
  Leukemia or neoplasm metastatic to bone marrow
  Infection
  Osteopetrosis
  Histiocytosis
  Myelofibrosis
  Storage diseases
Nutritional Deficiencies
  Iron deficiency
  Folate deficiency
  Vitamin B_{12} deficiency
Blood Loss
  Hemorrhage
  Bleeding disorder

Nonhematologic Causes

Infectious Causes
  Bacterial process leading
  to shock, anemia, or
  both
Toxic Causes
  Lead poisoning
Neoplastic Causes
  Pheochromocytoma
Traumatic Causes
  Head trauma resulting in
  a closed head injury or
  cerebral hemorrhage
Congenital Causes
  Constitutional skin color

Metabolic or Genetic Causes
  Hypoglycemia
Inflammatory Causes
  Atopic dermatitis
  Other chronic systemic
  diseases
Miscellaneous Causes
  Shock
  Skin edema (myxedema, as
  in thyroid disease)
  Uremia
  Cystic fibrosis
  Seizures
  Syncope
  Lack of sun exposure

DIFFERENTIAL DIAGNOSIS DISCUSSION

Blood Loss

Etiology

Blood loss, acute and chronic, is one of the most common causes of anemia in the pediatric patient. Chronic blood loss may be caused by **gastrointestinal bleeding, excessive menstrual bleeding, or a bleeding disorder** characterized by frequent bleeding episodes.

Clinical Features

Patients with chronic blood loss may present with **pallor,** usually noted by an observer who has not seen the child recently. **Chronic blood loss** may be **difficult to recognize** because the hemoglobin level diminishes slowly.

Evaluation

Initial laboratory studies should include a **complete blood count (CBC), blood type and cross-match, prothrombin time, and partial thrombo-plastin time.** In a patient with anemia secondary to **chronic blood loss,** a peripheral smear shows **hypochromic, microcytic RBCs** from iron deficiency. In a patient with **acute blood loss,** it shows **normocytic, nor-mochromic RBCs.**

Treatment

If bleeding is **massive or life threatening, intravenous access should be estab-lished, active bleeding controlled, and type O-negative, uncross-matched** packed RBCs should be transfused. Rarely, in the previously transfused, alloimmunized child, minor blood group antigen incompatibility results in severe delayed hemolytic transfusion reactions following the administration of O-negative uncross-matched packed cells.

Iron-Deficiency Anemia

 HINT: Nutritional deficiencies may be caused by decreased oral intake, increased requirements, decreased absorption, or ineffective transport or metabolism of the element. The specific deficiency should be determined as well as the underlying cause to provide optimal treatment.

Etiology

Iron deficiency, which is the most common cause of anemia in childhood, can occur at any age, although children between 6 and 36 months of age and girls between 11 and 17 years of age are at increased risk. Iron deficiency in childhood is caused by **rapid growth in the presence of inadequate dietary intake, chronic or massive blood loss, or poor gut absorption.** Infants with iron deficiency usually have a history of **consuming large amounts of cow's milk** and other food substances low in iron.

HINT: Iron deficiency is less common in breast-fed infants. Although the iron content of breast milk is lower than that of a formula based on cow's milk, iron absorption is improved.

HINT: Pica may be a symptom of iron deficiency or a risk factor for iron deficiency. Children who eat dirt should be evaluated for lead poisoning.

Clinical Features

Children with severe iron deficiency are commonly **pale, irritable, and have little appetite.** In addition to signs of anemia, **spooning of the nails, angular stomatitis, and splenomegaly** may be present.

Laboratory Evaluation

The degree of iron deficiency can be estimated by the abnormalities found on laboratory studies. The following laboratory abnormalities occur progressively: decreased serum ferritin, decreased serum iron, increased microcytosis, and decreased hemoglobin with a normal or decreased reticulocyte count. The red (blood cell) distribution width (index) is increased. The platelet count may be markedly increased. The peripheral blood smear shows hypochromic, microcytic RBCs with increased variation in RBC size (anisocytosis) and shape (poikilocytosis). Increased numbers of elliptocytes and ovalocytes may be noted.

Treatment

Treatment of iron deficiency includes iron supplementation, as well as treatment of the underlying cause with nutritional counseling when appropriate. Oral iron replacement is achieved with ferrous sulfate (3 to 6 mg/kg per day of elemental iron in two or three divided doses). Although absorption is better on an empty stomach, gastric irritation is lessened if the iron is given with meals.

In patients with severe anemia, the hematologic response to ferrous sulfate administration can be documented by obtaining a reticulocyte count within 7 to 10 days. The reticulocyte count increases earlier than the hemoglobin level, which may not reach a normal level until 2 months after starting iron therapy, depending on the degree of anemia.

Many physicians believe that because iron deficiency is so common, the healthy child or adolescent with a microcytic, hypochromic anemia is appropriately managed using a trial of iron supplementation without additional laboratory evaluation. If a patient is managed this way, close follow-up should be provided. If the microcytic anemia persists, a comprehensive evaluation for other causes (e.g., thalassemia, anemia of chronic disease, chronic blood loss, sideroblastic anemia) should be performed.

Megaloblastic Anemias

Etiology

Megaloblastic anemias are often caused by folate and vitamin B_{12} deficiencies, which result in abnormal DNA synthesis. Folate deficiency in the United States is primarily caused by malabsorption of folate, increased RBC turnover, and drugs. Vitamin B_{12} deficiency may be caused by malabsorption or pernicious anemia, a rare disease caused by an inability to secrete the intrinsic factor required for normal vitamin B_{12} absorption.

Evaluation

Megaloblastic anemias are characterized by macrocytic RBCs and a mean corpuscular volume (MCV) value >95 fL. The reticulocyte count is low, and in advanced cases pancytopenia may exist. Analysis of a bone marrow aspirate and biopsy shows dyssynchrony between nuclear and cytoplasmic maturation with increased cellularity.

Serum folate may be decreased, but measurement of **RBC folate levels** provides a more accurate picture of chronic folate deficiency. In pernicious anemia, **serum vitamin B$_{12}$ levels are reduced** and **intrinsic factor antibodies may be positive.**

Therapy

Therapy includes **supplemental folate or vitamin B$_{12}$** administration, as well as **treatment of the underlying cause** of the deficiency.

Transient Erythroblastopenia of Childhood

Clinical Features

Transient erythroblastopenia of childhood is characterized by the **acute onset of anemia** in a previously healthy child **between 6 months and 4 years of age.** There may be a history of a **viral prodrome.** The physical examination is normal except for signs of anemia.

Evaluation

The hemoglobin and reticulocyte values vary according to the stage of disease. **Early in the illness,** the **hemoglobin and reticulocyte count are low,** whereas **in the recovery stage** the hemoglobin may be low but the **reticulocyte count is increasing.** Therefore, **serial reticulocyte counts** should be used **in conjunction with serial hemoglobin values** to clarify the stage of disease.

Other laboratory findings include **neutropenia** (25% of patients) and a **normal platelet count.** The bone marrow aspirate shows a marked **decrease in erythroid precursors** early in the disease.

Treatment

Because of the potential severity of the anemia and the need for serial testing, these patients are initially managed more appropriately in a **hospital inpatient setting.** Transient erythroblastopenia of childhood usually **resolves in 1 to 2 months.** No medications accelerate bone marrow recovery. **RBC transfusion** is sometimes necessary.

Diamond-Blackfan Anemia (Congenital Hypoplastic Anemia)

Etiology

Diamond-Blackfan anemia is a **congenital disorder** characterized by **pure RBC aplasia.**

Clinical Features

Most patients become anemic within the first 6 months of life. **Congenital anomalies** occur in 25% of patients, including **radial anomalies** (triphalangeal thumbs); **short stature;** and **eye, palate, heart, and kidney anomalies.**

Evaluation

The disease is characterized by a **macrocytic anemia,** although a normocytic anemia with a decreased reticulocyte count is seen early in life. Bone marrow aspirate may show **normal cellularity** with isolated **decreased RBC precursors. Hemoglobin F is increased** in a heterogeneous fashion and erythrocyte adenosine deaminase levels are elevated. Some patients have RPS19 gene mutations.

Treatment

Approximately 60% to 70% of patients with Diamond-Blackfan anemia respond to corticosteroids and do not require chronic transfusions. Steroid-unresponsive patients receive **RBC transfusions** each month and have a poorer prognosis because of the long-term complications associated with chronic blood transfusion (e.g., iron overload). **Splenectomy** has also been attempted in steroid-unresponsive patients with mixed success. Some patients are cured by **bone marrow transplantation.**

Congenital Hemolytic Anemia with Aplastic Crisis

Etiology

Children with congenital hemolytic anemias can experience a **transient aplastic crisis as a result of human parvovirus B19 infection.**

Evaluation

Transient erythroblastopenia of childhood, Diamond-Blackfan anemia (congenital pure red cell aplasia), **and an aplastic episode** in the presence of a previously undiagnosed hemolytic anemia can be **difficult to distinguish** from one another. Children with congenital hemolytic anemia may have the following:

- A history of intermittent scleral icterus with intercurrent illnesses.
- **Family members with anemia** or family members **who have required splenectomy or cholecystectomy** before adulthood. Children with transient erythroblastopenia of childhood or Diamond-Blackfan anemia do not have this history as frequently.
- **Splenomegaly** on physical examination, which is absent in patients with transient erythroblastopenia of childhood but may be present in those with Diamond-Blackfan anemia.
- Peripheral RBC morphology that suggests the diagnosis of hereditary spherocytosis, hereditary elliptocytosis, or sickle cell disease (SCD).

If the RBC morphology is normal but the history is suspicious for a congenital hemolytic anemia, hemoglobin electrophoresis, measurement of RBC enzyme levels, and evaluation of membrane abnormalities should be performed (prior to transfusing the patient).

Children with congenital hemolytic anemia and aplastic crisis usually have a **febrile viral prodrome** and may have **profound anemia and reticulocytopenia.** Serum should be obtained for human parvovirus B19 titers (see Chapter 40, "Hemolysis").

Aplastic Anemia

Etiology

Aplastic anemia (i.e., bone marrow failure characterized by decreased bone marrow cellularity and pancytopenia) is **usually acquired.** However, congenital causes are not uncommon in children. Acquired aplastic anemia may be idiopathic or secondary to a number of processes (Table 57-1). Idiopathic aplastic anemia is more common because 30% to 50% of the patients have no antecedent cause. Most reported pediatric cases of aplastic anemia with definable causes result from **exposure to drugs, chemicals, or other toxic substances.**

TABLE 57-1 Causes of Severe Aplastic Anemia
Drugs
Chloramphenicol
Sulfa drugs
Anticonvulsants
Cancer chemotherapeutic agents
Chemicals
Benzenes
Gold
Insecticides (DDT)
Lindane (active ingredient in shampoos used to treat pediculosis)
Pregnancy
Viral Infection
Hepatitis A, hepatitis B, hepatitis C
Epstein-Barr virus
Radiation
Paroxysmal Nocturnal Hemoglobinuria
Inherited Disorders
Fanconi anemia
Dyskeratosis congenita
Reticular dysgenesis
Shwachman-Diamond syndrome
Immunologic Disorders
Severe combined immunodeficiency disorder with graft-versus-host disease
Systemic lupus erythematosus
Eosinophilic fasciitis
Thymoma
Hypogammaglobulinemia

Clinical Features

Patients with aplastic anemia usually present with signs of **thrombocy-topenia** (e.g., petechiae, ecchymoses, abnormal bleeding); however, signs of **anemia** may be present as well. Hepatosplenomegaly and lymphadenopathy are usually absent on physical examination.

Evaluation

Laboratory findings demonstrate **moderate to severe anemia, thrombocytopenia, and neutropenia. Reticulocytopenia** occurs with corrected reticulocyte counts <2%.

Analysis of a bone marrow aspirate and biopsy sample is necessary to establish a diagnosis. Bone marrow aspirate shows a paucity of RBC, white blood cell (WBC), and platelet precursors, as well as an absence of bone marrow infiltration with malignant cells. Bone marrow biopsy shows a decrease in overall bone marrow cellularity and replacement with fatty tissue. A bone marrow biopsy that demonstrates normal cellularity does not eliminate the possibility of aplastic anemia because these patients may have patchy foci of normal bone marrow activity. In these patients, magnetic resonance imaging may be useful to demonstrate bone marrow replacement with fat, especially in the spine. Evaluation should include tests to determine congenital causes of bone marrow failure as well.

Treatment

Once the diagnosis of aplastic anemia is established and a full evaluation performed to identify possible causes, potential treatment options should be evaluated. Initial management of the pediatric patient with pancytopenia should be directed toward **treating life-threatening bleeding, infection, and anemia-related congestive heart failure.** Supportive measures include **irradiated RBC and platelet transfusions** (when necessary) and **antimicrobial administration** to treat or prevent severe infections.

The majority of cases of aplastic anemia can be **cured by bone marrow transplantation or pharmacologic regimens.** Any patient with severe aplastic anemia and an **HLA-identical sibling** should first be evaluated for bone marrow transplantation. If there is no HLA-identical sibling, pharmacological treatment includes the administration of immunosuppressive agents such as **antithymocyte globulin, cyclosporine, and corticosteroids.** Other options include **androgens and growth factors.** Despite therapeutic interventions, a small number of patients with aplastic anemia do not respond or they develop leukemia.

Bone Marrow Infiltration

Etiology

Malignant diseases that can infiltrate or replace bone marrow include leukemia, rhabdomyosarcoma, neuroblastoma, retinoblastoma, Ewing sarcoma, lymphoma, and histiocytosis syndromes. Nonmalignant diseases that infiltrate and replace bone marrow include storage diseases, osteopetrosis, infections such as tuberculosis, and fibrous tissue replacement.

Evaluation

Bone marrow infiltration with malignant or abnormal cells can cause pancytopenia. Peripheral blood smears may show predominant teardrop-shaped RBCs and increased RBC and WBC precursors.

Treatment

Treatment is directed toward management of the causative disorder. Supportive measures include antibiotic therapy and RBC and platelet transfusions.

EVALUATION OF PALLOR (TABLE 57-2)

Patient History

The following information should be sought:

- Patient's age. The differential is slightly different for neonates (Table 57-3).
- A complete prenatal history, birth history, and family history, including information regarding the need for transfusion, a childhood history of splenectomy or cholecystectomy, or abnormal bleeding (if excessive blood loss is the cause of anemia)
- Signs of anemia (e.g., pallor with or without scleral icterus)
- Symptoms of cardiovascular compromise (e.g., easy fatigability; shortness of breath, at rest or with exercise; orthopnea; headache; mental status changes)
- Presence of other systemic symptoms (e.g., fever)
- History of chronic disease
- History of seizures, syncope, or head trauma
- Dietary history

Physical Examination (Table 57-2)

In addition to a general physical examination, care should be taken to examine the skin and mucosa. In a dark-skinned child, pale conjunctivae, palmar creases, nail beds, and oral mucosa help confirm the presence of pallor.

TABLE 57-2 **Clinical Evaluation of Pediatric Patients with Pallor**

Question	If the Answer is "Yes," Consider...
History	
Has the child been lethargic with a sudden onset of pallor?	An acute process such as head trauma, bacterial infection, hypoglycemia, or an acute anemia
Has the child had a slow onset of pallor with other major systemic symptoms?	A chronic illness such as cystic fibrosis, nephrotic syndrome, malignancy
Does the child have a known chronic disease?	Anemia of chronic disease
Is the child an infant whose diet primarily consists of cow's milk?	Iron-deficiency anemia
Is the child African American?	G6PD deficiency, SCD, thalassemia syndromes
Is the child of Mediterranean or Asian descent?	G6PD deficiency, thalassemia syndromes
Are the child's parents pale without a history of anemia?	Constitutional pallor
Is the child a neonate?	Acute or chronic blood loss, hemolytic disease of the newborn
Physical Examination	
Are there tongue abnormalities?	Nutritional deficiencies
Are there congenital anomalies?	Fanconi anemia, Diamond-Blackfan anemia, congenital infections
Is the child ill appearing with lymphadenopathy and hepatosplenomegaly?	Chronic systemic illness, congenital infection, malignancy
Does the child have jaundice and hepatosplenomegaly?	A hemolytic process
Does the child have petechiae, ecchymoses, or excessive bleeding?	A platelet or coagulation disorder
Does the child have hepatomegaly or a gallop on cardiovascular examination?	Congestive heart failure
Laboratory Studies	
Is the MCV low for age?	Iron-deficiency anemia, thalassemia, sideroblastic anemia, anemia of chronic disease
Is the MCHC low with microcytic, hypochromic RBC morphology?	Iron-deficiency anemia, thalassemia, sideroblastic anemia, anemia of chronic disease
Is the MCV elevated?	Megaloblastic anemia, reticulocytosis, hypothyroidism, trisomy 21, liver disease
Is there a normocytic, normochromic anemia?	Acute or chronic blood loss, hemoglobinopathies, early iron-deficiency anemia, infection, RBC membrane or enzyme abnormalities, hypersplenism
Is there an elevated RDW?	SCD, iron-deficiency anemia, megaloblastic anemias, thalassemia
Are the BUN and creatinine levels elevated?	Uremia, hemolytic uremic syndrome
Are there prominent target cells?	Liver disease, thalassemia, hemoglobinopathies

(Continued)

TABLE 57-2 Clinical Evaluation of Pediatric Patients with Pallor (*Continued*)

Question	If the Answer is "Yes," Consider...
Are there prominent burr cells?	Liver disease, renal disease, dehydration, pyruvate kinase deficiency, artifact
Are there prominent schistocytes?	Severe hemolytic anemia, microangiopathic hemolytic process, Kasabach-Merritt syndrome, hemolytic uremic syndrome, thrombotic thrombocytopenic purpura
Are there prominent elliptocytes?	Hereditary elliptocytosis, iron-deficiency anemia, normal variant
Is there prominent basophilic stippling?	Consider iron-deficiency anemia, lead poisoning, thalassemias, unstable hemoglobins
Are there prominent blister cells?	G6PD deficiency
Are there prominent Howell-Jolly bodies?	Postsplenectomy patient, megaloblastic anemia

BUN = blood urea nitrogen; *G6PD* = glucose-6-phosphate-dehydrogenase; *MCHC* = mean corpuscular hemoglobin concentration; *MCV* = mean corpuscular volume; *RBC* = red blood cell; *RDW* = red (blood cell) distribution width (index); *SCD* = sickle cell disease.

TABLE 57-3 Causes of Anemia in Neonates

Blood Loss

Fetomaternal hemorrhage
Placental abnormalities
   Abruptio placentae
   Placenta previa
Twin-to-twin transfusion
Excessive blood loss caused by a coagulation disorder
Cord abnormalities
Hemorrhage
   Cephalohematomas
   Hepatic hematomas
   Intracerebral hemorrhage
   Delivery trauma involving the placenta, the umbilical cord, or both

Hemolytic Anemia

Blood group incompatibility
Red blood cell membrane or enzyme abnormalities
Hemoglobinopathies
Microangiopathic processes

Hypoplastic Anemia

Infections
   Cytomegalovirus infection
   Syphilis
   Toxoplasmosis
   Rubella
   Severe bacterial infections
Diamond-Blackfan anemia

Cardiovascular findings often include tachycardia and a systolic ejection (flow) murmur. Signs of congestive heart failure caused by severe anemia include extreme tachycardia, a third heart sound (S_3) cardiac gallop, rales, hepatomegaly (possibly accompanied by splenomegaly), pedal edema (rare), and shock. Congenital anomalies suggest a congenital bone marrow failure syndrome.

Laboratory Studies (See Table 57-2)

Appropriate laboratory studies may include the following:

- CBC
- Reticulocyte count
- Peripheral blood smear
- Blood type and cross-match
- Bone aspirate and/or biopsy
- Serum electrolyte panel
- Blood urea nitrogen (BUN) and creatinine levels
- Glucose level
- Blood culture

> **HINT:** Pallor caused by anemia (i.e., a decrease in RBC mass) can only be confirmed by a CBC, which includes estimates of the RBC mass: the volume of packed RBCs, the hematocrit, and the hemoglobin level. Because expansion of the intravascular volume can decrease the hematocrit or hemoglobin levels, these values should be interpreted with the patient's intravascular volume status in mind.

APPROACH TO THE PATIENT

A child who presents with pallor and appears ill could have a **potentially life-threatening illness**. Most patients with **shock** are **pale, lethargic, and often have cool extremities.** After the patient is stabilized, **routine blood work** should be obtained, including a CBC; serum electrolyte panel; serum BUN, creatinine and glucose levels; blood culture; and blood type and cross-match. The brief history should **focus on head trauma** and the presence of **seizures, syncope, prior illness, or fever.** A more extensive history should be obtained after the child is stable.

A child who is pale and well appearing should also have a **CBC, reticulocyte count, and a serum chemistry panel, including bilirubin.** If the hemoglobin is low, the reticulocyte count is high, and the indirect bilirubin fraction is high, then a hemolytic anemia is very likely. A **Coombs or direct antibody test** should be obtained to determine whether the hemolysis is immune-mediated.

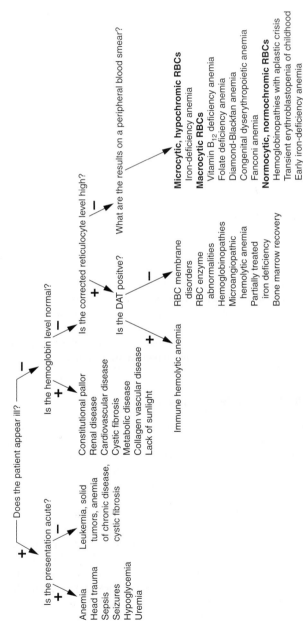

Figure 57-1 ■ Evaluation of a patient with pallor
DAT = direct antibody test; *RBC* = red blood cell

A **peripheral blood smear** should be examined in all children with anemia. Variations in the RBC shape (poikilocytosis) and size (anisocytosis) should be documented. Laboratory values such as the **MCV and mean corpuscular hemoglobin** should be included in the assessment. The **RBC distribution width** confirms the degree of anisocytosis and is increased in patients with iron-deficiency anemia, SCD, and megaloblastic anemias.

Once the differential diagnosis is narrowed (Figure 57-1), specific tests should be obtained as necessary. For example, iron studies should be obtained for a well-appearing, milk-drinking toddler with a microcytic, hypochromic anemia. Children with a **chronic anemia,** a **severe anemia** with no cause, or an **anemia that is unresponsive** to definitive therapy should be referred to a **pediatric hematologist.**

Suggested Readings

Cohen AR: Pallor. In *Pediatric Emergency Medicine*, 5th ed. Edited by Fleisher GR, Ludwig S, Henretig F. Baltimore, Williams & Wilkins, 2006, 535–543.

Graham EA: The changing face of anemia in infancy. *Pediatr Rev* 15:175–183, 1994.

Molteni RA: Perinatal blood loss. *Pediatr Rev* 12:47–54, 1990.

Richardson M: Microcytic anemia. *Pediatr Rev* 28:5–14, 2007.

Segel GB, Hirsh MG, Feig SA: Managing anemia in pediatric office practice: part 1. *Pediatr Rev* 23:75–83, 2002.

Segel GB, Hirsh MG, Feig SA: Managing anemia in pediatric office practice: part 2. *Pediatr Rev* 23:111–121, 2002.

chapter 58

Paraplegia

Amy R. Brooks-Kayal

INTRODUCTION

Paraplegia is any **weakness of the lower extremities** caused by dysfunction of the nervous system at the level of the peripheral nerves, spinal cord, or brain. Some paraplegias have **congenital causes** (tethered cord, syringomyelia, familial spastic paraparesis, spastic diplegia). Those that are **acquired** are grouped by timing of onset:

- **Acute** (evolving over minutes to hours)—trauma, spinal cord infarction
- **Subacute** (evolving over hours to days)—transverse myelitis, viral myelitis, epidural abscess, Guillain-Barré syndrome
- **Chronic** (evolving over weeks to months)—tumors

DIFFERENTIAL DIAGNOSIS LIST 🔓

Infectious Causes
Epidural abscess
Viral myelitis
Diskitis
Polyradiculoneuropathy
Tubercular osteomyelitis

Neoplastic Causes
Astrocytoma
Ependymoma
Neuroblastoma
Other (e.g., glioma, gangli-
oglioma, meningioma,
neurofibroma)

Traumatic Causes
Contusion
Transection
Epidural hematoma

Congenital or Vascular Causes
Spastic diplegia
Cord infarction

Arteriovenous malformation
Congenital malformations—
myelomeningocele, tethered
cord, syringomyelia

Genetic/Metabolic Causes
Familial spastic paraparesis
Adrenal myeloneuropathy
(rarely presents in childhood)

Inflammatory Causes
Transverse myelitis
Guillain-Barré syndrome
(acute inflammatory demyelinating polyneuropathy)
Chronic inflammatory
demyelinating polyneuropathy

Psychosocial Causes
Conversion disorder

DIFFERENTIAL DIAGNOSIS DISCUSSION

Trauma

Etiology

Spinal cord injury is usually associated with major force, such as occurs with **significant trauma**. The most common causes of traumatic paraplegia are **motor vehicle accidents** and **sports-related injuries**, although **gunshot injuries** are increasingly more common. Trauma can result in contusion, acute edema, compression secondary to epidural hematoma, or actual transection.

Clinical Features

Initial examination shows **weak, flaccid muscles, absent reflexes,** and **sensory loss** below the level of the lesion (spinal shock). **Bowel and bladder dysfunction** is typical. Autonomic disturbance (e.g., sweating, piloerection) is usually found below the level of the lesion. Over a period of weeks to months, **flaccidity evolves into spasticity, hyper-reflexia,** and **extensor plantar responses.**

Evaluation

The **neck must be stabilized** in a cervical collar until the stability of the cervical spine is established. **Magnetic resonance imaging (MRI)** should be done to differentiate contusion or transection from epidural hematoma. Plain radiographs or **computed tomography** of the spine may also be helpful to evaluate for vertebral fractures and dislocations.

Treatment

- **Spinal-dose steroids** (i.e., intravenous methylprednisolone, 30 mg/kg over 1 hour) should be initiated immediately (within 8 hours of injury). The initial dose is followed with 5.4 mg/kg per hour for 24 hours (if treatment is initiated <3 hours after injury) or 48 hours (if treatment is initiated 3 to 8 hours after injury).
- **Neurosurgical intervention** may be required for decompression of epidural hematomas or reduction and stabilization of vertebral fracture.
- **Meticulous supportive care,** including good bowel and bladder management and deep venous thrombosis (DVT) prophylaxis with sequential compression stockings, is essential. Subcutaneous heparin, 5000 U twice a day, or low-molecular-weight heparin may be added in patients at particularly high risk for DVT.

Spinal Cord Infarction

Etiology

Spinal cord infarction is usually the result of **occlusion** of the **anterior spinal artery,** which supplies blood to the ventral two thirds of the cord.

The most common causes in children are dissection secondary to **trauma, infection, emboli** in patients with cardiac disease, or **thrombosis** in patients with hypercoagulable states.

Clinical Features

Patients with spinal cord infarction present with **flaccid motor paralysis, areflexia,** and **dissociated sensory loss** (loss of pain and temperature sensation with sparing of vibration and position sense) below the level of arterial occlusion. **Bowel and bladder dysfunction** are usual. **Back pain** is sometimes present. Over weeks to months, **flaccidity evolves** into **spasticity,** with hyperreflexia, clonus, and extensor plantar responses.

Evaluation

An **MRI** of the spine should be performed to look for evidence of cord infarction. A **spinal arteriogram** should also be considered. Evaluations for cardiac disease and hypercoagulable states should be performed if there is no obvious cause for the occlusion.

Treatment

Intravenous corticosteroids should be administered early to minimize cord edema, which may result in additional ischemia. **Anticoagulation** should be considered in **selected patients,** including those with hypercoagulable states, cardiogenic emboli, or vascular dissection.

Transverse Myelitis

Etiology

Transverse myelitis is an **acute inflammatory, demyelinating disorder** of the cord. It can occur as a complication of systemic **viral infections** (infectious mononucleosis [EBV], varicella, mumps, rabies, rubella, rubeola, influenza, HIV) or **bacterial infections** (cat-scratch disease, *Mycoplasma pneumoniae*), **autoimmune disorders** (lupus), **immunizations** (rare), and **multiple sclerosis** (MS).

Clinical Features

The mean age of onset is 9 years. The patient presents with **thoracic back pain, lower extremity numbness, leg weakness** (symmetric or asymmetric), and **progressive urinary retention or incontinence.** Initial findings include weak, flaccid muscles (symmetric or asymmetric); absent reflexes; and sensory loss below the level of the lesion. Optic disc swelling and decreased vision or vision loss are often present in patients with Devic disease (i.e., transverse myelitis accompanied by optic neuritis), although the ocular symptoms may occur after the onset of spinal symptoms. Spasticity, hyperreflexia, clonus, and extensor plantar responses are seen later in the course of the disease.

Evaluation

A **lumbar puncture (LP)** should be performed to check for cerebrospinal fluid (CSF) opening pressure (normal to slightly elevated), protein level (usually increased) and electrophoresis (looking for oligoclonal bands), and cell count (usually a mixed pleocytosis of <200 cells/mm^3). **Spinal MRI** often shows swelling and abnormal signal at the level of the lesion. **Head MRI** should also be performed to look for other areas of demyelination suggestive of MS. **Viral serologies** (including HIV) may be helpful in identifying a triggering viral infection. **Antinuclear antibody panel and complement levels** should be considered as a screen for an autoimmune disorder.

Treatment

Usual therapy is a 3- to 5-day course of **high-dose intravenous methylprednisolone** (15 mg/kg per day, maximum 1 g/day) followed by a **4-week prednisone taper.** Use of intravenous immunoglobulin is also reported. **Supportive care** and intensive **physical therapy** are critical.

Viral Myelitis

Etiology

Viral myelitis is the **acute segmental infection of anterior horn cells.** Viruses most commonly responsible include poliovirus, group B coxsackievirus, and echoviruses.

Clinical Features

The patient usually has a history of **malaise, myalgias, low-grade fever,** and **upper respiratory tract symptoms progressing to severe headache** and **nuchal rigidity. Areflexia** and **flaccidity** and weakness of the muscles (usually asymmetric) are often heralded by pain in the spine and affected limbs. **Bulbar weakness** may also be present. There are usually no sensory symptoms.

Evaluation

The **most important diagnostic test is the LP,** which demonstrates pleocytosis (50 to 200 cells/mm^3). The predominance of polymorphonuclear cells is replaced by lymphocytes after the first week. CSF protein may be normal or slightly elevated, and CSF glucose is usually normal. **Viral isolation from CSF, stool, and nasopharyngeal swabs,** as well as **acute and convalescent viral titers,** can help confirm the diagnosis.

Treatment

Treatment of viral myelitis is **supportive.**

Epidural Abscess

Etiology

Epidural abscess is most commonly caused by the hematogenous spread of **bacteria,** usually *Staphylococcus aureus* in older children. The most common location is the **dorsal surface** of the **midthoracic** or **lower lumbar spine.**

Clinical Evaluation

Characteristically, the history includes **severe, localized back pain** (worse with cough or flexion) and **fever,** often associated with **headache, vomiting,** and a **stiff neck. Radiating pain** begins 3 to 6 days after the onset of back pain, followed by progressive **paraplegia** and **bladder dysfunction.** Examination shows localized spinal tenderness, lower extremity hyperreflexia, and spasticity (in patients with thoracic lesions) or hyporeflexia and decreased tone (in patients with lower lumbar lesions).

Evaluation

If epidural abscess is suspected, LP should not be performed because it can result in iatrogenic meningitis. **MRI,** however, is safe and demonstrates the lesion well.

Treatment

Initial treatment is with a **broad-spectrum intravenous antibiotic** with antistaphylococcal activity. Once a specific organism has been identified and sensitivities established, antibiotic therapy can be tailored to the patient. **Surgical drainage** may be required if there is evidence of cord compression.

Guillain-Barré Syndrome

Etiology

Guillain-Barré syndrome is an immune-mediated, acute, **inflammatory demyelinating polyneuropathy.** Approximately 50% of patients with Guillain-Barré syndrome have a history of antecedent viral infection.

Clinical Features

The syndrome can present at any age, but is **uncommon in children** <3 years. Often the first symptoms are **transient dysesthesias** and **muscle aches.** A typical feature is rapidly progressive, symmetric motor weakness beginning distally and ascending proximally. **Areflexia** is the rule and may precede significant weakness (e.g., biceps and triceps jerks may be lost while the arms are only minimally weak). **Facial weakness** and other cranial nerve involvement may be present in up to half of patients. Weakness can progress to include **respiratory muscles** with resultant hypoventilation. Although mild, symmetric, length-dependent sensory changes are common, extensive sensory loss or a sensory level should not be present. **Autonomic instability** (e.g., unstable blood pressure, cardiac arrhythmia) may occur.

Evaluation

On **LP,** patients with Guillain-Barré syndrome demonstrate **elevated CSF protein** with a paucity of cells (seen after the first week of illness). **Nerve conduction studies** show **reduced nerve conduction velocities** and **motor conduction block.** Vital capacity and **negative inspiratory potentials** should be monitored closely as indicators of impending respiratory failure.

Treatment

Meticulous **supportive care** (particularly of **respiratory function**) is critical. **Plasmapheresis** or **intravenous immune globulin** (2 g/kg divided over 2 to 5 days) is indicated if the patient loses the ability to ambulate independently.

> **HINT:** Initially, it can be very difficult to distinguish transverse myelitis, viral myelitis, epidural abscess, and Guillain-Barré syndrome from one another. It may not be possible to get a good sensory examination in an uncooperative child, and all four disorders can initially present with flaccid weakness and areflexia in the lower extremities. Furthermore, many of the diagnostic tests are not helpful until approximately 1 week into the course of the disease; for example, nerve conduction studies and CSF protein levels can both be normal for up to 1 week in Guillain-Barré syndrome. Although the following clues may help, ultimately the "tincture of time" and repeating studies after 1 week may be required to make a definitive diagnosis.

- A high fever, severe back pain or tenderness, and an **increased peripheral white blood cell count** are suggestive of epidural abscess.
- **Reflexes.** If the reflexes are down in the arms as well as the legs, think Guillain-Barré syndrome. Mild symmetric facial weakness (facial diplegia) and diminished gag reflex may also be present in Guillain-Barré syndrome but should not be seen in a spinal cord process.
- **Distribution of weakness.** The weakness in viral myelitis is often asymmetric, whereas Guillain-Barré syndrome and transverse myelitis usually cause symmetric weakness. In transverse myelitis, there is often a complete, uniform paralysis below the level of the lesion; in Guillain-Barré syndrome, the distal muscles tend to be weaker than the proximal muscles.

- **Bowel and bladder dysfunction** are suggestive of epidural abscess or transverse myelitis first, but remember that patients with Guillain-Barré syndrome occasionally also have bowel and bladder involvement.

Tumors

Etiology

Astrocytomas and **ependymomas** are the most common intrinsic spinal cord tumors, and **neuroblastoma** is the tumor that most commonly results in extrinsic cord compression (from extension of a paraspinal tumor through the neural foramen).

Clinical Features

Paraplegia caused by tumors presents with **slowly progressive leg weakness, gait difficulty,** and **sensory loss.** Often there is associated **back pain** and **bowel and bladder dysfunction.** Findings on physical examination depend on the location of the tumor: Thoracic lesions produce spastic paraplegia with hyperreflexia; tumors involving the conus medullaris and cauda equina produce weak, flaccid muscles with decreased or absent reflexes. **Sensory loss** is present below the level of the tumor. **Scoliosis** is frequently seen in association with intrinsic cord tumors.

Evaluation

Spinal MRI is the diagnostic test of choice for detection of tumors.

Treatment

Initial therapy consists of **dexamethasone** (0.25 mg/kg every 6 hours) to decrease surrounding edema. Definitive treatment depends on the type, extent, and location of the tumor but usually consists of some combination of **surgery, radiation,** and **chemotherapy.**

Tethered Cord

Etiology

In pediatric patients with tethered cord, the **conus medullaris** is **anchored** to the **base of the vertebral column** by a thickened filum terminale, lipoma, dermal sinus, or other site of traction. As the child grows, the spinal cord is stretched and lumbosacral segments become increasingly ischemic.

Clinical Features

Symptoms can occur at any time between infancy and young adulthood. Typical symptoms are **progressive clumsiness of gait, constipation,** and **urinary incontinence.**

Evaluation

Findings on general examination may include **scoliosis, stunted leg growth,** or **foot deformity** (pes cavus), **pigmentation, tufts of hair,** or a **deep dermal sinus** over the **lower spine.** On neurologic examination, **spastic leg weakness, hyperreflexia,** and **extensor plantar responses** are present.

Treatment

Surgery is required to release the cord.

Syringomyelia

Etiology

Syringomyelia is a **cavity within the spinal cord,** usually resulting from a congenital neural tube malformation. This condition most commonly occurs in the cervical and lumbar spinal cord segments.

Clinical Features

Syringomyelia often presents in adolescence or later with **progressive weakness** and **sensory loss.** Motor examination results depend on the **location of the lesion. Cervical lesions** show flaccid paralysis and hyporeflexia of the arms with spasticity and hyperreflexia in the legs; **lumbar lesions** present with flaccid paralysis of the legs with hyporeflexia, fasciculations, and muscle atrophy. Interruption of the **crossing spinothalamic fibers** in the central cord produces a "cape distribution" of pain and temperature sensation loss with relative sparing of light touch and proprioception.

Evaluation

The diagnostic test of choice is an **MRI.**

Treatment

Symptomatic congenital cord malformations are treated **surgically.**

Familial Spastic Paraparesis

Etiology

Familial spastic paraparesis is an **inherited progressive spastic paraparesis.** The genetics are complex, with autosomal dominant transmission seen in 70% of patients, but autosomal recessive and X-linked recessive transmission also reported. The mean age of onset in childhood type I familial spastic paraparesis is 11 to 16 years.

Clinical Features

Toe walking and **slowly progressive gait disturbance** are typical. A third of patients present with **urinary symptoms.** On examination, **spasticity** is out of proportion to weakness. **Hyperreflexia** involves all four extremities, and **ankle clonus** may be present. A third of patients have pes cavus deformity. The autosomal recessive form can also be associated with ataxia, sensory neuropathy, and pseudobulbar palsy.

Evaluation

Genetic testing for familial spastic paraparesis is of limited clinical utility at present. **Exclusion** of other, treatable disorders is critical. **MRI** of the spine can be useful to rule out structural disorders (e.g., vascular malformation, tumor, syringomyelia) or demyelination. **Vitamin B$_{12}$, vitamin E,** and **very-long-chain fatty acid levels** should be obtained. Eliciting a **family history** of similarly affected individuals is critical.

Treatment

No **specific treatment** is available.

Spastic Diplegia
Etiology

In this form of cerebral palsy, **all four extremities** are involved to some degree; however, the lower extremities are affected much more significantly than the upper extremities.

Clinical Features

In early infancy (<4 months of age), muscle tone is usually normal or hypotonic. Between 4 months and 1 year of age, there is an **insidious onset of lower extremity spasticity,** often associated with delay in sitting, crawling, and walking. **Toe walking** is common. On examination, there is **spasticity** and **hyperreflexia,** involving the legs more than the arms. **Scissoring** of the legs, ankle clonus, and extensor plantar responses are common.

Evaluation

Historical information suggesting premature birth or possible perinatal injury could be significant. **Brain MRI** may demonstrate evidence of periventricular leukomalacia or other evidence of perinatal injury.

Treatment

Supportive therapy often includes **physical and occupational therapy, bracing,** and, if needed, **botulinum toxin injections** or **surgical release** for treatment of contractures.

EVALUATION OF PARAPLEGIA

Patient History

The history should include the following information:

- Timing of onset of symptoms (acute, subacute, or chronic)
- Trauma

- Fever
- Back pain
- Changes in sensation—if so, in what distribution?
- Bowel and bladder dysfunction
- Visual problems—past or present
- Previous weakness, numbness, or other neurologic symptoms
- Family history of leg weakness

Physical Examination

The following should be sought on physical examination:

- **General examination**—evidence of head, neck, or back trauma; scoliosis; stunted leg growth; foot deformity (pes cavus); or pigmentation, tufts of hair, or a deep dermal sinus over the lower spine.
- **Cranial nerve examination**—look for papillitis (associated with transverse myelitis in Devic disease); eye movement abnormalities (associated with transverse myelitis secondary to MS); Horner syndrome (associated with cervical cord trauma); facial diplegia and decreased gag reflex (associated with Guillain-Barré syndrome).
- **Motor strength, tone, and reflexes in arms and legs**—weak, flaccid leg muscles and absent reflexes (associated with acute cord processes and Guillain-Barré syndrome); spasticity, hyperreflexia, and extensor plantar responses (associated with chronic spinal cord processes).
- **Sensation to all sensory modalities**—a sensory level (associated with spinal cord problems); mild distal sensory changes (associated with Guillain-Barré syndrome).
- **Autonomic disturbances**—associated with cord processes (usually found below the level of the lesion) or Guillain-Barré syndrome.

Laboratory Studies and Diagnostic Modalities

The usual workup for a patient with paraplegic symptoms includes an **MRI**, an **electromyogram, nerve conduction velocity studies,** and an **LP.** Several timing factors may cause false-negative results (e.g., CSF protein levels and nerve conduction studies may be normal for up to 1 week in patients with Guillain-Barré syndrome; MRI may not demonstrate cord swelling or signal changes in the first 24 hours in patients with transverse myelitis or cord infarction).

TREATMENT OF ACUTE PARAPLEGIA

If there is any suspicion of cord trauma, the **neck should be stabilized** and spinal-dose **steroids** should be administered. **DVT prophylaxis with sequential compression stockings** is essential. **Subcutaneous heparin,** 5000 U twice a day, or low-molecular-weight heparin may be added in patients at particularly high risk of DVT but only after hemorrhage is

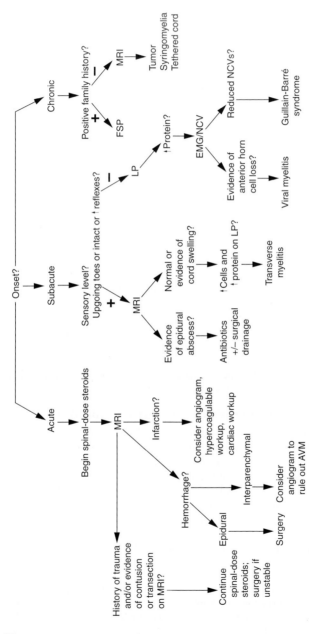

Figure 58-1 ■ Evaluation of a patient with paraplegia

AVM = arteriovenous malformations; *EMG* = electromyogram; *FSP* = familial spastic paraparesis; *LP* = lumbar puncture; *MRI* = magnetic resonance imaging; *NCVs* = nerve conduction velocities; ↑ = increased ruled out. Urinary retention is common, so an **indwelling bladder** (Foley) **catheter** should be placed or intermittent bladder catheterizations should be performed. **Histamine blockers** should be administered to prevent gastritis. Autonomic instability may be a problem, so careful monitoring of heart rate and **blood pressure** are essential.

APPROACH TO THE PATIENT (FIGURE 58-1)

Suggested Readings

Bracken MB, Shepard MJ, Holdrod TR, et al.: Administration of methylprednisolone for 24 or 48 hours or tirilazad mesylate for 48 hours in the treatment of acute spinal cord injury. *JAMA* 277:1597–1604, 1997.

Dias MS: Traumatic brain and spinal cord injury. *Pediatr Clin North Am* 51:271–303, 2004.

Hughes RAC, Wijdicks EFM, Barohn R, et al.: Practice parameter: immunotherapy for Guillain-Barré syndrome. *Neurology* 61:736–740, 2003.

Pidcock FS, Krishnan C, Crawford TO, et al.: Acute transverse myelitis in childhood. *Neurology* 68:1474–1480, 2007.

Renoux C, Vukusic S, Mikaeloff Y, et al.: Natural history of multiple sclerosis with childhood onset. *N Engl J Med* 356:2603–2613, 2007.

Sladky JT: Guillain-Barré syndrome in children. *J Child Neurol* 19:191–200, 2004.

Transverse Myelitis Consortium Working Group: Proposed diagnostic criteria and nosology of acute transverse myelitis. *Neurology* 59:499–505, 2002.

59

Pelvic Pain

Okeoma Mmeje and Jenell Coleman
Courtney Schreiber (Third Edition)

INTRODUCTION

Knowledge regarding the location of organs in the female pelvic region and how they may cause discomfort is key to the evaluation of pelvic pain in female patients. There may be distinct causes of pelvic pain depending on the timing and onset of pain. **Acute pelvic pain** is intense with a sudden and sharp onset that is short in duration. **Chronic pelvic pain** has been present for >6 months and severe enough to cause functional disability.

DIFFERENTIAL DIAGNOSIS LIST

Acute Pelvic Pain

Obstetric—ectopic pregnancy, abortion (threatened, missed or incomplete), labor

Gynecologic—endometriosis, adenomyosis, dysmenorrhea, mittelschmerz, pelvic adhesions, ovarian/adnexal torsion, stable/ruptured ovarian cyst, obstructive müllerian tract anomaly

Infectious—endometritis, pelvic inflammatory disease (PID), tubo-ovarian abscess

Gastrointestinal—gastroenteritis, appendicitis, Meckel diverticulitis, pancreatitis, inflammatory bowel disease (IBD), constipation, volvulus, intestinal obstruction, irritable bowel syndrome (IBS), Henoch-Schönlein purpura, mesenteric adenitis, regional enteritis

Genitourinary—cystitis, radiation cystitis, urinary tract infection, pyelonephritis, ureteral/renal lithiasis

Musculoskeletal—hernia, back pain, pelvic bone and joint infection, slipped femoral epiphysis, muscular strain/sprain

Other—falls, accidents, sexual abuse

Chronic Pelvic Pain

Obstetric—pregnancy

Gynecologic—obstructive müllerian tract anomaly, cervical stenosis, ovarian tumor, pelvic adhesions, endometriosis

Gastrointestinal—hernia, IBD, IBS, midgut malrotation, lactose malabsorption, chronic constipation

Genitourinary—ureteropelvic junction obstruction, detrusor

instability, pelvic kidney, cystitis
Musculoskeletal—scoliosis, kyphosis, fibromyalgia, abdominal wall trigger points

Neurologic—neurofibromatosis, nerve entrapment syndrome
Psychological—sexual abuse, emotional stress

DIFFERENTIAL DIAGNOSIS DISCUSSION

Ectopic Pregnancy

Etiology

An ectopic pregnancy is one in which a **fertilized ovum implants itself outside the uterine cavity (most often in the fallopian tube)** as a result of **delayed passage** of the fertilized ovum into the uterine cavity. **Abdominal, cervical, and ovarian ectopic pregnancies** can also occur. Delayed passage of the fertilized ovum into the uterine cavity usually results from a **condition that interferes with tubal structure or function** (e.g., chronic salpingitis, pelvic adhesive disease, tubal surgery, congenital abnormalities of the fallopian tube, intrauterine devices).

Clinical Features

The **classic triad of symptoms** consists of **abdominal pain, amenorrhea, and vaginal bleeding,** which is present in about 50% of patients. The abdominal pain may develop **suddenly or gradually.** In **unruptured ectopic pregnancies,** the pain tends to be **unilateral, colicky, and localized** to the involved adnexa. If **rupture** has occurred, the pain becomes **diffuse and intense. Referred shoulder pain** may occur in the presence of hemoperitoneum. **Dizziness and syncope** are the result of anemia and hypotension.

Evaluation

- **Abdominal examination.** Localized tenderness may be revealed in the lower quadrant. With rupture and intra-abdominal bleeding, rebound tenderness and guarding may be elicited. On pelvic examination, the cervix and uterus may be soft and tender from the effects of pregnancy hormones. Adnexal fullness or a discrete, tender mass may be noted in some patients.
- **Complete blood count (CBC).** The hemoglobin and hematocrit values may be low in patients with acute or gradual intraperitoneal hemorrhage; in the absence of bleeding, they are usually normal.
- **Type and screen.** Rh status is assessed in case blood replacement is necessary.
- **A pregnancy test.** A quantitative beta human chorionic gonadotropin (β-hCG) should be drawn.

- **Vaginal ultrasonography** can detect an intrauterine gestational sac as early as 4 weeks of gestation when the quantitative β-hCG is >1500 to 2000 mIU/mL. In addition, it may show an adnexal mass or complex free fluid in the pelvis. An adnexal mass seen on ultrasound further substantiates the diagnosis of an ectopic pregnancy. Free fluid in the cul-de-sac seen on ultrasound suggests hemoperitoneum and the necessity of early surgical intervention.

> **HINT:** A quantitative β-hCG >1500 to 2000 mIU/mL and an empty uterus by vaginal ultrasound is presumptive evidence of an ectopic pregnancy.

Treatment

Surgical diagnosis and treatment via **laparoscopy or laparotomy** is almost always indicated to manage an ectopic pregnancy with a tubal mass >3.5 cm. Medical treatment with **methotrexate** can be considered when an intrauterine pregnancy is absent, no adnexal mass is present, or the mass is <3.5 cm in the setting of a positive β-hCG. **Early gynecology consultation** is highly recommended.

Dysmenorrhea

Etiology

- Primary dysmenorrhea is **painful menstruation with no demonstrable cause.** Patients with primary dysmenorrhea have a greater endometrial production of prostaglandins, which cause uterine contractions, uterine ischemia, and pelvic pain.
- **Secondary dysmenorrhea** results from various pathologic conditions (e.g., endometriosis, salpingitis, or congenital müllerian anomalies).

Clinical Features

Symptoms of **primary dysmenorrhea** usually begin 1 to 2 years after menarche when ovulatory cycles are established. The pain is described as **crampy, lower abdominal pain,** starting within **several hours of the onset of menses.** The pain usually lasts for **2 to 3 days.** Associated symptoms include **headache, nausea, vomiting, diarrhea, and backache.** The symptoms of **secondary dysmenorrhea** are **similar** to those described for primary dysmenorrhea, although it develops years after menarche.

Evaluation

In patients with **primary dysmenorrhea** the **physical examination is normal.** Findings in **secondary dysmenorrhea** are related to the underlying cause. A CBC and **screening tests for *Neisseria gonorrhoeae*** and *Chlamydia trachomatis* are obtained to evaluate for possible infection. A **pregnancy test** is obtained to rule out pregnancy. **Pelvic ultrasonography** is useful for delineating the internal pelvic anatomy and evaluation of adnexal pathology. **Magnetic resonance imaging (MRI)** is helpful in the diagnosis of müllerian abnormalities.

Treatment

If the pelvic examination is normal, treatment is aimed at **symptomatic relief. Nonsteroidal anti-inflammatory drugs (NSAIDs)** should be initiated 1 day prior to expected menses and continued for 2 to 3 days. If dysmenorrhea persists, a trial of **combination oral contraceptives** may be initiated. When the pain is refractory to all medical therapy, a **diagnostic laparoscopy** is warranted to evaluate for pelvic pathology, such as endometriosis, adhesions, or ovarian cysts.

Adnexal Torsion

Etiology

Adnexal torsion is the **twisting of a fallopian tube or both the fallopian tube and the ovary on its pedicle.** This may result in **vascular occlusion, ischemia, and tissue death.** Usually, a normal tube or ovary doesn't "twist" without **predisposing factors** (e.g., ovarian cysts, tumors, tubal neoplasm, parovarian cysts, or pregnancy). The risk of ovarian torsion is greatest if there is an ovarian cyst >5 cm.

Clinical Features

Abdominal pain may develop **suddenly or gradually.** It is usually **paroxysmal and intermittent.** It tends to be **unilateral** and **localized** to the involved adnexa. If ischemia occurs, the **pain worsens and becomes persistent.** Associated symptoms include **nausea, vomiting, anorexia, and a sense of fullness in the lower abdomen.**

Evaluation

The patient usually appears in **acute distress. Mild tachycardia** and a **slight elevation of temperature** may be present. The abdominal examination may reveal **tenderness in the iliac fossa.** With increasing ischemia and peritoneal irritation, **guarding, rebound tenderness, and decreased bowel sounds** may be noted. On pelvic examination, a **tender adnexal mass** may be noted.

The white blood cell count is normal or slightly elevated as a marker of an inflammatory process or stress response. Urinalysis is normal. **Pelvic ultrasonography** reveals an **adnexal mass** and Doppler flow may or may not be present, depending if twisting is intermittent.

Treatment

Evidence of an acute surgical abdomen warrants **laparoscopy** and possibly **exploratory laparotomy.** A conservative approach is paramount and every effort should be made to preserve the adnexa. Recent studies have shown that necrotic-appearing ovaries may still be viable and functional. Despite theoretical concerns, studies have not demonstrated an increase in thromboembolic events after untwisting the adnexa.

Ovarian Cysts

Etiology

During **puberty,** gonadotropin-releasing hormone (GnRH) secretion from the hypothalamus resumes and **levels of the gonadotropins** (follicle-stimulating hormone and luteinizing hormone) **rise.** The surge in gonadotropins usually is **not cyclical** in adolescents, as it is in adults. The **constant stimulus of gonadotropins on the ovaries results in multiple follicles or cysts** that may range from a few millimeters to 8 cm. Pain is caused by follicular distention, rupture, hemorrhage, ovarian torsion, or peritoneal irritation after rupture.

Clinical Features

Most follicular cysts are **asymptomatic. Large follicular cysts** may cause a **vague, constant, dull sensation or a heaviness in the pelvis. Extreme distention with rupture or torsion of the cyst and ovary** may result in **acute, severe pelvic pain.**

Evaluation

Tender, slightly enlarged ovaries may be appreciated. Rarely, a large cystic ovary is identified. A **CBC** is obtained to **rule out rupture and internal hemorrhage.** A **pregnancy test** is ordered to rule out pregnancy. **Pelvic ultrasound** may reveal ovarian cysts or fluid in the cul-de-sac.

Treatment

For **mildly symptomatic** patients, **reassurance** may be all that is necessary. The cyst should be observed using **serial ultrasounds,** typically at 3-month intervals, to monitor for resolution. Most follicular cysts resolve before the first repeat ultrasound; however, it is not uncommon to require several months for cyst resolution. **NSAIDs** may be prescribed for pain management and **oral contraceptives** to suppress new cyst formation. **Laparoscopy** is indicated in the presence of a ruptured hemorrhagic cyst accompanied by severe anemia, ovarian torsion, or a persistent cyst.

Congenital Obstructive Müllerian Malformations

Etiology

The differentiation and development of the urogenital system in the embryo and fetus is complex. Developmental errors may occur along this sequential process, resulting in distinctive structural abnormalities. Obstructive müllerian malformations include **imperforate hymen, transverse vaginal septum, and various types of uterine anomalies.**

Clinical Features

Often obstructive müllerian abnormalities are **asymptomatic** and not diagnosed **until an adolescent girl presents with primary amenorrhea and recurrent pelvic pain.** The obstruction, leading to **increasing collection of menstrual fluid,** causes **distention of the uterus and vagina** and results in **monthly cyclic pain.**

Evaluation

A **genital or rectal examination** is essential whenever a child complains of pelvic or abdominal symptoms. A **pediatric otoscope or vaginal speculum** (Huffman "virginal," pediatric regular, and pediatric narrow) may be used to visualize the vagina and cervix. The child can be examined in either the **lithotomy or knee-chest position.** An **imperforate hymen** is diagnosed by **simple inspection.** In infants and children, the hymen may be **bulging and distended by mucus.** In adolescents, menstrual blood fills the vagina. The **transverse vaginal septum** may be **complete or incomplete** and is recognized on vaginoscopy. Uterine anomalies are more difficult to detect unless an abnormally shaped uterus or pelvic mass is noted on examination.

> **HINT:** Prior to puberty, rectal examination is often the best method for evaluation of the upper genital tract.

Laboratory studies are nondiagnostic. **Abdominopelvic MRI** is the most useful in the detection of uterine anomalies. Because the embryonic differentiation and development of the urologic system occurs around the same time as that of the genital system, **errors in development of the urologic system** must be sought using **intravenous pyelography.**

Treatment

An imperforate hymen is **opened surgically. In infants,** the hymenal membrane is tented and excised centrally with scissors. **In postmenarchal patients,** a portion of the membrane should be excised. In complete transverse vaginal septum, a simple incision is made to allow the egress of secretions in premenarchal patients. The **definitive surgical treat-ment,** which involves excision of the vaginal septal membrane with a surrounding ring of dense connective tissue, should be **delayed until after puberty** because technical difficulties may be encountered if the surgery is performed on immature structures. **Anomalies of the uterus** (e.g., a blind rudimentary uterine horn) **should not be resected until the patient is postmenarchal.**

Endometriosis

Etiology

Endometriosis is the presence of **endometrial tissue outside of the uterus.** Theories of pathogenesis include retrograde menstruation, direct implantation, coelomic metaplasia, and lymphatic and hematoge-nous spread. A polygenic multifactorial mode of inheritance has also been demonstrated. The risk of endometriosis is 7 times greater if a first-degree relative is affected. The major distinction between endometriosis in adolescents and adults is its **association with con-genital anomalies of the reproductive tract in the pubertal patient.** Premenarchal patients are not affected by this disease because the **onset of menses must precede the development of endometriosis.**

Clinical Features

Characteristically, the pelvic pain is described as **cramping in the pelvic or sacral region** that is **aggravated during menstruation.** The pain may also be **intermittent, chronic, and not related to the menstrual cycle.** Other features in the adolescent may include **dyspareunia, gastrointesti-nal symptoms, and urinary complaints.**

Evaluation

Examination under anesthesia may be necessary for an adequate pelvic examination **in the virginal adolescent.** A search for **anomalies of the hymen, vagina, cervix, uterus, and adnexa is mandatory.** In **older patients,** the finding of **pain on palpation of the adnexa** (i.e., the ovary and fallopian tube), **in the cul-de-sac, or along the uterosacral ligaments** suggests the possibility of endometriosis. Occasionally, **enlargement of the ovary, fixation of the pelvic organs as a result of adhesions,** or decreased mobility of pelvic organs on bimanual exam may be noted.

Screening tests (either **endocervical or urine based) for N. gonor-rhoeae and C. trachomatis** are obtained to rule out the possibility of pelvic infection. A **pregnancy test** is obtained to rule out pregnancy.

Pelvic ultrasonography is useful when examination is difficult and indi-cated when a palpable pelvic mass is noted. **MRI** is helpful in delineating the pelvic anatomy and establishing the diagnosis of congenital müllerian anomalies. **Diagnostic laparoscopy with visualization and biopsy** of endometrial implants is essential to confirm the diagnosis.

Treatment

NSAIDs remain the first line of medical therapy for pain control; **narcotics** are reserved for severe cases. If pain persists, **combination oral contraceptives** may be prescribed in a continuous fashion to suppress ovulation and promote endometrial atrophy. Alternatively, Depo-Provera may be administered. GnRH agonists can cause osteoporosis and should not be prescribed to girls who have not reached their maximal bone density. When medical therapy fails, **laparoscopy** is indicated to **fulgurate, laser vaporize, or excise** endometrial implants and **perform lysis of adhesions.**

Pelvic Inflammatory Disease

PID is discussed in Chapter 70, "Sexually Transmitted Diseases."

Constipation

Constipation is discussed in Chapter 22, "Constipation."

EVALUATION OF PELVIC PAIN

There are various causes of acute and chronic pelvic pain (Tables 59-1 and 59-2). The most important tool for making the correct diagnosis is

TABLE 59-1 Age-related Prevalence of Principal Laparoscopic Findings in 121 Adolescent Females 11 to 17 Years Old with Acute Pelvic Pain (The Children's Hospital, Boston, 1980–1986)

Diagnosis	Number of Patients		
	Age 11–13	Age 14–15	Age 16–17
Ovarian cyst	12 (50%)	16 (35%)	19 (37%)
Acute pelvic inflammatory disease	4 (17%)	7 (16%)	10 (19%)
Adnexal torsion	0 (0%)	7 (16%)	2 (4%)
Endometriosis	0 (0%)	2 (4%)	4 (7%)
Ectopic pregnancy	0 (0%)	3 (7%)	1 (2%)
Appendicitis	3 (13%)	4 (9%)	6 (12%)
No pathology	5 (20%)	6 (13%)	10 (19%)
Total	24 (20%)	45 (37%)	52 (43%)

Reprinted from Goldstein DP: Acute and chronic pelvic pain. *Pediatr Clin North Am* 36(3):576, 1989.

TABLE 59-2 Age-Related Incidence of Laparoscopic Findings in 129 Adolescent Females 11 to 21 Years Old with Chronic Pelvic Pain (The Children's Hospital, Boston, 1980–1983)

Diagnosis	Number of Patients				
	Age 11–13	Age 14–15	Age 16–17	Age 18–19	Age 20–21
Endometriosis	2 (12%)	9 (28%)	21 (40%)	17 (45%)	7 (54%)
Postoperative adhesions	1 (6%)	4 (13%)	7 (13%)	5 (13%)	2 (15%)
Serositis	5 (29%)	4 (13%)	0 (0%)	2 (5%)	0 (0%)
Ovarian cyst	2 (12%)	2 (6%)	3 (5%)	2 (5%)	0 (8%)
Uterine malformation	1 (6%)	0 (0%)	1 (2%)	0 (0%)	1 (0%)
Others	0 (0%)	1 (3%)	2 (4%)	1 (3%)	0 (0%)
No pathology	6 (35%)	12 (37%)	19 (36%)	11 (29%)	3 (23%)

Reprinted from Goldstein DP: Acute and chronic pelvic pain. *Pediatr Clin North Am* 36(3):580, 1989.

a **detailed history**, physical examination, and laboratory and radiographic evaluation. The following information should be sought:

Patient History

- Medical, surgical, sexual, gynecologic history; including method of contraception in postmenarchal patients.
- Psychosocial history (to assess the possibility of stress, substance abuse, or sexual or physical abuse)
- Pain history (mnemonic: **OLD CAARTS**)
  - Onset: When and how did the pain start? Did it change over time?
  - Location: Localize specifically. Can you put a finger on it?
  - Duration: How long does it last?
  - Characteristics: Cramping, aching, stabbing, burning, tingling, itching?
  - Alleviating/Aggravating Factors: What makes it better (medication, stress reduction, heat/ice, position change) or worse (specific activity, stress, menstrual cycle)?
  - Associated symptoms: Gynecologic—dyspareunia, dysmenorrhea, abnormal bleeding, discharge, infertility. Gastrointestinal—constipation, diarrhea, bloating, gas, rectal bleeding. Genitourinary—frequency, dysuria, urgency, incontinence.
  - Radiation: Does it move to other areas?
  - Temporal: What time of day? Relation to menstrual cycle and activities of daily living?
  - Severity: Scale of 0 to 10

Physical Examination

The following should be sought on physical examination:

- Structural abnormalities
- The reproduction of pain on palpation of specific abdominopelvic structures
- Signs of peritonitis (guarding, rigidity, rebound tenderness)

Laboratory Studies

In the patient with a suspected acute abdomen, the following laboratory studies should be considered:

- CBC with differential
- Blood electrolytes
- Blood type and screen
- Pregnancy test (β-hCG)
- Urinalysis
- Urine culture
- Testing for *N. gonorrhoeae* and *C. trachomatis*

Radiographic Studies

- Pelvic ultrasound
- Abdominal/pelvic computed tomography scan or MRI (if indicated)

Suggested Readings

Arbel-DeRowe Y, Tepper R, Rosen DJ, et al.: The contribution of pelvic ultrasonography to the diagnostic process in pediatric and adolescent gynecology. *J Pediatr Adolesc Gynecol* 10(1):3–12, 1997.

Carrico CW, Fenton LZ, Taylor GA, et al.: Impact of sonography on the diagnosis and treatment of acute lower abdominal pain in children and young adults. *Am J Roentgenol* 172(2):513–516, 1999.

Goldstein DP: Acute and chronic pelvic pain. *Pediatr Clin North Am* 365:573–580, 1989.

Khoiny FE: Pelvic inflammatory disease in the adolescent. *J Pediatr Health Care* 3(5):230–236, 1989.

Laufer MR, Goitein L, Bush M, et al.: Prevalence of endometriosis in adolescent girls with chronic pelvic pain not responding to conventional therapy. *J Pediatr Adolesc Gynecol* 10:199–202, 1997.

Ozaksit G, Caglar T, Zorlu CG, et al.: Chronic pelvic pain in adolescent women: diagnostic laparoscopy and ultrasonography. *J Reprod Med* 40(7):500–502, 1995.

Propst AM, Laufer MR: Endometriosis in adolescents: incidence, diagnosis, and treatment. *J Reprod Med* 44:751–758, 1999.

Rapkin AJ, Howe CN: Chronic pelvic pain: a review. *Family Practice Recertification.* 28:59–67, 2006.

Reese KA, Reddy S, Rock JA: Endometriosis in an adolescent population: the Emory experience. *J Pediatr Adolesc Gynecol* 9(3):125–128, 1996.

Sanfilippo JS: Dysmenorrhea in adolescents. *Female Patient* 18:29–33, 1993.

Seeber BE, Barnhart KT: Suspected ectopic pregnancy. *Obstet Gynecol* 107(2):399–413, 2006.

Vercellini P, Fedele L, Arcaini L, et al.: Laparoscopy in the diagnosis of chronic pelvic pain in adolescent women. *J Reprod Med* 34(10): 827–830, 1989.

chapter 60

Pleural Effusions
Amy H. Schultz

INTRODUCTION

A pleural effusion is an **accumulation of fluid between the parietal and visceral pleura.** Normally, fluid is produced by the capillaries of the parietal pleura and absorbed by the capillaries of the visceral pleura; only a trivial amount of fluid is left within the pleural space. The Starling relationship governs the net flow of fluid at each capillary bed:

$$F = k[(Pcap - Ppl) - \sigma(\Pi cap - \Pi pl)]$$

Where:

  F = the rate of fluid movement
  P = the hydrostatic pressure
  Π = the oncotic pressure
  k = the filtration coefficient
  σ = the osmotic reflection coefficient for protein

A larger difference between capillary and pleural hydrostatic pressure, or a smaller difference between capillary and pleural oncotic pressure, results in a larger amount of fluid left in the pleural space. Lymphatic drainage normally removes excess fluid from the pleural space. Accumulation of a pleural effusion may result from **increased capillary hydrostatic pressure, decreased hydrostatic pressure in the pleural space, decreased capillary oncotic pressure, capillary leak, lymphatic obstruction, movement of fluid from the peritoneal space,** or a combination of these factors.

Pleural effusions are classified according to their etiology as **transudative or exudative.** Pleural fluid analysis can often distinguish a transudate from an exudate and serves as the first step in the differential diagnosis.

- **Transudative effusions** are usually secondary to increased hydrostatic pressure or decreased oncotic pressure. The differential diagnosis is relatively straightforward.
- **Exudative effusions** are typically seen in diseases that injure the capillary membrane, result in increased capillary permeability, or impair lymphatic drainage. A broad differential diagnosis is implied by an exudative effusion and may require more extensive workup.

DIFFERENTIAL DIAGNOSIS LIST

Transudative Effusion

Cardiac
Congestive heart failure
Increased pulmonary arterial pressure (left-to-right shunt)
Pulmonary or systemic venous hypertension
Superior vena caval obstruction
Constrictive pericarditis

Pulmonary
Acute atelectasis

Hepatic
Cirrhosis with ascites
Hypoalbuminemia

Renal
Peritoneal dialysis
Nephrotic syndrome
Urinothorax

Iatrogenic
Extravasation from subclavian or jugular central venous lines

Exudative Effusions

Infectious
Bacterial infection—parapneumonic effusion/empyema, upper abdominal abscess
Viral infection (e.g., adenovirus)
Mycoplasma infection
Mycobacterial infection—*Mycobacterium tuberculosis*, atypical *Mycobacterium*
Legionella infection
AIDS-related infection
Fungal infection (e.g., *Aspergillus, Coccidioides,*
Histoplasma, Cryptococcus; latter seen most often in immunocompromised patients)
Parasitic *Echinococcus granulosus, Pneumocystic carinii* infection (e.g., *Paragonimus westermani, Entamoeba histolytica*)

Neoplastic
Hematologic neoplasm—acute lymphoblastic leukemia, lymphoma, malignant histiocytosis
Cervical teratoma
Pleural mesothelioma
Pheochromocytoma
Wilms tumor
Metastatic sarcoma—Ewing sarcoma, rhabdomyosarcoma, clear cell sarcoma
Squamous cell carcinoma
Bronchogenic carcinoma

Gastrointestinal Disease
Esophageal rupture
Subdiaphragmatic abscess
Pancreatic pseudocyst
Acute pancreatitis
Intrahepatic abscess

Pulmonary Disease
Pulmonary embolism and infarction (e.g., sickle cell disease)
Trapped lung
Acute respiratory distress syndrome
Chronic atelectasis
Hemothorax

Collagen Vascular Disease
Rheumatologic—Rheumatoid arthritis,

lupus pleuritis, sarcoidosis,
    Wegener granulomatosis
Sjögren syndrome
Lymphatic
    Chylothorax—postsurgical,
        traumatic
    Obstruction of lymphatic
        drainage caused by
        malignancy
    Congenital lymphangiectasis
    Noonan syndrome
    Lymphedema

Iatrogenic
    Radiation therapy
    Surgery (e.g., post lung
        transplantation)
    Esophageal sclerotherapy
    Feeding tube placement into
        mediastinal pleural space
    Extravasation from subcla
        vian or jugular central
        venous lines

DIFFERENTIAL DIAGNOSIS DISCUSSION

If the etiology of the effusion is unclear, the distinction should be made between a transudate and an exudate by thoracentesis and pleural fluid analysis.

Transudative Effusions

Transudative effusions usually resolve with treatment of the underlying disease process.

Exudative Effusions: Infectious Causes

Parapneumonic Effusions

A parapneumonic effusion is any effusion that occurs in the presence of pneumonia, lung abscess, or bronchiectasis. Between 50% and 70% of pleural effusions in hospitalized children are parapneumonic.

Bacterial Infections

The most common bacterial causes of parapneumonic pleural effusions and empyema (gross pus in the pleural space) are *Streptococcus pneumoniae*, *Staphylococcus aureus*, and *Streptococcus pyogenes*. *Haemophilus influenza* type B was a major cause of infection in the preimmunization era. Oral anaerobes can be causal in neurologically impaired children. Gram-negative rods are seen in neonates and chronically ventilated children.

A minority of bacterial parapneumonic effusions progress to empyema, leading to deposition of fibrin in the pleural space and loculation of the effusion. Loculation of the effusion makes clearance of infection difficult and ultimately results in the development of a fibroblast "peel" on the visceral and parietal pleural surfaces. Parapneumonic effusions are classified as uncomplicated, those that will resolve with systemic antibiotic therapy alone, and complicated, those that require

TABLE 60-1 Causes of Pleural Effusions in Hospitalized Children

Cause	Alkrinawi and Chernick[*] n = 127 Number (%)	Hardie et al.[†] n = 210 Number (%)
Parapneumonic	64 (51%)	143 (68%)
Congenital heart disease	22 (17%)	23 (11%)
Malignancy	13 (10%)	10 (5%)
Renal	11 (9%)	
Liver failure		7 (3%)
Trauma	9 (7%)	
Sickle cell disease		7 (3%)
Ruptured appendix		6 (3%)
Miscellaneous	8 (6%)	14 (7%)

[*]Alkrinawi S, Chernick V: Pleural fluid in hospitalized pediatric patients. *Clin Pediatr* 35:5–9, 1993.
[†]Hardie W, BoKulic R, Garcia VF, et al.: Pneumococcal pleural empyemas in children. *Clin Infect Dis* 22:1057–1063, 1996.

drainage for resolution. Pleural fluid analysis can be helpful in predicting which parapneumonic effusions are likely to be complicated.

Viral Infections

Pleural effusions occur in 10% to 15% of patients with viral lower respiratory tract infections. **Adenoviral infection** is the most common cause of virus-related effusions. Effusions rarely occur with influenza, cytomegalovirus, herpes simplex virus, Epstein-Barr virus, or hepatitis virus infections. An effusion usually **resolves spontaneously** within a few weeks.

Other Causes

Table 60-1 lists the frequency of various causes of a pleural effusion in two hospital-based series.

APPROACH TO THE PATIENT WITH PLEURAL EFFUSION

Physical Examination

The clinical findings in a patient with a pleural effusion vary, depending on the size and cause of the effusion. With **small effusions,** patients may be **asymptomatic** or have a **cough, chest pain, fever,** or a combination of the three. Patients with moderate effusions may develop **shallow, rapid respirations** as the lung becomes compressed. With **large effusions, cyanosis** may be seen as intrapulmonary shunting occurs.

Examination of the chest reveals **decreased breath sounds** and **dullness to percussion** on the affected side. If the lung is compressed by the effusion, **egophony** ("E to A" changes) may also be noted.

Diagnostic Modalities

In chest radiographs, pleural fluid is best seen on an **upright posteroanterior and lateral film or a decubitus film.** A supine film may show only a hazy lung field. With **small effusions,** only **blunting of the costophrenic angle** may be seen. A **subpleural effusion** may simulate an **elevated hemidiaphragm.** As **fluid accumulates** the hemithorax begins to opacify. Pleural fluid **layers out** on a lateral decubitus film, allowing as little as 50 mL to be seen. If the opacity does not layer out, a loculated effusion, empyema, or lobar consolidation should be considered. An **ultrasound or computed tomography (CT) scan** may be useful in distinguishing consolidation from effusion and identifying loculations within the fluid.

Laboratory Studies

Thoracentesis and Pleural Fluid Analysis

Thoracentesis can be performed when there is **>10 mm of fluid layered on a lateral decubitus radiograph.** Thoracentesis should be performed if the cause of the effusion is unclear, to determine the need for drainage in a parapneumonic effusion, or if the pleural effusion is causing respiratory distress. If the **effusion is small or loculated, ultrasound or CT-guided thoracentesis** may be necessary.

Classification of Transudates Versus Exudates

Pleural fluid should be sent for analysis of **pH, lactate dehydrogenase (LDH), and total protein** with concurrent determination of **serum LDH and total protein.** The **Light criteria define an effusion as an exudate** if it fulfills **at least one of the following criteria.** In adult studies, this definition is 98% sensitive and 83% specific for an exudate.

- Pleural fluid-to-serum protein ratio >0.5
- Pleural fluid LDH >200 IU/L
- Pleural fluid-to-serum LDH ratio >0.6

Table 60-2 lists other studies that may be helpful in the differential diagnosis of an exudate.

Unexplained exudates require further workup beyond the scope of this chapter.

TREATMENT OF PLEURAL EFFUSION

In all cases, the underlying disease-stimulating effusion formation should be treated. The patient's respiratory status should be monitored closely. If the effusion significantly compromises the patient's respiratory status, **therapeutic thoracentesis or chest tube placement** is indicated.

TABLE 60-2 Other Pleural Fluid Studies That May Be Helpful in the Differential Diagnosis of an Exudate

Test	Comments
White blood cell count and differential	Lymphocyte predominance in neoplastic processes, tuberculosis, chylothorax, or certain fungal infections
	Segmented neutrophil predominance in bacterial infections, connective tissue disease, pancreatitis, or pulmonary infarction
	Eosinophil count may be elevated in patients with bacterial infections, a neoplastic process, or a connective tissue disease
Red blood cell (RBC) count	RBC count $>100,000/mm^3$: consider trauma, neoplasia, or pulmonary infarction
Microbiologic studies	Consider the clinical context
■ Gram stain and fluid culture for aerobes and anaerobes ■ Acid-fast bacillus smear and culture ■ Viral culture ■ Fungal culture	
Cytology	May reveal malignant cells
Rheumatoid factor, lupus erythematosus preparation, and antinuclear antibody levels	Useful if a collagen vascular disorder is suspected
Amylase	Elevated in pancreatitis or esophageal rupture
Triglycerides	>110 mg/dL in chylothorax
Cholesterol	May be markedly elevated in certain inflammatory conditions, especially tuberculosis and rheumatoid arthritis

Rarely, **pleurodesis with a sclerotic agent** (e.g., tetracycline) is used to fibrose the two pleural linings to prevent fluid reaccumulation.

The management of parapneumonic effusions has attracted much attention because of the risk of empyema, and variations in the management approach exist.

- **An uncomplicated parapneumonic effusion** is defined as one that will resolve with systemic antibiotic therapy alone.
- **A complicated parapneumonic effusion** requires chest tube or surgical drainage for resolution.

Chest radiographs including lateral decubitus views should be obtained. A chest ultrasound should be obtained to evaluate for loculation. **Diagnostic thoracentesis** in patients with an effusion ≥ 10 mm deep on a lateral decubitus film may be helpful. A pleural fluid **pH <7.0, glucose <40 mg/dL or LDH $>1,000$ UI/L predicts a complicated effusion** and is an **indication for tube drainage**. In addition, a **positive Gram** stain or culture or the presence of pus is an indication for tube drainage. Of note, British Thoracic Society guidelines do not rely on biochemical parameters but recommend tube drainage of any significant pleural effusion associated with infection. **Intrapleural fibrinolytic therapy** is useful in patients with loculated pleural effusions. **Video-assisted thoracoscopic debridement (VATS) or open drainage** is used for patients with loculated effusions or for those who do not respond to tube drainage. Some authors advocate earlier, more universal use of VATS in complicated parapneumonic effusion, but this approach remains controversial. **Surgical decortication** has been used in the organized stage of empyema.

Suggested Readings

Jahani IA, Fakhoury K: Management and prognosis of parapneumonic effusion and empyema in children. UpToDate [serial online], accessed November 28, 2007.

Montgomery M, Sigalet D: Air and liquid in the pleural space. In *Kendig's Disorders of the Respiratory Tract in Children*, 7th ed. Edited by Chernick V, Boat TF. Philadelphia, WB Saunders, 2006, 368–387.

Precocious Puberty

Marta Satin Smith
Paul S. Thornton (Third Edition)

INTRODUCTION

Normal Pubertal Development

Girls

In girls, **puberty** usually begins at 10.5 to 11 years with a range of **9 to 11 years.** Breast development (thelarche) is usually the **first sign** of normal sexual development; however, in a small number of girls, pubic hair development may precede breast development by 6 months. **Pubic hair development (adrenarche)** usually **follows thelarche** by 6 months and **axillary hair** 12 to 18 months later. The **growth spurt occurs early** in pubertal development in girls at a mean age of 11.5 years (between Tanner stages 2 to 3; see Chapter 2, "The Physical Examination," Table 2-6. **Menses (menarche)** begin 18 to 24 months after thelarche and become ovulatory in most girls within 18 months. Puberty is completed within 1.5 to 6 years. Pubertal growth in girls contributes 25 cm to overall height.

Breast development and cornification of the vaginal mucosa are controlled primarily by **ovarian estrogens,** which are influenced by follicle-stimulating hormone (FSH). Pubic and axillary hair growth is stimulated primarily by **adrenal androgens,** although there may also be an ovarian contribution.

Boys

In boys, puberty usually begins at age 11.5 to 12 years with a range of **10 to 14 years.** **Testicular enlargement** occurs first, followed by the **development of pubic hair** approximately 6 months later. **Phallic enlargement** usually begins 12 months after testicular size begins to increase. The pubertal **growth spurt** in boys occurs between Tanner stages 3 and 4, with progression of male pubertal development occurring over 2 to 4.5 years (see Chapter 2, "The Physical Examination," Table 2-5). The average growth during puberty is 28 cm. Onset of **spermatogenesis** occurs early in puberty with the mean age of conscious ejaculation of 13.5 years (range 12.5 to 15.5 years).

The virilizing changes seen at puberty are mainly the result of **testosterone secretion** from the testes. Growth of the penis and pubic hair are stimulated primarily by **testicular androgens;** however, **adrenal androgens** also contribute. Luteinizing hormone (LH) stimulates Leydig cell production of testosterone, whereas FSH supports spermatogenesis. It is now clear that peripheral **conversion of testosterone to estrogen** is important in bone growth and maturation in males.

Precocious Puberty

Precocious puberty is defined as the development of secondary sexual characteristics <6 years of age in African American girls and <7 years in white American girls, and <9 years of age in boys regardless of race. These age limits in girls are based on a large study completed in 1997 within the Pediatric Research in the Office Setting network. This recommendation has been somewhat controversial because Tanner staging of breast development was done visually and not by palpation. With increasing obesity in the pediatric population, it has been argued that their data may have been skewed because of the inability to distinguish fat from true breast tissue by inspection only. Many experts still recommend evaluation, including magnetic resonance imaging (MRI) of the head, in girls with premature onset of puberty >6 years of age if the tempo of pubertal progression is unusually rapid; bone age is >2 years advanced; predicted height is <150 cm, or if neurologic signs or symptoms are detected. Precocious puberty is classified as either **central (gonadotropin-dependent)** precocious puberty (CPP), which is caused by an elevation of FSH and LH, or **peripheral (gonadotropin-independent)** precocious puberty (PPP), which is caused by an elevation of sex steroids.

DIFFERENTIAL DIAGNOSIS LIST

Central (Gonadotropin-Dependent) Precocious Puberty (CPP)

Infectious Causes
Brain abscess
Meningitis—viral or bacterial
Encephalitis
Granulomatous disease
Tuberculosis, sarcoidosis, or histiocytosis
Toxic Causes
Chronic exogenous androgen or estrogen exposure (initially presenting as peripheral precocious puberty)
Brain Tumor
Glioma
Astrocytoma
Ependymoma
Hypothalamic hamartoma

Brain Injury
Head trauma
Brain surgery
Cranial irradiation
Hemorrhage and stroke
Congenital Causes
Central nervous system (CNS) malformation
Suprasellar cyst
Hydrocephalus
Idiopathic precocious puberty
Constitutional precocious puberty

Peripheral (Gonadotropin-Independent) Precocious Puberty (PPP)

Toxic Causes
Exogenous estrogens—face creams, breast-enlarging

creams, contraceptive pill, and vaginal creams
Excess ingestion of phyto-estrogens in soy products
Exogenous androgens—transdermal testosterone gel, anabolic steroid abuse
Neoplastic causes
Boys
Human chorionic gonadotropin (hCG)-secreting tumors—brain, liver choriocarcinomas
Leydig cell tumor
Virilizing adrenal tumor
Girls
Ovarian tumors
Adrenal tumors
Congenital Causes
Congenital adrenal hyperplasia (CAH)
Familial gonadotropin-independent Leydig cell maturation—testitoxicosis
McCune-Albright syndrome
Ovarian follicular cysts

DIFFERENTIAL DIAGNOSIS DISCUSSION

Central (Gonadotropin-Dependent) Precocious Puberty

Etiology

CPP, or true precocious puberty, refers to sexual precocity **secondary to elevations in the gonadotropins (FSH and LH).** CPP arises from early activation of the hypothalamic-pituitary-gonadal axis. CPP is investigated five times more often in girls than in boys.

In most cases of CPP, especially in girls, **no cause is identified** (idiopathic precocious puberty). The younger the onset, the more likely an etiological factor will be found. Other cases involve various forms of **CNS pathology,** including malformations and benign or malignant tumors. **Hamartomas of the tuber cinereum** are the CNS tumors most frequently identified as causing precocious puberty. These tumors contain ectopic gonadotropin-releasing hormone (GnRH) neurosecretory cells. The pulsatile release of GnRH from these cells stimulates the pituitary gland. These hamartomas may be associated with gelastic (involving emotional features) seizures. CPP has also developed after **cranial irradiation therapy** for CNS tumors and after **head trauma.** Children with malformations of the CNS, such as septo-optic dysplasia and hydrocephalus, also have an increased incidence of precocious puberty.

Clinical Features

As with children progressing through normal puberty, the first physiologic change is an increase in the amplitude and frequency of hypothalamic GnRH pulses. This causes **increased FSH and LH secretion** from the pituitary gland, **maturation of the gonads,** and **increased release of sex steroids.**

TABLE 61-1 Normal Ranges for Gonadotropin and Sex Steroid Levels: Females

	LH (mIU/mL)	FSH (mIU/mL)	Estradiol (ng/dL)	Testosterone (ng/dL)
0–1 yr	0.02–7.0	0.24–14.2	0.5–5.0	<10
Prepubertal	0.02–0.3	1.0–4.2	<1.5	<3–10
Tanner 2	0.02–4.7	1.0–10.8	1.0–2.4	7.0–28
Tanner 3	0.10–12.0	1.5–12.8	0.7–6.0	15–35
Tanner 4	0.4–11.7	1.5–11.7	2.1–8.5	13–32
Tanner 5	0.4–11.7	1.0–9.2	3.4–17.0	20–38
Adult	—	—	—	10–55
Follicular phase	2.0–9.0	1.8–11.2	3.0–10.0	—
Midcycle	18.0–49	6.0–35.0	—	—
Luteal phase	2.0–11.0	1.8–11.2	7.0–30.0	...

FSH = follicle-stimulating hormone; *LH* = leuteinizing hormone.

Evaluation

Boys have pubertal FSH and LH levels, a pubertal response to GnRH, and a pubertal value of **testosterone. Girls** have pubertal FSH and LH levels, a pubertal response to GnRH, and a pubertal value of **estradiol** (Tables 61-1 and 61-2). The diagnosis of **CPP in boys is almost always serious** and necessitates a search for a **CNS tumor.** Unfortunately, GnRH, which was considered the gold standard stimulation test for diagnosis of CPP, is no longer available. Alternative methods of diagnosis include stimulation tests using nafarelin or leuprolide, ultrasound evidence of ovarian and uterine enlargement, and ultrasensitive assays for LH and estradiol.

Treatment

CNS tumors associated with CPP are rarely completely resectable because of their proximity to vital structures. Therefore, a **joint medical and surgical approach** is required. Usually a **biopsy** is performed and treatment is determined based on the results.

TABLE 61-2 Normal Ranges for Gonadotropin and Sex Steroid Levels: Males

	LH (mIU/ml)	FSH (mIU/ml)	Estradiol (ng/dl)	Testosterone (ng/dl)
0–1 yr	0.02–7.0	0.16–4.1	1.0–3.2	<10
Prepubertal	0.02–0.3	0.26–3.0	<1.5	<3–10
Tanner 2	0.2–4.9	1.8–3.2	0.5–1.6	18–150
Tanner 3	0.2–5.0	1.2–5.8	0.5–2.5	100–320
Tanner 4	0.4–7.0	2.0–9.2	1.0–3.6	200–620
Tanner 5	0.4–7.0	2.6–11.0	1.0–3.6	350–970
Adult	1.5–9.0	2.0–9.2	0.8–3.5	350–1030

FSH = follicle-stimulating hormone; *LH* = leuteinizing hormone.

Hamartomas of the tuber cinereum are benign tumors of the hypothalamus that are usually asymptomatic, except for causing precocious puberty and gelastic seizures. Surgical treatment is not indicated for these hamartomas; treatment is directed at **medically halting the puberty.**

The treatment of choice for CPP is a **synthetic GnRH agonist,** which, when administered chronically, suppresses gonadotropin secretion and gonadal steroid output. Several different forms of GnRH analogs are available, including long-acting forms that can be administered monthly. In 2007, a subdermal implant containing histrelin was approved for treatment of CPP after a multicenter study. The implant needs to be replaced annually and is as effective as the monthly injections of GnRH analogs.

Peripheral (Gonadotropin-Independent) Precocious Puberty

Etiology

The secondary sexual development in PPP results from circulating sex steroids that originate independently of gonadotropin stimulation. Possible sources of sex steroids are the following:

- The **gonads** (e.g., ovarian cysts, ovarian tumors, and testicular tumors)
- The **adrenal glands** (e.g., CAH, adrenal tumors)
- **Exogenous administration** in the form of estrogen creams, birth control pills, or anabolic steroids

Isosexual precocity occurs when the hormonal changes are consistent with gender (e.g., excess estrogens in a female), and **heterosexual precocity** occurs when the hormonal changes are of the opposite gender (e.g., adrenal carcinoma-producing androgens in a female).

PPP may develop in boys via **autonomous secretion of sex steroids** or as a result of **hCG secretion,** which stimulates testosterone secretion from the Leydig cells. **Autonomous androgen secretion** can result from adrenal 21-hydroxylase deficiency or 11-β-hydroxylase deficiency, adrenal carcinomas, interstitial cell tumors of the testes, or premature Leydig cell maturation. **Tumors that secrete hCG** include hepatomas; hepatoblastomas; teratomas; chorioepitheliomas of the gonads, mediastinum, retroperitoneum, or pineal gland; and germinomas of the pineal gland.

PPP can develop in girls from **ovarian or adrenal estrogen secretion** or from **exogenous estrogen.** Follicular ovarian cysts, granulosa cell tumors, gonadoblastomas, lipoid tumors, and ovarian carcinomas can all secrete estrogen.

Of note, certain forms of PPP, such as poorly controlled CAH, can eventually activate the hypothalamic-pituitary-gonadal axis and therefore initiate true precocious puberty via central mechanisms.

Clinical Features

The hypothalamic-pituitary-gonadal axis has not been activated and therefore the sexual characteristics that are manifested are limited to those stimulated by the elevated sex steroid level (e.g., breast development following estrogen production). Adrenal tumors can produce excessive androgens or estrogens, resulting in **virilization** or **feminization.** Ovarian abnormalities can also produce both androgens and estrogens. The classical features of PPP in boys are **development of the penis without testicular enlargement.**

Evaluation

If sex steroid levels are elevated but gonadotropin levels are decreased, the diagnosis is likely PPP. LH cross-reacts with hCG on some radioimmunoassays; therefore, **measurement of hCG** along with **LH, FSH, and testosterone** should be done to rule out an hCG-secreting tumor in boys. An **ultrasound evaluation** of the pelvis should be performed if ovarian pathology is suspected.

Treatment

Treatment of PPP is dictated by the cause. In the case of steroid-producing tumors, **surgery, chemotherapy,** or both may be indicated. PPP has been treated with **ketoconazole** (steroidogenesis inhibitor), **tamoxifen,** and a combination of **spironolactone** (androgen receptor inhibitor) **and testolactone and anastrozole** (aromatase inhibitors).

Premature Adrenarche

Etiology

Premature adrenarche, the **isolated appearance of sexual hair** <6 or 7 years of age in girls or 9 years of age in boys, is the most common cause of premature pubic hair development. Premature adrenarche, which is more common in girls, is a **benign condition** that appears to be secondary to premature increased secretion of adrenal androgens or increased end-organ sensitivity, or both.

Clinical Features

Affected children may have only pubic hair, or they may also have **axillary hair, acne, perspiration,** and **body odor.** There is no premature growth spurt. Girls do not have associated clitoromegaly. **Repeat observation** is the most important evaluation and diagnostic tool.

Evaluation

The need for laboratory studies is dictated by the **degree of concern** raised by the results of complete and repeated examinations and by the **bone age.** Premature adrenarche is usually slowly progressive.

Dehydroepiandrosterone sulfate levels are modestly elevated in patients with premature adrenarche. Plasma levels of gonadotropin and gonadal steroids are normal. Measurements of 17-α-hydroxyprogesterone, androstenedione, and testosterone are indicated to differentiate premature adrenarche from true precocious puberty (in boys) and from adrenal tumors or adrenal hyperplasia (in boys and girls). The bone age is often mildly advanced but not significantly advanced. Beware the patient with **rapidly progressive pubic hair development and normal bone age.** This may suggest an aggressive androgen-producing tumor.

Treatment
Because there are no long-term sequelae other than progression into central puberty, **observation** is the only necessary treatment.

Premature Thelarche
Etiology
Premature thelarche refers to **isolated breast development,** which usually appears in the first 3 years of life. It is felt to be secondary to episodic formation of ovarian cysts or increased sensitivity of the breasts to estradiol.

Clinical Features
Affected children have **unilateral or bilateral** premature breast development. There are **no other signs of estrogen effect** or precocious puberty (e.g., vaginal cornification, pubic hair, or growth spurt).

Evaluation
As with premature adrenarche, **regular examinations** for several months should precede any laboratory or radiologic evaluations. **Plasma levels of FSH, LH, and estradiol** should be obtained if significant progression or signs of other estrogen effects develop with repeat observations. Gonadotropin levels, estradiol levels, and bone age are usually normal. **Continued observation** is necessary because this may be the first sign of CPP or PPP.

Treatment
Because there are no long-term sequelae, **observation** is the only necessary treatment.

EVALUATION OF PRECOCIOUS PUBERTY

Patient History
The following information should be sought:

- History of accelerated growth
- Behavioral changes

- CNS infections or trauma
- Use of steroid medications
- Family history of precocious puberty

> **HINT:** Ask specifically about the presence of estrogen- or testosterone-containing preparations in the house.

Physical Examination

- Breast, genital, and sexual hair development should be carefully assessed and Tanner staged.
- Special measuring devices such as testicular volume beads (Prader orchidometer) may be useful.
- Skin should be examined for acne, oiliness, and hirsutism (signs of androgen secretion), and café-au-lait spots (McCune-Albright syndrome).
- Funduscopic and neurologic evaluations should be performed to investigate the possibility of intracranial lesions.

Laboratory Studies

Initial laboratory and radiologic evaluations should be guided by the history and physical examination findings. In general, **blood work** should include determination of LH, FSH, estradiol, testosterone, and adrenal steroid levels. If these initial studies are abnormal or equivocal, **provocative testing with synthetic GnRH or leuprolide** may be indicated. Normal pubertal children and children with true precocious puberty have a mature LH response to exogenous GnRH administration. Normal ranges for gonadotropin and sex steroid levels are presented in Table 61-1 (girls) and Table 61-2 (boys). β-HCG should be measured in boys with signs of puberty. Thyroid function tests should also be drawn because hypothyroidism can be associated with central precocious puberty.

Imaging Studies

The **bone age** should be determined. If indicated, **ultrasound of the ovaries and adrenal glands** should be performed. The need for additional studies, such as an **MRI scan** of the head to investigate the cranial cavity and pituitary fossa, is dictated by the results of these initial studies.

> **HINT:** Small cysts on the ovaries are not uncommon in girls who have no clinical evidence of puberty.

APPROACH TO THE PATIENT

Treatment options for precocious puberty are dictated by the cause. However, while the inciting cause of the precocious pubertal development is being sought and treated, the physician must also focus on the **long-term consequences of the physical changes** that are occurring. **Short stature** is the most obvious result of early pubertal development. The advanced skeletal maturity associated with some forms of precocious puberty results in a child who initially is taller and stronger than his or her peers but who, ultimately, if the disorder is untreated, loses years of growth potential as a result of fusion of the epiphyseal growth plates.

Suggested Readings

Cesario SK, Hughes LA: Precocious puberty: a comprehensive review of literature. *J Obstet Gynecol Neonatal Nurs* 36(3):263–274, 2007.

Eugster EA, Clark W, Kletter GB, et al.: Efficacy and safety of histrelin subdermal implant in children with central precocious puberty: a multicenter trial. *J Clin Endocrinol Metab* 92(5):1697–1704, 2007.

Haddad N, Eugster E: An update on the treatment of precocious puberty in McCune-Albright syndrome and testotoxicosis. *J Pediatr Endocrinol Metab* 20(6):653–661, 2007.

Kaplowitz P: Precocious puberty: update on secular trends, definitions, diagnosis, and treatment. *Adv Pediatr* 51:37–62, 2004.

Muir A: Precocious puberty. *Pediatr Rev* 27(10):373–381, 2006.

Nathan BM, Palmert MR: Regulation and disorders of pubertal timing. *Endocrinol Metab Clin North Am* 34 617–664, 2005.

Tato L, Savage MO, Antoniazzi F, et al.; International Workshop on Management of Puberty for Optimum Auxological Results: optimal therapy of pubertal disorders in precocious/early puberty. *J Pediatr Endocrinol Metab* 14(Suppl 2):985–995, 2001.

INTRODUCTION

Proteinuria, the presence of excessive protein in the urine, is a **common finding in school-age children.** As many as 10% of children test positive for proteinuria (**≥1+ on urine dipstick**) at some time (Table 62-1). The prevalence of proteinuria increases with age and **peaks during adolescence.** Although most proteinuria is transient or intermittent, it is the most **common laboratory finding indicative of renal disease.** The challenge is to differentiate proteinuria caused by renal disease from that associated with benign conditions. Normal urinary protein excretion in adults is <150 mg/day, whereas in children it is <4 mg/m² per hour (Table 62-2).

DETECTION OF PROTEINURIA

Qualitative

The **dipstick measures the concentration of protein in urine.** It is impregnated with tetrabromophenol blue, which changes color in the presence of albumin when the pH is in the normal range. A urine sample is considered positive for protein if it measures ≥1+ when the specific gravity of urine is <1.015, or ≥2+ when the specific gravity is >1.015. A child is said to have persistent proteinuria if the dipstick is **positive for protein** on **two of three random urine samples** collected at least a week apart.

Although not as convenient as dipstick analysis, a reagent called **sulfosalicylic acid detects all forms of proteinuria.** False-positive results by this method may result from radiographic contrast material, penicillins, cephalosporins, sulfonamides, and high uric acid concentrations.

> **HINT:** The following can cause false-positive results on dipstick analysis: alkaline urine (pH >7.0), prolonged immersion, placing the strip directly in the urine stream, cleansing of the urethral orifice with quaternary ammonium compounds prior to collecting the sample, pyuria, and bacteriuria. False-negative results can occur when the urine is too dilute (i.e., the specific gravity is <1.005) or when the patient excretes abnormal amounts of proteins other than albumin.

TABLE 62-1 Qualitative Evaluation of Proteinuria by Dipstick

Grade	Protein Concentration (mg/dL)
Trace	10–20
1+	30
2+	100
3+	300
4+	1000–2000

Quantitative

A timed urine collection for protein quantitation is essential to establish the degree of proteinuria. A **24-hour urine collection** can be done by asking the child to void as soon as he wakes up and discarding the specimen; then every void should be collected for the next 24 hours including the first void the next morning. In clinical practice, it is difficult to obtain timed urine collections in children. A **random urine specimen** can be analyzed for protein and creatinine concentration, and the ratio of the urine protein (in milligrams) to urine creatinine (in milligrams) can be used as a measure of 24-hour urine protein. The normal ratio of urine protein to urine creatinine in children >2 years is 0.2 and in children < years is 0.5. Multiplying the random protein-to-creatinine ratio by 0.63 gives an actual 24-hour total protein content in g/m^2 per day.

Microalbuminuria

It is recommended that children with diabetes of more than 5 years' duration have their urine checked for microalbuminuria to monitor them for signs of chronic kidney disease. First-morning collections are optimal to avoid a confounding effect of postural proteinuria. A value of <30 mg albumin per gram creatinine is normal. A level between 30 and 300 mg/g creatinine is consistent with microalbuminuria and a level >300 mg/g indicates clinical proteinuria. Both microalbuminuria and clinical proteinuria necessitate further evaluation by a nephrologist because they signal early diabetic nephropathy.

TABLE 62-2 Quantitative Evaluation of Proteinuria by Timed 24-Hour Urine Collection

Normal	<4 mg/m²/hr
Abnormal	4–40 mg/m²/hr
Nephrotic range	>40 mg/m²/hr

DIFFERENTIAL DIAGNOSIS LIST

Transient Proteinuria
Fever
Dehydration
Exercise
Cold exposure
Congestive heart failure
Seizures
Emotional stress
Epinephrine administration

Isolated Proteinuria
Orthostatic proteinuria
Persistent asymptomatic
  isolated proteinuria (PAIP)

Glomerular Disease
Minimal change nephrotic
  syndrome (MCNS)
Focal segmental
  glomerulosclerosis (FSGS)
Postinfectious
  glomerulonephritis
Membranoproliferative
  glomerulonephritis
Membranous nephropathy

Immunoglobulin A
  nephropathy
Henoch-Schönlein purpura
Hemolytic uremic syndrome
Hereditary nephritis
Systemic lupus erythematosus
  (SLE)
Diabetes mellitus
Sickle cell disease
HIV-associated nephropathy

Tubulointerstitial Disease
Reflux nephropathy
Pyelonephritis
Interstitial nephritis
Fanconi syndrome—cystinosis,
  tyrosinemia, Lowe syndrome
Toxins—drugs
  (aminoglycosides, penicillins,
  heavy metals)
Ischemic tubular injury
Renal hypoplasia or dysplasia
Polycystic kidney disease

DIFFERENTIAL DIAGNOSIS DISCUSSION

Transient Proteinuria

Transient proteinuria is **unrelated to renal disease** and resolves when the inciting factor disappears. It is rarely >2+ on the dipstick. **Febrile proteinuria** usually appears with the onset of fever and resolves by 10 to 14 days. Proteinuria that occurs **after exercise** usually abates 48 hours after cessation of exercise. Transient proteinuria seen with fever, exercise, and congestive heart failure is caused by hemodynamic alterations in glomerular blood flow.

Orthostatic Proteinuria

Etiology and Incidence

Orthostatic proteinuria is abnormal protein excretion that **occurs only when the patient is in an upright position.** Although the exact mechanism is unclear, orthostatic proteinuria is most likely the result of excessive glomerular filtration of protein. Orthostatic proteinuria is the most common form, accounting for **60% of all proteinuria in children**. The prevalence is even higher among **teenagers**, especially **girls**. Orthostatic proteinuria is an incidental finding, and there are no specific clinical features.

Evaluation

The diagnosis of orthostatic proteinuria can be made if urinary protein excretion is abnormal in samples obtained while the patient is upright but normal in samples obtained when the patient is recumbent. Total protein excretion should be <1 g/day. In some patients, orthostatic proteinuria is reproducible; in others, it is intermittent. There are three approaches to evaluating orthostatic proteinuria:

■ **Dipstick analysis of first-morning (recumbent) and daytime (upright) random urine samples.** Negative or trace protein in the first-morning sample with a ≥1+ protein in the daytime urine sample is suggestive of orthostatic proteinuria.
■ **Quantitative evaluation of proteinuria in a split collection.** Urine samples may be collected at timed intervals while recumbent as well as while ambulating, and evaluated quantitatively for protein excretion (see Table 62-2). The timed urine samples should be collected by asking the child to void and discard the urine just prior to going to bed. Collect the void into a container marked "recumbent" immediately on arising. Then collect all the urine during the day including the specimen voided just prior to going to bed in a separate container labeled "ambulatory." In orthostatic proteinuria, the amount of protein in the ambulatory collection should be 2 to 4 times that of the recumbent collection.
■ **Calculation of the urine protein-to-urine creatinine ratio.** The urine protein-to-urine creatinine ratio is calculated on first-morning and upright random urine samples.

The prognosis for orthostatic proteinuria is thought to be very good.

Persistent Asymptomatic Isolated Proteinuria

Etiology

PAIP is defined as proteinuria **detected in >80% of the urine specimens taken,** including recumbent samples, in an **otherwise healthy child,** which persists for 3 months. The prevalence in school-age children is 6%. It is usually <2 g/day and is never associated with edema. Numerous studies have revealed that children with PAIP have normal histology or mild nonspecific glomerular abnormalities. Other studies have reported divergent results with a significant number of patients having glomerular abnormalities such as focal sclerosis. Children with

PIAP form a heterogeneous group, and in the absence of large prospective studies, the prognosis of PAIP should be viewed with caution.

Nephrotic Syndrome

Nephrotic syndrome is defined by the presence of proteinuria, edema, hypercholesterolemia, and hypoalbuminemia.

Etiology

Nephrotic syndrome can be **primary** (isolated to the kidney) or **secondary** (part of a systemic disease, such as SLE). Glomerular diseases that can cause primary nephrotic syndrome include MCNS (77%), FSGS (10%), membranoproliferative glomerulonephritis (5%), diffuse mesangial proliferation (3%), crescentic glomerulonephritis (3%), and membranous nephropathy (2%).

Clinical Features

Edema is the cardinal finding in nephrotic syndrome. One of the most common manifestations is periorbital edema on awakening, which is sometimes mistaken for an allergic reaction. The **edema increases over time,** and the child may develop ascites, pleural effusion, and labial or scrotal edema.

Clinical features that favor a diagnosis of MCNS are **male gender,** age **<6 years** at onset of disease, **absence of hypertension,** and possibly a **small degree of hematuria.**

Evaluation

Evaluation should include a **urinalysis,** a **serum albumin level,** and a **serum cholesterol level.** Nephrotic syndrome is characterized by proteinuria >40 mg/m^2/hour, a serum albumin level of <2.5 g/dL, and hypercholesterolemia.

A biopsy is indicated for patients who.

■ Are <1 year or >10 years.
■ Have manifestations of nephritis (hematuria with red blood cell casts), azotemia, hypertension.
■ Fail a 4-week course of prednisone.

Treatment

More than 80% of patients with nephrotic syndrome and approximately 95% of children with MCNS respond favorably to **corticosteroid therapy.** Corticosteroids are generally started in a dose of 2 mg/kg per day (to a maximum dose of 80 mg/day), administered in two divided doses, and tapered over 4 to 8 weeks, after the urine is free of protein. The taper should be gradual enough to reduce the rate of relapse, without causing side effects (e.g., growth retardation).

Approximately 80% of the children who initially respond to prednisone **relapse.** Those who do not respond or those with frequent relapses (more than three relapses per year) are candidates for additional **immunosuppressive medications,** such as cyclophosphamide or cyclosporine A.

> **HINT:** Most children with MCNS have fewer relapses as they grow older and generally do well.

Proteinuria Caused by Structural Abnormalities

Damage to the glomerulus or tubules can cause proteinuria. Proteinuria from glomerular insult can be in the nephrotic range (Table 62-2), whereas proteinuria from tubular injury rarely exceeds 1 g/day.

EVALUATION OF PROTEINURIA

Once abnormal proteinuria is found and confirmed, a stepwise workup can be initiated.

Phase I Workup

The initial workup of proteinuria should begin with a complete history and physical examination. The physician should elicit history of **recent infections** (streptococcal, impetigo), **urinary tract infections, oliguria/ hematuria,** and **family history** of renal disease. The physical examination should be focused on looking for **hypertension** (glomerulonephritis), **edema** (nephrotic syndrome), **rash/arthritis** (vasculitis), and **short stature** (chronic renal disease). Laboratory investigations in this phase should include a **urine dipstick** (ambulatory and recumbent), a **urine analysis** including microscopic examination, and a **urine protein-to-creatinine ratio.**

Phase II Workup

Laboratory tests for serum electrolytes, creatinine, albumin, cholesterol, blood urea nitrogen, antistreptococcal antibodies, complement levels, and antinuclear antibodies should be done. A **renal ultrasound** should be performed to look for abnormalities of size and structure in the kidney. **Timed 12-hour urine protein quantitation** should be done for recumbent and upright samples to look for orthostatic proteinuria, and a **24-hour urinary protein level** should be obtained.

Phase III Workup

If the initial workup suggests the presence of an underlying renal disease, a **referral to a pediatric nephrologist** should be made. A referral should be made in the following situations:

- Persistent fixed (i.e., nonorthostatic) proteinuria
- Family history of glomerulonephritis
- Systemic complaints (e.g., fever, rash, arthralgias)
- Hypertension
- Edema
- Cutaneous vasculitis or purpura
- Hematuria
- Abnormal renal function
- Abnormal ultrasound
- Increased parental anxiety

The nephrologist may perform a renal biopsy to define the etiology of proteinuria in some of these situations.

Most cases of proteinuria in children can be managed by a primary care physician at times in consultation with a pediatric nephrologist. **Long-term follow-up** is important because prognosis in some of the conditions is not well-defined.

APPROACH TO THE PATIENT (FIGURE 62-1)

Figure 62-1 ■ Approach to the patient with proteinuria
ANA = antinuclear antibody; *ASO* = antistreptolysin-O;
BUN = Blood urea nitrogen

Suggested Readings

Bergstein JM: A practical approach to proteinuria. *Pediatr Nephrol* 13:697–700, 1999.

Ettenger RB: The evaluation of the child with proteinuria. *Pediatr Ann* 23(9):486–494, 1994.

Hogg RJ, Portman RJ, Milliner D, et al.: Evaluation and management of proteinuria and nephrotic syndrome in children: recommendations from a pediatric nephrology panel established at the National Kidney Foundation Conference on Proteinuria, Albuminuria, Risk, Assessment, Detection and Elimination (PARADE). *Pediatrics* 105:1242–1249, 2000.

Roy S: Proteinuria *Pediatr Ann* 25(5):277–278, 281–282, 1996.

Yoshikawa N, Kitagawa K, Ohta K, et al.: Asymptomatic constant isolated proteinuria in children. *J Pediatr* 119(3):375–379, 1991.

Pruritus
Janet H. Friday

INTRODUCTION

Pruritus, simply defined, means "itching." Pruritus that is **persistent and severe** requires further investigation. Pruritus usually has a primary **dermatologic** cause but may also be **drug induced** or caused by **systemic disease**.

DIFFERENTIAL DIAGNOSIS LIST

Infectious Causes
Varicella
Enterovirus
Pinworms
Scabies
Pediculosis
Trichinosis
Hookworms

Toxic Causes
Scombroid ingestion
Opiates
Barbiturates
Aminophylline
Aspirin
Erythromycin
Griseofulvin
Isoniazid
Phenothiazines
Vitamin A

Neoplastic Causes
Malignancy

Traumatic Causes
Overbathing, dry heat, harsh detergents
Healing wounds
Irritant-mediated contact dermatitis
Ultraviolet or chemical burns
Insect bites
Coelenterata envenomation

Foreign body (cactus spines or fiberglass)

Congenital or Vascular Causes
Congenital ectodermal dysplasia
Erythropoietic protoporphyria
Urticaria pigmentosa
Mastocytosis
Neurofibromatosis

Metabolic or Genetic Causes
Hypothyroidism or hyperthyroidism
Diabetes mellitus
Hypercalcemia
Hyperparathyroidism

Inflammatory Causes
Atopic dermatitis
Contact dermatitis, allergen mediated
Urticaria
Systemic lupus erythematosus
Juvenile rheumatoid arthritis

Neurologic and Psychiatric Causes
Cholestasis
Postherpetic pruritus
Spinal cord tumors
Delusional parasitosis

Miscellaneous Causes

Uremia
Iron-deficiency anemia
Polycythemia
Pityriasis rosea
Psoriasis

Seborrheic dermatitis
Acropustulosis of infancy
Lichen planus
Pregnancy
Nummular eczema

DIFFERENTIAL DIAGNOSIS DISCUSSION

Any skin condition comprising exudation, lichenification, and pruritus falls under the broad category of eczema. Two common forms of eczema, atopic dermatitis and contact dermatitis, are considered, and other common causes of pruritus are discussed.

Atopic Dermatitis

Etiology

Although it is one of the **most common causes of pruritus** in children, this condition is **poorly understood.** Characterized by **inflammatory hyperreactivity,** the disease is currently believed to be caused by aberrancies in T-cell function, with immunoglobulin E overproduction and cell-mediated immune dysfunction.

Clinical Features and Evaluation

Most children with atopic dermatitis have a **family history of atopic disease** (asthma, hay fever, or atopic dermatitis). Many children also have or later develop **asthma or hay fever.** The rash usually appears in susceptible patients during the first year of life, and involves the **face, neck, and trunk.** Distribution in older children is typically in **flexor creases of the elbows and knees.** The eruption consists of **erythematous, poorly demarcated patches,** and **initially is exudative, later forming crusts.** There may be **associated papules or vesicles.** With the **scratching** that ensues, the lesions become **thickened or lichenified** and may develop a **surface scale. Pigmentation changes** are common complications. Atopic dermatitis has a **chronic, recurrent, or recalcitrant nature.**

> **HINT:** It may be difficult to differentiate seborrheic dermatitis from atopic dermatitis in infants. Classically, seborrheic dermatitis appears in the first 2 months of life, whereas atopic dermatitis may appear later. The scale of seborrhea is yellow and greasy and is often seen behind the ears. The diagnosis of atopic dermatitis may be delayed until repeated outbreaks occur.

Treatment

Treatment focuses on **moisturizing the skin, avoiding overdrying, and eliminating possible irritants.** Increasing hydration by means of **bathing followed by application of a hydrophobic barrier** is essential. A **topical steroid,** such as 1% hydrocortisone cream, is used initially to control flares. Unresponsive cases may require treatment with more potent steroids or pimecrolimus (Elidel) or tacrolimus (Protopic), which inhibit cytokines. Although these are immunosuppressive agents, the topical forms are not systemically absorbed and are safe in children. The patient with severe atopic dermatitis is at risk for **secondary skin infections** with staphylococci, extensive primary herpes (eczema herpeticum), and varicella zoster infection.

Contact Dermatitis

Etiology

Contact dermatitis can be mediated by irritants or allergens.

- **Primary irritant dermatitis** is a direct response of the skin to an irritant. The most common irritants are soaps, bubble baths (may cause severe vaginal pruritus in prepubertal girls), saliva, urine, feces, perspiration, citrus juice, chemicals (creosote, acids), and wool.
- **Allergic contact dermatitis** requires reexposure to the allergen and is characterized by a delayed hypersensitivity reaction. The most common allergens implicated include poison ivy, poison oak, and poison sumac (rhus dermatitis) (Figure 63-1); jewelry (nickel); cosmetics

Figure 63-1 ■ Rhus dermatitis (poison ivy), an example of allergic contact dermatitis
(Reprinted with permission from Avery ME, First LR: Pediatric Medicine, 2nd ed. Baltimore, Williams & Wilkins, 1994.)

(causing eyelid involvement) and nail polish; topical medications (neomycin, thimerosal, calamine, para-aminobenzoic acid); shoe materials (rubber, tanning agents, dyes); and clothing materials (elastic or latex compounds).

Clinical Features and Evaluation

In either case, the **rash is the key to diagnosis**, being **most prominent in the areas of direct approximation to the trigger.** It may appear as erythematous papules, vesicles, bullae, or patches.

Treatment

The cornerstone of treatment is **removal of the offending agent.** A short course of **topical steroids** may help speed recovery. **Failure to respond** to these measures **indicates possible misdiagnosis.**

Xerosis

Etiology

Xerosis refers to **dryness of the skin** and may be the diagnosis of exclusion in common pruritus. Children of any age may be affected.

Clinical Features and Evaluation

The rash often has a **fine, flaky, white, diffuse scale,** which may be **excoriated from scratching.** The **lower legs** are commonly involved. The **hands** may also be afflicted in older children, especially when exposed to frequent handwashing or dishwashing. The condition is **made worse by dry heat, frequent bathing in hot water, and wool fabrics.**

Treatment

Treatment with **emollients** and **cessation of causative behaviors** are effective.

Scabies

Etiology

Scabies is caused by an **infestation with the mite** *Sarcoptes scabiei.* The mites burrow into the stratum corneum and deposit eggs and feces, which cause the itching.

Clinical Features

Lesions may be **papules, pustules, or vesicles** (Figure 63-2). Fewer than 15% of patients have the classic S-shaped burrows. The **rash distribution on infants** (neck, face, scalp, axilla, and groin) **differs from that of older children** (wrists, axilla, interdigital webs, intragluteal web, and belt line).

Figure 63-2 ■ Erythematous papules, pustules, vesicles, and crusted lesions of scabies
(Reprinted with permission from Avery ME, First LR: Pediatric Medicine, 2nd ed. Baltimore, Williams & Wilkins, 1994.)

Evaluation

Skin scrapings from an unscratched burrow in immersion oil under 10 × magnification should reveal the female mite, her eggs, and her feces.

Treatment

Permethrin 5% cream is applied to the entire body and left on for 12 hours. This treatment may be repeated in 2 weeks if necessary. Because the infestation is highly contagious, household contacts should also be treated. Bedding and clothing may harbor the mites and should be laundered; the dryer heat kills the remaining animals.

Bedbugs

Etiology

The bedbug (*Cimex lectularius*) has reemerged as a cause of pruritus. The insect is 5 mm with a brown body that turns mahogany red after feeding. It emerges during the night. The insect attaches itself to the skin and injects an enzyme, anticoagulant, and vasodilator. Following feeding, it returns to **dark crevices of mattresses, furniture, wallpaper, and suitcases.** Unlike mosquitoes, **bedbugs are not known to transmit diseases.**

Clinical Features

Most patients present with pruritic **macules that become papular, erythematous, and indurated.** The lesions may be in linear groups ("breakfast, lunch, and dinner"). **Bullous lesions, wheals, and anaphylactoid reactions** are also reported. Younger patients may develop **papular urticaria.** When healed, the lesions may be hypopigmented.

Evaluation

History and physical should suggest the diagnosis. Frequently, **small dark brown stains on the bedding** can be a clue. **Recent travel** may precede the infestation. A **careful search of the bedroom,** including turning the mattress over, may reveal the culprit.

Treatment

Local care of the lesions, with twice-daily cleansing and application of topical antibiotic ointment is usually all that is necessary. **Eradication** of the insect from the home usually requires an **exterminator** and **may be difficult** because of the multiple stages of insect larvae.

Varicella

Etiology

Varicella is caused by **primary infection with varicella zoster virus,** usually from droplet contact with a primarily infected individual. It is contagious from several days before the outbreak of lesions until all of the lesions are crusted over. Children who have received the varicella vaccine may exhibit milder symptoms.

Clinical Features

The rash is characterized by a **progression of lesions from erythematous macules, to papules, to fluid-filled vesicles, to crusted lesions.** Crops of lesions appear on the **face, trunk, and scalp,** with minimal involvement of the distal extremities. The **mucous membranes** are often involved; commonly, superficial ulcerations appear on the oral mucosae after the vesicles rupture. The clinician should always look for lesions in the **scalp, mouth, and vaginal areas.** Classically, lesions in various stages of evolution are simultaneously present. **Fever and malaise** may accompany the rash.

Treatment

Treatment is **supportive,** including attempts to **alleviate the itching** and **avoidance of secondary bacterial infections. Antiviral agents** (e.g., acyclovir) are effective only in shortening the course of illness **if given within 24 hours** of the onset of lesions.

> **HINT:** Aspirin use in patients with varicella is associated with Reye syndrome and is contraindicated. Immunocompromised hosts and neonates warrant special precautions and consultation with infectious disease specialists.

Drug Reaction Pruritus

Etiology

Although many medications cause pruritus, in an otherwise ill patient, **iatrogenic effects** may be **difficult to separate from the disease** process. The pruritus may be caused by **drug-induced intrahepatic cholestasis** (from erythromycin, oral contraceptives, anabolic steroids, phenothiazines) or **mast cell degranulation** (from codeine, aspirin, penicillin).

Treatment

If clinically feasible, a **trial period** during which the **patient is off medication** should be attempted. Relief of pruritus should occur **within several days if it is histamine mediated** but can take **several weeks to resolve if it is caused by cholestasis**.

Urticaria

Etiology

This classic pruritic rash is a manifestation of **immediate hypersensitivity reaction**, which may or may not be allergen mediated. The most common triggers are **foods** (nuts, berries, shellfish, dairy products), **plants, viral infections** (enterovirus, hepatitis), **group A streptococci, and drug reactions** (codeine, aspirin, penicillin). Intravenous injection of **radiopaque contrast material or blood products** may cause **severe reactions**. Less commonly, the trigger may be **cold, heat, tactile stimuli, or sunlight**.

Clinical Features and Evaluation

Diagnosis is made clinically. The classic appearance of urticaria is a **rash of erythematous raised, often evanescent, wheals** scattered over the body.

Treatment

Treatment may begin with **subcutaneous injection of epinephrine**, which usually clears the rash temporarily. Signs of **systemic progression** such as **laryngospasm, wheezing, and hypotension** warrant **more aggressive treatment. Antihistamines** are commonly prescribed to help alleviate itching and should be continued for 7 to 10 days. Attempts should be made to **identify and remove the trigger,** although often none can be found. The patient should be counseled that the rash may persist for days to weeks.

EVALUATION OF PRURITUS

Patient History

Key complaints are the presence of rash, fever, or both. Answers to the following questions should be sought:

- Are there any new or unusual exposures?
- What is the patient's drug history?
- Are any household contacts also suffering from similar symptoms?
- What is the patient's past medical history, including renal and hepatic disorders, atopic disease, psychiatric disorders, and autoimmune diseases?

Physical Examination

Physical examination findings that may point to the diagnosis include wheezing, oral lesions, organomegaly, ascites, and any abnormal skin findings. The pattern of distribution should be noted.

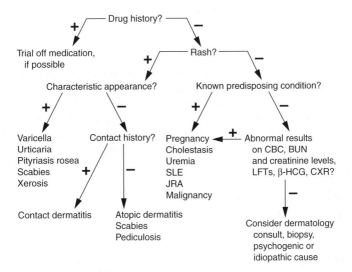

Figure 63-3 ■ Evaluation of a patient with pruritus
If the diagnosis remains elusive, refer the patient to a dermatologist. β-HCG = β-human chorionic gonadotropin; BUN = blood urea nitrogen; CBC = complete blood count; CXR = chest radiograph; JRA = juvenile rheumatoid arthritis; $LFTs$ = liver function tests; SLE = systemic lupus erythematosus.

Laboratory Studies and Diagnostic Modalities

Appropriate laboratory studies and diagnostic modalities may include the following:

- Complete blood count
- Blood urea nitrogen and creatinine levels
- Liver function tests
- β-Human chorionic gonadotropin level
- Chest radiograph
- Skin biopsy
- Microscopic examination of skin scrapings
- Chest radiograph

TREATMENT OF PRURITUS

If **urticaria** is present, the patient should be **urgently assessed for airway compromise, breathing, and circulation** because **airway edema and shock** can rapidly progress. If the rash is thought to be urticarial, a **rapid improvement after subcutaneous epinephrine administration** confirms this suspicion. Treatment with **intravenous antihistamines and steroids** is indicated if any **systemic signs** or symptoms are present.

APPROACH TO THE PATIENT (FIGURE 63-3)

Suggested Readings

Angel TA, Nigro J, Levy ML: Infestations in the pediatric patient. *Pediatr Dermatol* 47(4):921–935, 2000.

Boguniewicz M: Atopic dermatitis: beyond the itch that rashes. *Immunol Allergy Clin North Am* 25(2):333–351, 2005.

Frieden IJ, Resnick SD: Childhood exanthems: old and new. *Pediatr Clin North Am* 38(4):859–887, 1991.

Hurwitz S: *Clinical Pediatric Dermatology: A Textbook of Skin Disorders of Childhood and Adolescence,* 2nd ed. Philadelphia, WB Saunders, 1993.

Raimer SS: New and emerging therapies in pediatric dermatology. *Dermatol Clin* 18(1):73–78, 2000.

Ter Poorten MC, Prose NS: The return of the common bedbug. *Pediatr Dermatol* 22(3):183–187, 2005.

DIFFERENTIAL DIAGNOSIS LIST

Rash Accompanied by a Fever

Bacterial Causes
Scarlet fever
Staphylococcal scalded skin syndrome
Toxic shock syndrome
Acute meningococcemia
Rocky Mountain spotted fever

Viral Causes
Herpes simplex
Varicella
Roseola infantum
Erythema infectiosum
Enteroviruses
Measles
Rubella
Lyme disease

Miscellaneous
Juvenile idiopathic arthritis
Kawasaki disease

Rash in a Neonate

Erythema toxicum neonatorum
Transient neonatal pustular melanosis
Miliaria
Infantile seborrheic dermatitis
Candidiasis
Neonatal acne
Acropustulosis of infancy

Eczematous Dermatitis

Atopic dermatitis
Contact dermatitis
Nummular dermatitis
Asteatotic eczema
Id reaction

Papulosquamous Disease

Psoriasis
Lichen planus
Seborrheic dermatitis
Tinea (dermatophyte) infections
Tinea versicolor
Pityriasis rosea
Secondary syphilis
Pityriasis lichenoides et varioliformis acuta
Acrodermatitis enteropathica
Exfoliative dermatitis

Vesiculobullous Disease

Herpes simplex
Herpes zoster
Varicella
Rhus dermatitis (poison ivy)
Contact dermatitis
Insect bite or poapular urticaria
Urticaria pigmentosa

Annular Erythema

Lyme disease
Erythema multiforme

Papular Eruptions

Scabies
Papular acrodermatitis of childhood (Gianotti-Crosti syndrome)
Papular urticaria
Molluscum contagiosum
Warts

DIFFERENTIAL DIAGNOSIS DISCUSSION

Scarlet Fever

Etiology

Scarlet fever is caused by **group A β-hemolytic *Streptococcus.***

Clinical Features

Illness begins with **fever and pharyngitis** followed in 24 to 48 hours by an **enanthem and exanthem.**

The face appears flushed, except for circumoral pallor. The tongue initially has a white coating (**white strawberry tongue**) that is gone by the fourth day, revealing a very erythematous tongue with prominent papillae (**red strawberry tongue**). Cervical and submandibular lymphadenopathy are noted.

The rash appears as a **diffuse erythema;** small fine papules give it a **sandpaperlike** quality. The rash begins on the neck and spreads rapidly to the trunk and extremities. It is accentuated in the intertriginous areas (i.e., the axillae and antecubital, inguinal, and popliteal creases), and the palms and soles are spared. The rash resolves in 4 to 5 days with **fine peeling** of the skin. Peeling begins on the face, spreading to the trunk and extremities. On the hands and feet, peeling in large sheets may occur.

> **HINT:** Petechiae may occur on the soft palate and uvula or in streaks in the intertriginous areas (Pastia lines).

Evaluation

Diagnosis is by **culture or rapid test of a pharyngeal swab. Antistreptolysin-O titers** or **antideoxyribonuclease B titers** may also be used to indicate recent infection.

Treatment

Treatment of choice is with **penicillin, amoxicillin,** or a **first-generation cephalosporin. Erythromycin** can be used in penicillin-allergic patients.

Staphylococcal Scalded Skin Syndrome

Etiology

Staphylococcal scalded skin syndrome is caused by an **epidermolytic toxin, exfoliatin,** which is produced by some strains of *Staphylococcus aureus.*

Clinical Features

Staphylococcal scalded skin syndrome typically occurs in children <5 years of age. The illness begins with **fever and/or irritability** after an

Figure 64-1 ■ Crusted superficial erosions favoring intertriginous sites in staphylococcal scalded skin syndrome.

episode of conjunctivitis, rhinitis, or an upper respiratory tract infection. The skin initially becomes **erythematous** and **tender.** The eruption usually begins around the **nose and mouth** and **spreads to the trunk.** The rash is most **prominent in the flexures** and can involve the hands and feet. After 1 to 2 days, the **skin develops bullae** and begins **peeling in sheets.** After 2 days, the involved **skin surfaces become crusted** and then begin to **develop scaling,** which lasts up to 5 days (Figure 64-1).

Evaluation

S. aureus can sometimes be isolated by **bacterial culture of the nose,** nasopharynx, throat, conjunctiva, or perianal area.

> **HINT:** Periocular and perioral crusting in association with tender erythema and blisters and/or superficial erosions that favor intertriginous areas (the neck, axillae, groin, and perineum), is characteristic of this disease.

Treatment

Treatment is with a **penicillinase-resistant antibiotic** such as **nafcillin** or **oxacillin** (parenteral) or **dicloxacillin** or **amoxicillin-clavulanate** (oral). **Clindamycin** reduces the bacterial production of the toxin and is increasingly used because of concern about methicillin-resistant *Staphylococcus aureus.*

Toxic Shock Syndrome

Etiology

Toxic shock syndrome (TSS) is a multisystem disease caused by **exotoxin-producing strains** of either *S. aureus* (TSS) or *Streptococcus pyogenes* (STSS). These exotoxins—toxic shock syndrome toxin-1 (TSST-1) in the case of *S. aureus* and most commonly streptococcal pyrogenic exotoxin-A (SPE-A) in the case of *S. pyogenes*—function as superantigens and stimulate the release of massive amounts of proinflammatory cytokines, including tumor necrosis factor-alpha and interleukin-1. Although **classic TSS** is seen in association with **menstruation,** nonmenstrual TSS is now more common. STSS is usually seen as a complication of a **wound infection.**

Clinical Features

The association of **fever, rash, and hypotension** is the hallmark of TSS. Involvement of other organ systems may present as **myalgias, acute renal failure, encephalopathy, disseminated intravascular coagulopathy, diarrhea, metabolic acidosis, and/or hepatitis.** The rash may appear **morbilliform** (resembling measles) or as **confluent erythema** (erythroderma). Involvement of the **palms and soles** is common, and late **desquamation** of these areas is a key feature (Figure 64-2). A **strawberry tongue** is also characteristic.

Figure 64-2 ■ Desquamation of the palms in toxic shock syndrome.

> **HINT:** The presence of fever, hypotension and an erythematous rash in combination with dysfunction of at least three organ systems is diagnostic of TSS.

Evaluation

Blood cultures should be sent, although they are not always positive. Culture of any **cutaneous wounds** should also be performed. Evaluation for systemic involvement should include complete blood counts, serum chemistries, liver function tests, urinalysis, creatine kinase, and coagulation studies. Other diagnostic tests that may be helpful when indicated include electrocardiogram, echocardiography, and chest radiography. Skin biopsy is rarely needed.

Treatment

Appropriate antibiotic therapy should be promptly initiated. Use of an agent that is effective against both *S. aureus* and *S. pyogenes* is required if the causative agent is unknown. Initial choices include use of **oxacillin** or **vancomycin.** Addition of **clindamycin** is recommended as an adjunct to decrease toxin production.

Meningococcemia

Etiology

Meningococcemia is caused by *Neisseria meningitidis.* Asymptomatic nasopharyngeal carriage occurs and transmission occurs via respiratory droplets.

Clinical Evaluation

The illness begins with symptoms of a **mild upper respiratory tract infection,** followed by **fever, malaise, headache,** and the development of a **petechial eruption** on the skin and mucous membranes. In addition, patients can have **erythematous macules, papules, and urticarial lesions.** In severe cases, the purpura can involve **large areas that eventually necrose.**

Many patients develop meningitis, disseminated intravascular coagulation, and hypotension.

> **HINT:** Always think of meningococcemia when a patient presents with fever and petechiae.

Evaluation

Cultures of blood and cerebrospinal fluid are indicated. The organism can sometimes be recovered from a small petechial lesion if a **biopsy of**

the lesion is performed and cultured. A **Gram stain** of a scraping of a petechial lesion may reveal organisms.

Treatment

Initial treatment is with a **broad-spectrum antibiotic;** once the diagnosis is confirmed, the patient can be treated with **penicillin, ceftriaxone, or cefotaxime.**

Rocky Mountain Spotted Fever

Etiology

Rocky Mountain spotted fever is caused by *Rickettsia rickettsii,* which is transmitted by **ticks.**

Clinical Features

After a prodrome characterized by **headache, malaise, photophobia, and joint and muscle pain,** the patient develops a **fever** followed on the **fourth day** by a **rash.**

The rash begins on the **wrists and ankles** as small erythematous macules that eventually become petechial or purpuric. The rash then spreads to the trunk and within 2 days is generalized, with involvement of the palms and soles.

Other findings may include **generalized edema** (especially affecting the periorbital area in children), **severe muscle tenderness, photophobia, and hyponatremia.**

> **HINT:** Consider Rocky Mountain spotted fever in any patient with fever and a petechial eruption involving the palms and soles.

Evaluation

Diagnosis is with the detection of **rickettsial-specific antibodies.** Indirect immunofluorescence antibody, enzyme immunoassay, and indirect hemaglutination are the most sensitive and specific diagnostic tests. Direct immunofluorescence of a skin lesion biopsy specimen and serum polymerase chain reaction (PCR) are useful for confirming a clinical diagnosis but not widely available.

Treatment

The treatment of choice for all patients is a **tetracycline derivative.**

Herpes Simplex Virus

Herpes simplex virus is discussed in Chapter 70, "Sexually Transmitted Diseases."

Varicella (Chickenpox)

Varicella is discussed in Chapter 63, "Pruritus."

Roseola Infantum

Etiology

Roseola is caused by **human herpes virus-6** (HHV-6) infection. Transmission occurs through saliva.

Clinical Features

Usually seen in infants, roseola classically present with **3 days of high fever,** followed by rapid defervescence. **Febrile seizures** are common. After the fever abates, a **diffuse, faint, blanchable, erythematous reticulated rash** appears. It lasts for several days. An **enanthem** characterized by erythematous macules on the soft palate and uvula may also develop.

Evaluation

The diagnosis is usually made clinically, although serology and/or serum PCR for HHV-6 DNA may be performed if the diagnosis is unclear.

Treatment

The disease is self-limiting.

Erythema Infectiosum

Etiology

Erythema infectiosum is caused by infection with parvovirus B19. Transmission occurs via respiratory droplets.

Clinical Features

Erythema infectiosum is seen predominantly in **school-age children.** Prodromal symptoms such as **fever, pharyngitis, malaise, or coryza** may occur, followed by the development of the classic **"slapped cheek" erythema.** A **lacy, reticulated, erythematous exanthem** then develops most commonly on the extremities. It may wax and wane over several weeks. Older children and adults may complain of **arthralgias or arthritis.**

Evaluation

The diagnosis is usually made clinically. Serologic tests and serum PCR for parvovirus B19 DNA may be performed if the diagnosis is unclear.

Treatment

The disease is self-limiting.

Enterovirus

Etiology

Several human enteroviruses are capable of causing disease with cutaneous manifestations. **Coxsackievirus A 1-10, 16, and 22** are common causes of **herpangina. Coxsackievirus B16** is the most common cause of **hand-foot-mouth disease.** Other enteroviruses may cause pustular, morbilliform, vesicular, or papular exanthems.

Clinical Features

Prodromal symptoms such as **fever, malaise, headache, pharyngitis, or diarrhea** may be present. Herpangina presents with **small gray-white vesicles and erosions with an erythematous ring on the uvula, soft palate, and tonsils.** Hand-foot-mouth disease presents with similar **vesicles and erosions that favor the hard palate, buccal mucosa, tongue, and gingiva.** Small oval vesicles with an erythematous ring are seen on the lateral aspects of the **hands and feet,** as well as on the palms and soles. Papules and vesicles may also be seen on the buttocks. Many patients with herpangina or hand-foot-mouth disease have significant oral pain and decreased oral intake; young infants are at risk for dehydration.

Evaluation

The diagnosis is usually made clinically.

Treatment

Enterovirus infections are self-limiting. Intravenous hydration and analgesics may be required in severe cases.

Juvenile Rheumatoid Arthritis

Juvenile rheumatoid arthritis is discussed in Chapter 47, "Joint Pain."

Kawasaki Disease

Etiology

The cause of Kawasaki disease is **unknown.**

Clinical Features

The patient must present with five of the following six criteria to make the diagnosis of typical Kawasaki disease. Atypical cases of Kawasaki disease are increasingly recognized and an approach to these cases has been summarized in recent practice guidelines (see references):

- Fever ≥5 days
- Bilateral nonpurulent conjunctivitis
- Erythema and crusting of the lips

- Edema or erythema of the palms and soles with subsequent desquamation
- Rash
- Cervical adenopathy

The **rash** can have many different forms, including **generalized erythema, scarlatiniform lesions, erythema multiforme, and pustular lesions.** The **lips** are usually **bright red** with some **crusting,** and the patient may have a **strawberry tongue.**

> **HINT:** An important cutaneous finding is that of fine desquamation of the perineal area early in the course of the disease.

Evaluation

Thrombocytosis is present by the second week of illness. Sterile pyuria, hyponatremia, hypoalbuminemia, elevated erythrocyte sedimentation rate, anemia, and leukocytosis may be seen. An **echocardiogram** should be performed to look for coronary artery aneurysmal dilation.

Treatment

Treatment is with **intravenous gamma globulin** and **aspirin.**

Erythema Toxicum Neonatorum

Etiology and Clinical Features

The cause of erythema toxicum neonatorum is **unknown.** Affected infants appear healthy. The rash develops **within 3 to 4 days of birth** and is characterized by **erythematous macules and patches, some with a central papule or pustule.** The rash may occur **anywhere on the body except for the palms and soles.** There may be **few or several hundred lesions.**

Clinical Evaluation

A **smear** of a pustule reveals **clusters of eosinophils;** Gram staining is negative for bacteria. As many as 15% of patients have **peripheral eosinophilia.**

Treatment

No treatment is needed. The eruption generally resolves by the time the patient reaches 2 weeks of age.

Transient Neonatal Pustular Melanosis

Etiology and Clinical Features

The cause of transient neonatal pustular melanosis is **unknown.** This condition is more commonly seen in **African American infants** and is characterized by **pustules, vesicles, and hyperpigmented macules** that are **present at birth.** Pustules **rupture,** leaving a **fine white collarette of scale.** The eruption **resolves within several days,** most of the time leaving pigmented macules. The eruption can appear **anywhere on the body, including the palms and soles.** A **smear** of the pustules shows neutrophils.

Evaluation and Treatment

Gram stain, a Tzanck preparation, and potassium hydroxide preparation are negative for infection. **No treatment** is needed.

Miliaria

An **eruption,** characterized by **small nonfollicular, erythematous papules,** is caused by **sweat retention in eccrine ducts.** The rash is most commonly seen in the **intertriginous or flexor regions** of the body but can appear anywhere. There is no evidence of infection. Treatment entails **avoidance of excessive heat, humidity, and friction.**

Infantile Seborrheic Dermatitis

Etiology

The cause is **unknown** but may be related to **maternal hormonal stimulation.**

Clinical Features

The eruption often begins during the **first 12 weeks of life** with **scaling of the scalp,** sometimes associated with **erythema ("cradle cap");** the eruption generally **clears by 1 year of age.** The eruption is characterized by **greasy yellow scales** associated with **patches of erythema, fissuring, and occasional oozing** on the **scalp, face, ears, trunk, and intertriginous areas.**

Treatment

Parents should be advised to **gently loosen the scale with a soft comb or brush.** Application of **baby oil** to the scalp prior to shampooing may be helpful. A **low-potency topical corticosteroid** (i.e., hydrocortisone) may be applied to acutely inflamed areas.

Candidiasis

Etiology

Cutaneous candidiasis is common in neonates and infants. It is most commonly caused by infection with the yeast **Candida albicans,** although other Candida species are also implicated. Transmission usually occurs during or after delivery. Congenital candidiasis, which results from antepartum infection, is rare.

Clinical Features

The presence of **superficial erythematous papules and pustules,** often with a **collarette of scaling,** is seen. Involvement of the **diaper area** and other **intertriginous areas such as the neck** is common. Congenital candidiasis may present with more diffuse erythema and pustules.

Evaluation

The diagnosis is usually clinical. **Microscopic examination of a potassium hydroxide preparation** of a skin scraping may demonstrate **budding yeast.** A **fungal culture** can be performed if the diagnosis is unclear.

Treatment

Use of a topical antifungal cream or ointment such as nystatin or clotrimazole is effective. Affected areas should be kept dry, and frequent diaper changes should be performed.

Neonatal Acne

The cause is **unknown,** but the condition is probably related to **stimulation of sebaceous glands** by maternal and infant **androgens.** Neonatal acne is **more commonly seen in boys** and is reported in as many as 20% of newborns. **Closed comedones (whiteheads)** are most common, but **open comedones, inflammatory papules, and pustules** may also be noted. **No treatment** is necessary for most patients; patients with **moderate to severe cases** should be **referred to a pediatric dermatologist.**

Atopic Dermatitis and Contact Dermatitis

Atopic dermatitis and contact dermatitis are discussed in Chapter 63, "Pruritus."

Nummular Dermatitis

The cause of nummular dermatitis is **unknown,** although it tends to be a manifestation of **dry skin and ichthyosis.** The **rash** is characterized by **coin-shaped lesions** with **vesicles, papules, erythema, and scaling that enlarge by confluence** or peripheral extension. Lesions are treated with **midpotency topical steroids.**

> **HINT:** Nummular dermatitis lesions may be confused with impetigo or tinea corporis.

Id reaction

Etiology

An id reaction is a **reactive inflammatory dermatitis** that develops in response to a primary infection, often a **cutaneous dermatophyte (tinea)**

Figure 64-3 ▪ Id reaction in tinea capitis.

or bacterial infection, or an eczematous dermatitis such as a **contact dermatitis.**

Clinical Features

Patients present with an **acute, pruritic rash** characterized by a **symmetric eruption of multiple small papules and/or vesicles** (Figure 64-3). Sites of predilection include the **face, ears, and extremities,** although any area may be involved.

Evaluation

The diagnosis is usually made clinically. Patients should be examined for evidence of an associated dermatophyte infection such as tinea corporis or tinea capitis, impetigo, or contact dermatitis.

Treatment

Most patients respond to treatment of the underlying infection or eczematous dermatitis. The use of **topical corticosteroids** and **systemic antihistamines** may afford symptomatic relief.

Psoriasis

Etiology

The cause is **unknown,** although some evidence indicates a **genetic** component. An **immune defect** may be a primary or secondary factor.

Clinical Features

Psoriasis is characterized by **erythematous plaques with silvery scale** located **symmetrically** on the **elbows, knees, extensor surfaces of the wrist, genitalia, and scalp.** Children may present with **guttate (teardrop-like) plaques on the trunk** (Figure 64-4). Patients can also present with **large plaques, pustular plaques, or as an erythroderma,** whereby most of the body's skin is erythematous and scaling. **Nail changes include pitting** on some or all of the fingers **and onycholysis** (i.e., separation of the nail plate from the nail bed).

Evaluation

Psoriasis is a **clinical diagnosis,** but if there is doubt, a **skin biopsy** may be beneficial.

Figure 64-4 ■ Guttate psoriasis.

Treatment

Midpotency topical steroids, topical retinoids, topical calcipotriene (a vitamin D derivative), tar preparations, and antiseborrheic shampoos are useful. Patients with severe cases may require **ultraviolet light therapy** or **systemic medication.** Referral to a **pediatric dermatologist** is recommended for all patients with psoriasis, except those with very mild cases.

> **HINT:** Guttate psoriasis may be triggered by an antecedent Group A α-hemolytic streptococcus infection.

Lichen Planus

Etiology and Clinical Features

Lichen planus is a dermatologic disorder with lesions characterized by the "five Ps"—**pruritic, polygonal, purple, planar, papules** located on the **flexor surfaces, genitalia, mucous membranes, scalp, and nails** (Figure 64-5). The cause is **unknown.** The disease can eventually lead to **scarring of the scalp and nails.**

Figure 64-5 ■ Polygonal, pruritus, and purple papules of lichen planus.

Evaluation

A **skin biopsy** confirms the diagnosis when the clinical lesions do not conform to the classic description.

Treatment

Initial treatment is with **mid- to high-strength topical steroids.** Some patients may require oral corticosteroids or phototherapy; these patients are best managed by a dermatologist.

Seborrheic Dermatitis

Etiology

The cause is **unknown,** although there appears to be a relation to the yeast *Pityrosporum ovale.* In addition, there may be a **hormonal component** because it usually appears in neonates or after the onset of puberty.

Clinical Features

Typically, **scalp scaling** is present and may be associated with **erythema and pruritus.** In addition, **erythematous patches with greasy scaling** may be present **behind the ears, on the forehead and eyebrows, and in the nasolabial folds.** The eruption can occasionally be seen in the **presternal area, axillae, and inguinal folds.**

> **HINT:** Seborrheic dermatitis is usually not seen in patients between 1 year of age and puberty. In patients in this age group, one must always think of the possibility of dermatophyte (tinea) infections.

Treatment

Treatment entails **frequent shampooing with antidandruff shampoo** and the application of **low-potency topical steroids.**

Tinea (Dermatophyte) Infections

Etiology

Tinea infections are caused by superficial cutaneous infection with one of many species of **dermatophyte molds.** They may be transmitted from other persons, animals, or the environment.

Clinical Features

Infection may involve the **body (tinea corporis), face (tinea facie), hands (tinea manuum), feet (tinea pedis), groin (tinea cruris), scalp (tinea capitis), or nails (onychomycosis).** Cutaneous involvement usually presents with **pruritus and scaly erythematous papules and annular plaques.** Tinea capitis may present as **scalp scaling, erythematous papules and** pustules, hair loss, or painful, boggy, scaling plaques (kerion). Cervical lymphadenopathy may be prominent in tinea capitis. Onychomycosis presents with brittle, thickened, discolored nails. One or several nails may be involved.

Evaluation

Microscopic examination of a **potassium hydroxide preparation** of a skin scraping may demonstrate **fungal hyphae. Fungal culture** from skin or scalp scrapings or from nail clippings is the diagnostic test of choice and can identify the causative species of mold.

Treatment

A variety of topical antifungal agents, such as **clotrimazole, naftifine, and ketoconazole,** are appropriate for the treatment of cutaneous infection. Treatment of tinea capitis requires the use of a systemic antifungal, usually **griseofulvin.** Adjuvant therapy with antifungal shampoo such as ketoconazole or selenium sulfide is recommended to decrease shedding of spores. Treatment of onychomycosis also requires the use of a systemic antifungal agent such as **terbinafine.**

Tinea Versicolor

Etiology and Clinical Features

Tinea versicolor is caused by superficial infection with the mold *Malassezia furfur.*

Tinea versicolor presents with **hypopigmented or hyperpigmented round, oval, coalescent macules** with **slight superficial scale** on the chest, back, abdomen, or proximal extremities. It is usually asymptomatic.

Evaluation

The diagnosis is usually made clinically. **Microscopic examination of a potassium hydroxide preparation** of a skin scraping may demonstrate **fungal spores and hyphae** with a characteristic **"spaghetti and meatballs"** appearance.

Treatment

Intermittent use of a topical antifungal shampoo or cream such as **keto-conazole** or **selenium sulfide** is usually effective.

Pityriasis Rosea

Etiology and Clinical Features

Pityriasis rosea is an **acute, self-limited eruption.** The cause is **unknown.** Most cases start with a **single, large, oval, scaling plaque** known as a **herald patch.** Within 1 week of the initial lesion, crops of **small, pink,**

Figure 64-6 ■ Oval scaling macules arranged along skin tension lines in pityriasis rosea.

finely scaled plaques develop on the **trunk** (Figure 64-6). These lesions have a tendency to follow **skin cleavage lines,** creating a **"Christmas tree" pattern.** The rash usually **spares the face, except in children,** in whom facial involvement is common. The eruption may be associated with **moderate pruritus.**

> **HINT:** The eruption of secondary syphilis can mimic pityriasis rosea and should be considered in sexually active adolescents.

Treatment
Topical steroids and oral antihistamines can help alleviate the itching.

Lyme Disease
Etiology
Lyme disease is a tick-borne illness caused by the spirochete *Borrelia burgdorferi.* It is most commonly seen in the northeastern United States.

Figure 64-7 ■ Annular patch of erythema with central clearing (erythema chronicum migrans) in Lyme disease.

Clinical Features

The most characteristic finding is the presence of an **expanding annular patch of erythema with central clearing** (erythema chronicum migrans) at the site of the tick bite (Figure 64-7). Early symptoms may include **fever, myalgias, arthralgias, headache, and fatigue.** Late manifestations include arthritis, carditis, and neurologic abnormalities such as aseptic meningitis and Bell palsy.

Evaluation

Serologic testing of acute and convalescent sera is helpful. Skin biopsy is rarely needed.

Treatment

The treatment of choice for early Lyme disease in children >8 years of age is **doxycycline.** In younger children, use of **amoxicillin** is appropriate.

Erythema multiforme

Etiology

Erythema multiforme (EM) is a reactive, inflammatory dermatosis. It usually occurs in response to an antecedent infection, although medications may also trigger the reaction. The most common cause is a **herpes simplex virus (HSV) infection,** although other viruses as well as bacteria and fungi are reported to cause EM. Recurrent episodes are often associated with HSV infection.

Figure 64-8 ▪ Classic acral "target lesions" of erythema multiforme.

Clinical Features

The characteristic rash is the **target lesion,** which is characterized by a central area of **dusky erythema, surrounded by a ring of pallor (edema) and a peripheral ring of erythema** (Figure 64-8). Common sites of involvement are the **palms and extremities,** although any area may be involved. Some patients complain of pruritus or burning. Mucous membrane involvement of the lips or oropharynx may be seen but is generally mild. Associated symptoms are generally mild and may include **fever, fatigue, or pharyngitis.** Stevens-Johnson syndrome is a more severe form of this entity with mucosal involvement.

> **HINT:** Erythema multiforme may be confused with annular forms of urticaria. Urticaria presents with transient pruritic annular and polycyclic plaque characterized by erythematous lesions with central clearing.

Evaluation

The diagnosis is usually made clinically. Skin biopsy is rarely needed.

Treatment

The use of **topical steroids** and **systemic antihistamines** may be helpful. Systemic steroids may be required for more extensive cases. Analgesics, emollients, and oral hygiene may be required for painful oral lesions. The condition is self-limited.

Scabies

Scabies is discussed in Chapter 63, "Pruritus."

Papular Acrodermatitis of Childhood (Gianotti-Crosti Syndrome)

Etiology

Papular acrodermatitis of childhood is associated with many viruses, most commonly **Epstein-Barr virus** in the United States. In Europe, there is a strong association with nonicteric hepatitis B virus infection.

Clinical Features

The patient presents with **skin-colored to erythematous flat-topped papules** that are found on the **face, extremities, and buttocks,** with the trunk usually spared (Figure 64-9). **Pruritus** is sometimes associated with the eruption. **Hepatomegaly and lymphadenopathy** are occasionally present.

Evaluation and Treatment

Liver function tests may be abnormal in those patients with hepatomegaly. Usually, there is no need to do any laboratory tests

Figure 64-9 ■ Acrally located papular rash of Gianotti-Crosti syndrome.

because the diagnosis can be made clinically and the eruption is **benign and self-limiting,** usually resolving in 3 to 6 weeks.

Papular Urticaria

Etiology and Clinical Features

Papular urticaria, caused by a **hypersensitivity reaction to insect bites,** is characterized by **intensely pruritic wheals** (5 to 10 mm in diameter) **and papules** that contain a **central punctum.** Many times, the central punctum cannot be seen secondary to excoriation. Mosquitoes, fleas, and bedbugs are the most common exposures.

Lesions can be seen on any part of the body but are typically observed on exposed areas such as **the extremities, head, neck, and shoulders.** The eruption can **persist for months** and lesions can become **secondarily infected.** Extremely sensitive patients can develop **bullous lesions.** Fully resolved lesions tend to develop **temporary hyperpigmentation.**

> **HINT:** Always consider an insect bite reaction when a patient presents with grouped urticarial papules that occur only on exposed areas.

Evaluation

The **history and physical examination** are diagnostic.

Treatment

In patients with prolonged episodes, it is important to **identify the arthropod exposure. Pets** should be **treated for infestations.** An exterminator may need to inspect the home. Secondarily infected lesions should be treated with the appropriate topical or systemic **antibiotics.**

Molluscum Contagiosum

Etiology

Molluscum contagiosum is caused by cutaneous infection with the molluscum virus, a poxvirus. It may be spread by close physical contact, sharing of fomites such as towels, and autoinoculation.

Clinical Features

Infection is most commonly seen in school-age children. From several to tens of **small pearly, umbilicated papules** develop. Involvement may occur anywhere, but involvement of the face is common. Lesions are usually asymptomatic. During the resolution of individual lesions, an intense inflammatory reaction with surrounding erythema may develop. The condition is self-limited and generally resolves over 9 to 15 months.

Evaluation

The diagnosis is made clinically.

Treatment

Because the infection is self-limited, no treatment is required. When treatment is considered, therapeutic options include topical application of **cantharidin**, a blistering agent; **cryotherapy**; **curettage**; and **topical retinoids**.

EVALUATION OF RASH

Patient History

Ask about **associated symptoms** such as fever, pharyngitis, and malaise. It is important to ascertain **how the rash has evolved** and if any **topical or systemic treatment** has been rendered. A **complete drug and immunization history** should be obtained.

TABLE 64-1 Topical Corticosteroids

Class	Generic Name	Brand Name	Formulation
1: Highest potency	Clobetasol propionate 0.05%	Temovate	Cream, ointment
	Betamethasone dipropionate 0.05%	Diprolene	Cream, ointment
	Diflorasone diacetate 0.05%	Psorcon	Ointment
2: High potency	Fluocinonide 0.05%	Lidex	Cream, ointment, gel
	Desoximetasone 0.25%	Topicort	Cream, ointment
3: Mid- to high potency	Triamcinolone acetonide 0.5%	Aristocort	Cream, ointment
	Mometasone furoate 0.1%	Elocon	Cream, ointment
	Betamethasone valerate 0.1%	Valisone	Ointment
4: Midpotency	Triamcinolone acetonide 0.1%	Aristocort	Ointment
	Mometasone furoate 0.1%	Kenalog	Ointment
	Fluocinolone acetonide 0.025%	Elocon	Cream
	Desoximetasone 0.05%	Topicort LP	Cream
5: Low to midpotency	Alclometasone dipropionate 0.05%	Aclovate	Cream, ointment
	Betamethasone valerate 0.1%	Valisone	Cream, lotion
	Fluocinolone acetonide 0.025%	Synalar	Cream
	Hydrocortisone valerate 0.2%	Westcort	Cream, ointment
6: Low potency	Triamcinolone acetonide 0.025%	Aristocort	Cream
	Desonide 0.05%	DesOwen	Cream
	Fluocinolone acetonide 0.01%	Synalar	Cream, lotion
7: Lowest potency	Hydrocortisone 1%	Numerous over-the-counter preparations	Cream, ointment
	Hydrocortisone 2.5%		

Physical Examination

Important features include the **morphology** of the eruption and its **distribution**. A complete examination of the **skin, hair, nails, and mucous membranes** should be performed.

TREATMENT OF RASH

Table 64-1 summarizes commonly used topical corticosteroids but is not all inclusive. In general, the use of class 1 and 2 topical steroids are best avoided in children.

Suggested Readings

Gable EK, Liu G, Morrell DS: Pediatric exanthems. *Prim Care* 27(2): 353–369, 2000.

Nelson JS, Stone MS: Update on selected viral exanthems. *Curr Opin Pediatr* 12(4):359–364, 2000.

Newburger JW, Takahashi M, Gerber MA, et al.: Diagnosis, treatment, and long-term management of Kawasaki disease. American Heart Association Scientific Statement. *Circulation* 110:2747–2771, 2004. Available at: http://www.circ.ahajournals.org/cgi/content/full/110/17/2747.

Wagner A: Distinguishing vesicular and pustular disorders in the neonate. *Curr Opin Pediatr* 9(4):396–405, 1997.

INTRODUCTION

Red eye may refer to **erythema of the ocular adnexa, conjunctiva, sclera, or cornea,** or **inflammation of deeper structures.**

DIFFERENTIAL DIAGNOSIS LIST

Ocular Adnexa

Infectious Causes
Hordeolum and chalazion
Dacryocystitis
Molluscum contagiosum
Blepharitis
Phthiriasis (louse)
Frontal sinus infection or
other sinusitis
Periostitis of orbital bones
Orbital cellulitis, periorbital
cellulitis
Dental abscess

Neoplastic Causes
Neuroblastoma
Leukemia
Neurofibroma

Traumatic Causes
Insect bites
Basilar skull fracture
Trauma to eyelid or nose

Miscellaneous Causes
Frequent eye rubbing
Cavernous sinus thrombosis
Prolonged crying
Contact dermatitis
Seborrhea

Conjunctiva

Infectious Causes
Bacteria
Viruses

Fungi
Protozoans
Helminths—onchocerciasis
(river blindness)

Toxic Causes
Atropine, scopolamine
Irritants—makeup, smoke,
smog, chemicals, contact
lenses, caterpillar hair,
wind, ultraviolet light,
tobacco

Neoplastic Causes
Orbital tumors—
retinoblastoma

Traumatic Causes
Foreign body
Entropion, ectropion
Child abuse
Blunt or penetrating trauma
Traumatic glaucoma
Subconjunctival hemorrhage

Immunologic Causes
Allergic/inflammatory
conjunctivitis
Keratoconjunctivitis sicca
and other dry eye disorders
Nasal inflammation
Sjögren syndrome and other
collagen vascular diseases
Kawasaki syndrome
Stevens-Johnson syndrome
Inflammatory bowel disease

Juvenile rheumatoid
  arthritis
Graves disease
Miscellaneous Causes
  Bone marrow transplant
  Ectodermal dysplasia
  Subconjunctival hemorrhage
    (secondary to severe cough,
    bacteremia, blood dyscrasia,
    or vomiting)

Cornea

Infectious Causes
  Keratitis
  Syphilis
Traumatic Causes
  Contact lenses

Corneal ulcer
Corneal abrasion
Chemical irritant

Uveal Tract

Iridocyclitis
Reiter syndrome

Sclera

Episcleritis
Scleritis
Collagen vascular disease

Pupil

Hyphema
Globe
Glaucoma

DIFFERENTIAL DIAGNOSIS DISCUSSION

Neonatal Conjunctivitis

Etiology

Neonatal conjunctivitis is most often **secondary to infection or chemical irritation.**

- **Infection.** Causes of infectious conjunctivitis in the neonate include sexually transmitted and nonsexually transmitted organisms. Sexually transmitted agents, in order of decreasing frequency, are *Chlamydia trachomatis, Neisseria gonorrhoeae,* and herpes simplex virus (HSV), usually type 2. *Staphylococcus aureus* is the most common nonsexually transmitted infectious pathogen. Other bacterial causes include enteric Gram-negative rods.
- **Chemical irritation.** Silver nitrate is the most common cause of neonatal chemical conjunctivitis, although other antibiotics used for prophylaxis can also cause conjunctivitis.

Clinical Features

Conjunctivitis that presents in the **first 24 hours of life** is most likely **secondary to chemical irritation,** unless there was prolonged rupture of membranes before delivery.

- **Gonococcal conjunctivitis,** which presents 2 to 6 days after birth, is an acute to hyperacute infection that causes edema of the eyelids and conjunctiva (chemosis), local pain, and a copious purulent discharge.

Swelling and discharge can be so extensive that the orbit is difficult to view. Often there is a palpable preauricular node, a finding otherwise uncommon in bacterial conjunctivitis.

■ **Chlamydial conjunctivitis** has a slightly later onset than gonococcal conjunctivitis but can be symptomatic as early as 4 to 5 days after birth. Modest purulent drainage and mild to moderate inflammation are seen. As with gonococcal conjunctivitis, the preauricular lymph node may be tender.

■ **Herpes simplex conjunctivitis** is associated with clusters of vesicles on the face, eyelids, and mucous membranes.

> **HINT:** Chlamydial conjunctivitis, in general, is markedly less acute and impressive than gonococcal conjunctivitis.

> **HINT:** Chlamydial pneumonitis occurs in as many as a one-third of infants with chlamydial conjunctivitis, although it presents later, typically at 3 to 16 weeks of age.

Evaluation

Bacterial culture, including **chocolate agar or Thayer-Martin plates** and **Gram stain of the purulent material,** should be obtained. In up to 95% of cases of gonococcal conjunctivitis, Gram-negative intracellular diplococci are identified by Gram stain.

Chlamydia culture and a rapid assay should be obtained on **conjunctival scrapings** (not purulent material). In patients with suspected herpes simplex conjunctivitis, conjunctival scrapings reveal mononuclear cells and giant multinucleated epithelial cells.

Treatment

■ **Chlamydial conjunctivitis.** Hospitalization is not necessary. Treatment consists of 14 days of oral erythromycin combined with topical erythromycin.

■ **Gonococcal conjunctivitis.** Hospitalization and consultation with an ophthalmologist are required. The eye should be irrigated every 1 to 2 hours to reduce bacterial load and local irritation. Improperly treated gonococcal conjunctivitis can quickly damage vision. Intravenous therapy for 7 days is indicated for disseminated infection, and up to 14 days for meningitis; one dose is adequate for isolated conjunctivitis. Cefotaxime or ceftriaxone are appropriate until sensitivities are known.

■ **Herpes simplex conjunctivitis.** Patients must be followed by an ophthalmologist to minimize the chance of permanent scarring and damage to vision.

Infectious Conjunctivitis
(Outside the Neonatal Period)

Etiology

The most common bacterial cause of conjunctivitis is *S. aureus,* which affects all age groups. *Haemophilus influenzae* and *Streptococcus pneumoniae* are common causes of conjunctivitis in **young children.** Adolescents can also present with **gonococcal** conjunctivitis **secondary to sexual contact.**

Epidemic keratoconjunctivitis, the name given to rapidly spreading viral conjunctivitis, most often occurs secondary to adenoviral infection. **HSV, types 1 and 2,** and **varicella-zoster virus** are more serious causes of viral conjunctivitis; these organisms are associated with **corneal destruction** (keratitis) and **loss of vision.** Herpes simplex keratitis is the most common infectious cause of corneal blindness in developed countries.

Protozoal infections, specifically *Acanthamoeba,* are seen almost exclusively in **contact lens wearers.**

> **HINT:** Contact lens wearers are more susceptible to virulent Gram-negative infections and unusual fungal infections of the conjunctiva.

Clinical Features (Table 65-1)

The clinical signs and symptoms of **bacterial** conjunctivitis include **tearing, purulent discharge, conjunctival hyperemia, and foreign body sensation.**

TABLE 65-1　Differentiation of Conjunctivitis (Outside the Neonatal Period)

Clinical Findings	Viral	Bacterial	Chlamydial	Allergic
Itching	Minimal	Minimal	Minimal	Severe
Hyperemia	Generalized	Generalized	Generalized	Generalized
Tearing	Profuse	Moderate	Moderate	Moderate
Exudation	Minimal	Profuse	Profuse	Minimal
Preauricular node	Common	Uncommon*	Inclusion conjunct	None
Stained scraping	Monocytes	Bacteria, PMNs	PMNs, plasma cells	Eosinophils
Sore throat/ fever?	Occasionally	Occasionally	Never	Never

*Except in gonococcal conjunctivitis.
Modified with permission from Schwab I, Dawson C: Conjunctiva. In *General Ophthalmology*, 14th ed. Edited by Vaughan D, Ashbury T, Riordan-Eva P. Norwalk, CT, Appleton & Lange, 1995, 98.
PMNs = polymorphonuclear cells.

The **eyelids** are often **crusted closed** on arising in the **morning.** *H. influenzae* and *S. pneumoniae* conjunctival infections are often associated with **subconjunctival hemorrhage.** Infection is often **bilateral.**

The physical findings of **nonherpetic viral** conjunctivitis include a **serous or lightly purulent discharge, minimal to moderate eyelid swelling, a unilateral or bilateral presentation,** and occasional systemic symptoms (e.g., malaise, fever, or sore throat). **Profuse tearing** is often present. Viral conjunctivitis is much more likely than bacterial infection to be associated with **tender preauricular adenopathy.**

HINT: Subconjunctival hemorrhage may point to adenoviral conjunctivitis.

In patients with **herpetic viral** conjunctivitis, the **initial HSV infection** is clinically **indistinguishable from other causes of viral conjunctivitis,** with the exception that it is almost always **unilateral.** Herpetic recurrences are unilateral in 96% of patients, are often **corneal** (keratitis), and produce the classic **dendritic lesion of the cornea best seen with fluorescein.**

Evaluation

Culture is necessary only **if an unusual or serious pathogen** is suspected. Although recovery of the offending organism is difficult once antibiotic therapy has been initiated, cultures are also recommended **if treatment failure occurs.** Culture recovery of HSV is successful in only 70% of patients with herpetic conjunctivitis.

Treatment

Viral and bacterial conjunctivitis are **self-resolving** illnesses **except for herpes simplex** conjunctivitis and conjunctivitis caused by **varicella zoster virus.** Because it is **impossible clinically to differentiate viral and bacterial** conjunctivitis with certainty, **nonherpetic viral** conjunctivitis is **treated in the same fashion as bacterial** conjunctivitis. Treatment involves instillation of **antibiotic drops and periodic removal of eye discharge with warm wet washcloths.** Improvement usually occurs within 3 to 4 days. Without treatment, bacterial conjunctivitis usually resolves within 2 weeks. In the event of **treatment failure,** a **second antibiotic** with a significantly **different spectrum** from the first antibiotic should be prescribed.

Any child with a **prior history of herpetic conjunctivitis** who presents with red eye should be assumed to have **recurrent herpes infection** and must be **referred to an ophthalmologist urgently. Steroid use** in all types of conjunctivitis is best **left to an ophthalmologist** because **serious harm** can result if steroids are inadvertently prescribed for a patient with herpetic conjunctivitis.

Allergic Conjunctivitis

Etiology

Common environmental allergens (e.g., animal dander, dust, molds, grass, pollens) can cause allergic conjunctivitis. Antibiotic drops and facial creams or lotions are also implicated.

Clinical Features

The hallmark of allergic conjunctivitis is **pruritus.** There can be significant erythema and swelling of the eyelids, most often in a bilateral distribution. These symptoms can be confused with those of periorbital or orbital cellulitis; however, a lack of tenderness and the absence of systemic symptoms make cellulitis unlikely. Conjunctival hyperemia is diffuse. Discharge is moderate in volume and clear. Adenopathy is not found.

The onset of symptoms can be abrupt, after acute exposure to the offending agent, or chronic, with repeated or continuous exposure. Symptoms may show a seasonal variation, commonly worsening in the spring. Rhinitis and other allergic symptoms may also be present.

Treatment

Treatment depends on the age of the child and the subjective symptoms. Erythema alone does not warrant intervention. Cold compresses are effective for short-term relief of pruritus. Topical vasoconstrictors and antihistamines are the first-line medications if treatment is undertaken. If unsuccessful, topical steroids may be required. Systemic antihistamines and nasal steroids often provide relief.

Chalazia and Hordeola

Etiology

A chalazion is a chronic inflammatory lipogranuloma of the meibomian gland resulting from obstruction of the gland duct. Secondary infection is common. An infected chalazion is sometimes referred to as an internal hordeolum.

An external hordeolum (stye) is a purulent, usually staphylococcal, infection of the follicle of an eyelash or its associated sebaceous or sweat gland.

Clinical Features and Evaluation

Uninfected chalazia are characterized by gradual, painless swelling in the body of the eyelid. Chalazia that become secondarily infected usually point and drain on the inside of the eyelid (the conjunctival side).

Hordeola present with **swelling, induration, and purulent drainage** at or near the margin of the eyelid. Hordeola tend to **point and drain outward.** Hordeola often occur in **groups,** following the spread of infection from one follicle to another.

Both chalazia and hordeola may be **unilateral or bilateral.** The child with either a hordeolum or an infected chalazion is **afebrile and appears otherwise well.**

Treatment

Small, uninfected chalazia may **resolve spontaneously. Large chalazia** must be **surgically removed. Infected** chalazia require **medical management.**

Hordeola and infected chalazia are treated identically. **Warm to hot compresses** should be applied to the affected eye for **20 minutes, four times per day,** to encourage spontaneous drainage of the purulent collections. Some advocate daily **cleaning of the lid margins, using baby shampoo and water on a washcloth** rubbed on the lid margin with the eyes held shut. **Topical antibiotic ointment or drops** should be instilled daily. Attention to **general hygiene** keeps recurrences to a minimum.

Corneal Abrasion

Etiology

Corneal abrasions result from **traumatic removal of part of the corneal epithelium.**

Clinical Features

The signs and symptoms seen with corneal abrasion often mimic those of infectious conjunctivitis—**diffuse injection of the conjunctiva, watery discharge, pain,** and, often, **decreased visual acuity.** The main difference is found in the history—**trauma,** even if apparently minor, **immediately precedes the onset of symptoms** in patients with corneal abrasion.

Evaluation

Patients presenting with **red eye** and any **history of trauma** should have a **fluorescein examination of the eye** to rule out an abrasion. The eye should be carefully examined to **exclude** the possibility of a **retained foreign body** or a **deeper injury.** This includes performing a **maneuver to flip the upper lid and inspect the inner surface.** If the **pain** persists for **>24 hours** after the initial trauma, **referral to an ophthalmologist** should be made.

Treatment

The primary goal of treatment is to **prevent further injury. Foreign bodies** should be **removed by irrigation** with sterile saline solution. If this is ineffective, an **ophthalmologist** should be **consulted** for removal. Many authors recommend **topical antibiotic eyedrops.** For large abrasions or those involving the visual axis, the eye should be **examined daily** until fully healed.

> **HINT:** Topical anesthetics should never be given to a patient for repeated home instillation after corneal injury. Their use delays healing, masks damage, and can lead to permanent corneal scarring.

Orbital and Periorbital Cellulitis

Etiology

Periorbital cellulitis refers to **infection of the tissues anterior to the globe.** Infection occurs either via **hematogenous spread or local trauma.** In the past, hematogenously spread disease was most often caused by *H. influenzae,* but *S. pneumoniae* and other organisms are becoming more prevalent as a result of the success of the universal *H. influenzae* type B vaccination. In patients with a **history of local trauma,** *S. aureus* and *Streptococcus* are the most common pathogens.

Orbital cellulitis most commonly results from **direct spread of infection from the sinuses.** The infectious process in orbital cellulitis involves the retrobulbar tissues, including the **ocular muscles, orbital fat, and bone.**

Clinical Features

Periorbital cellulitis is a unilateral disease that presents with **significant swelling, induration, tenderness, and erythema of the eyelids** and a variable amount of **purulent discharge. Fever** is common.

Orbital cellulitis presents with a clinical picture **similar to** that of periorbital cellulitis. In addition, orbital cellulitis is characterized by a **decreased range of motion of ocular muscles, proptosis, changes in vision, and papilledema.**

Evaluation

Children with periorbital or orbital cellulitis may be **bacteremic,** and **blood cultures** should be considered in highly febrile patients. **Computed tomography** should be used whenever **orbital** cellulitis is considered.

Treatment

Hospitalization and the intravenous administration of antibiotics is indicated for patients with orbital cellulitis. **Ampicillin-sulbactam, oxacillin or ceftriaxone** are appropriate antibiotic choices, although coverage for methicillin-resistant *S. aureus* (**MRSA**) should also be considered. **Surgical drainage** may be required. Patients with periorbital cellulitis often require hospitalization, but outpatient therapy can be considered if they are older (generally >2 years), afebrile, well appearing, and have close follow-up with their primary care physician. **Amoxicillin-clavulanic acid or cefuroxime axetil** are appropriate antibiotic choices.

Patients with **orbital** cellulitis should be seen by an **ophthalmologist** because orbital cellulitis carries **a significant risk for damage to the visual axis**—specifically, **optic neuritis with atrophy. Significant extraocular complications** are also associated with orbital cellulitis, including **cavernous sinus thrombosis, meningitis, and brain abscess.**

Suggested Readings

Block SL, Hedrick J, Tyler R, et al.: Increasing bacterial resistance in pediatric acute conjunctivitis (1997–1998). *Antimicrob Agents Chemother* 44(6):1650–1654, 2000.

King RA: Common ocular signs and symptoms in childhood. *Pediatr Clin North Am* 40:753–766, 1993.

Leibowitz HM: The red eye. *N Engl J Med* 343(5):345–351, 2000.

Limberg M: A review of bacterial keratitis and bacterial conjunctivitis. *Am J Ophthalmol* 112:2S–9S, 1991.

Roy FH: *Ocular Differential Diagnosis,* 6th ed. Baltimore, Williams & Wilkins, 1996.

Respiratory Distress

Laura Mulreany
Burton Lesnick (Second Edition)

INTRODUCTION

Respiratory distress may be defined as **increased work of breathing** that causes the patient to have a **sense of altered well-being.** Symptoms may include shortness of breath, chest tightness, chest pain, cough, and even mental status changes in later stages.

DIFFERENTIAL DIAGNOSIS LIST

Infectious Causes

Peritonsillar abscess
Retropharyngeal abscess
Epiglottitis
Croup (viral laryngotracheo-bronchitis)
Bacterial tracheitis
Bronchiolitis
Pertussis
Pneumonia

Structural Lesions

Laryngeal lesions/masses
Laryngomalacia
Vocal cord paralysis
Subglottic stenosis
Tracheomalacia
Bronchomalacia
Lobar emphysema
Bronchogenic cyst
Vascular ring, other aberrant vessels
Mediastinal or other intrathoracic mass (cystic hygroma, teratoma, cystic adenomatoid malformation, neuroblastoma, diaphragmatic hernia or eventration)

Toxic Causes

Carbon monoxide poisoning
Methemoglobinemia

Neoplastic Causes

Hemangioma
Papilloma
Brainstem tumor

Traumatic Causes

Foreign body aspiration
Aspiration caused by gastroesophageal reflux disease
Pneumothorax

Metabolic or Genetic Causes

Metabolic acidosis
Cystic fibrosis

Psychosocial Causes

Psychogenic hyperventilation

Neuromuscular Disorders

Respiratory muscle weakness, myopathy
Duchenne muscular dystrophy
Spinal muscle atrophy
Prune-belly syndrome
Werdnig-Hoffmann disease

Miscellaneous Causes

Anaphylaxis
Asthma
Atelectasis
Pleural disease (effusion, empyema)

Pulmonary hemorrhage
Pulmonary edema
Pulmonary embolism

Sickle cell crisis—acute chest
 syndrome
Vocal cord dysfunction

DIFFERENTIAL DIAGNOSIS DISCUSSION

Infectious Causes

Infections causing respiratory distress may be **bacterial or viral** and may **affect any part of the respiratory tract.** Some infections are more common in different age groups, aiding in the diagnosis. In addition to the symptoms of respiratory distress mentioned earlier, the patient may have **congestion** or **rhinitis** or a variety of constitutional symptoms such as **fever, malaise, poor appetite, or body aches.** The causative agent may be identified by cultures of the nasopharynx, pharynx, or sputum.

Epiglottitis
Etiology

Infection of the epiglottis is most commonly caused by *Haemophilus influenzae* type B and results in **rapid swelling and airway compromise,** creating a **medical emergency.** Fortunately, near universal use of the *H. influenzae* type B vaccine has dramatically reduced the incidence of this disease in children. Other pathogens that may cause epiglottitis include *Streptococci, Staphylococci,* and *Candida albicans.*

Clinical Features

Epiglottitis is most common in children **between the ages of 3 and 6** years who have not been vaccinated against *H. influenzae* type B. Symptoms develop over several hours and include **high fever, dysphagia, drooling, inspiratory stridor, and holding the head in an upright "sniffing" position,** with the neck extended and the jaw protruding.

Evaluation

When the history is suggestive, **the child should not be excessively disturbed.** Attempts to visualize the pharynx directly may result in **complete occlusion** of the airway and **respiratory arrest.** Vaccination status of a patient with suspected epiglottitis must be assessed, although a positive history of vaccination does not rule out the possibility of epiglottitis. A **lateral neck radiograph** should not be attempted until a secure airway is established if the diagnosis is strongly suspected. A **characteristic "thumbprint" epiglottis** (the epiglottis is swollen) is diagnostic.

A blood culture drawn after an airway is established may help determine the causative bacteria.

Treatment

The most experienced staff available should establish an artificial airway under controlled circumstances, preferably by an otolaryngologist in an operating room with the support of an anesthesiologist. When intubation of the trachea cannot be accomplished, **tracheostomy** is indicated. **Broad-spectrum antibiotics** are then administered **intravenously**.

Croup (Viral Laryngotracheobronchitis)
Etiology

Most cases of croup are caused by **parainfluenza virus types 1 and 3,** although other pathogens have been encountered. **Inflammation of the larynx, trachea, and bronchi** results in increased airway resistance and obstruction. Rarely, airway obstruction is so severe that cardiopulmonary arrest ensues.

Clinical Features

Patients are usually <3 years old (typical range is 6 months to 6 years of age), and the presence of typical symptoms in the first few months of life should prompt evaluation for congenital anomalies. Patients with mild cases may demonstrate a **bark-like cough, nasal congestion, and fever**. Typically, a mild cough with intermittent stridor **progresses to continuous stridor, especially at night.** Many patients improve after exposure to humidified air or cool night air.

Evaluation

Critical airway narrowing is denoted by severe retractions, inspiratory stridor, and decreased air entry on physical examination. In patients with severe airway obstruction, **cyanosis and weakness** may be noted. **Cyanosis, tachycardia, and mental status changes** may accompany hypoxia. **Lateral and anteroposterior neck radiographs** can help differentiate croup from epiglottitis, although radiographs should not be required in typical presentations. A characteristic **"steeple sign"** is often seen in the subglottic airway in croup, and the epiglottis is normal.

Treatment

An **artificial airway** should be established for patients with impending respiratory failure. Therapeutic strategies include the following:

- **Humidified oxygen.** Cool, humidified oxygen is the best treatment for patients with mild to moderate cases of croup, although this practice is not clearly supported in randomized clinical trials.
- **Racemic epinephrine.** Patients with severe cases may temporarily benefit from the inhalation of racemic epinephrine. These patients may need to be hospitalized to observe for rebound effects, which

may occur within 1 to 4 hours after the administration of racemic epinephrine.

- **Intravenous fluids.** Fluids are helpful to maintain adequate hydration in patients with severe tachypnea.
- **Steroids.** The use of systemic or inhaled steroids in treating croup has been controversial; although according to recent studies, a single dose of oral dexamethasone is helpful in reducing respiratory symptoms even in mild cases.
- **Antibiotics.** Unless a secondary bacterial infection is suspected, antibiotics are not indicated.

Bronchiolitis
Etiology

Viruses (e.g., respiratory syncytial virus [RSV], parainfluenza viruses, and adenoviruses) infect the **lining of the small airways (bronchioles),** resulting in **mucosal edema and intraluminal accumulation of mucus and cellular debris.** Infants <2 years are predominantly affected because the small caliber of their airways predisposes them to the development of increased airway resistance with even mild airway narrowing.

Clinical Features

A **prodrome of nasal congestion and coryza** lasting several days is usual. **Fever and anorexia** may be present, particularly in young infants with severe nasal congestion who may have difficulty feeding. Often, another family member has a mild upper respiratory tract infection. **Respiratory distress** usually **develops gradually** and is characterized by a worsening cough and wheezing. Typically, the **symptoms are worse at night.**

Evaluation

On physical examination, infants may be **tachypneic,** with a respiratory rate of 60 to 80 breaths/minute. The **expiratory phase is usually prolonged,** and **diffuse wheezing** is often present. **Breath sounds** may be diminished in severe cases. **Severe retractions and the use of accessory muscles** are common. Lung hyperinflation and depression of the diaphragm typically result in a **palpable liver and spleen.** A **chest radiograph** shows hyperinflation, peribronchial thickening, and, in many patients, subsegmental atelectasis. The diagnosis of bronchiolitis is a clinical one, although **nasopharyngeal swab** or washing for RSV may help support the diagnosis in some cases.

Treatment

Supportive care entails administration of **humidified oxygen** and positioning of the infant with the **head and neck slightly elevated.** Frequent

nasal suctioning is often helpful. **Intravenous fluids** are useful in maintaining hydration in the presence of tachypnea and decreased oral intake. The use of nebulized medications has been studied extensively, with inconclusive and variable results. **Nebulized albuterol** is not effective in most cases, but **nebulized racemic epinephrine** in some studies was more beneficial. Systemic corticosteroids also show variable results in clinical trials, although they are not currently recommended for routine use. **Sedatives should not be used,** and antibiotics are generally not helpful. In infants with a severe course, or those with underlying cardiac or pulmonary disease, **ribavirin** may have a role in treating bronchiolitis caused by RSV.

> **HINT:** Very young infants and infants with a history of premature birth (with or without associated lung disease) or chronic heart or lung disease are at greater risk for apnea and poor outcome. A monoclonal antibody (Palivizumab), given in monthly intramuscular injections through the typical RSV season, is available for patients who meet high-risk criteria.

Pertussis
Etiology
The classic causative organism is *Bordetella pertussis*, but *Bordetella parapertussis* and adenovirus infection can also cause pertussis, which is characterized by **necrosis** and desquamation of the superficial epithelium of the pharynx. Children **<2 months** are most at risk, even if immunized. Adolescents and adults are often first affected because of waning immunity, and the diagnosis should be entertained in a younger child if an adult contact has a prolonged coughing illness.

Clinical Features
- **A catarrhal stage,** consisting of symptoms of an upper respiratory tract infection, lasts 1 to 2 weeks.
- **A paroxysmal stage** follows and is characterized by a distinctive, repeated, staccato cough that occurs during a single expiration, often emptying the lungs of all their vital capacity. In the following inspiration, a "whoop" sound is produced as the edematous, narrowed glottis oscillates between the open and closed position, causing the column of inspired air to vibrate. Whoops are not always present; rather some patients demonstrate posttussive emesis at the end of a paroxysm. Patients are usually well between paroxysmal attacks.

  With repeated coughing, facial redness or cyanosis and neck vein distension may occur. Petechiae of the head and neck and conjunctival hemorrhages may develop after severe coughing. Infants may develop respiratory distress, apnea, or both.

- **During the convalescent stage,** the frequency of paroxysms gradually decreases, although the cough often persists for several months (called the "100-day cough"). Habitual (or psychogenic) coughing may result in a few patients.

Evaluation

During the early paroxysmal phase, a **complete blood cell count may** reveal lymphocytosis. **Chest radiographs** may show perihilar infiltrates and subsegmental atelectasis. **Fluorescent antibody staining** can be performed on pharyngeal swabs to detect *B. pertussis*. A positive culture is necessary to confirm the diagnosis. Many states require notification to the department of health, and contacts may warrant prophylaxis.

Treatment

Erythromycin estolate can help reduce the spread of infection but does not shorten the disease once it progresses to the paroxysmal phase. Alternative therapy with clarithromycin or azithromycin may be effective and is more likely to be tolerated based on frequency of dosing, duration of therapy, and side effects. Supportive care consists of maintaining adequate **hydration,** administering **supplemental oxygen** for patients with respiratory distress, and **suctioning nasal secretions** in infants. **Inhaled bronchodilators** may help reduce coughing paroxysms. Cough suppressants are generally not helpful or recommended in young children, although they may sometimes be considered at bedtime in older patients with significant sleep disruption.

Structural Lesions

Structural lesions may occur at any point along the respiratory system and may cause respiratory symptoms any time from the early neonatal period onward. The symptoms may worsen in the face of an intercurrent acute respiratory illness such as a viral infection or asthma exacerbation. Treatment for lesions may involve **observation, medical therapy, or surgical intervention.**

Laryngomalacia, Tracheomalacia, and Bronchomalacia
Etiology

Weakened or softened underlying cartilaginous and/or muscular infrastructure of the airway results in **collapse of the airway** and **luminal narrowing.** The process may be **primary or secondary,** often caused by insults such as prolonged mechanical ventilation in the premature newborn or recurrent aspiration from gastroesophageal reflux disease.

Clinical Features

The patient may demonstrate **stridor if the lesion is extrathoracic** or **wheezing if the lesion is intrathoracic.** The wheeze is often homophonous and vibratory. The symptoms may be accentuated during crying or agitation or during an intercurrent acute respiratory illness.

Evaluation

The history and physical examination are often highly suggestive of the diagnosis. Confirmation requires visualization by **endoscopy.** Radiography, with lateral neck radiographs and/or airway fluoroscopy, are less helpful, although anterior and lateral chest films should be performed to evaluate for other causes of respiratory symptoms.

Treatment

Because airway collapsibility improves with increasing age, malacia usually **resolves spontaneously by 15 to 18 months of age.** Some children with tracheomalacia continue to have a characteristic loud or barky "smoker's" cough well into school age. Intercurrent acute illnesses should be managed accordingly, and causative diseases, such as reflux, should be treated appropriately. In severe cases, **positive airway pressure** (either noninvasively or invasively through a tracheostomy) or **surgical procedures** may be needed. Poor feeding, poor growth, cyanotic spells or recurrent apparent life-threatening events, or failure to follow a typical course of spontaneous improvement and resolution should all prompt further evaluation and intervention.

Traumatic Causes

Foreign Bodies
Etiology

Foreign bodies may be **inhaled into the airway,** or they may get **caught in the esophagus** and externally compress the trachea. Foreign body aspiration is more common in toddlers and infants, who tend to put objects in their mouths. Parents may even recall the exact time of the start of symptoms, and the symptoms often start suddenly without a prodrome of infection symptoms.

Clinical Features

If the object is **in the esophagus, drooling, dysphagia, and anorexia** may accompany **respiratory distress.** Respiratory symptoms may be **acute or chronic,** with a history of **chronic cough** unresponsive to other treatments.

Evaluation

A **monophonic wheeze or absent breath sounds on one side** may be noted on chest examination.

Chest and neck radiographs with lateral views may be helpful in identifying the location of an object. **Inspiratory and expiratory lateral**

decubitus films may denote an area of hyperinflation. Fluoroscopy may be used to show abnormal inflation or deflation in real-time. Retained foreign bodies, if small and not obstructing the larger airways, may result in chronic infection with persistent opacification on plain films and later bronchiectasis.

Arterial blood gas analysis (to establish the adequacy of gas exchange) is indicated when the patient is in severe distress.

Treatment

- If the child is calm with good air exchange, removal of the foreign body should take place under controlled circumstances because manipulation may change the position of the object, inducing more severe obstruction.
- If the child is in significant distress, back blows and chest thrusts may be performed as per the standard technique for cardiopulmonary resuscitation. **Emergency tracheostomy** may be necessary.

Aspiration Caused by Gastroesophageal Reflux Disease
Etiology

Gastroesophageal reflux disease (GERD) may cause respiratory symptoms from **large bolus aspiration, recurrent microaspiration, or reflex laryngospasm or bronchospasm.** Patients with underlying neurologic disorders are at increased risk for aspiration, although GERD may be found in children of all ages in the absence of other predisposing conditions.

Clinical Features

Patients may or may not have a history of **overt reflux with vomiting followed by coughing or choking.** Some patients may simply have **recurrent cough** (especially at night), **frequent stomachaches, heartburn or chest pain, globus, or sour burps.** With aspiration pneumonitis, significant **respiratory distress and hypoxemia** may occur as well as **fever.**

Evaluation

GERD is often clinically diagnosed by symptom recognition and trial of GERD therapy. Diagnostic procedures include **radionucleotide scan** (milk scan), **pH probe, and impedance pH testing.** To ensure the absence of an anatomic abnormality causing the reflux, an **upper gastrointestinal series** is often performed prior to the initiation of therapy. After aspiration, a **chest radiograph** may show a consolidation in the affected area.

Treatment

Aspiration pneumonitis requires **antibiotic therapy,** usually intravenous antibiotics until fever and significant respiratory symptoms have resolved.

GERD is usually treated with feeding precautions (liquid volume limitation, positioning) as well as **an H$_2$ blocker or proton pump inhibitor**, sometimes in combination with a **prokinetic agent**. In severe reflux that does not respond to medical therapy, **surgical treatment** (fundoplication) may be necessary.

Pneumothorax
Etiology

Trauma to the chest, foreign body aspiration (with a ball-valve effect), **severe underlying pulmonary disease, or idiopathic bulla formation** may result in the entry of air into the potential space between the parietal and visceral pleurae, impairing the ability of the chest wall to inflate the lung parenchyma adequately on the affected side. Patients with **asthma, cystic fibrosis, and connective tissue diseases** (e.g., Marfan syndrome) may be at **increased risk for pneumothorax**. Often, the precipitating event is a **Valsalva maneuver,** which causes a transient elevation of intrathoracic pressure. **Commercial air travel** in pressurized cabins and **scuba diving** are also risk factors.

Tension pneumothorax (a life-threatening event that results from the rapid filling of the pleural space by gas under pressure) can **distort the vascular flow** via compression and **cause rapid death.** Patients undergoing positive-pressure mechanical ventilation are at risk for tension pneumothorax.

Clinical Features

Symptoms are usually **abrupt in onset** and consist of **pleuritic chest pain, tachypnea, and hypoxemia.** With large pneumothoraces, **cough and cyanosis** may be seen as well. Shoulder pain may be a more subtle presenting symptom.

The degree of distress is related to the size of the pneumothorax, usually described as a percentage of the thoracic volume on the affected side. Small pneumothoraces may be asymptomatic.

Evaluation

A **history** of trauma, underlying lung disease, or past pneumothoraces from bullae should be elicited. **Chest examination** demonstrates **decreased breath sounds** on the affected side and **tympany** to percussion. **Heart tones may be shifted** toward the affected side (as a result of lung collapse) or away from the affected side (in patients with tension pneumothorax). **Transillumination of the chest** is helpful in demonstrating pneumothorax in young infants. **Chest radiographs** should be done in the expiratory phase to accentuate areas of hyperlucency. **Arterial blood gas analysis** may help establish the degree of ventilatory compromise. Chest computed tomography (CT) may be performed to evaluate for the presence of bullae, especially in spontaneous pneumothorax.

Treatment

Tension pneumothorax is a **medical emergency.** **Thoracentesis** should be attempted by placing a needle at the second anterior intercostal space at the midclavicular line. Care must be taken not to puncture the underlying lung. For large pneumothoraces, **tube thoracostomy** may be necessary to drain the air until the visceral pleura can repair itself. Occasionally, in patients with recurrent pneumothoraces, **sclerosing the pleura by chemical or physical means** to the internal chest wall is necessary to allow the lung to remain reexpanded. **Supplemental oxygen** should be given to hypoxemic patients. Inhalation of **100% oxygen can displace the nitrogen** in the gas that forms the pneumothorax, although this practice is not supported in research trials. Because oxygen is more readily absorbed by the body, displacement of nitrogen with oxygen can hasten resolution of the pneumothorax. A history of pneumothorax may result in delayed airplane travel and is considered a contraindication to scuba diving.

Neuromuscular Disorders
Etiology

Respiratory muscle weakness accompanies skeletal muscle weakness, and this weakness results in failure of the respiratory pump that functions in ventilation. Patients with neuromuscular diseases also may have a **weak cough** resulting in impaired airway clearance, potentially causing recurrent infections or atelectasis. Progressive muscular disease may result in the development of chronic respiratory insufficiency and failure. In the face of an acute respiratory illness, these patients are at risk for significant respiratory decompensation and acute respiratory failure.

Clinical Features

The patient may demonstrate **shallow, rapid respiratory pattern and a weak cough.** With worsening chronic respiratory failure, **morning headaches** and **poor sleep quality** may be present. **Hypoxemia and respiratory distress** may accompany an acute illness.

Evaluation

Pulmonary function testing, including spirometry, lung volumes, and maximal respiratory pressures, should be measured on a regular basis to follow the patient's trend. **End tidal carbon dioxide level** may indicate worsening ventilatory failure. **Overnight polysomnography** is used to evaluate sleep pattern, respiratory events, and oxygenation and ventilation during sleep.

Treatment

Aggressive airway clearance and assisted coughing, on a regular basis as well as during an acute illness, are the mainstays of therapy. **Early**

recognition of impending chronic respiratory failure should be followed by early **initiation of nocturnal noninvasive ventilation.** Some patients progress to needing 24-hour support, which warrants consideration for invasive chronic mechanical ventilation via **tracheostomy.**

Miscellaneous Causes

Asthma

The triggers for asthma are discussed in Chapter 23, "Cough." This discussion focuses on asthma as a cause of respiratory distress and impending respiratory failure.

Clinical Features

Important differential diagnoses include **anaphylaxis and foreign body aspiration.** A thorough history should be taken, including the **duration, frequency, and severity of attacks;** the **medications** the patient uses acutely and chronically, as well as any used during this particular exacerbation; **peak flows** (if the patient keeps a log); and the **family history.** On physical examination, the **expiratory phase is prolonged. Breath sounds are often tubular or decreased** at the bases. **Heterophonous wheezing** is usually appreciated diffusely, but it may be absent when air exchange is severely affected.

Evaluation

A **pulsus paradoxus** may be measured. If the patient is severely affected, **arterial blood gases** can be ordered to assess oxygenation and carbon dioxide elimination. Table 66-1 lists the normal values. **Pulse oximetry** is useful for determining oxygenation status. **Spirometry** may be helpful in patients with mild to moderate symptoms but should not be performed in the presence of significant distress.

> **HINT:** A near-normal carbon dioxide tension in the presence of significant tachypnea heralds impending respiratory failure.

Treatment

- **Oxygen** should be administered to all patients with evidence of hypoxemia.
- **Bronchodilation.** Patients with mild symptoms may improve with the inhalation of a β-agonist, such as albuterol. The continuous use of nebulized albuterol (administered at a rate of 10 to 40 mg/hour) in severely affected patients with impending respiratory failure is often necessary. Care must be taken to monitor for hypokalemia, a side

TABLE 66-1 Normal Blood Gas Values from the Children's Hospital of Philadelphia Blood Gas Laboratory

Parameter	Age of Patient	Normal Value
pH	1 day	7.29–7.45
	3–24 months	7.34–7.46
	>7 years	7.37–7.41
P_{CO_2}	1 day	27–40 mm Hg
	3–24 months	26–42 mm Hg
	>7 years	34–40 mm Hg
P_{O_2}	1 day	37–97 mm Hg
	3–24 months	88–103 mm Hg
	>7 years	88–103 mm Hg
Base excess	1 day	>8–(–2)
	3–24 months	–7–0
	>7 years	–4–(+2)
HCO_3	1 day	19 mmol/L
	3–24 months	16/24 mmol/L
	>7 years	22–27 mmol/L
O_2 saturation	—	94%–99%
Venous pH	—	7.32–7.42
Venous CO_2	—	25–47 mm Hg
Venous O_2	—	25–47 mm Hg

CO_2 = carbon dioxide; HCO_3 = bicarbonate; O_2 = oxygen; P_{CO_2} = carbon dioxide tension; P_{O_2} = oxygen tension.

effect of high-dose albuterol therapy. Intravenous bronchodilators, such as terbutaline, may also be considered in severe patients.

■ **Fluids and steroids.** Patients with severe symptoms may benefit from intravenous fluids because patients are often dehydrated from the underlying viral illness or from increased fluid loss caused by the work of breathing. Oral or intravenous steroids (usually prednisone or methylprednisolone sodium succinate, 1 to 2 mg/kg per day) are vitally important in the management of an asthma exacerbation to treat the inflammation.

■ **Aminophylline.** The intravenous administration of aminophylline may be helpful in some patients, but constant cardiac monitoring is indicated. Although terbutaline and aminophylline are equally effective in continuous infusion, aminophylline has significantly worse side effects.

■ **Magnesium.** Intravenous magnesium has been shown to improve pulmonary function in severe exacerbations.

Atelectasis
Etiology
Partial or complete collapse of normally aerated pulmonary parenchyma can result from an **intraluminal obstruction, extrinsic compression of the airway, or decreased respiratory muscle strength.** Loss of gas-exchanging regions of the lung may lead to **ventilation-perfusion mismatching** and **respiratory distress.**

Atelectasis is common in **postoperative patients** with impaired respiratory drive or muscle strength, **patients with infection or bronchospasm** leading to airway plugging, and **patients with alterations in the normal airway structure** as a result of congenital lesions, bronchopulmonary dysplasia, or recurrent aspiration.

Evaluation

Breath sounds may be decreased in the affected area. Anteroposterior and lateral **chest radiographs** help delineate the affected region. Volume loss results in displacement of fissures or hemidiaphragm toward the area of atelectasis.

Treatment

Definitive treatment entails eliminating the pathologic process that is responsible for the atelectasis. **Chest physiotherapy** and **postural drainage** combined with **bronchodilator therapy** can help reexpand atelectatic areas. In refractory cases, **bronchoscopy** may help remove a particularly tenacious mucus plug. **Supplemental oxygen** is indicated for patients with hypoxemia. In the postoperative period, **early incentive spirometry, early ambulation, and good pain control** are helpful in preventing atelectasis.

Vocal Cord Dysfunction
Etiology

Vocal cord dysfunction (VCD) is a paradoxical closure of the vocal cords (of unclear etiology) during periods of high-flow breathing (such as exercise or hyperventilation). It is often misdiagnosed as asthma, but it is unresponsive to typical bronchodilator therapy or even long-term controller therapy with inhaled corticosteroids. Although most often seen in competitive athletes and high-performing individuals, it often develops as a somatic manifestation of **psychosocial stress** in preadolescents and adolescents.

Clinical Features

The **associated cough and respiratory distress are real** and a result of paradoxical vocal cord movement. Stridor or difficulty inspiring may be noted, especially during sporting events or stressful activities. Sour taste or heartburn, caused by GERD, may also be noted before or at the same time as the respiratory difficulty.

Evaluation

Consideration should be made in the patient diagnosed with asthma who does not respond to appropriate asthma therapy, especially if the patient has a competitive, high-achieving, or anxious temperament.

An attempt should be made to **identify significant psychosocial stressors** in the patient's life. Sometimes sports and exercise are withheld by parents and/or coaches until a diagnosis is confirmed. On physical examination, **wheezing is absent** or a monophonic inspiratory wheeze is heard on auscultation of the neck. **Flow-volume loops** performed as part of pulmonary function testing may show **flattening of the inspiratory curve.** **Exercise testing** may reproduce symptoms or demonstrate flattening of the inspiratory loop, often without reduction in spirometry flows seen with exercise-induced asthma.

Flexible laryngoscopy can sometimes identify paradoxical vocal cord movement.

Treatment

Vocal cord muscle relaxation exercises, taught by an experienced speech pathologist, are often very effective. **Psychological counseling and/or biofeedback** may be appropriate if symptoms persist. Many patients with VCD also have true **asthma;** for these patients, appropriate asthma therapy is indicated. A protocol often is provided for the patient to use for relief of symptoms in cases where both VCD and asthma exist. With therapy, the patient should be able to continue or resume sports and other activities that triggered the symptoms.

APPROACH TO THE PATIENT

The physician should consider typical and common illnesses for the patient's age and underlying medical conditions. A focused history should be taken, with special attention to onset of symptoms, presence of prodromal symptoms of infection, course and duration of symptoms, and response to therapies tried. A detailed history may be postponed in the case of severe respiratory distress, so emergency life support measures may be performed. On physical examination, one may note **tachypnea, tachycardia, decreased oxyhemoglobin saturation, positioning with the neck hyperextended, cyanosis, nasal flaring, retractions or accessory muscle use, grunting, wheezing, or stridor.** Helpful diagnostic studies include **arterial blood gas, radiographic studies** (chest radiograph, chest CT scan, upper airway films, fluoroscopy, barium swallow, bronchogram, pulmonary arteriogram, ventilation perfusion scan), **endoscopy, and pulmonary function testing.** Some procedures may need to be delayed in severe distress. The underlying cause of respiratory distress should be sought and treated, if possible. In some cases, supportive care is the only recommended option for treatment. Hallmarks of therapy include **maintaining airway patency, oxygenation, and circulation** first and foremost. Continuing care may involve a variety of medical treatments, including **bronchodilators, anti-inflammatories, airway clearance, antimicrobials,** analgesia, and even invasive or noninvasive **mechanical ventilation.** Surgical procedures, such as **airway endoscopy, thoracentesis** or **lung biopsy,** may be necessary for diagnosis or treatment. Untreated respiratory distress may advance to respiratory failure, in which oxygenation and ventilation are impaired.

Suggested Readings

American Academy of Pediatrics Subcommittee on Diagnosis and Management of Bronchiolitis: Diagnosis and management of bronchiolitis. *Pediatrics* 118(4):1774–1793, 2006.

Bent J: Pediatric laryngotracheal obstruction: current perspectives on stridor. *Laryngoscope* 116(7):1059–1070, 2006.

Lichenstein R, Suggs AH, Campbell J: Pediatric pneumonia. *Emerg Med Clin North Am* 21(2):437–451, 2003.

National Asthma Education and Prevention Program: Expert Panel Report 3. NIH Publication No. 08-4051. Bethesda, MD. See www.nhlbi. nih.gov/guidelines/asthma

Panitch HB: Respiratory issues in the management of children with neuromuscular disease. *Respir Care* 51(8):885–893; discussion 894–895, 2006.

Rafei K, Lichenstein R: Airway infectious disease emergencies. *Pediatr Clin North Am* 53(2):215–242, 2006.

Sanchez I, Navarro H, Mendez M, et al.: Clinical characteristics of children with tracheobronchial anomalies. *Pediatr Pulmonol* 35(4):288–291, 2003.

Werner HA: Status asthmaticus in children: a review. *Chest* 119(6): 1913–1929, 2001.

INTRODUCTION

When evaluating a patient with acute scrotal pain, **testicular torsion** should be considered **the diagnosis until proven otherwise.** This complaint must be **evaluated in person;** telephone consultation for such symptoms is dangerous because valuable time may be wasted, leading to testicular loss. Approximately 25% of males presenting with acute scrotal pain to a hospital emergency department prove to have testicular torsion. This represents a **surgical emergency** because **testicular viability is compromised beyond 8 hours** of warm ischemia time. Therefore, patients presenting with this complaint must be given high priority in an acute-care setting.

Another inherent danger in evaluating this complaint is the definition of "acute" because the patient's time frame is often different from that of the clinician. **Adolescent patients are especially at risk** because the **symptoms are often denied** for some time before treatment is sought. This may account for the fact that the salvage rate is lowest in this age group. It is also important that the clinician not be led astray by a **history of trauma** because this history **can mask a serious testicular problem.**

DIFFERENTIAL DIAGNOSIS LIST

Testicular torsion
Torsion of the appendix testis
Epididymitis
Hernia/hydrocele
Trauma
Varicocele

Tumor
Bites and stings
Henoch-Schönlein purpura
Mumps orchitis
Vasculitis
Ureteral colic (referred pain)

DIFFERENTIAL DIAGNOSIS DISCUSSION

Common Causes

Of the entities shown in the differential diagnostic list, 95% fall into one of the top-four categories. In one study, almost 70% of all cases of acute scrotal pain were classified as either a testicular torsion or torsion of the appendix testis.

Testicular Torsion

Testicular torsion results from a **complete twist of the testis on its vascular pedicle.** The **resulting ischemia** produces **pain** that can be **constant** or, at times, colicky. The **sudden onset of pain** is often accompanied by **nausea and vomiting.** The testis in question **is pulled up high in the scrotum** (secondary to the twists in the spermatic cord). In the majority of cases, **no cremasteric reflex** can be elicited. A strong 2- to 4-cm testicular excursion during a cremasteric reflex usually rules out acute testicular torsion, although this sign is less reliable in delayed presentations. Because the cremasteric reflex is not always present, especially in older males, **absence of a cremasteric reflex does not invoke a diagnosis** of testicular torsion.

Testicular torsion is felt to occur **secondary to a congenital anatomic malpositioning of the testis,** termed the **bell-clapper deformity.** A normal testis and its blood supply are attached to the tunica vaginalis posteriorly. However, with the bell-clapper deformity, **no such posterior attachment exists to anchor the testis** and prevent it from twisting completely around its blood supply. Establishing this **diagnosis early on is crucial,** for the situation presents a **surgical emergency;** the longer the delay in diagnosis, the lower the chances for testicular salvage.

Torsion of the Appendix Testis

Torsion of the appendix testis results when this tiny müllerian remnant twists around its base and ischemia results. The typical presentation is characterized by a **gradual onset of pain,** and patients often note significant **scrotal swelling** and **erythema** secondary to a **reactive hydrocele.** The appetite is unaffected and nausea and vomiting are rare. It is often possible to elicit a **strong cremasteric reflex,** which greatly aids in distinguishing this condition from torsion of the testis. If the patient presents early on, **point tenderness** is noted **on the upper outer pole.** Some patients have a **blue dot on the scrotum.** Once the diagnosis is established, treatment consists of **nonsteroidal anti-inflammatories and rest.** Over a 1-week period, 90% to 95% of these patients improve with no need for further treatment. In about 5% to 10% of cases, the **appendix torses intermittently,** and **surgical excision of the appendix testis** is warranted.

Epididymitis

This diagnosis is **extremely rare in the prepubertal boy.** A true bacterial epididymitis in a prepubertal boy is usually secondary to a urethral stricture or posterior urethral valve. In the adolescent male, the usual causes of bacterial epididymitis are **chlamydia or gonorrhea.** However, at times the adolescent male may present with a **normal urinalysis and a tender and inflamed epididymis.** Often these patients present **following a period of heavy physical exertion** such as weight lifting. It is believed that **reflux of sterile urine via the prostatic ducts under pressure** sets up an **inflammation** within the epididymis. Regardless of etiology, the diagnosis of epididymitis is established by the history and physical findings. The **onset of pain is slow,** and the **appetite is preserved.**

A history of **urethral discharge and/or dysuria** may be noted. The physical examination demonstrates a **nontender testis,** with a **large and very tender epididymis** palpable posteriorly.

Hernia/Hydrocele

Patients may present with an acute herniation that produces **significant pain.** This is because the hernia sac represents an extension of the peritoneal cavity, which, when suddenly distended, can cause pain. The findings of an **enlarged scrotum** that transilluminates in conjunction with a **thickened inguinal bulge** provide evidence for a **patent processus vaginalis.** This allows for **peritoneal fluid to roll down and pool within the scrotum.** The **testis is not tender** in this setting. On occasion the patent processus vaginalis expands from a **small tunnel** that only allows for **passage of fluid to a much larger diameter** that enables **bowel or omentum to herniate** into the sac. Presence of bowel or omentum produces a **thicker spermatic cord.** On occasion the bowel or omentum becomes **inflamed,** causing pain, and becoming more difficult to reduce. At this point **surgical consultation** is required.

EVALUATION OF ACUTE SCROTAL PAIN

Despite technological advances in Doppler sonography, the vast majority of patients presenting with scrotal pain may be accurately diagnosed with a **complete history and physical examination,** especially when patients present early in the course of their symptoms. **After 8 to 12 hours of inflammation,** it becomes much more difficult to distinguish the individual scrotal contents, and it is in this setting that **Doppler sonography** becomes especially useful. Table 67-1 summarizes the diagnostic features for acute scrotal pain.

Patient History

The history provides valuable clues to the cause of acute scrotal pain. Answers to the following specific questions should be sought:

- Has the patient ever experienced pain like this before? Often patients with torsion have had several episodes of intermittent torsion preceding the current presentation.
- Was the onset sharp and acute in onset, or slow and gradual? Patients with testicular torsion may be able to note the time of day when the pain began. In some instances, the pain awakens the patient from sleep.
- Has there been nausea or vomiting? The presence of these symptoms is often seen with testicular torsion. In contrast, boys presenting with a torsed appendix testis often are hungry.
- Is the patient having difficulty finding a position of comfort? In testicular torsion, parents describe their child as restless and writhing.

TABLE 67-1 Diagnostic Features of Acute Scrotal Pain

	Testicular Torsion	Torsed Appendix	Epididymitis	Hernia/ Hydrocele
History				
Sudden onset	+	+/−	−	+/−
Nausea/vomiting	+	−	−	−
Altered gait	−	+	−	−
Prior episodes	+	−	+/−	+
Physical Examination				
High riding	+	−	−	−
Transilluminates	−	+/−	−	+
Cremasteric reflex	−	+	+	+/−
Laboratory				
Urine dipstick	−	−	+/−	−
Radiology				
Doppler flow	−	+	+	+
Radionuclide perfusion	−	+	+	+

Patients with a torsed appendix testis prefer to lie still, and parents may describe a change in their child's gait while walking. This wide-based gait (cowboy gait) produces less parietal irritation of the inflamed tunica vaginalis and tunica albuginea.

Physical Examination

Observation of the patient provides useful clues. The patient who is in obvious pain and writhing at times has a higher likelihood of having testicular torsion. In contrast, the patient with a torsed appendix testis prefers to lie still. The appearance of the scrotum is also helpful, for if one testis is high riding, this clue favors testicular torsion. This is because the torsed testis has a shorter spermatic cord because of the twisting that has produced the ischemia. A major component of the physical examination is the eliciting of the cremasteric reflexes. A brisk stroking of the inner thigh should result in a rise in the testis that is prominent (at least 2 cm). Such a brisk cremasteric reflex is not seen in cases of testicular torsion in which the twisted cord precludes such movement.

> **HINT:** A high-riding testis and absent cremasteric reflex are strong signs suggesting that testicular torsion is present.

An effort should be made to distinguish pain within the testis from pain in the epididymis or an inflamed appendix testis. With a gentle touch it is often possible to isolate the localized point tenderness associated with an early torsed appendix testis, which is always located on the upper outer pole. If the examiner's large fingers diminish such accuracy, the use of a **pencil eraser** can be helpful in locating the **exact point of discomfort.** Doppler stethoscopes were recommended in the past to diagnose torsion, but false-positive and false-negative results have rendered this test ineffective. However, the sound of the Doppler and the distraction it provides make it useful while probing for point tenderness.

Finally, note that **manual detorsion of a torsed testis** can be **diagnostic** as well as **temporarily therapeutic.** Early on in the course of testicular torsion, the testis can be rotated laterally in a series of 180° flips. Because 80% of all torsions occur with a medial rotation of the testes, detorsion should **first be tried with a lateral rotation.** Once the critical turns are reached, the **relief of pain is instantaneous.** If the pain subsides, this can be diagnostic. If access to the operating room or surgical subspecialist is limited, manual detorsion can be a valuable maneuver. However, the patient must be **explored as soon as possible,** for **retorsion** may occur, and despite relief of symptoms, there may still be a **residual twist** in the cord producing venous stasis.

Laboratory Studies

A **urine dipstick test** should be performed to assist in the workup of epididymitis, **especially important in adolescent males.** If a urethral discharge is present, swabs should be sent for **gonorrheal cultures** as well as **chlamydia** screening.

Imaging Studies

Scrotal pain lasting **>12 hours** is often associated with **significant inflammation and edema** that renders the physical examination less accurate. The **exquisite point tenderness** seen with a torsed appendix testis **becomes less prominent as a reactive hydrocele forms,** and the **tunica vaginalis and albuginea become inflamed.** Surprisingly, many teenagers have stoically dealt with their pain and the physical examination reveals only mild discomfort with palpation.

In this kind of setting, **Doppler ultrasound** has become the imaging modality of choice. This noninvasive test is readily available and provides a quick answer as to whether or not blood flow is present within the testis itself. This **spatial localization of blood flow is crucial** because the handheld Doppler stethoscope often picks up arterial flow within the scrotal wall. The spatial localization of flow (or lack thereof) makes Doppler sonography far more accurate. The role of **nuclear scintigraphy** has faded because procuring of isotope during off-peak hours can be a rate-limiting step. As such this test takes longer to perform in the scenario of a diagnosis in which time is of the essence. In some institutions, this may still remain the diagnostic test of choice, and it remains an accepted and valid measure of testicular perfusion.

As accurate as such technology might be, it is **critical to remember that the image is but one moment in time.** Cases are reported in which flow was present at one time and subsequent exploration demonstrated testicular torsion. This serves as a reminder that **intermittent testicular torsion** is a real phenomenon, and on occasion urologists recommend **surgical correction even in the presence of blood flow,** based on the **history alone.**

Surgery

When there is doubt about the diagnosis of testicular torsion, it is prudent to perform **exploratory surgery.** If a surgical team is 100% accurate in their diagnosis of the acute scrotum, they are missing the occasional case of torsion. It is **never wrong to operate and establish an exact diagnosis** of the acute scrotum by ruling out torsion. Although it is true that Doppler sonography has made negative exploratory surgery more rare, the fact remains that the study is not perfect. **Testes may torse and detorse** to a point **allowing for arterial inflow at the time of the actual study.** The best way to establish the diagnosis is by examining the patient at the time of symptom occurrence. However, occasionally physicians are asked to assess the patient who has pain of short duration without classic symptoms. This patient may have **intermittent torsion** and could benefit from elective orchiopexies. Such patients should still be **referred for urologic evaluation** and are advised to **keep a diary** of such episodes, noting their **frequency, degree of pain, and duration.**

Suggested Readings

Barada JH, Weingarten JL, Cromie WJ: Testicular salvage and age-related delay in the presentation of testicular torsion. *J Urol* 142:746–747, 1989.

Cattolica EV: Preoperative manual detorsion of the torsed spermatic cord. *J Urol* 133:803–804, 1985.

Cronan KM, Zderic SA: Manual detorsion of the testes. In *Textbook of Pediatric Emergency Procedures.* Edited by Henretig FM, King C. Baltimore, Williams & Wilkins, 1991, 1003–1006.

Kadish HA, Bolte RG: A retrospective review of pediatric patients with epididymitis, testicular torsion, and torsion of testicular appendages. *Pediatrics* 102:73–76, 1998.

Kass EJ, Lundak B: The acute scrotum. *Pediatr Clin North Am* 44(5): 1251–1266, 1997.

Lewis AG, Bukowski TP, Jarvis PD, et al.: Evaluation of acute scrotum in the emergency department. *J Pediatr Surg* 30(2) 277–282, 1995.

Siegel A, Snyder H, Duckett JW: Related epididymitis in infants and boys: underlying urogenital anomalies and efficacy of imaging modalities. *J Urol* 133:1100–1103, 1987.

INTRODUCTION

A seizure is a spell characterized by altered behavior, consciousness, sensation, or autonomic function caused by hypersynchronous excessive firing of neurons. **Generalized** seizures initially involve the entire cortex, and consciousness is generally lost. **Partial** seizures begin in one portion of the brain with symptoms related to that region's function. They may either remain restricted to that location without affected alertness (**simple partial** seizure), spread to involve adjacent regions such that consciousness is affected (**complex partial** seizures), or may spread widely to involve the entire cortex (**secondary generalization**). Seizures may occur in an individual with an underlying tendency to have seizures (**epilepsy**) or may be secondary to an ongoing process that primarily or secondarily affects the central nervous system (CNS) (acute **symptomatic seizures**). The initial evaluation of a patient with a seizure must focus on identifying and treating any underlying condition that may be causing seizures. Prolonged or multiple recurrent seizures without return to baseline mental status is called **status epilepticus**. Seizures are described by the behavioral manifestations.

Epilepsy is defined by recurrent unprovoked seizures. It is one of the most common neurologic conditions with a pediatric incidence of about 75 per 100,000 children. Epilepsy may be **symptomatic** (an underlying cause is known), **cryptogenic** (an underlying cause is suspected but not identified, as in a child with chronic static encephalopathy of unknown etiology that includes seizures as a manifestation), or **idiopathic** (presumed genetic etiology). Table 68-1 lists common terms related to seizures and epilepsy, and Table 68-2 lists events that may mimic seizures. In some patients, the clinical history, age, seizure type, and electroencephalogram (EEG) findings can be grouped into an epilepsy syndrome that can guide management and suggest prognosis (see Tables 68-3 and 68-4).

> **HINT:** Consider acute symptomatic etiologies when evaluating a patient with a first seizure. Unprovoked seizures (epilepsy) is a diagnosis of exclusion.

TABLE 68-1 Common Terms Used to Describe Seizures and Epilepsy

Aura. Symptom felt by patient because of a seizure such as sensory symptoms (abdominal discomfort, abnormal smell), psychic symptoms (déjà vu, sudden fear).

Automatism. Coordinated, involuntary movements during a period of altered consciousness

Complex seizure. Focal seizure with altered consciousness.

Cryptogenic epilepsy. Suspected to be symptomatic but no identified etiology on imaging and other testing.

Epilepsy. Chronic disorder of the brain characterized by a disposition toward recurrent unprovoked seizures.

Epilepsy syndrome. Combination of seizure type, EEG findings, clinical information and often other information that allows for more specific treatment and prognostication.

Generalized epilepsy. Epilepsy in which seizures initially involve both hemispheres.

Ictal. Seizure.

Idiopathic epilepsy. Unknown cause, generally used to describe genetic epilepsies.

Localization-related epilepsy. Epilepsy with partial onset seizures (also called focal epilepsy).

Postictal. Period immediately following a seizure.

Prodrome/Premonition. Vague sense or agitation patient may feel before seizure.

Reflex epilepsy. Seizures precipitated by a stimulus (reading, eating, startle).

Seizure. Sudden spell characterized by altered behavior, consciousness, sensation, or autonomic function because of hypersynchronous excessive firing of neurons.

Semiology. Clinical seizure manifestations.

Simple seizure. Focal seizure with no change in consciousness.

Symptomatic. Seizure with an identified cause.

Acute symptomatic. Seizure caused by ongoing medical condition (infection, hypoglycemia.)

Remote symptomatic. Seizure caused by remote brain lesion (poststroke, postinfection).

TABLE 68-2 Nonseizure Etiologies of Transient Neurologic Events

Neurologic

Stroke/Transient ischemic attack
Migraine headache
Movement disorders
Reflex movements

Cardiac

Vasovagal syncope (which may be followed by a seizure in syncopal convulsion)
Arrhythmia
Hypotension

Endocrine/Metabolic

Hypoglycemia
Hyponatremia

(Continued)

TABLE 68-2 *(Continued)*

Sleep Disorders

Hypnic jerks
Benign sleep myoclonus
Parasomnias
Narcolepsy/Cataplexy

Psychological

Nonepileptic psychogenic seizures (pseudoseizures)—conversion disorder

Other

Breath holding
Masturbation
Gastroesophageal reflux
Behavior
Apparent life-threatening event

DIFFERENTIAL DIAGNOSIS LIST

Neurological Etiologies

Neurovascular
  Ischemic stroke
  Sinovenous thrombosis
  Intracerebral hemorrhage
  Subarachnoid hemorrhage
  Arteriovenous malformation
  Hyperperfusion syndrome
Tumor
  Primary
  Metastatic
Infection
  Meningitis
  Encephalitis
  Abscess
  Cat-scratch disease
  Tick-borne disorders
Inflammatory
  Acute disseminated
    encephalomyelitis
  Vasculitis
  Lupus cerebritis
  Rasmussen syndrome

TABLE 68-3 Classification of Epileptic Seizures

Generalized

Typical absence
Atypical absence
Myoclonic
Tonic
Clonic
Tonic-clonic
Atonic
Infantile spasms

Partial/Focal/Localization Related

Simple
Complex
Secondarily generalized

TABLE 68-4 International Classification of Epilepsy Syndromes

Neonates

Benign familial seizures
Early myoclonic encephalopathy
Ohtahara syndrome
Migrating partial seizures of infancy

Infants

West syndrome
Aicardi syndrome
Benign myoclonic epilepsy of infancy
Severe myoclonic epilepsy of infancy (Dravet syndrome)
Benign infantile seizures

Children

Benign childhood epilepsy with centrotemporal spikes (Rolandic epilepsy)
Early-onset benign childhood occipital epilepsy (Panayiotopoulos syndrome)
Late-onset childhood occipital epilepsy (Gastaut syndrome)
Epilepsy with myoclonic absences
Myoclonic-astatic epilepsy of childhood
Lennox-Gastaut syndrome
Landau-Kleffner syndrome
Epilepsy with continuous spike and waves during slow wave sleep (ESES)
Childhood absence epilepsy
Progressive myoclonic epilepsies
Lafora body disease
Unverricht-Lundborg syndrome (Baltic myoclonus)
Neuronal ceroid lipofuscinosis
Myoclonic epilepsy with ragged red fibers (MERRF)
Sialidoses

Juvenile/Adult

Idiopathic generalized epilepsies
    Juvenile absence epilepsy
    Juvenile myoclonic epilepsy
    Epilepsy with generalized tonic-clonic seizures only
Reflex epilepsies
    Idiopathic photosensitive occipital lobe epilepsy
    Primary reading epilepsy
    Startle epilepsy

Trauma
  Contusion
  Epidural hematoma
  Subdural hematoma
  Subarachnoid hemorrhage
  Depressed skull fracture
Neurosurgery
Inherited
  Neurodegenerative disorders

Congenital and Intrauterine
  Brain malformations
  Neonatal hypoxic ischemic
    injury
  Congenital infections
Primary Epilepsy

Systemic Etiologies

Hypoxia-Ischemia
Drug Toxicity

Amphetamines
Cocaine
Phencyclidine (PCP)
Local anesthetics
Antipsychotics
Antidepressants
Immunosuppressants
Antibiotics
Drug Withdrawal
Benzodiazepines
Barbiturates
Opioids
Alcohol
Febrile Infection (not involving the CNS)
Metabolic Abnormalities
Hypoglycemia
Hyponatremia
Hypophosphatemia
Renal dysfunction
Hepatic dysfunction
Metabolic Disorders
Urea cycle disorders
Aminoacidopathies
Organic acidurias
Mitochondrial encephalopathies
Storage diseases
Vitamin B_6 (pyridoxine) deficiency
Folinic acid responsive seizures
Nonketotic hyperglycinemia

DIFFERENTIAL DIAGNOSIS DISCUSSION

Benign Childhood Epilepsy with Centrotemporal Spikes (Rolandic Epilepsy)

Benign childhood epilepsy is one of the most common idiopathic focal epilepsy syndromes of childhood. Onset is typically between 2 and 13 years of age, most often between 5 and 10 years of age. It most often presents with predominantly **nocturnal** seizures that include salivation, clonic mouth movements, and gurgling sounds. Daytime seizures are less common and generally consist of speech arrest and face/arm clonic movements with preserved consciousness. Normal cognitive function and neurologic examination are present. EEG demonstrates sharp waves in one or both centrotemporal regions. **Antiepileptic drug (AED)** treatment is considered optional, and it is usually easy to control seizures if treatment is initiated. The syndrome is often outgrown by adolescence.

Juvenile Myoclonic Epilepsy

Juvenile myoclonic epilepsy is another idiopathic generalized epilepsy syndrome that generally starts somewhat later in the early teenage years. It is characterized by **myoclonic seizures seen soon after awakening** with involvement of the **upper extremities.** This condition is often misconstrued as morning clumsiness. Patients usually come to medical attention with generalized tonic-clonic seizures. These adolescents have normal cognitive function and neurologic examinations. EEG may be entirely normal in the waking state but typically shows irregular fast spike and wave pattern during sleep and occasionally precipitated by photic stimulation. Seizures may be exacerbated by sleep deprivation, stress, and alcohol consumption. Although seizures are usually easily treated, they often recur if treatment is discontinued, so individuals must prepare for the possibility of lifelong therapy.

Childhood Absence Epilepsy

Childhood absence epilepsy is the most common idiopathic generalized epilepsy syndrome of childhood with a typical onset between 4 and 10 years of age with a **peak at 5 to 7 years of age.** Most children have normal cognitive function and neurologic examination, although associated behavioral impairments (e.g., attention deficit hyperactivity disorder) is overly represented. Seizures are brief (4 to 10 seconds), with frequent (>10/day) arrest of activity with **loss of awareness.** They may occur hundreds of times per day (often far more often than recognized by caregivers) and thus may **interfere with learning.** EEG demonstrates 3-Hz generalized spike and waves provoked by hyperventilation. Seizures are usually easily treated and often remit by adolescence.

Juvenile Absence Epilepsy

Juvenile absence epilepsy is very similar to childhood absence epilepsy, but this idiopathic generalized epilepsy syndrome has a later onset at 10 to 17 years of age with a **peak at 12 to 14 years of age.** Normal cognitive function and neurologic examination are usually present. **EEG** demonstrates generalized spike-wave discharges at 3.5 to 4.5 Hz. Seizures are much less frequent, often less than a few per week, also brought out by fatigue and hyperventilation. They are also usually easily treated but often recur if treatment is discontinued, so lifelong therapy may be required. Some develop generalized tonic-clonic seizures.

West Syndrome

West syndrome is an age-related epileptic encephalopathy with typical onset between **4 and 12 months of age.**

Only one third of these individuals are neurologically and developmentally normal before onset (idiopathic); two thirds have preexisting **abnormalities (symptomatic). West syndrome is defined by the triad of infantile spasms, mental** retardation **and hypsarrhythmia on EEG.** Infantile spasms describe the seizure type, which can be flexor or extensor (also referred to as jackknife seizure or **"salaam"** attacks). They tend to occur on sleep-wake transition in clusters. The EEG pattern is hypsarrhythmic (irregular, high amplitude, disorganized spikes and slow waves). Etiologies vary widely from neonatal hypoxic ischemic injury or infection to brain malformations, tuberous sclerosis, and Down syndrome. Evaluation for etiology generally includes magnetic resonance imaging (MRI) and sometimes metabolic testing. About half progress to Lennox-Gastaut syndrome. Only about 10% have good outcome, mostly those in the idiopathic group.

Treatment is usually **adrenocorticotropic hormone** given in low dose in a daily intravenous injection; it is important to rule out infections before initiating treatment and monitory closely for side effects. **Vigabatrin** may be especially useful in patients with tuberous sclerosis. Standard AEDs (especially topiramate) may be appropriate with symptomatic etiology.

Lennox-Gastaut Syndrome

This devastating seizure syndrome is a triad of diffuse **slow spike waves on EEG, mental retardation,** and multiple types of **generalized seizures.** Onset is usually from 2 to 8 years of age. It can appear de novo or evolve from West syndrome. Common seizure types include atypical absence, tonic, and atonic seizures. Remission is rare; severe cognitive impairment is common.

Landau-Kleffner Syndrome

Insidious onset of **aphasia** at 3 to 8 years of age (typically progressive verbal auditory agnosia) may mimic autistic regression. Most have seizures preceding or with the onset of language problems, although epilepsy is generally mild with seizures that are easy to control. **EEG** demonstrates bilateral temporal or parieto-occipital spikes and spike waves that are dramatically activated during slow-wave sleep. It is called **electrical status epilepticus of sleep** if a substantial portion of the record contains epileptiform discharges. Although seizures are usually controlled by medication, language disorder may be more difficult to treat and persists in half of affected children.

Febrile Seizures

Febrile seizures are the most common cause of seizures in children, occurring in 2% to 4% of those between **6 months and 5 years of age. Simple** febrile seizures are seizures that occur associated with **fever** in children **without an underlying neurologic disorder;** they are **generalized,** last **<15 minutes,** and there is only **one seizure in 24 hours.** With simple febrile seizures, there is up to a 30% to 50% risk of recurrence, but only a 2% to 3% risk of epilepsy. There is no effect on development or cognition. **Complex** febrile seizures are those which are focal, >15 minutes, or recurrent in 24 hours. If all three characteristics are present, then there is a 50% risk of epilepsy. Research is ongoing, but at this time it is unclear whether prolonged febrile seizures cause mesial temporal sclerosis. MRI should be performed if there are focal features. Diagnostic evaluation begins with identification and treatment of the source of fever. Common etiologies are similar to those seen with fever without seizure (see Chapter 33, "Fever"). Because seizure can be the initial manifestation of CNS infection, one should consider **lumbar puncture (LP)** in an infant <12 to 18 months of age in whom CNS infection may be difficult to rule out by clinical examination or if an older patient remains lethargic, irritable, or does not return to baseline. Neuroimaging and EEG are generally not required if the seizure was simple. Only phenobarbital and valproate have shown efficacy in clinical trials, but neither is generally indicated. Antipyretics are not effective in preventing the recurrence of febrile seizures, which often occur at the onset of fever.

Neonatal Seizures

Seizures in the first weeks of life are usually subtle rather than well-localized partial or symmetric, generalized tonic-clonic seizures. Typically they show lip smacking, eye deviation, focal motor, autonomic variability or myoclonus. Most neonatal seizures are in **response to injury** from an identifiable cause (60% hypoxic-ischemic injury, 20% intracerebral hemorrhage or infarction, 5% to 10% infections, and 5% to 10% other disorders including metabolic disease). In the first 3 days of life, one should primarily consider hypoxic-ischemic encephalopathy, intracranial hemorrhage, metabolic abnormalities, pyridoxine dependency, nonketotic hyperglycinemia, local anesthetic intoxication, sepsis, and meningoencephalitis. After 3 days of life one needs to consider more likely metabolic disease, brain malformations, "fifth day fits" (healthy term infant with seizures on about day of life 5 that resolve by about 2 weeks and carry a good prognosis), benign (nonepileptic) neonatal sleep myoclonus, and familial neonatal seizures (autosomal dominant, seizures often persisting for 1 to 6 months with a good prognosis). Prognosis depends on underlying etiology.

Specific Disorders to Consider

Pyridoxine-sensitive seizures may respond to pyridoxine (vitamin B_6) or pyridoxal phosphate administration. GLUT-1 deficiency (low cerebrospinal fluid [CSF] glucose) may be treated with the ketogenic diet.

Routine evaluation includes blood sugar, electrolytes, arterial blood gas, ammonia, drug screen, LP, computed tomography [CT]/MRI, blood and CSF cultures, EEG, and pyridoxine trial. Additional evaluation, if indicated, may include plasma amino acids, urinary organic acids, very-long-chain fatty acids, lysosomal enzymes, CSF as well as blood lactate/pyruvate, and CSF glycine.

Initial treatment is generally **phenobarbital** (20 mg/kg intravenously [IV]), which can be repeated if needed to achieve serum levels of 20 to 40 µg/mL. Persistent seizures can be treated with phenytoin (20 mg/kg IV) with additional doses if needed to achieve serum levels of 15 to 20 µg/mL.

Subclinical seizures are extremely common, so continuous EEG monitoring may be indicated. If seizures are completely controlled for 1 to 2 weeks and the underlying acute etiology is stable or resolved, it is reasonable to discontinue AEDs.

HINT: There is almost always an underlying cause for neonatal seizures. It is essential to identify and treat the underlying etiology, in addition to managing seizures.

Posttraumatic seizures

Seizures can occur as an acute consequence of blunt or penetrating head trauma or as a delayed posttraumatic consequence.

- **Impact** seizures occur within an hour of head trauma and may or may not be associated with associated brain injury. They are the least likely type of trauma-related seizures to persist.
- **Early posttraumatic** seizures occur within 1 week of the injury and are associated with cerebral edema, epidural, subdural, and intracerebral hematomas, and traumatic subarachnoid hemorrhages. Neuroimaging is indicated. These are not associated with future epilepsy.
- **Late posttraumatic** seizures (after 1 week) are considered remote symptomatic seizures, and recurrent spells should be treated.

EVALUATION OF A PATIENT WITH A FIRST SEIZURE

It should be assumed that there is an acute symptomatic etiology for an initial seizure to avoid missing treatable causes. Unprovoked recurrent seizures (i.e., idiopathic epilepsy) can only be diagnosed after symptomatic etiologies are ruled out. All children deserve a detailed history and physical examination. They should have **blood glucose and electrolyte** evaluation if they do not quickly return to baseline alertness and neurologic status or if they develop recurrent seizures. A **CT** scan should be performed emergently in children with risk factors including head trauma, focal (partial) seizure, seizure >15 minutes, focal postictal deficits (Todd paralysis), persistently altered level of consciousness, sickle cell disease, bleeding disorders, malignancy, and HIV infection. **MRI** is more sensitive than CT in detecting abnormalities related to seizures and thus is preferred to CT when nonurgent imaging is required. Nonurgent MRI should be considered if the child is <1 year old, has focal seizures, has focal neurologic examination signs, or has other motor/cognitive deficits. CNS infection must be ruled out with an LP if infection is suspected. A **toxicology screen** should be performed if ingestion is possible. Neonates and infants can present with seizures as the initial manifestation of CNS infections, so absence of fever or clear encephalopathy should not preclude LP in these young children if infection is suspected. If the child has returned to baseline and the history is not suggestive of an underlying disorder, then laboratory testing, LP, and neuroimaging are generally not indicated.

TABLE 68-5 History Taking in a Patient with Seizure

Patient History
  Birth history
  History of febrile seizures
  Neurologic problems
  Developmental problems
  Psychiatric problems
  Medication use
Related to Suspected Seizure Event
  Precipitating factors
  Factors lowering seizure threshold (sleep deprivation, alcohol, systemic infection, fever)
  Preceding symptoms
  Duration of symptoms
  Motor and sensory symptoms
  Level of awareness and responsiveness
  Injury
  Incontinence
  Breathing or skin color changes
  Duration of event
  Duration and description of time after the event.
Related to the Pattern of Events
  Frequency of events
  Stereotyped quality or variable
  Family History
  Social History: Household medications/toxins

Immediate EEG is indicated for **persistently altered mental status or movements of unclear etiology to evaluate for subclinical** seizures (i.e., nonconvulsive status epilepticus). Otherwise, emergent EEG is not needed because soon after a seizure the EEG shows nonspecific slowing. An EEG can generally be performed nonurgently to help determine the seizure type and identify any underlying epilepsy syndrome.

Table 68-5 lists useful history questions regarding seizures, and Figure 68-1 presents an algorithm for epilepsy evaluation and classification.

MANAGEMENT OF SEIZURES

Antiepileptic Drugs

When seizures are provoked by an acute condition, it is essential to treat the underlying condition, but AEDs are generally not indicated. AEDs may be used for several weeks or months as a bridge when recurrent seizures complicate an acute condition or if additional seizures might threaten the neurologic status (as in posttraumatic seizures further increasing intracranial pressure).

If a first seizure is unprovoked, only **20% to 40%** of children have a second seizure, and thus AEDs are not generally initiated after a first unprovoked seizure. Statistics are different after a second unprovoked seizure because most children will have a third unprovoked seizure;

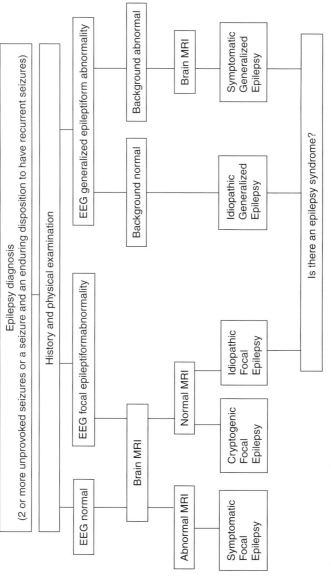

Figure 68-1 ■ Epilepsy evaluation. *EEG* = electroencephalogram; *MRI* = magnetic resonance imaging. (From Sullivan J, Dlugos D: Anti-epileptic drug monotherapy: pediatric concerns. *Sem Pediatr Neurol* 12:88–96, 2005.)

therefore, AEDs are often initiated after a second unprovoked seizure. Decisions regarding whether to initiate AED therapy also take into account the child's age, an identifiable epilepsy syndrome, EEG findings, and the duration between subsequent seizures.

Table 68-6 summarizes the commonly used antiepileptic drugs. Medication choices are based on epilepsy classification, seizure frequency, efficacy data, possible adverse reactions, titration schedule, dosing schedule, and the availability of pediatric-friendly formulations (liquids, sprinkle capsules).

Diastat (preloaded syringe of rectal diazepam) is approved for use in children with repetitive seizures. Evidence indicates that it is also effective in terminating prolonged seizures. It is generally administered for **cluster** seizures or if a seizure persists >5 minutes. Not every child with a seizure needs rectal diazepam, but it should be considered in all children with a history of prolonged seizures, for those who live far from medical attention, or any child whose caregivers would benefit from the ability to intervene actively to stop seizures.

Other Treatment Modalities

- **Ketogenic diet.** This employs a high-fat, low-carbohydrate regimen. Common adverse events to consider include hypoglycemia and nephrolithiasis. If IV fluids are required, they should be dextrose free.
- **Vagal nerve stimulator.** This surgically implanted device can be set to cycle continuously but also can be programmed to provide a higher current over a longer time course that can be used to abort seizures. It must be turned off prior to MRI scans.
- **Epilepsy surgery.** Options include resective surgery including standard temporal lobectomy and tailored cortical resection to hemispherectomy as well as corpus callosotomy and multiple subpial transections. Outcomes are best for lesional epilepsy with concordant EEG and imaging findings.

Discontinuing AEDs

One should consider an attempt to discontinue AEDs once the child is seizure free for 2 years because more than half will continue to do well without medication. Predictors of successful discontinuation include 2 years of seizure freedom, normal EEG, normal examination, and a single seizure type.

Epilepsy Patient with Increased Seizure Frequency

When seizures suddenly increase in frequency or severity, one must consider epilepsy exacerbation, but more frequently worsening is caused by missed medication doses, recent growth leading to lower AED levels, and exacerbation caused by **intercurrent infection** (with or without

TABLE 68-6 Anti-Epileptic Medications

AED	Indications	Advantages	Side Effects
Phenobarbital	Focal epilepsy; initial monotherapy (but no longer used as first line in children)	IV formulation; quick load and bolus; available as suspension	Cognitive concerns; hepatic enzyme induction; rash and hypersensitivity reactions; rapid administration may cause hypotension and reduced respiratory rate; long-term use: Osteoporosis.
Phenytoin (Dilantin)	Focal epilepsy; initial monotherapy (but no longer used as first line in children)	IV formulation; quick load and bolus; available as suspension	Hepatic enzyme induction; rash and hypersensitivity reactions; unpredictable pharmacokinetics; may cause cardiac arrhythmias; long-term use: gingival hyperplasia and osteoporosis.
Carbamazepine (Tegretol, Carbatrol)	Focal epilepsy; initial monotherapy	Possible mood stabilization; available as suspension and sprinkles	Hepatic enzyme induction; rash and hypersensitivity reactions; idiosyncratic leukopenia and aplastic anemia; long-term use: osteoporosis.
Valproate (Depakote, Depakene)	Broad spectrum	IV formulation; available as suspension and sprinkles	Hepatic enzyme inhibition; idiosyncratic pancreatitis and hepatic failure (especially in young children, polypharmacy, metabolic disease); dose-related thrombocytopenia; long-term use: weight gain, hair loss, tremor, menstrual irregularities; highly teratogenic.

(Continued)

789

TABLE 68-6 Anti-Epileptic Medications (Continued)

AED	Indications	Advantages	Side Effects
Ethosuximide (Zarontin)	Absence epilepsy	Available as suspension	Idiosyncratic rash and leukopenia.
Felbamate (Felbatol)	Broad spectrum; intractable epilepsy	Available as suspension	Idiosyncratic aplastic anemia and hepatic failure; frequent blood tests and consent form.
Gabapentin (Neurontin)	Focal epilepsy	Neuropathic pain; available as suspension	Prolonged use: weight gain.
Lamotrigine (Lamictal)	Broad spectrum	Possible mood stabilization; available as a chew tablet	Slow titration; rash and hypersensitivity reactions; interacts with Valproate, rash (especially with rapid titration).
Levetiracetam (Keppra)	Broad spectrum	IV formulation; available as suspension	May exacerbate behavior problems.
Oxcarbazepine (Trileptal)	Focal epilepsy; initial monotherapy	Available as suspension	Rash and hypersensitivity reactions; hyponatremia.
Topiramate (Topamax)	Broad spectrum; initial monotherapy	Migraine prevention; no weight gain; available as sprinkle	Word-finding difficulty; weight loss; nephrolithiasis; hypohidrosis (overheating); metabolic acidosis; acute angle closure glaucoma.
Zonisamide (Zonegran)	Broad spectrum	No weight gain	Weight loss; nephrolithiasis; hypohidrosis (overheating); metabolic acidosis.

IV = intravenous.

TABLE 68-7 Status Epilepticus Protocol

Stage	Management

Impending SE
 <5 min
	Out of hospital: Consider buccal midazolam or rectal diazepam.
	 Benzodiazepines
	     Lorazepam, 0.1 mg/kg IV (max 5 mg), over 1 min
	     Diazepam, 0.2 mg/kg IV (max 10 mg), over 1 min
	 Allow 5 minutes to determine whether seizure terminates.
	 Give oxygen. Stabilize airway, respiration, and hemodynamics as needed. Obtain IV access. Check bedside glucose. Begin ECG monitoring.

Established SE
 5–10 min
	Repeat benzodiazepine administration.
	 Do not wait for seizure termination.
	 Administer fosphenytoin 20 mg/kg phenytoin equivalents IV at 2 mg/kg/min (max 150 mg/min).
	 (or phenytoin, 20 mg/kg IV, at 1 mg/kg/min [max 50 mg/min])
	 If <2 years, consider pyridoxine 100 mg IV push.
	 If hypoglycemic, administer bolus of 2 mL/kg 50% glucose.
	 Testing:
	     Bedside glucose, CBC, cultures
	     BMP, Mg, Phos, LFT, toxicology (serum, urine)
	     AED levels, PT, PTT
	     Head CT
	 Draw phenytoin level (10 min after infusion)
	 Support airway, respiration, hemodynamics as needed.
	 Continuous vital sign and ECG monitoring.
	 Consult neurology service.

Initial Refractory SE	If seizure continues 10 minutes after fosphenytoin infusion, then patient has refractory SE regardless of time elapsed.
	 Third-line medications to consider:
	 -Levetiracetam, 40 mg/kg IV, at 5 mg/kg/min (max 3 g)
	 -Valproate, 20 mg/kg, at 5 mg/kg/min
	     Contraindicated if liver/metabolic disease.
	 -Phenobarbital, 30 mg/kg IV, at 2 mg/kg/min (max rate 60 mg/min).
	     Carefully monitor and prepare to support ventilation and blood pressure.

Later Refractory SE	Admit to PICU. Prepare to secure airway, mechanically ventilate, and obtain central venous access and continuous hemodynamic monitoring through arterial line. Once clinical seizure terminates will likely need EEG monitoring to assess for subclinical seizures.
Coma Induction	If seizure continues, then initiate coma with midazolam, 0.2 mg/kg bolus (max 10 mg), over 2 min, and then initiate infusion at 0.1 mg/kg/hr. If clinical seizures persist 5 min after initial midazolam bolus, then administer additional midazolam bolus of 0.2 mg/kg bolus. Continue infusion. Titrate up as needed to terminate seizures and generally to achieve a burst suppression pattern on EEG. If seizure persists at maximum midazolam (generally 2 mg/kg/hr) or midazolam infusion is not tolerated, then consider transition to isoflurane. Also consider pentobarbital, topiramate, valproic acid, or levetiracetam.

AED = antiepileptic drug; *BMP* = basic metabolic profile; *CBC* = complete blood count; *CT* = computed tomography; *ECG* = electrocardiogram; *EEG* = electroencephalogram; *IV* = intravenous; *LFT* = liver function test; *max* = maximum; *PICU* = pediatric intensive care unit; *PT* = prothrombin time; *PTT* = partial thromboplastin time; *SE* = status epilepticus.

fever). On occasion, one must consider acute symptomatic etiologies because children with preexisting epilepsy can also develop additional CNS disorders such as infection and stroke. If a bridge medication is needed for acute exacerbation (e.g., during an intercurrent infection), consider administering a long-acting benzodiazepine such as **clorazepate** for several days.

STATUS EPILEPTICUS

Status epilepticus is a life-threatening emergency characterized by prolonged or recurrent seizures without return to baseline mental status. The older definition of status epilepticus is 30 minutes of persistent seizure activity (or 30 minutes of recurrent seizures without full recovery of consciousness). However, given the compelling evidence that most seizures stop spontaneously within 5 minutes, prolonged seizures become harder to terminate, and prolonged seizures are associated with worse outcome, treatment is now typically initiated at **5 to 10 minutes**. Status epilepticus may be convulsive or nonconvulsive (requiring EEG for detection). In patients with preexisting epilepsy, common etiologies include poor compliance with medication, recent medication changes, benzodiazepine or barbiturate withdrawal, or exacerbation by intercurrent infection. Acute **symptomatic etiologies** predominate in first attacks of status epilepticus. One must consider meningoencephalitis, stroke, intracranial hemorrhage, acute head injury, cerebral neoplasm, demyelinating disorders, metabolic disorders, and medication/drug overdose. Evaluation and treatment must focus on terminating the seizure and treating the underlying condition. Particular attention to traditional resuscitation issues (airway, breathing, circulation: the ABCs) is important because abnormalities may worsen or cause secondary brain injury. Table 68-7 presents a status epilepticus guideline.

> **HINT:** Convulsive and most nonconvulsive status epilepticus is an emergency that requires rapid and aggressive treatment.

Suggested References

Hirtz D, Berg A, Bettis S, et al.: Practice parameter: treatment of the child with a first unprovoked seizure. *Neurology* 60:166–175, 2003.

Riviello J, Holmes G: The treatment of status epilepticus. *Sem Pediatr Neurol* 11(2):129–139, 2004.

Waruiru C, Appleton R: Febrile seizures: an update. *Arch Dis Child* 89:751–756, 2004.

INTRODUCTION

Child sexual abuse is defined as the involvement of children in sexual activities that they cannot understand, are not developmentally prepared for, cannot give informed consent to, and that violate societal taboos. "Sexual abuse" is a general term that includes a broad range of activities, including **noncontact activities** (e.g., pornography, either in its production or in its viewing; inappropriate observation of the child while dressing, toileting, or bathing; and perpetrator exhibitionism directed at the child) and **contact activities.** Sexual abuse **frequently occurs over time** as the perpetrator gains the trust of the child, and it can progress from noncontact to contact forms of abuse.

DIFFERENTIAL DIAGNOSIS LIST

Child sexual abuse can have various presenting signs and symptoms. The following are physical signs associated with sexual abuse and the differential diagnosis for each.

Vaginal or Penile Discharge

Infectious Causes
  Sexually transmitted
    infections (STIs)—
    Neisseria gonorrhoeae,
    Chlamydia trachomatis,
    Trichomonas vaginalis
    Group A streptococcus
    Haemophilus influenzae
    Staphylococcus aureus
    Corynebacterium diphtheriae
    Mycoplasma hominis
    Gardnerella vaginalis
    Shigella
  Anatomic Causes
    Ectopic ureter
    Rectovaginal fistula
    Draining pelvic abscess

Traumatic Causes
  Foreign body
  Chemical irritation (e.g.,
    bubble bath)
  Tight, nonporous clothing
Miscellaneous Causes
  Nonspecific vulvovaginitis
  Leukorrhea

Genital Bleeding

Infectious Causes
  Urinary tract infection with
    gross hematuria
  Vaginitis
Anatomic Causes
  Vaginal polyp
  Urethral prolapse
  Vulvar hemangioma

Traumatic Causes
  Straddle injuries (usually
    anterior lacerations)
  Impaling (penetrating)
    injuries
  Foreign body (e.g., toilet
    paper, small toys)
Dermatologic Causes
  Lichen sclerosus et
    atrophicus (girls)
  Balanitis xerotica obliterans
    (boys)
Endocrinologic Causes
  Neonatal estrogen
    withdrawal
  Precocious puberty
Neoplastic Causes
  Sarcoma botryoides
  Vaginal rhabdomyosarcoma
  Estrogen-producing tumors

Genital Inflammation or Pruritus

Infectious Causes
  Nonspecific vulvovaginitis
  STIs—*N. gonorrhoeae*,
    C. trachomatis, T. vaginalis
  Pinworms
  Scabies
  Vaginal candidiasis
  Group A streptococcal
    perianal cellulitis
Traumatic Causes
  Poor hygiene
  Poorly ventilated or tight
    underwear
  Chemical irritation
  "Sandbox" vaginitis
Dermatologic Causes
  Atopic dermatitis
  Contact dermatitis
  Seborrhea
  Diaper dermatitis
  Psoriasis

  Lichen sclerosus et
    atrophicus (girls)
  Balanitis xerotica obliterans
    (boys)
Systemic Causes
  Urticaria
  Crohn disease
  Kawasaki syndrome
  Stevens-Johnson syndrome

Bruising

Infectious Causes
  Purpura fulminans
  Disseminated intravascular
    coagulation (DIC)
Traumatic Causes
  Straddle injuries
  Accidental penetrating
    injuries
Dermatologic Causes
  Lichen sclerosus et
    atrophicus (girls)
  Balanitis xerotica obliterans
    (boys)
  Erythema multiforme
  Mongolian spots
  Vascular nevi
Hematologic Causes
  Idiopathic thrombocy-
    topenic purpura
  Leukemia
  Vitamin K deficiency
  Coagulopathies
  DIC
Metabolic Causes
  Ehlers-Danlos syndrome
  Osteogenesis imperfecta
Autoimmune Causes
  Henoch-Schönlein purpura
  Vasculitis

Anatomic Variations

Acquired
  Labial agglutination

Hair thread tourniquet
  syndrome
Phimosis
Paraphimosis
Urethral prolapse
Congenital
  Septate hymen
  Cribriform hymen

Microperforate hymen
Imperforate hymen
Urethral caruncles
Vestibular bands
Median raphe
Ectopic ureterocele

DIFFERENTIAL DIAGNOSIS DISCUSSION

A few diagnoses are commonly mistaken for sexual abuse and deserve comment.

Lichen Sclerosus et Atrophicus

Etiology

Lichen sclerosus et atrophicus, a **dermatologic condition,** generally affects **prepubertal and postmenopausal women** and is characterized by **thin, atrophic vulvar skin that is easily injured.** The atrophic skin typically involves the labia majora, perineum, and perianal area in an hourglass configuration. The hymen is not usually involved.

Clinical Features and Evaluation

Leukoplakia and hemorrhagic bullae may develop. Children often present with **pruritus and vaginal bleeding after minimal trauma.** The diagnosis is usually made clinically, although biopsy is sometimes required.

Treatment

Treatment is usually **symptomatic, with attention to hygiene.** Hydrocortisone can be used to relieve irritation and pruritus.

Straddle Injuries

Etiology

Straddle injuries, common injuries to the genitalia of both boys and girls, result from the **crushing of the genital tissues between the bony pelvis and a solid structure** (e.g., a bicycle bar or the arm of a chair).

The term "straddle injury" is also used to describe **accidental penetrating trauma to the genitals.** These injuries can occur in any area of the genitalia and in girls can potentially lead to injury of the hymen. Accidental penetrating injuries to the genitals are far less common than straddle injuries and should be accompanied by a history that confirms an impaling injury.

Clinical Features

In girls, most nonpenetrating straddle injuries cause **ecchymosis and/or lacerations of the anterior vulva,** often involving the labia minora. Because of its posterior location and recessed position, the hymen is not typically involved. **In boys,** straddle injuries commonly cause **scrotal and penile lacerations or ecchymoses.** These injuries **heal quickly** and usually no treatment is needed other than **sitz baths.** Some lacerations or impaling injuries require **surgical repair,** with the patient under general anesthesia.

Vulvovaginitis

Etiology

There are many causes of vulvovaginitis in children, many of which do not relate to sexual abuse. In **adolescent females,** most cases of vulvovaginitis are caused by a **specific infectious organism.** The most common type of vulvovaginitis in **prepubertal children,** however, is **nonspecific vulvovaginitis,** which results from a combination of **anatomic, physiologic, and hygienic factors.** Vulvovaginitis may also result from **sexual abuse,** either as a result of mechanical trauma and irritation or from STIs.

Clinical Features

The **discharge** associated with nonspecific vulvovaginitis is **generally chronic, intermittent, scant to moderate,** and may or may not be seen in the introitus during the examination.

Evaluation

The laboratory evaluation of a genital discharge in a child can include **cultures for *N. gonorrhoeae, C. trachomatis,* and *T. vaginalis,* a general vaginal culture, antigen testing for *T. vaginalis*** and **"clue cells"** (vaginal epithelial cells with adherent bacteria), a **Gram stain** of the discharge, and a **potassium hydroxide preparation** for *Candida.* A **whiff test** is done by mixing a sample of the **vaginal discharge** with a **small amount of potassium hydroxide;** an amine-like odor is present in **bacterial vaginosis** as well as in **trichomoniasis.** Nucleic amplification tests that identify *N. gonorrhoeae* and *C. trachomatis* have gained popularity in recent years, but they are **not yet approved for use in prepubertal children.**

Treatment

The treatment of **nonspecific vulvovaginitis** is aimed at **modifying hygiene practices** (e.g., wiping front to back after a bowel movement; wearing loose-fitting clothing and white cotton underwear). The treatment of vulvovaginitis caused by STIs and other infectious pathogens is detailed in Chapter 70, "Sexually Transmitted Diseases."

EVALUATION OF CHILD SEXUAL ABUSE

Discovery of sexual abuse is usually by one of the following mechanisms:

- The child discloses abuse.
- A third party discovers the abuse (e.g., a sibling walks in the room during an assault).
- The child presents with physical injuries.
- The child develops an STI.

Many sexually abused children **do not have physical injuries at the time of an examination,** either because the child did not sustain physical injury during the abuse or the injuries have healed. The evaluation of a patient in whom sexual abuse is suspected therefore requires **careful attention to the history, physical examination, and laboratory specimen collection** and must include **meticulous documentation** of both historical and physical findings.

Patient History

Complaints may be related to physical injuries or STIs, but, more commonly, the signs and symptoms of sexual abuse are nonspecific and are **manifestations of the psychological stress** associated with the abuse. These include **nonspecific behavioral complaints** (e.g., hypersexualized behaviors, phobias, sleep disturbances, poor school performance, runaway behaviors, truancy, aggressive behavior, symptoms and signs of depression) as well as **nonspecific physical complaints** (e.g., enuresis—secondary, day or night; encopresis; headaches; abdominal, genital, and/or rectal pain; dysuria; vaginitis; genital erythema; vaginal or penile discharge; genital and/or rectal bleeding; pregnancy). Information related to both physical and behavioral symptoms of abuse should be explored.

In most cases, the diagnosis of child sexual abuse depends on the **history obtained from the child.** Ideally, the **interview** of the child is **conducted by a professional** familiar with the dynamics of sexual abuse, knowledgeable about child development, and comfortable with speaking to children about these issues. **Joint interviews** (with a representative from Child Protective Services and a law enforcement official) are **recommended,** although in the medical setting, this is often not possible. The child should be **interviewed with the parents absent** because some children are hesitant to talk with a parent present, and others may be overly coached by anxious parents.

The child should be asked **nonleading questions,** although specific questions to clarify statements are necessary of course. It is best to start the interview with an **open-ended question** such as "Can you tell me why you were brought here today?" The interviewer should ask **developmentally** appropriate questions. For example, a young child's sense of dates and time is best approximated by references to seasons, holidays, and other important events in the child's life. Statements made by the child should be **recorded verbatim** in the medical record if possible.

It is important to try and elicit the following information:

- Identity of the alleged perpetrator and his or her relationship to the child
- The time of the last contact
- The reason why the child chose to disclose the incident at this time
- The frequency of abuse (one time versus chronic)
- The specific types of sexual contact included in the abuse
- History of perpetrator ejaculation
- Whether threats were made to the child by the alleged perpetrator
- Whether prior official reports of the abuse have been made

Physical Examination

The type of examination performed depends on the age of the child. **Adolescent girls or children with suspected intravaginal injury** may require a **full pelvic examination,** whereas **most children** usually require only **careful inspection of the vulva.** Common positions used for examination of children include the supine, frog-leg position with labial traction (young girls), lithotomy position (adolescent girls), knee-chest position, and lateral decubitus position.

Few physical findings are pathognomonic of sexual abuse. Many genital findings are nonspecific but with a history may support the diagnosis of sexual abuse. **Definitive findings** of sexual abuse include the **finding of semen or sperm. In pregnant patients and those with STIs** or injuries **without a history of sexual activity, sexual abuse is a very likely possibility.** Further investigation is warranted for patients with **suspicious injuries or anatomic variants** (e.g., posterior angular concavities or transections of the hymen). **Less serious vaginal problems** (e.g., infections, adhesions) are **common in children** and do not independently suggest sexual abuse. Perianal erythema or hyperpigmentation are examples of nonspecific changes.

The decision to complete a "rape kit" is **determined by clinical presentation.** Recent research suggests that forensic evidence collection can be limited to children who present for medical evaluation **within 24 hours of the last assault** or those who have **injury or bleeding** on examination. Local crime laboratories have different protocols for collection of evidence. In general, the following evidence may be collected:

- **Victim's clothing.** Clothing provides the highest yield of forensic evidence in child sexual assault and should be vigorously sought.

The clothing the child was wearing at the time of the assault is collected by having the child undress while standing on a sterile sheet and placing all items into a clean paper bag. (Plastic bags should not be used because they may be airtight; the buildup of heat and moisture can degrade evidence.) Police should be notified of unwashed clothing at home that might provide forensic evidence.

- **Swabs for semen, sperm, acid phosphatase, P30 analysis and DNA analysis.** Moist secretions should be collected from the oral cavity (e.g., the pharynx, gum line), vagina, and rectum with a swab and allowed to air-dry before packaging. Swabs may also be collected from areas of the body that appear to have dried secretions, either by scraping a dry sample into a paper envelope or using a swab slightly moistened with sterile water, which is then allowed to air-dry.
- **Fingernail scrapings for foreign debris** should be placed into a paper envelope.
- **Pubic hair collection.** Collect combed pubic hairs into a paper envelope.
- **Foreign debris.** Any suspicious foreign debris found on the victim should be placed in a paper envelope.
- **Victim identification samples.** Collect a saliva sample and a blood sample from the victim to be used for identification of secretor status of the patient or for later DNA analysis.

Laboratory Studies

Laboratory evaluation is not universally required. When indicated, recommended tests to screen for STIs include the following:

- Culture of the cervix, vagina, or urethra; rectum; and pharynx for *N. gonorrhoeae*
- Culture of the cervix/vagina/urethra and rectum for *C. trachomatis*
- Wet preparation of vaginal secretions for *T. vaginalis*
- Culture of lesions for herpes simplex virus
- Serology for syphilis
- Serology for HIV, based on the prevalence of infection and suspected risk (should be repeated 3 and 6 months after last assault; obtain written consent)
- Gram stain and general culture of any vaginal, urethral, or anal discharge
- Nucleic acid amplification techniques are now approved for use in adolescent and adult women for STI screening, although appropriate confirmation is required for positive screening tests.

Documentation

A **detailed medical record** is imperative to ensure that the best interests of the child are served. A well-documented medical evaluation in the

medical record can serve as the basis for future discussion of the case. The physician should not rely on memory alone to reconstruct what occurred. The following hints are offered as a quick reference:
Do:

- Describe findings simply.
- Be aware of the child's developmental status.
- Use the child's words, defining the child's language if necessary.
- Ask nonleading questions.
- Record questions asked and specific answers given.
- Use diagrams and photographs to supplement the written record.

Do not:

- Use leading questions if at all possible.
- Use the terms "virginal" or "intact hymen" because these terms are imprecise and can be problematic during the legal investigation of the case.
- State conclusions in absolute terms; rather, describe findings and comment if they are consistent with expectations based on information known at that time.

TREATMENT OF CHILD SEXUAL ABUSE

Medical treatment is guided by the **specific injuries or infections.** Hospitalization of sexually abused children is rarely required and, in general, is limited to children with severe genital trauma or systemic manifestations of STIs. Victims of sexual abuse, nonoffending parents, and perpetrators may all benefit from **therapy,** and referrals for patients should be made.

APPROACH TO THE PATIENT

All cases of suspected sexual abuse must be reported to Child Protective Services (for abuse committed by a caretaker or household member), **law enforcement, or both.** Each state has laws that define child sexual abuse, and physicians should be aware of the laws operating in their state of practice. Individual institutions often have policies or guidelines regarding the evaluation of abuse, and some hospitals have a multidisciplinary team with expertise in recognizing and evaluating child abuse. Physicians who report suspected abuse "in good faith" are given immunity should a suit be brought against a physician for "false reports." **Parents should be informed of the need to report** before doing so.

Suggested Readings

Adams JA, Harper K, Knudson S, et al.: Examination findings in legally confirmed child sexual abuse: it's normal to be normal. *Pediatrics* 94:310–317, 1994.

American Academy of Pediatrics: Guidelines for the evaluation of sexual abuse of children. *Pediatrics* 103:186–191, 1999.

Berenson AB, Chacko MR, Wiemann CM, et al.: A case-control study of anatomic changes resulting from sexual abuse. *Am J Obstet Gynecol* 182:820–834, 2000.

Christian CW, Lavelle JM, De Jong AR, et al.: Forensic evidence findings in prepubertal victims of sexual assault. *Pediatrics* 106:100–104, 2000.

Heger AH, Tiscon L, Guerra L, et al.: Appearance of the genitalia in girls selected for nonabuse: review of hymenal morphology and nonspecific findings. *J Pediatr Adolesc Gynecol* 15:27–35, 2002.

Kellogg ND, Menard SW, Santos A: Genital anatomy in pregnant adolescents: "normal" does not mean "nothing happened." *Pediatrics* 113(1 Pt 1):e67–e69, 2004.

Kellogg ND, Parra JM, Menard S, et al.: Children with anogenital symptoms and signs referred for sexual abuse evaluations. *Arch Pediatr Adolesc Med* 153:634–641, 1998.

Sexually Transmitted Diseases

Lisa K. Tuchman

Marina Catallozzi, Jonathan Pletcher, and Joseph Zorc (Third Edition)

INTRODUCTION

Over a third of sexually transmitted diseases (STDs) are diagnosed in patients <19 years of age. The rates of many STDs are **highest among adolescents** (e.g., gonorrhea in 15- to 19-year-old females, chlamydia prevalence, and human papillomavirus [HPV] infections). Adolescents are at such high risk for STDs because of developmental behavioral factors, biologic susceptibility to infection, and the myriad health-use issues they face.

The majority of STDs in adolescents are asymptomatic, and therefore clinical presentation can be protean. Females may present with **vaginal discharge, abnormal vaginal bleeding, vaginal itching, dysuria, or pain** (lower abdominal, right upper quadrant, or rectal). **Males** may present with **urethral discharge, dysuria, testicular pain or swelling, or rectal pain.** Presentation can also include rash, pharyngitis, arthralgia or arthritis, and inguinal adenopathy.

Clinicians can **educate adolescents about the transmission and importance of protecting oneself from contracting an STD. Primary prevention** includes helping guide the development of healthy sexual behaviors and providing accurate sexual and reproductive health information as well as access to reproductive health resources. There are limited exceptions, but, in general, adolescents in the United States can consent to the **confidential diagnosis and treatment of STDs** so that medical care for STDs can be provided to adolescents without parental consent or knowledge. Providers should respect confidentiality of adolescents and should follow policies that comply with state laws to ensure the confidentiality of STD-related services provided to adolescents.

Appropriate treatment of the patient and partner is essential.

DIFFERENTIAL DIAGNOSIS LIST

Bacterial Infection

Chancroid (*Haemophilus ducreyi*)

Gonorrhea (*Neisseria gonorrhoeae*)

Granuloma inguinale (*Calymmatobacterium granulomatis*)

Lymphogranuloma venereum (*Chlamydia trachomatis*)

Shigella species

Syphilis or condyloma latum
(*Treponema pallidum*)

Ureaplasma urealyticum

Bacterial vaginosis
(*Gardnerella vaginalis*)

Parasitic Infection

Pubic lice (*Phthirus pubis*)

Scabies (*Sarcoptes scabiei*)

Protozoal Infection

Trichomonas vaginalis

Entamoeba histolytica

Giardiasis (*Giardia lamblia*)

Viral Infection

Cytomegalovirus infection

Hepatitis A, B, or C

Herpes simplex virus (HSV)
infection

HIV

HPV (genital warts, condyloma
acuminatum)

Molluscum contagiosum

DIFFERENTIAL DIAGNOSIS DISCUSSION

Selected Diseases That Cause Genital Lesions

Syphilis

Etiology

Syphilis is caused by the spirochete *T. pallidum*.

Clinical Features

- **Primary syphilis** is characterized by a painless ulcer or chancre at the site of inoculation.
- **Most children and adolescents present with secondary syphilis.** Most commonly, a maculopapular rash involving the palms and soles is the presenting complaint. Other symptoms include mucocutaneous lesions (condyloma lata) and systemic symptoms (e.g., adenopathy, fever, pharyngitis, malaise).
- **Tertiary syphilis** includes aortitis, neurologic dysfunction, and gummatous lesions of the bone, kidney, and liver.
- **Latent syphilis** describes disease in patients who have no symptoms of infection. Early latent syphilis refers to infection within the past year. Late latent syphilis and syphilis of unknown duration make up the remainder of this category.

Evaluation

The diagnosis of syphilis is generally made by using a **nonspecific** (nontreponemal) **antibody test** such as the **Venereal Disease Research Laboratory (VDRL) test** and the **rapid plasma reagent test.** The specific tests for treponemal antibody, fluorescent treponemal antibody, absorbed (FTA-ABS) or the *T. pallidum* particle agglutination (TP-PA) test, remain positive for life; therefore, they do not denote activity. Nontreponemal tests can be quantified by **testing serial dilutions of** serum. **Quantification is important** because the appearance of clinical lesions correlates with a rise in titers. These titers diminish with appropriate treatment and can be used to follow response to therapy.

> **HINT:** **FTA-ABS or TP-PA help differentiate infections from diseases such as lupus that produce a false-positive VDRL. However, these tests are positive in Lyme disease, which does not have a positive VDRL.**

- *T. pallidum* cannot be cultured in artificial media but **darkfield examination and direct fluorescent antibody tests** of lesion exudate or tissue are definitive ways to diagnose syphilis.

Treatment

Parenteral penicillin G is the treatment of choice for all stages of syphilis (see Table 70-1 for details).

Treatment may be complicated by an acute febrile syndrome known as the Jarisch-Herxheimer reaction. This reaction resolves within 24 hours.

The expected serologic response to treatment is a minimum fourfold decrease in nontreponemal test titers within 6 months.

Herpes Genitalis
Etiology

Most recurrent cases of herpes genitalis result from **herpes simplex virus-type 2 (HSV-2)**, although up to 50% of primary cases of genital herpes are caused by **HSV-1**, the type more commonly associated with stomatitis. These viruses account for up to 90% of all ulcerative lesions of the genitalia and are highly contagious; as many as 90% of women exposed to infected men develop genital herpes. Transmission can occur in patients who are asymptomatic and often unaware that they are infected.

Clinical Features

Primary infection is characterized by **single or multiple vesicles** that may appear anywhere on the genitalia. These vesicles **spontaneously rupture to form shallow ulcers,** which are exquisitely **painful** but **resolve spontaneously** without scarring. Some cases of primary genital herpes are severe enough to require **hospitalization.** Mild to severe **systemic symptoms** may accompany the genital lesions. The mean duration of the initial episode of HSV is 12 days.

Recurrent infections, which occur in some patients, are less painful and of shorter duration, lasting 4 to 5 days.

Evaluation

Viral culture allows detection of the virus in 1 to 3 days. New vesicles are unroofed and scraped for inoculation of viral media. The yield of

TABLE 70-1 Selected Sexually Transmitted Diseases (STDs)

Etiology	Disease	Diagnostic Tests	Treatment
Treponema pallidum	Syphilis[a]	Darkfield microscopy or direct fluorescent antibody	
		Serology	
		Nontreponemal (VDRL, RPR)	
		Treponemal (TP-PA, FTA-ABS)	
	Primary: chancre		Benzathine penicillin G, 2.4 million U IM × 1.
	Secondary: rash adenopathy, fever		Benzathine penicillin G, 2.4 million U IM × 1.
	Tertiary: cardiac, gummatous		Benzathine penicillin G, 2.4 million U IM weekly × 3.
	Neurosyphilis		Aqueous penicillin G, 18–24 million U daily for 10–14 days.
	Early latent		Benzathine penicillin G, 2.4 million U × 1.
	Late latent or latent of unknown duration		Benzathine penicillin G, 2.4 million U IM weekly × 3.
Herpes simplex virus	Herpes[b]	Culture	
		Rapid fluorescent antibody test	
	Primary: painful genital mucosal lesions, mild systemic symptoms		Acyclovir, 400 mg PO three times daily or 200 mg PO 5 times daily for 7–10 days.
			Famciclovir, 250 mg PO three times daily for 7–10 days.
			Valacyclovir, 1 g PO twice daily for 7–10 days.
	Secondary: less severe recurrence		Acyclovir, 400 mg PO three times daily or 800 mg PO twice daily or
			800 mg PO 3 times daily for 5 days.
			Famciclovir, 125 mg PO twice daily for 5 days or 1 g PO twice daily for 1 day.
			Valacyclovir, 500 mg PO twice daily for 3 days or 1 g PO once daily for 5 days.
Trichomonas vaginalis	Trichomoniasis: vaginal discharge, dysuria, local irritation	Wet mount	Metronidazole, 2 g PO × 1, or Tinidazole, 2 g orally in a single dose.
		Culture	
Human papilloma virus	Condyloma acuminata (genital warts)[c]	Visual inspection	Patient applied:
			Podofilox, 0.5% solution or gel. Apply twice daily for 3 days then 4 days off up to four cycles.
			Imiquimod, 5% cream. Apply three times weekly up to 16 weeks. Wash off after 6–10 hours.

(Continued)

TABLE 70-1 Selected Sexually Transmitted Diseases (STDs) (*Continued*)

Etiology	Disease	Diagnostic Tests	Treatment
Chlamydia trachomatis	Uncomplicated cervicitis Urethritis Epididymitis Proctitis	NAAT (urethral, cervical, urine) culture	Azithromycin, 1 g PO × 1, or Doxycycline, 100 mg PO twice daily for 7 days. In pregnant women: Azithromycin, 1 g PO × 1, or Amoxicillin, 500 mg PO 3 times daily for 7 days.
	Neonatal conjunctivitis or pneumonia		Neonatal: Erythromycin, 50 mg/kg/day, in four doses for 14 days.
Neisseria gonorrhoeae	Uncomplicated cervicitis Urethritis Pharyngitis Epididymitis Proctitis	NAAT (urethral, cervical, urine) Culture Gram stain (urethral discharge)	Ceftriaxone, 125 mg IM, × 1 or Cefixime,[d] 400 mg PO × 1. *Quinolones[e] are no longer recommended as first-line therapy because of increasing resistance and should only be used in culture-proven quinolone sensitive strains. Ceftriaxone, 1 g IM × 1; consider eye lavage with saline.
	Conjunctivitis Disseminated disease		Ceftriaxone,[f] 1 g IV every 24 hr.

FTA-ABS = fluorescent treponemal antibody, absorbed (test); *IM* = intramuscularly; *IV* = intravenously; *NAAT* = nucleic acid amplification test; TP-PA = *Treponema pallidum* particle agglutination; *PO* = orally; *VDRL* = Venereal Disease Research Laboratory (test).

[a]All doses listed for adolescents and adults. Doses for children and alternative regimens for persons with penicillin allergies can be found in Centers for Disease Control and Prevention: Sexually transmitted diseases treatment guidelines 2006. *MMWR Recomm Rep* 55(RR-11):1–94, 2006.

[b]Regimens for suppressive therapy for recurrent genital herpes can be found in Centers for Disease Control and Prevention: Sexually transmitted disease treatment guidelines 2006. *MMWR Recomm Rep* 55(RR-11):1–94, 2006.

[c]Exact regimens for the treatment of external genital warts and future inflammation in treatment of cervical warts can be found in Centers for Disease Control and Prevention: Sexually transmitted diseases treatment guidelines 2006. *MMWR Recomm Rep* 55(RR-11):1–94, 2006.

[d]The tablet form of cefixime is currently not available in the United States.

[e]Fluoroquinolones have not been recommended for persons <18 years of age because of possible damage to articular cartilage. Because of the lack of data the CDC recommends any adult regimens for patients >45 kg.

[f]See the 2006 CDC STD guidelines for other treatment options for disseminated gonorrhea. The parenteral regimens can be switched to oral regimens for 7 days after 24 to 48 hours of improvement.

culture diminishes over time. **Direct fluorescent antibody tests** are available and are rapid and highly sensitive. Serologic testing is available but is of limited value in the management of the patient.

Treatment

- **Management of a first episode** of genital herpes includes antiviral therapy and counseling regarding the natural history of genital herpes with particular emphasis on potential recurrent episodes, asymptomatic viral shedding, sexual transmission, risk for neonatal infection for women of childbearing age, and risk reduction. Acyclovir, famciclovir, and valacyclovir can all be used. Analgesics as well as local care (e.g., sitz baths, barrier creams) may offer some relief. Herpes proctitis may require higher doses of antiviral medication.

- **For recurrent disease,** acyclovir is most beneficial if initiated within 1 day of the onset of lesions. It may be administered as 800 mg orally twice daily for 5 days. Famciclovir and valacyclovir have also been effective in decreasing the severity and length of recurrent infection. In patients who have frequent recurrences (at least six per year) the physician may want to consider suppressive oral therapy, which requires continuous treatment with antiviral agents.

Human Papilloma Virus
Etiology

There are more than **30 types of HPV** that can infect the genital tract. Although most HPV infections are asymptomatic, types 6 and 11 are implicated with **visible genital warts** and types 16, 18, 31, 33, and 35 have been strongly **associated with cervical dysplasia.** The virus is **transmitted by direct contact.** The incubation period can be as long as 20 months. **In children, the presence of genital warts** can be secondary to **vertical transmission at birth or sexual abuse.**

Clinical Features

Warts can be **asymptomatic or symptomatic** and are found in a variety of locations, including the uterine cervix, vagina, urethra, anus, and extragenital areas (conjunctival, nasal, oral, laryngeal). Depending on the location and size of the warts, they can be **painful, friable, and pruritic.**

Evaluation

Identification of the characteristic lesion is diagnostic. Application of **3% acetic acid** produces a **classic acetowhite appearance.** Depending on the location and appearance, condyloma acuminatum can be confused with urethral prolapse, syphilis, vulvar tumors, and sarcoma botryoides.

Treatment

Because there are no currently available treatments that eradicate or affect the natural history of HPV infection, the primary goal of treating genital warts is the **removal of symptomatic or visible warts.** Treatment often induces wart-free periods but does not necessarily decrease infectivity. There is no known effect of treatment on the subsequent development of cervical cancer. Without treatment, genital warts can resolve on their own, stay unchanged, or increase in both size and number.

Because none of the available treatments is superior, treatment should be guided by the preference of the patient and the experience of the health care provider. Medical and surgical treatments are available. Treatments include patient-applied therapies (e.g., podofilox and imiquimod) and provider-administered therapies (e.g., cryotherapy, podophyllin resin, trichloroacetic acid, interferon, and surgery). Warts on moist surfaces respond better to topical treatment. The treatment modality should be changed if a patient does not have significant improvement after three provider-administered treatments. Recurrences are most common in the first 3 months after treatment. Although the presence of genital warts is not an indication for cervical colposcopy, regular surveillance and cytologic screening is recommended, given the association of HPV with cervical dysplasia.

> **HINT:** The quadrivalent HPV vaccine is a prophylactic immunization and only protects against strains of HPV to which one has not been exposed prior to receiving the vaccination; there are no therapeutic benefits if someone has already been infected with a particular stain of HPV.

Selected Diseases that Cause Mucopurulent Discharge

Chlamydia Trachomatis
Etiology

C. trachomatis is a Gram-negative, intracellular organism. Prevalence rates of chlamydia genital infections are as high as 25% in sexually active individuals between 15 and 24 years of age.

Clinical Features

In females, *C. trachomatis* can cause **cervicitis, urethritis, or pelvic inflammatory disease (PID).** Although the majority of **females** are asymptomatic or mildly symptomatic (vaginal discharge, dysuria, dyspareunia, urinary frequency), serious sequelae include **PID, ectopic pregnancy, and potential tubal fertility difficulties.**

Like females, chlamydia infection is often asymptomatic in males but can result in urethritis, epididymitis, proctitis, or prostatitis. Clinical signs of epididymitis are pain and swelling of the epididymis; for prostatitis the patient has pain in the testicles and scrotum; for proctitis the patient complains of rectal pain on defecation or of tenesmus.

Reiter syndrome (conjunctivitis, dermatitis, urethritis, and arthritis) or reactive arthritis can occur in males or females.

Evaluation

In symptomatic females, genitourinary examination is vital. Nucleic acid amplification tests (NAATs) are highly sensitive and specific permitting collection of less invasive specimens for testing. Urine or swabs from the endocervical or vaginal canal can be used. The cervix can appear normal or be friable with the presence of mucopurulent discharge. Cervical cultures range in sensitivity from 50% to 85% and should be used if NAAT testing available to the provider is unreliable in the presence of gross blood, if the sample is being obtained in a prepubertal girl, or in case of specimen collection in medicolegal cases.

In males, urine or urethral swab can be sent for chlamydia NAAT.

The Centers for Disease Control and Prevention (CDC) does not recommend that a chlamydia test be performed for a "test of cure" after completing treatment unless there are persistent symptoms or suspicion of reinfection. Testing with NAAT that is done <3 weeks after completion of therapy may give false-positive results because of detection of nonviable organisms.

Because of high reinfection rates secondary to partners not being treated and the increased risk of PID with repeat infection, women with chlamydia infections should be rescreened 3 to 4 months after treatment.

Treatment

Most recommended regimens include either **azithromycin or doxycycline**. In the past, given high coinfection rates with gonococcal infection, presumptive treatment for chlamydia was ubiquitously recommended. Given the high sensitivity of NAATs, patients with a negative chlamydia and a positive gonorrhea NAAT result need only be treated for gonorrhea. If a non-NAAT assay is performed or chlamydial infection is not ruled out, presumptive treatment for coinfection is appropriate. Empirical treatment is indicated for patients who may not return for test results. See Table 70-1 for treatment regimens.

Partners with sexual contact within 60 days preceding symptoms or diagnosis should be evaluated, tested, and treated. Patients should abstain from sexual intercourse until 1 week after they and their partners have completed treatment.

Gonorrhea

Etiology

Gonorrhea is caused by a Gram-negative diplococcus, *N. gonorrhoeae*. In the United States, approximately 600,000 new infections occur each year. Because gonococcal **infections in women** are often asymptomatic and **can lead to PID, tubal scarring, and subsequent tubal infertility or ectopic pregnancy,** screening is of utmost importance in women younger than 25 years.

Clinical Features

In **premenarchal females,** the **vagina** is the primary site of infection, whereas in **postmenarchal females** the organism can cause **endocervicitis, urethritis, bartholinitis, perihepatitis, or upper genital tract disease.** Common presentations include vaginal discharge, dysuria, labial swelling and tenderness, abnormal vaginal bleeding, or abdominal pain. Only about 50% of women with gonorrhea are symptomatic.

In males, *N. gonorrhoeae* infection can cause **urethritis, prostatitis, or epididymitis.**

In both **males and females,** infection in **extragenital sites** includes **pharyngitis, conjunctivitis, or disseminated infection** presenting as meningitis, septic arthritis, osteomyelitis, or septic shock. Gonococcal endocarditis and pericarditis have been described but are rare. **Adolescents** commonly have **migratory arthritis or tenosynovitis.** The two patterns of arthritis are the **arthritis-dermatitis syndrome** and **monoarticular arthritis.** The arthritis-dermatitis syndrome, characterized by fever, chills, and arthritis or tenosynovitis, is accompanied by skin lesions that affect approximately 50% of patients. There are usually <20 lesions, which are small tender papules or pustules on the distal extremities. The remainder of patients with gonococcal arthritis have a monoarticular arthritis affecting, in order of frequency, the knees, elbows, ankles, wrists, and small joints of the hands and feet.

Evaluation

Culture and Gram stain have been the mainstays of diagnosis for gonorrhea in symptomatic patients, but **NAATs** are now available for detection of genital *N. gonorrhoeae* infection. Diagnosis of the gonococcal infection depends on the location and circumstances of the infection.

- In males, a Gram stain of the urethral exudates (revealing typical Gram-negative intracellular diplococci) is sufficient for the diagnosis of gonorrhea, but, in the absence of urethral exudate, cultures or preferably NAAT specimens from urine or **anterior urethra** swab should be obtained to rule out a gonorrheal infection.

- In female patients depending on available NAAT assays, the presence of blood may necessitate testing with cultures from the endocervix. Otherwise, NAAT can be used. Endocervical Gram stain is not helpful in females.
- In patients with gonococcal arthritis-dermatitis syndrome, blood cultures may be positive.
- In patients with gonococcal monoarticular arthritis, joint fluid culture may be positive; blood cultures are usually negative.

Treatment

Given the **high coinfection rates of N. gonorrhoeae with C. trachomatis**, patients who are treated empirically for gonococcal infection are also routinely treated with a regimen effective against uncomplicated genital C. trachomatis infection. See Table 70-1 for details of treatment.

Pelvic Inflammatory Disease
Etiology

The term PID refers to a spectrum of infections of the **upper female genital tract** including endometritis, salpingitis, tubo-ovarian abscess, and pelvic peritonitis. Although C. trachomatis and N. gonorrhoeae are the most important causative organisms of PID, it should be managed as a **polymicrobial infection** of microorganisms that are part of the **vaginal flora** (e.g., anaerobes, G. vaginalis, H. influenzae, enteric Gram-negative rods, and Streptococcus agalactiae) as well as other organisms (e.g., M. hominis, Mycobacterium genitalium, U. urealyticum).

Risk factors for PID include age (highest rate in 15- to 19-year-olds), increased number of sexual partners, previous history of PID, sexual partner with an STD, and socioeconomic factors such as drug use, youth with behavioral and emotional problems, and disadvantaged youth.

Clinical Features

The wide variety of signs and symptoms plus many asymptomatic patients make the **diagnosis of PID difficult.** PID is more likely to present during the first half of the menstrual cycle. **Bilateral lower abdominal pain** is the most common presenting symptom. Other associated symptoms include abnormal vaginal discharge, abnormal uterine bleeding, dysuria, dyspareunia, nausea, vomiting, and fever. Because of this presentation, **other common causes of lower abdominal pain** (e.g., ectopic pregnancy, ovarian torsion, acute appendicitis, urinary tract infection, and functional pain) **must be considered and ruled out.**

Evaluation

Given the potential for **devastating sequelae if left untreated,** the diagnosis of PID should be **considered in any female of child-bearing age**

TABLE 70-2 Criteria for the Diagnosis of Acute Pelvic Inflammatory Disease

Minimum criteria (initiate empirical treatment if present and no other causes):
  Uterine/adnexal tenderness **OR**
  Cervical motion tenderness
Additional criteria to support a diagnosis of pelvic inflammatory disease:
  Abnormal cervical or vaginal mucopurulent discharge
  Presence of white blood cells on saline microscopy of vaginal secretions
  Elevated erythrocyte sedimentation rate
  Elevated C-reactive protein
  Laboratory documentation of cervical infection with *Neisseria gonorrhoeae* or *Chlamydia trachomatis*
  Temperature >101°F (38°C)

who has pelvic pain. As noted earlier, history can be very helpful and information should be obtained regarding past episodes of PID (increased risk for recurrent PID) and date of last menstrual cycle. Because visualization of the pelvic structures for inflammation by laparoscope, the gold standard, is almost never practical, the diagnosis is made on clinical evidence. Most women with PID have pelvic tenderness in addition to either mucopurulent discharge or evidence of white blood cells (WBCs) in saline preparation of vaginal fluid. Table 70-2 reviews the criteria for the diagnosis of acute PID.

Important laboratory testing includes a **pregnancy test** (to rule out pregnancy or complications of pregnancy), **complete blood cell count (CBC) with differential, erythrocyte sedimentation rate (ESR), NAAT** (or cultures) for *N. gonorrhoeae* and *C. trachomatis*, **urinalysis, and urine culture. Blood cultures** should be obtained in septic-appearing patients. **Pelvic ultrasonography (with Doppler if ovarian torsion is suspected)** should be considered in all adolescents with the diagnosis of PID because a tubo-ovarian abscess (TOA) may not be noted on the examination, and physical examination and laboratory findings are not sensitive or specific for the diagnosis of TOA. **Ultrasonography** can also help to rule out acute appendicitis and torsion. **Transvaginal sonography** may show thickened fluid-filled tubes with or without free pelvic fluid or tubo-ovarian complex in cases of PID. **Laparoscopy** is only indicated when the diagnosis of PID is uncertain or for patients with a diagnosis of PID who have recurrent abdominal pain.

Treatment

Because even mild disease can result in long-term sequelae, clinicians should have a **low threshold for making the diagnosis** and initiating treatment.

TABLE 70-3 Regimens for the Treatment of Pelvic Inflammatory Disease in Adolescents

Outpatient Regimens
 Ceftriaxone, 250 mg IM once
 OR
 Cefoxitin, 2 g IM once WITH probenecid, 1 g PO once
 OR
 Other parenteral third-generation cephalosporin (e.g., ceftizoxime or cefotaxime)
 PLUS
 Doxycycline, 100 mg PO twice daily for 14 days, WITH or WITHOUT metronidazole, 500 mg orally twice daily for 14 days

Inpatient Regimens
 Regimen A
  Cefoxitin, 2 g IV every 6 hours
  OR
  Cefotetan, 2 g IV every 12 hours
  PLUS
  Doxycycline, 100 mg orally or IV every 12 hours
 Regimen B
  Clindamycin, 900 mg IV every 8 hours
  PLUS
  Gentamicin, 2 mg/kg IV loading dose, followed by a maintenance dose of 1.5 mg/kg every 8 hours

IM = intramuscularly; *IV* = intravenously; *PO* = orally.
Adapted from Centers for Disease Control and Prevention: Sexually transmitted diseases treatment guidelines 2006. *MMWR Recomm Rep* 55(RR-11):1–94, 2006. Published by the United States Centers for Disease Control and Prevention.
Note: Parenteral therapy can be discontinued 24 hours after clinical improvement with continuation of PO doxycycline 100 mg twice daily or clindamycin 450 mg PO four times daily (preferred when tubo-ovarian abscess is present) to complete a 14-day course.

PID treatment regimens must provide empirical **broad-spectrum coverage** of likely pathogens. Coverage should include *N. gonorrhoeae, C. trachomatis*, anaerobes, Gram-negative facultative bacteria, and streptococci. Table 70-3 reviews appropriate antibiotic regimens for the treatment of PID.

The CDC recommends considering **hospitalization when the diagnosis is unclear, the possibility of surgical emergencies** (e.g., appendicitis, ectopic pregnancy) **cannot be excluded, the patient is pregnant, the patient has a TOA,** the patient has severe illness (severe nausea and vomiting or high fever), or there is **intolerance or failure of an outpatient regimen** (after 72 hours). Because there are no data to suggest that either adolescent women or women with HIV infection benefit from hospitalization for PID treatment, clinical judgment and an assessment of the patient's compliance is recommended based on the previously described considerations. All patients treated as outpatients should be reevaluated within 72 hours to ensure clinical improvement.

EVALUATION OF SEXUALLY TRANSMITTED DISEASES

Patient History

Important questions to ask include:

- Are there other common symptoms consistent with infection (e.g., presence of abnormal vaginal discharge or bleeding, dysuria, abdominal pain, genital lesions)?
- Is there testicular pain or swelling?
- What type of birth control method is used?
- Is the person currently trying to get pregnant?
- Is there a previous history of STDs or known exposure to an infected partner?
- What was the beginning date of the last menstrual period?
- Is there a history of pregnancy or abortion?
- When was the last pelvic examination?

Physical Examination

In all patients, when there is concern about an STD, the **external genitalia** must be examined. In sexually active adolescent females, the **internal genitalia** should be examined by bimanual examination; using a speculum is indicated if cervical cultures need to be collected. In males, the **penis, testes, scrotum, and rectum** should be examined. Vaginal or meatal discharge, skin lesions, lacerations, contusions, epididymal or testicular tenderness, or inguinal adenopathy should be noted.

> **HINT:** Avoid using lubricant for speculum insertion because the lubricant may interfere with cultures. Instead, rinse the speculum with warm water before inserting.

Laboratory Studies

- **Cultures or NAAT** should be performed on samples from the endocervical canal, vagina, or urine (for females) and from the urethra or urine (for males) if chlamydia or gonorrhea is suspected.
- **Wet mount.** In females, a wet mount should be done if Trichomonas is suspected. Some centers may have access to rapid trichomonas polymerase chain reaction testing, which is preferred over direct visualization.
- **Gram stain** of a vaginal specimen should be done if vaginal candidiasis or bacterial vaginosis is suspected and to assess for WBCs.
- **Gram stain** of urethral discharge can be useful in diagnosing gonococcal urethritis in males.

- **Blood tests.** In females with suspected upper genital tract disease, a CBC and ESR or C-reactive protein should be considered.
- **Urinalysis.** In males, a urinalysis should be performed. A positive leukocyte esterase in men has a good negative predictive value (97%) for *C. trachomatis.*

> **HINT:** In prepubertal girls, Dacron swabs are gently inserted approximately 1 inch into the vagina and gently rotated for a few seconds to obtain a specimen for NAAT or culture.

> **HINT:** In a prepubertal boy, specimens are obtained by swabbing the urinary meatus only. In postpubertal boys, the swab is inserted into the urethra a short distance (i.e., approximately 1 inch [2.5 cm]) and rotated for a few seconds.

TREATMENT OF SEXUALLY TRANSMITTED DISEASES

Females

Empirical therapy for gonorrhea and chlamydia should be instituted **for patients with a mucopurulent cervical or vaginal discharge** while awaiting results of cultures or NAAT. Additionally, empirical therapy is warranted **if the partner** (or perpetrator, in the case of suspected sexual abuse) **has been diagnosed** with an STD. In most other patients, treatment can be deferred until the results of testing are available, provided appropriate follow-up is feasible.

Males

Empirical therapy for gonorrhea and chlamydia should be **considered in males with a urethral discharge.** In patients with dysuria or an abnormal urinalysis, further workup for STD is warranted prior to treatment.

SCREENING, PROPHYLAXIS, AND PREVENTION OF SEXUALLY TRANSMITTED DISEASES

The consideration of an STD in a sexually active adolescent or young adult serves as an important opportunity to **initiate STD screening, prophylaxis**, and a discussion about **prevention.**

Screening

All patients diagnosed with an STD should be **screened for syphilis and offered HIV antibody testing.**

Yearly screening for chlamydia and gonorrhea by culture or NAAT should be considered for all sexually active males and females. For females with a history of an STD, more frequent screening (every 3 to 4 months) is indicated.

Pap smear should be performed yearly on **all females who have been sexually active for at least 3 years or who are at least 21 years old. Pap smears do not need to be obtained** in the presence of an STD. Routine pap smears should be deferred until symptoms of vaginitis/cervicitis resolve. Although some providers perform anal pap smears on MSMs (men who have sex with men), the CDC currently does not recommend this type of screening.

Prophylaxis

- **Hepatitis B.** Effective prophylaxis for hepatitis B can be accomplished with the hepatitis B vaccine. The vaccine should be considered in all sexually active individuals without hepatitis B disease or prior vaccination.
- **HIV.** There is no consensus on the use of antiretroviral medications for HIV-negative patients with sexual exposure to an HIV-infected or suspected HIV-infected individual. In certain settings, however, post-exposure prophylaxis may be considered for HIV.
- **HPV.** The quadrivalent HPV vaccine confers prophylactic protection against the high-risk strains 16 and 18 and those most commonly associated with genital warts, strains 6 and 11. The vaccine is recommended for all females ages 9 to 26 years old regardless of sexual activity status. This vaccine is not approved for use in males.
- **Hepatitis A (HAV).** Vaccination is important to prevent fecal-oral transmission during sexual contact, with the majority of cases reported in MSMs.

Prevention

Information regarding major STDs should be **provided to all adolescents and individuals diagnosed with an STD.**

Education on the correct use and efficacy of condoms in preventing pregnancy and STDs should be given to all patients, male and female, diagnosed with an STD or engaging in sexual activity. The **limitations of condoms should also be stated,** namely, that they may not prevent many cases of HPV, HAV, and some cases of HSV. Providers should advocate for dual contraception.

Treatment of partners of patients with chlamydia, gonorrhea, syphilis, and trichomonas is an effective means of preventing symptomatic disease in the partner. It also minimizes the risk of reinfection in the patient and future infection of other sexual partners. Understanding the complex developmental and biologic issues that contribute to adolescents' risk for STDs is an important first step in providing sexual and reproductive health care for this population.

Suggested Readings

Banikarim C, Chacko MR: Pelvic inflammatory disease in adolescents. *Adolesc Med* 15:273–285, 2004.

Catallozzi M, Rudy BJ: Lesbian, gay, bisexual, transgendered, and questioning youth: the importance of sensitive and confidential sexual history in identifying the risk and implementing treatment for sexually transmitted infections. *Adolesc Med* 15:353–367, 2004.

Centers for Disease Control and Prevention: Quadrivalent human papilloma virus vaccine. Recommendations of the Advisory Committee of Immunization Practice (ACIP). *MMWR Recomm Rep* 56(RR-2): 1–24, 2007.

Centers for Disease Control and Prevention: Sexually transmitted diseases treatment guidelines 2006. *MMWR Recomm Rep* 55(RR-11): 1–94, 2006. See: www.cdc.gov/std/treatment

English A, Ford CA: The HIPAA Privacy Rule and adolescents: legal question and clinical challenges. *Perspect Sex Reprod Health* 36:80–86, 2004.

Ford CA, English A, Sigman G: Confidential health care for adolescents: position paper of the Society for Adolescent Medicine. *J Adolesc Health* 35:160–167, 2004.

Ikeda MK, Jenson HB: Evaluation and treatment of congenital syphilis. *J Pediatr* 117:843–852, 1990.

Neinstein LS: Sexually transmitted diseases. In *Adolescent Health Care: A Practical Guide,* 4th ed. Edited by Neinstein LS. Baltimore, Williams & Wilkins, 2002.

Shafii T, Burstein GR: An overview of sexually transmitted infections among adolescents. *Adolesc Med* 15:201–214, 2004.

Shrier LA: Sexually transmitted diseases in adolescents: biologic, cognitive, psychologic, behavioral, and social issues. *Adolesc Med* 15: 215–234, 2004.

Spigarelli MG, Biro FM: Sexually transmitted disease testing: evaluation of diagnostic tests and methods. *Adolesc Med* 15:287–299, 2004.

Trager JDK: Sexually transmitted diseases causing genital lesions in adolescents. *Adolesc Med* 15:323–352, 2004.

Tramont EC: *Treponema pallidum* (syphilis). In *Principles and Practice of Infectious Diseases,* 4th ed. Edited by Mandell GL, Douglas RG, Bennett JE. New York, Churchill Livingstone, 1995, 2117–2133.

INTRODUCTION

Linear growth is an integral part of childhood development. Human growth generally occurs in a predictable pattern:

- Rapid growth of intrauterine life—how much the fetus grows is primarily determined by maternal health and nutrition.
- Less rapid growth of infancy—genetic factors gradually come into play and eventually outweigh the intrauterine conditions that initially determined fetal size; in practice, this means that infants often cross growth percentiles (channelize) to a percentile more in line with their genetic potential, whether tall or short. Growth gradually slows: Averages are 25 cm over the first year of life, 10 cm over the second year of life.
- Slow, relatively constant rate of growth of early to middle childhood—from 2 years of age to beginning of puberty: 4 to 6 cm/year.
- Growth acceleration of midpuberty—also known as the pubertal "growth spurt." Average rate of growth: 10 cm/year.
- Cessation of growth with epiphyseal (growth plate) fusion.

Deviations from this pattern may represent variants of normal growth, but may also be indicative of an underlying genetic abnormality, psychosocial or nutritional deprivation, or systemic illness. **Early detection** of any such deviations, with diagnosis and treatment of underlying illness (if any), is essential to maximizing potential adult height. Therefore, interval growth should be accurately assessed at each child-care visit, and any deviations from standard growth patterns should be evaluated. It is crucial to differentiate between **normal variants** of growth and **abnormal patterns** (i.e., between a healthy petite child and a child with an underlying systemic illness and/or other abnormality of growth).

> **HINT:** The more the child's growth pattern deviates from the usual pattern, the greater the chances of an underlying abnormality.

Definition of Important Terms

- **Short stature:** Because height is a continuous variable, the definition of "short" involves a selected cutoff; a height >2 standard deviations (SDs) below the mean for age and sex is the most commonly accepted threshold. Given the nature of bell curves, approximately 2% of the population (including a number of healthy children) are classified as short by definition. Thus **short stature may or may not be pathologic.** It is important to take the child's height and growth velocity in the context of the overall picture, including the variables discussed later.

- **Height/growth velocity:** The annualized rate of linear growth.
- **Growth failure:** A height velocity that is less than expected for a child's age, sex, genetic potential (as determined by parental heights—see later), and stage of puberty; alternately defined as the crossing downward of two or more major height percentiles (beyond 2 years of age) and/or dropping below the 3rd height percentile. **Growth failure is by definition pathologic.**
- **Chronological age:** Age in years.
- **Bone/skeletal age:** The stage of bone development or maturation as assessed by radiography.

Assessment of Growth

Length/Stature

Measurement of length/stature must be accurate and reproducible to assess the degree of interval growth correctly. Children <2 years should be measured supine, children >3 years should be measured standing, and children between 2 and 3 years of age can be measured either way, depending on the child's ability to stand erect for the time it takes to be measured. **Recumbent lengths should be recorded on the length (ages birth to 36 months) chart, and standing heights on the height (age 2 to 20 years) chart because they differ slightly.** Supine length is best measured with the child's head against an inflexible board in the Frankfurt plane (wherein the long axis of the trunk is perpendicular to the line formed by connecting the outer canthus of the eyes and the external auditory meatus), legs fully extended, and the feet placed perpendicularly against a movable foot board. To measure stature, a stadiometer fixed to the wall is most accurate. The child's feet are placed together parallel to each other, and the child's heels, buttocks, thoracic spine, and back of head should all be up against the stadiometer's vertical axis. The child should be standing fully erect, heels touching the ground, and the head must be in the Frankfurt plane.

Growth Charts

Evaluation of a child's current height and overall growth pattern occurs within the context of standards typical for the population. Most general pediatric and pediatric endocrine offices use the growth charts from the Centers for Disease Control and Prevention (CDC): percentile curves that illustrate the distribution, in U.S. children, of length or height, weight, head circumference (for ages birth to 3 years) and body mass index (BMI; weight [kg]/height [m^2]). The data used to construct the updated 2000 growth curves came from the National Health and Nutrition Examination Survey. The CDC growth curves were derived from cross-sectional population surveys, rather than longitudinal surveys that follow the same children over a course of years to determine their growth rates over time. Therefore, an individual's growth pattern may differ somewhat from the standardized pattern, especially during periods of rapid growth (infancy and the pubertal growth spurt).

Parental Heights

Because genetics play a large role in determining both the rate of maturation and the eventual target height, it is important to consider the heights of the biologic mother and father to place the child's current stature and predicted height in proper context. A **significant deviation from the familial growth pattern** should raise suspicion of possible pathologic processes.

Body Proportions

Several conditions underlying growth abnormalities cause disproportionate growth (e.g., extremities more shortened than trunk in *SHOX* insufficiency, skeletal dysplasias, and chondrodysplasias). Thus measurement of the following body proportions can aid the diagnosis of the underlying defect:

- Occipitofrontal head circumference
- Lower body segment: distance from top of pubic symphysis to the floor
- Upper body segment: distance from top of head to top of symphysis pubis
- Arm span: distance between the tips of the middle digits with both arms fully extended
- Published standards exist for each of these measurements relative to the child's age.

Skeletal Maturation (Skeletal or Bone Age)

The determination of bone age is predicated on the fact that ossification centers appear and progress in a predictable sequence in most children, so a radiograph may be compared to a standard. **The bone age, or skeletal age, is the only quantitative determination of somatic maturation; thus it mirrors the tempo of growth and maturation and gives an indication of the remaining growth potential.** Once the child is beyond infancy, an anteroposterior (AP) radiograph of the left hand and wrist is taken and compared to published standards (Greulich and Pyle or Tanner-Whitehouse); knee films can be used at ages when hand/wrist films are not yet too informative. Factors that impact the rate of skeletal maturation include genetic predisposition, thyroid hormone, growth hormone (GH), insulin-like growth factor (IGF)-1, glucocorticoids, and estrogens (in children of both sexes).

DIFFERENTIAL DIAGNOSIS LIST

Normal Variants

Familial (genetic) short stature (excluding genetic problems inherited in an autosomal dominant fashion, which can also cause short stature in successive family generations)

Constitutional delay of growth and puberty

Intrauterine Growth Retardation

Metabolic or Genetic Causes

Bone Disorders

Osteochondrodysplasias: Genetic abnormalities of cartilage and/or bone. Examples:

Achondroplasia and hypochondroplasia

Achondrogenesis

Mesomelic dysplasias

Epiphyseal and metaphyseal dysplasias

Osteogenesis imperfecta

Chromosomal Abnormalities

Trisomy 21

Turner syndrome

Trisomies 8, 13, 18

18q deletion

Other Genetic Conditions

Deletions of *SHOX* gene region of X chromosome

Polymorphism—chromosome 12q11, 1q12, 2q36

Russell-Silver syndrome

Prader-Willi syndrome

Noonan syndrome

Others (Cornelia de Lange syndrome, insulin receptor gene mutations [leprechaunism, or "Donovan" syndrome], Rubinstein-Taybi syndrome, Aarskog syndrome, Bloom syndrome, Cockayne syndrome, progeria, Seckel syndrome)

Inborn Errors of Metabolism

Glycogen storage diseases

Galactosemia

Mucopolysaccharidoses

Glycoproteinoses

Mucolipidoses

Malnutrition

Protein-calorie (kwashiorkor)

Generalized (marasmus)

Anorexia nervosa

Nutritional dwarfing and failure to thrive

Micronutrient deficiencies (especially iron, zinc)

Psychosocial (Deprivation) Dwarfism

Iatrogenic

Chronic glucocorticoid exposure (e.g., in severe asthma, inflammatory conditions)

Stimulant medications for attention deficit hyperactivity disorder (ADHD)

Chronic Systemic Diseases

Renal Disease

Fanconi syndrome

Renal tubular acidosis

Uremia/chronic renal failure

Heart Disease
  Congenital (especially
    cyanotic)
  Congestive heart failure
Malabsorption
  Celiac sprue
  Inflammatory bowel
    disease
  Short gut syndrome
Liver Disease
  Chronic liver disease and/or
    liver failure
Lung Disease
  Cystic fibrosis
Hematologic
  Profound anemia
  Thalassemia (especially if
    transfusion dependent)
  Hemosiderosis
Oncologic
  Primary malignancy
  Secondary to chemotherapy
  Secondary to irradiation

Collagen Vascular Diseases

Infectious
  AIDS or HIV (untreated)
  Tuberculosis
  Intestinal parasites

Endocrine Disorders
  Diabetes mellitus (Mauriac
    syndrome)
  Glucocorticoid excess
    (Cushing syndrome)
  Hypothyroidism
  Growth hormone deficiency
    (GHD)
  Primary IGF deficiency
    Growth hormone insensitiv-
      ity (Laron dwarfism)
    Post-GH receptor defects

Pseudohypoparathyroidism
Rickets
**Pituitary and/or hypothalamic
  dysfunction**
  Structural abnormalities
    associated with other
    midline defects (e.g., holo-
    prosencephaly, septo-optic
    dysplasia)
Isolated hypothalamic/pitu-
  itary malformation/s (e.g.,
  empty sella syndrome,
  ectopic neurohypophysis)
Trauma—generalized brain
  trauma or trauma specific to
  hypothalamus, pituitary
  stalk, or anterior pituitary
Surgical resection of pituitary
  and/or pituitary stalk
Inflammation of pituitary
  and/or hypothalamus
Brain and/or hypothalamic
  tumors (e.g., germinomas,
  gliomas)
Pituitary tumors (e.g., cranio-
  pharyngiomas, histiocytosis X)
Irradiation of brain and/or
  hypothalamus
Genetic causes:
Idiopathic GH deficiency
GHRH (growth hormone
  releasing hormone) receptor
  mutation
Isolated: *GH1* and *GH2*
  mutations, *CSHP1* mutation,
  CSH1 and *CSH2* mutations,
  idiopathic
GH secretagogue receptor
  mutation
Multiple pituitary hormone
  deficiencies: *HESX1* mutation, *PROP1* mutation,
  POUF1 mutation

DIFFERENTIAL DIAGNOSIS DISCUSSION

A comprehensive discussion of all the causes of short stature is beyond the scope of this chapter. The following is a focused review of a select number of normal variants and abnormal causes of short stature.

Familial Short Stature

Familial short stature (FSS) is a height that, although representing the lower end of the population norm, is nonetheless in keeping with the child's genetic potential. **This is usually a normal variant.** However, some causes of abnormal short stature such as GH gene deletions can be inherited in a dominant fashion, so even if there is a family history of short stature, taking a careful history, including heights and pubertal timing of parents, siblings, and extended family members, and performing a focused physical examination remain important.

Clinical Features

Both parents' heights are usually in the lower height percentiles, often below the 10th. The child's pattern of growth is **consistent** with that of his or her parents (and often siblings too). The child's growth velocity is usually normal, so the grow curve is low but parallel to the normal lines. The predicted adult height is in keeping with midparental target height. In the absence of a family history of delayed puberty, the timing of puberty is usually average.

Evaluation

The past medical history, review of systems, and physical examination are typically unremarkable, with no abnormalities of body proportions in either the patient or the parents. Because skeletal growth is not delayed, the bone age should be within the normal range. Laboratory workup, including growth factors and a chemistry panel, should be within the normal range. Abnormalities of history, physical examination, or laboratory studies should prompt the investigator to look for other causes of short stature.

Treatment

The child and family should be reassured **this is not a disease,** the child will likely enter puberty within the same average time frame as his or her peers, and the child's height will likely be in keeping with the family trend. **Because this is not a disease, treatment is not indicated.**

Constitutional Growth Delay

Constitutional growth delay is also known as constitutional delay of growth and puberty (CDGP) or constitutional delay of growth and maturation (CDGM). Delayed puberty is defined as the absence of secondary sexual characteristics by an age that is delayed by >2 to 2.5 SDs beyond the mean for the population: the absence of thelarche in girls >12 years, of signs of puberty in boys >13 years, or of menarche in girls >16 years (primary amenorrhea). CDGP represents the late end of the spectrum of pubertal development. Children with CDGP enter puberty later than most of their peers. Thus the pubertal growth spurt is also delayed, and these children continue to grow at the prepubertal rate of 4 to 6 cm/year while their peers' height velocity increases, resulting in a gap between the heights of children with CDGP and the heights of age-matched peers—a transient relative short stature.

Clinical Features

These children usually have a normal birth length, begin to cross height percentiles early in life, and settle in the lower percentiles by 2 years of age. Between the ages of 2 years and the onset of puberty in their peers, the children's height velocity usually places them along the lower margins of the growth curve (around or sometimes below the 5th to 10th percentile). Then, as their peers begin the pubertal growth spurt and the growth curve slope increases, the children with CDGP commonly fall further below the 5th percentile. They enter puberty spontaneously at a later-than-usual age and eventually attain an adult height within the normal range, although this height can fall short of the predicted adult height. There is often a family history of maternal and/or paternal relatives with similarly delayed puberty. CDGP can sometimes occur together with FSS, leading to pronounced short stature.

Evaluation

History, review of systems, and physical examination are usually normal except for short stature and the delayed pubertal status relative to age norms. Taking a detailed history and thoroughly reviewing the child's growth curve are essential steps to establishing this diagnosis; an isolated point on the growth curve at the time of the visit is insufficient. The differential diagnosis for CDGP includes Kallmann syndrome and partial gonadotropin deficiency; lack of anosmia can exclude the former, but only time can help distinguish between CDGP and the latter. Bone age is significantly delayed, enough so that the predicted adult height should be normal. Any abnormalities on physical examination or laboratory workup should suggest another diagnosis.

Treatment

After a thorough evaluation has excluded other causes of delayed puberty/abnormal growth, it is reasonable to reassure the child and family and monitor growth expectantly, given that spontaneous entry into puberty and attainment of a typical adult height are anticipated. However, because delayed puberty and consequent short stature in adolescence can have a significant social impact, it is also reasonable to offer a short course of low-dose androgens (for boys) or estrogen (for girls) to jump-start puberty. Low-dose, short-term courses are used to avoid acceleration of skeletal maturation and thus impairment of adult height from decreased time to grow. **This intervention only causes the child to enter puberty earlier; it does not increase the final adult height.** There are no data indicating that GH therapy increases final adult height.

Intrauterine Growth Retardation/Small for Gestational Age

Intrauterine growth retardation (IUGR) is defined as birthweight and/or length >2 SD below the mean for gestational age. Small for gestational age (SGA) is defined as birthweight <2,500 g at a gestational age of ≥37 weeks or length below the third percentile for gestational age. Affected infants are a diverse group because of a variety of maternal, placental, environmental, and intrinsic fetal causes that can lead to IUGR/SGA, including the following:

- Maternal causes: malnutrition, hypertension or preeclampsia, uterine malformations
- Placental abnormalities: two-vessel cord, vascular insufficiency or infarction, abnormal implantation
- Chromosomal disorders: trisomy 21
- Genetic disorders: Prader-Willi syndrome, Russell-Silver syndrome
- Congenital infections: rubella, varicella
- Intrauterine exposure to medications, drugs, or toxins: amphetamines, cocaine, nicotine, alcohol, propranolol, methotrexate
- IGF deficiency or resistance

Clinical Features

Most infants experience sufficient catch-up growth (i.e., an accelerated rate of weight gain and linear growth above the upper statistical limit for the child's age following a period of growth failure) in the first few years of life to place them on the normal height curve. However, a subset (10% to 25% in various studies) does not and remains below the 5th percentile throughout life. Children with IUGR who experience catch-up growth and, more importantly, accelerated weight gain are at higher risk of childhood obesity than children who were appropriate for gestational age (AGA) at birth. Children whose IUGR is caused by a genetic abnormality (e.g., Majewski osteodysplastic primordial dwarfism types I, II or III, or Russell-Silver syndrome) continue to have poor postnatal growth, a condition termed "primordial dwarfism."

Evaluation

The evaluation of a child with IUGR should begin with a careful history and physical examination. If the history or physical examination findings are suggestive of an intrinsic abnormality, the appropriate evaluation should be obtained (e.g., chromosomal analysis and/or referral to a geneticist to evaluate for a possible syndrome). If the limbs are disproportionate, skeletal radiographs should be obtained.

Treatment

GH improved final height prognosis in two large multicenter studies of short children who were SGA, and improved final adult height in another recent study of prepubertal children who were born SGA. Yet another study of GH administration, this one in young children (2 to 5 years of age) who were born SGA with continuing short stature, showed a significant increase in growth velocity in response to GH therapy without significant acceleration of bone age or side effects. Some caution in the interpretation of studies of GH in SGA children is indicated, however, for the following reasons:

- The group of SGA children is quite heterogeneous; there are a number of causes of SGA, and not all respond equally well to GH.
- Because GH is one of the counterregulatory hormones, GH therapy can increase insulin resistance, a particular concern in children born SGA who are at greater risk for developing obesity and insulin resistance later in childhood than children born AGA.

Each individual child should be carefully evaluated to see if he or she is a candidate for GH therapy, and the risks and benefits should be clearly explained to the family.

Osteochondrodysplasias

The osteochondrodysplasias are a diverse group of disorders whose common denominator is genetic abnormalities of cartilage and/or bone.

Clinical

Over 100 different conditions falling under this heading have been identified, each defined by specific skeletal and nonskeletal abnormalities and by radiographic features. These are the three broad groups:

- Defects of tubular and flat bones and/or axial skeleton (e.g., achondroplasia)
- Disorganized development of cartilaginous and fibrous components of the skeleton
- Idiopathic osteolyses

Nearly all children with a skeletal dysplasia grow slowly. If not, their growth is usually *disproportionate*—the **ratio of upper-to-lower (U:L)** body segment growth is abnormal, resulting in short limbs and/or trunks, and disproportionate rates of growth between limb segments (rhizomelic, mesomelic, or acromelic) are also frequently seen.

Evaluation

A careful family history should be obtained because the osteochondrodysplasias are hereditary (e.g., classical achondroplasia is an autosomal dominant disorder). However, many cases represent de novo mutations, so the absence of a family history does not rule out the possibility. A careful measurement of body proportions should be taken. Clinical and radiographic evaluation can determine what is primarily involved: long bones, vertebrae, and/or skull; and epiphyses, metaphyses, or diaphyses.

Treatment

GH therapy has been studied in several skeletal dysplasias. A few studies of GH in children with achondroplasia and hypochondroplasia showed an increase in height velocity (from 3.8 to 6.6 cm/year in one study in the first year, with a slight slowing of height velocity in subsequent years). A worsening of the disproportion between limb and trunk lengths in response to GH therapy was inconsistently seen.

Turner Syndrome

Turner syndrome, a disorder in females associated with the partial or complete absence of one X chromosome, is a relatively common condition, with a prevalence of 50 of 100,000 liveborn girls based on widespread genetic screening, or 32 of 100,000 liveborn girls based on clinical postnatal diagnosis. This discrepancy suggests the possibility of mild or even normal phenotype in girls with Turner syndrome. Short stature is the most common phenotypic manifestation of Turner syndrome in children and adults. The absence of two functional copies of the *SHOX* (short stature, homeobox-containing gene) appears to be the cause of the average 20-cm deficit in height observed for women with Turner syndrome.

Clinical

Turner syndrome may be recognized in infancy because of the characteristic webbed neck (formed following the resolution of cystic hygromas) and/or lymphedema of the extremities. Beyond infancy, the two most common features are short stature and sexual infantilism. Aside from short stature, other skeletal abnormalities may be seen, including relatively large hands and feet, a wide body, a short neck, cubitus valgus, genu valgum, and shortened fourth metacarpals. Madelung's deformity of the wrist (bilateral bowing of the radius with a dorsal subluxation of the distal ulna) is occasionally seen. Girls with Turner syndrome are at higher risk for developmental dysplasia of the hip in infancy and scoliosis during later childhood.

TABLE 71-1 Complications of Turner Syndrome

Cardiac (Seen in Approximately one third of all Patients with Turner Syndrome):

Coarctation of the aorta (about 10%)
Bicuspid aortic valve (increased incidence in patients with residual neck webbing at birth)
Aortic stenosis
Partial anomalous pulmonary venous connection
Conduction and repolarization anomalies (e.g., prolonged QT)
Increased risk of developing progressive aortic root dilation and, eventually, a dissecting aortic aneurysm: Careful monitoring throughout life is warranted.

Renal and Urinary Tract

Duplicated or cleft renal pelvis
Horseshoe kidney
Abnormal renal position or alignment
Increased risk of recurrent urinary tract infections

Reproductive Tract

Underdeveloped uterus, oviducts
Streak gonads
Although most women with Turner syndrome are infertile, up to 10% undergo some spontaneous pubertal development, and 2%–5% are able spontaneously to become pregnant.

Sensorineural Hearing Loss

Autoimmune diseases: Thyroiditis, celiac disease, Crohn's disease

Other physical examination findings may include ptosis, strabismus, low-set or deformed ears, micrognathia, high-arched palate, dental abnormalities, low posterior hairline, shield chest, hypoplastic areolae. Girls with Turner syndrome are at risk for a number of associated abnormalities of multiple organ systems (see Table 71-1 for more details.)

Evaluation

A careful physical examination may reveal some phenotypic features of Turner syndrome. However, not all girls with Turner syndrome manifest the classic phenotype, so the diagnosis should be considered in any female with unexplained short stature, and a standard karyotype should be sent (chromosomal analysis of 30 peripheral lymphocytes) to evaluate for possible mosaicism. Given the number of possible associated systemic problems, a comprehensive evaluation should be performed, including but not limited to the following:

- Echocardiogram at diagnosis to evaluate for cardiac anomalies; cardiac magnetic resonance imaging (MRI) later in life, to look for abnormalities of the aortic arch and descending aorta
- Renal and pelvic ultrasound to evaluate the kidneys and pelvocaliceal collecting system as well as the reproductive tract

- Auditory evaluation at diagnosis and every 1 to 5 years thereafter to look for possible sensorineural hearing loss
- Regular evaluation for hip dysplasia between infancy and 4 years of age, and evaluation for scoliosis in later childhood

Treatment

GH therapy is standard of care in pediatrics to improve final adult height in girls with Turner syndrome. **It is recommended that GH therapy be initiated as soon as growth failure is detected.** If pubertal development does not begin spontaneously, exogenous estrogen therapy should be initiated with the goal of reflecting as much as possible the process of normal puberty. If GH treatment is started young enough, sufficient growth is attained during the prepubertal years such that estrogen therapy need not be delayed as previously recommended.

Abnormalities of Growth Hormone/Insulin-like Growth Factor Axis

Background

Human GH is produced in and secreted by the somatotrophs of the anterior pituitary. Its secretion is regulated by GHRH and somatostatin, which stimulate and inhibit its release, respectively. Another hormone that may be involved in the regulation of GH release is ghrelin, a GH secretagogue produced in the stomach (primarily) and in the hypothalamus. Many, although not all, of GH's actions are mediated through the IGF peptides, in accordance with the somatomedin hypothesis. IGF-1 (also known as somatomedin-C), the primary IGF in humans, circulates in the bloodstream bound to IGF-binding proteins (especially IGFBP-3). IGF-1 then binds to IGF receptors, leading to activation of second messenger systems and multiple downstream effects, including insulin-like activity in extraskeletal tissue, promotion of incorporation of sulfate into cartilage, and stimulation of DNA synthesis. Other players in the growth system include insulin and IGF-2, which along with IGF-1 are the main mediators of fetal growth; androgens and estrogens, which induce the pubertal growth spurt and (estrogens only) epiphyseal fusion; and thyroid hormone, which has a permissive effect on GH secretion and exerts direct action on the growth plates.

Growth Hormone Deficiency and Related Conditions

Dysfunction may appear at a number of levels of the GH/IGF axis, including:

- Hypothalamic and higher centers
  - Congenital hypothalamic malformations
  - GHRH receptor mutations

- Trauma or inflammation of the brain and/or hypothalamus
- Central nervous system (CNS) and/or hypothalamic tumors
- Irradiation of brain and/or hypothalamus; chemotherapy
- GH neurosecretory dysfunction
- Pituitary
  - Absence of pituitary (empty sella syndrome) or other structural defects
  - Pituitary tumors (e.g., craniopharyngioma)
  - Hypophysitis
  - Genetic abnormalities of GH production or secretion (e.g., *PROP1* or *POU1F1* mutations, production of a bioinactive GH)
  - Pituitary trauma
  - Idiopathic GH deficiency
- GH insensitivity (e.g., caused by GH receptor defect—Laron dwarfism): high GH levels, but low IGF-1 levels, and, often, low GHBP levels
- Postreceptor signaling defects (e.g., primary IGF-1 deficiency)

A study of U.S. children with short stature found an incidence of GH deficiency of 1 of 3,500 children. Factors that should raise suspicion for GH deficiency include the following:

- Infants: A history of prolonged jaundice, hypoglycemia, microphallus, or traumatic delivery
- Craniofacial midline abnormalities (e.g., septo-optic dysplasia, holo-prosencephaly, central maxillary incisor)
- Consanguinity or family history of similar presentations
- History of a suprasellar tumor (e.g., craniopharyngioma)
- History of cranial irradiation, head trauma, or CNS infection/infarction

Clinical

Because insulin plays a large role in intrauterine growth, infants with congenital isolated GHD tend to have normal length and weight at birth. They may have a history of prolonged jaundice, microphallus, or hypoglycemia in infancy. Postnatal growth is overtly abnormal; in severe cases, growth failure is seen within the first months, and in less severe cases, poor linear growth manifests later. Other features of congenital GHD overlap with those of acquired GHD and include the following:

- Relatively normal skeletal proportions that correlate better with bone age than with chronologic age
- Increased adiposity (especially truncal) with poor lean body mass gain
- Growth deceleration and/or growth failure
- Standing height significantly below normal for the population and parental target height

- Delayed dentition
- Delayed average age of pubertal onset
- Depressed midfacial development, prominent forehead

Diagnosis of Growth Hormone Deficiency

A child suspected of having GHD should be referred to a pediatric endocrinologist for diagnostic evaluation. Because of the circadian rhythm of GH secretion, no one single test can definitively diagnose GH deficiency, so the workup involves a combination of different studies, including growth factors and provocative GH testing. Once the diagnosis of GH deficiency is established, **the child's ability to secrete other pituitary hormones must be evaluated (i.e., thyroid, adrenal, and, if age appropriate, gonadal function); there is an increased risk of mortality in patients with GHD because of underrecognized and undertreated central adrenal insufficiency.** Brain MRI with and without contrast, with special cuts of the pituitary and hypothalamus (which must be specifically requested), should be performed to evaluate for an intracranial tumor or structural abnormality as the cause of the GHD.

Recombinant Human Growth Hormone and Insulin-like Growth Factor-1 Treatment

GH and IGF-1 replacement therapy should be managed by pediatric endocrinologists. Doses and preparations vary. Recombinant human GH (rhGH) is administered as a daily subcutaneous injection. Those who care for patients on rhGH or rhIGF-1 therapy should be aware of the potential side effects; see Table 71-2 for more details.

TABLE 71-2 Possible Side Effects of Recombinant Human Growth Hormone and Recombinant Human Insulin-Like Growth Factor-1 Therapy

Possible Adverse Effects of rhGH Therapy

Pseudotumor cerebri
Slipped capital femoral epiphysis
Increased insulin resistance
Increased size and number of nevi (but no increased risk of malignancy)
Transient gynecomastia
Increased severity of scoliosis

Possible Adverse Effects of rhIGF-1 Therapy

Adenoidal hypertrophy
Hypoglycemia

Malignancy: Current Evidence Supports a Permissive Role, but not a Causal Role, for both GH and IGF-I in Cancer Development.

rhGH = recombinant human growth hormone; *rhIGF-1* = recombinant human insulin-like growth factor-1 therapy.

Current Non–Growth Hormone Deficiency Indications for Growth Hormone Therapy

- Chronic renal insufficiency
- Turner syndrome
- AIDS wasting syndrome
- Prader-Willi syndrome
- SGA/IUGR
- Idiopathic short stature
- *SHOX* deficiency
- Noonan syndrome (approved in 2007)

Chronic Systemic Illness

Many chronic illnesses are associated with short stature. The general mechanisms by which chronic illnesses lead to poor growth include the following:

- Anorexia/poor appetite/poor intake
- Malabsorption of nutrients
- Chronic acidosis
- Anemia
- Chronic hypoxemia
- Increased energy requirements
- Medical therapy for the condition (e.g., glucocorticoids)

These are some general categories of chronic illnesses associated with poor growth:

- Malabsorptive disorders—inadequate calorie or protein absorption leading to growth failure. **Abnormal growth can predate other disease manifestations.** In other words, dropping height and/or weight percentiles, even with a normal history, review of systems, and physical examination can be the first sign of a serious systemic illness. Examples: celiac sprue, inflammatory bowel disease (IBD), cystic fibrosis.
- Chronic renal insufficiency (CRI): decreased caloric intake, loss of electrolytes essential to growth, metabolic acidosis, protein-wasting, chronic anemia, deficiency of 1,25-dihydroxy vitamin D_3, and cardiac dysfunction can all play a role in the growth failure associated with CRI. Examples of diseases: Fanconi syndrome, renal tubular acidosis. GH accelerates growth in children with chronic renal failure prior to renal transplant, which is an indication approved by the Food and Drug Administration for GH therapy.
- Cardiovascular disease: Congestive heart failure and cyanotic heart diseases can both be associated with growth failure because of a

combination of the increased energy demands of the heart and to chronic hypoxia and with associated dysmorphic syndromes.

- Pulmonary disease: Chronic hypoxemia is associated with poor growth. The classical example is cystic fibrosis. Severe asthma can also be associated with growth failure; however, the chronic systemic glucocorticoids these children require also play a role in the growth failure.
- Chronic anemias: They can contribute to poor growth for a number of reasons:
  - Poor oxygen delivery to tissues
  - Increased cardiac work to maintain cardiac output
  - Higher energy needs because of increased hematopoiesis
  - In transfusion-dependent conditions such as thalassemias or severe sickle cell disease: the metabolic consequences of iron overload from chronic transfusion
- Chronic inflammation and infection: Poor growth in these conditions may be mediated in part by the inflammatory mediators; for example, interleukin-6 mediates a decrease in serum IGF-1 levels. Examples include AIDS and tuberculosis (the two top chronic illnesses causing growth failure worldwide) and intestinal parasites (e.g., hookworms). Growth failure can be the initial presentation of HIV infection in children.
- Diabetes mellitus (DM): Chronically poorly controlled DM can lead to growth failure in association with hepatomegaly because of excessive glycogen deposition. This condition is termed Mauriac syndrome. Insulin inhibits the transcription of IGF-binding protein-1 (IGFBP-1) in the liver. In the setting of insulin deficiency, IGFBP-1 synthesis increases, decreasing the bioavailability of serum IGF-1.
- Inborn errors of lipid, protein, or carbohydrate metabolism

Clinical

In most children with short stature caused by chronic illness, the weight tends to be depressed to a greater extent than the height, or there is a lag between the onset of weight deceleration and subsequent height deceleration. Bone age is usually delayed and approximates the height age.

Evaluation

A careful history and examination of the growth curve are important. The typical pattern is a period of normal growth followed by growth deceleration or even cessation, suggesting the onset of illness. Past medical history may reveal a previously diagnosed chronic illness, and review of systems may reveal features suggestive of certain illnesses (e.g., hematochezia and chronic abdominal pain in IBD). However, it is important to remember that growth failure can be the presenting sign of a chronic illness such as IBD; thus, even in the absence of concerning findings in the medical history or physical examination, the clinician should always consider and evaluate for chronic illnesses in children presenting for short stature evaluation.

Laboratory studies that screen for chronic illness include complete blood cell count (CBC), erythrocyte sedimentation rate (ESR), C-reactive protein (CRP), serum biochemistry profile, serum albumin level, celiac autoimmunity, and urinalysis. These preliminary screens may suggest the pathway for future diagnostic tests or procedures, such as endoscopy, small bowel biopsy, or renal biopsy.

Treatment

Once the underlying condition is treated, catch-up growth usually occurs.

Poor Nutrition

Optimal linear growth requires optimal nutrition. Globally, malnutrition is the most common cause of poor growth. Malnutrition affects the GH/IGF system. Total calorie and/or protein-calorie malnutrition cause decreased hepatic production of IGF-1. The lower IGF-1 levels provide decreased IGF-1-mediated negative feedback to the hypothalamus and pituitary, which can lead to increased GH production and secretion and thus higher than normal basal and stimulated serum GH levels.

Causes of malnutrition include social/societal (e.g., poverty, child neglect, societal upheaval), voluntary (e.g., anorexia nervosa), severe dietary restrictions (e.g., fear of obesity or of hypercholesterolemia), chronic illness, malformations of the oropharynx (e.g., Pierre Robin syndrome, cleft lip or palate), abnormal oral-motor function (e.g., pervasive developmental delay or severe cerebral palsy), or certain medications (e.g., stimulants for treatment of ADHD or chemotherapeutic agents). Isolated nutrient deficiencies, such as zinc, iron, and vitamin D (deficiency of which leads to rickets), can also cause short stature.

Clinical

Poor weight gain generally precedes the decrease and eventual failure of linear growth. The bone age is often delayed. With more advanced cases of malnutrition, signs of wasting may be seen on examination. Pubertal delay may be seen.

Evaluation

Taking a detailed dietary history is essential to establishing this diagnosis. A three-day diet log is a useful tool. Everything the child eats and drinks should be quantified and recorded. This record can be analyzed for intake of total calories, macronutrients, and micronutrients (i.e., sodium, potassium, iron, and zinc). Parental dietary recall is not sufficient because it is often inaccurate, although a 24-hour diet recall may shed some light during an initial clinic visit. Physical examination should look for the pubertal delay, evidence of malnutrition, and signs of systemic illness mentioned previously. Laboratory evaluations should include all those involved in the evaluation for chronic illness (see prior section).

Treatment

The treatment is **nutritional restitution.** Children unable to consume sufficient calories by mouth can be fed either enterally (via nasogastric or gastrostomy tube) or parenterally (partial or total parenteral nutrition). Chronically malnourished children provided with sufficient calories can experience catch-up growth.

Hypothyroidism

Growth failure is one of the most common and significant aspects of congenital and acquired hypothyroidism in children. Because of the significant cognitive consequences of hypothyroidism in the first 3 years of life, newborn screening now allows most cases to be diagnosed and treated early. Thus most cases of growth failure associated with hypothyroidism are caused by acquired hypothyroidism, which is most commonly owing to autoimmune Hashimoto's (chronic lymphocytic) thyroiditis or iodine deficiency. Growth retardation caused by acquired hypothyroidism can take several years to manifest clearly, although once clinically significant, it tends to be severe and progressive.

Clinical

Children with undiagnosed or untreated congenital hypothyroidism experience profound growth failure, delayed fontanel closure in infancy, and mental retardation (cretinism). Fortunately, most of these children are diagnosed by newborn screening and adequately treated, so this condition is now uncommon. Children with acquired hypothyroidism experience poor linear growth in the setting of excessive weight gain. They have immature body proportions, with an increased U:L body segment ratio, delayed dentition, and a profoundly delayed bone age. Puberty is often delayed, but precocious puberty can be seen as well.

Evaluation

Primary hypothyroidism is diagnosed by an elevated thyroid-stimulating hormone (TSH) level; total thyroxine (T4) level is normal in compensated hypothyroidism and low in uncompensated hypothyroidism. Autoimmune thyroiditis is confirmed by the presence of antithyroglobulin and/or antithyroid peroxidase antibodies. Secondary and tertiary hypothyroidism (of pituitary and hypothalamic etiologies, respectively) most often occurs with other pituitary hormone deficiencies and is best screened for with a free thyroxine (T4) level.

Treatment

The treatment of hypothyroidism is daily replacement with levothyroxine. Thyroid hormone replacement is associated with rapid catch-up growth.

EVALUATION OF SHORT STATURE

History

A careful history can uncover risk factors for short stature and signs or symptoms of underlying conditions or illnesses.

- Pregnancy History
    - Exposure to medications, drugs (e.g., alcohol, tobacco), or toxins
    - Maternal illnesses or pregnancy complications, especially infections or hypertension
    - History of any perinatal complications (e.g., traumatic delivery, perinatal asphyxia)
    - Birthweight and length (to see if child was an SGA infant)
- Growth Curve
    - Annualized growth velocity and any changes therein
    - Changes in height percentile
- Dietary History
    - Past Medical History
    - History of chronic/systemic illnesses or frequent hospitalizations (e.g., cystic fibrosis, IBD, or anemias requiring transfusion)
    - Medication history (e.g., history of systemic glucocorticoid therapy)
- Review of Systems
    - Symptoms suggestive of underlying illness (e.g., chronic diarrhea or abdominal pain, headache or visual disturbances, shortness of breath or lower extremity swelling, etc.)
    - Behavior problems or changes in school performance
    - Timing of pubertal onset and progression, if relevant (look for pubertal delay)
- Family History
    - Document heights of parents and other relatives (siblings, grandparents, aunts and uncles)
    - Determine if anyone in the family had a pattern of late growth and/or delayed puberty
    - Calculate midparental height: girls (mother's height in cm + father's height in cm – 13)/2; boys (mother's height in cm + 13 + father's height in cm)/2)

Physical Examination

- Measure and plot current and prior height and weight accurately; calculate height-to-weight ratio in younger children and BMI in older children to see if height or weight are disproportionately affected.
- General physical examination: Look for signs of underlying genetic abnormalities (e.g., dysmorphic features), midline defects suggestive of possible hypothalamic or pituitary malformations (e.g., central maxillary incisor), or systemic illness (e.g., aphthous ulcers, truncal adiposity, rachitic rosary, etc.).
- Dental examination: Dental maturation correlates well with skeletal maturation, so delayed dentition can be a clue to delayed bone age.
- Tanner staging: Look for pubertal delay (e.g., CDGP, Turner syndrome).
- Upper body segment-to-lower body segment ratio (normal ratio: 1.7 at birth, 1.3 at 3 years of age, and 1.0 by 7 years of age).
  - Abnormal ratio: possible rickets or skeletal dysplasia
- Arm span: less than the height before 8 years of age, equal to the height at 8 to 12 years of age, and greater than the height >12 years.

Laboratory Studies

- CBC: Look for anemia or other abnormalities.
- ESR and CRP: Elevated in inflammatory conditions.
- Serum electrolytes, blood urea nitrogen (BUN) and creatinine levels, calcium, phosphate, and alkaline phosphatase levels: Screen for renal dysfunction and calcium homeostasis.
- Total protein, albumin, prealbumin, and transaminase levels in evaluation of potential synthetic defects, inflammation/injury, and cholestasis.
- TSH and total T4 levels.
- IGF-1 and IGFBP-3 levels: Screen for GH deficiency and malnutrition.
- Urinalysis.
- Karyotype for females to evaluate for Turner syndrome.

Depending on the clinical diagnosis, other studies may be indicated, such as tissue transglutaminase immunoglobulin A (IgA) and immunoglobulin G to exclude celiac disease; 25-hydroxy and 1,25-dihydroxy vitamin D_3 levels to evaluate for vitamin D–deficiency rickets; sweat chloride analysis to exclude cystic fibrosis; tine testing or purified protein derivative to screen for tuberculosis; HIV testing; or screening for *SHOX* gene deletion.

Imaging Studies

- Bone age determination
  - AP left hand and wrist radiographs
  - AP and lateral knee radiographs, in children <2 years

- Skeletal survey, if indicated (suspected skeletal dysplasia)
- MRI of brain with pituitary cuts, if indicated (e.g., if neurologic symptoms or hypopituitarism)

PSYCHOSOCIAL RAMIFICATIONS OF SHORT STATURE

Many patient families seek evaluation and treatment of short stature to avoid the discrimination against shorter individuals, a phenomenon termed heightism. Although there is general agreement that short stature is associated with psychosocial stressors, whether they significantly impact the psychosocial function of the short individual remains controversial. The results of studies of the social function of children with short stature vary depending on the study population; children from a sample referred for medical evaluation of short stature are more likely to demonstrate problems than a population-based sample. The psychosocial, anthropological, historical, and biologic aspects of short stature are comprehensively reviewed in the book by Stephen Hall (see Suggested Readings).

Social pressures for tallness seem to affect males more than females in U.S. society. This has led to a referral bias for short stature evaluations. However, because growth failure can be the only presenting sign of an underlying health problem, the evaluation of short stature should receive equal import in both girls and boys. The primary job of the evaluating physician is to distinguish healthy variants from pathologic growth.

APPROACH TO THE PATIENT WITH SHORT STATURE

Short stature is a relatively common complaint in the pediatric patient population and one of the most common reasons for referral to a pediatric endocrinologist. A careful history can uncover the cause in many cases. The growth curve must be evaluated to determine patterns of growth and whether height and weight are equally affected. Other key components of the evaluation include a detailed dietary history to evaluate for malnutrition, a thorough physical examination (including evaluation of dentition, pubertal status, and body proportions), laboratory studies, and bone age radiographs. Children with growth failure who fall into certain categories—for example, Turner syndrome, chronic renal failure, GH deficiency—qualify for rhGH therapy and should be referred to pediatric endocrinologists to initiate the process. Clinicians should be aware of the possible adverse effects of rhGH therapy (pseudotumor cerebri, slipped capital femoral epiphysis, insulin resistance), and screen for those possibilities in patients receiving rhGH who develop worrisome symptoms.

Suggested Readings

AACE Growth Hormone Task Force; American Association of Clinical Endocrinologists: Medical guidelines for clinical practice for growth hormone use in adults and children—2003 update. *Endocr Pract* 9(1):64–76, 2003.

CDC Growth Charts, United States: Available at: http://www.cdc.gov/growthcharts.

Clayton PE: Management of the child born small for gestational age through to adulthood: a consensus statement of the International Societies of Pediatric Endocrinology and the Growth Hormone Research Society. *J Clin Endocrinol Metab* 92(3):804–810, 2007.

Grimberg A, Kutikov JK, Cucchiara AJ: Sex differences in patients referred for evaluation of poor growth. *J Pediatr* 146:212–216, 2005.

Growth Hormone Research Society: Consensus guidelines for the diagnosis and treatment of growth hormone (GH) deficiency in childhood and adolescence: summary statement of the GH Research Society. *J Clin Endocrinol Metab* 85(11):3990–3993, 2000.

Hall SS: *Size Matters: How Height Affects the Health, Happiness, and Success of Boys—and the Men They Become.* Boston, Houghton Mifflin, 2006.

Nathan BM, Palmert MR: Regulation and disorders of pubertal timing. *Endocrinol Metab Clin North Am* 34(3):617–641, ix, 2005.

Tanner JM, Goldstein H, Whitehouse RH: Standards for children's height at ages 2–9 years allowing for height of parents. *Arch Dis Child* 45:755–762, 1970.

INTRODUCTION

Sore throat is one of the most common reasons children are brought to medical attention. Most often, this complaint is part of an **upper respiratory tract infection.** Because children experience an average of five to seven upper respiratory tract infections per year, health care providers must be familiar with the evaluation and treatment of sore throat. In addition, **misdiagnosis** or inadequate treatment of a sore throat caused by certain bacterial pathogens **can result in serious complications.**

DIFFERENTIAL DIAGNOSIS LIST

Infectious Causes
Nasopharyngitis
Pharyngitis
Peritonsillar abscess or
  cellulitis
Retropharyngeal abscess or
  cellulitis
Parapharyngeal abscess
Tonsillitis
Laryngitis
Uvulitis
Epiglottitis
Lemierre syndrome
Laryngotracheobronchitis
  (croup)
Herpangina
Herpetic gingivostomatitis
Hand-foot-and-mouth disease
Cervical adenitis (referred
  pain)
Acute otitis media (referred
  pain)
Dental abscess (referred pain)
Scarlet fever
Kawasaki disease
Tularemia (*Francisella
  tularensis* infection)

Toxic Causes
Caustic or irritant ingestions
  (e.g., acid, lye)
Inhaled irritant (e.g., tobacco
  smoke)

Neoplastic Causes
Leukemia
Lymphoma
Rhabdomyosarcoma

Traumatic Causes
Foreign body
Intraluminal tear
Gastroesophageal reflux
  disease
Vocal abuse (e.g., shouting)
External neck trauma (e.g.,
  strangulation, child abuse)

Congenital or Vascular Causes
Branchial cleft cyst
Thyroglossal duct cyst

Inflammatory Causes
Autoimmune disorders
Allergy
Postradiation

Psychosocial Causes

Psychogenic pain (globus
hystericus)

Miscellaneous Causes

Cyclic neutropenia
Periodic fever, aphthous
stomatitis, pharyngitis,
cervical adenitis (PFAPA)
syndrome

Vitamin deficiency—A, B
complex, C
Dehydration
Pharyngeal irritation from
breathing dry, heated air

DIFFERENTIAL DIAGNOSIS DISCUSSION

Nasopharyngitis

Etiology

Most cases of nasopharyngitis, also known as the **common cold or upper respiratory tract infection,** are caused by **viral** agents. There are more than 200 serologically different causative agents. The most common are rhinoviruses, coronaviruses, parainfluenza virus, enteroviruses (coxsackievirus A and B, echovirus, polio virus), adenovirus, influenza virus A and B, and respiratory syncytial virus.

Clinical Features

The clinical picture typically includes **fever, runny nose, sneezing,** and **nasal congestion** with clear or purulent nasal secretions, a **sore throat** lasting for several days, and a self-limited clinical course of 4 to 10 days. Infection caused by group A beta hemolytic streptococcus (GABHS) may present as a seromucoid rhinitis in toddlers.

Associated symptoms may include irritability, restlessness, muscle aches, cough, eye discharge, vomiting, or diarrhea, depending on the causative agent. Otitis media with effusion, laryngotracheobronchitis, or bronchiolitis may be present.

Complications are typically attributable to **bacterial superinfection** and include sinusitis, cervical adenitis, mastoiditis, peritonsillar and periorbital cellulitis, acute otitis media, and pneumonia.

Evaluation

The patient or parent should be asked about **associated symptoms** and about **ill contacts** at home, school, or child care. A **complete physical examination** should be performed, paying particular attention to the patient's overall **appearance** and **hydration** status.

Treatment

The treatment of nasopharyngitis consists of **bed rest,** increased intake of **fluids,** and the administration of **acetaminophen or ibuprofen** for pain and fever. Because of the **risk of Reye syndrome** with influenza infection, **aspirin and aspirin-containing products should be avoided.** Oral decongestants (e.g., pseudoephedrine), **oral antihistamine** agents, and **phenylephrine drops** may be used for **older children. Saline drops** and **nasal suctioning** are appropriate for **infants** with nasal obstruction. **Humidifiers and vaporizers** may be useful to prevent drying of secretions.

Pharyngitis

Etiology

Most cases of acute pharyngitis are caused by **viruses**—most commonly, **adenoviruses.** Other viral causes include influenza viruses A and B; parainfluenza viruses 1, 2, and 3; Epstein-Barr virus (EBV); human metapneumovirus and enteroviruses. Bacterial causes include GABHS (15% to 30% of all acute pharyngitis in children), group C streptococci, group G streptococci, *Mycoplasma pneumoniae, Corynebacterium diphtheriae, Arcanobacterium hemolyticum, Neisseria gonorrhoeae, Neisseria meningitides, Yersinia enterocolitica, Yersinia pestis, and Francisella tularensis.*

Clinical Features

- **Viral pharyngitis (caused by viruses other than EBV)** is characterized by the gradual onset of a sore throat, fever, hoarseness, and halitosis (in some patients), and an erythematous throat with or without exudate. Follicular and ulcerative lesions, mild cough, rhinorrhea, conjunctivitis, diarrhea, enanthem, or exanthem suggest a viral cause. Cervical adenopathy (tender or nontender) and poor intake of solid foods and decreased appetite are seen. The clinical course is self-limited and lasts 1 to 5 days.
- **Although infectious mononucleosis is rare before 4 years of age, young children may experience pharyngitis caused by EBV.** Clinical features include fever and a sore and erythematous throat with or without exudate. Palatal petechiae, poor intake of solid foods, posterior cervical and generalized adenopathy, hepatosplenomegaly, and fatigue may be seen.
- **Many experts consider pharyngitis caused by GABHS and rheumatic fever to be uncommon in children <3 years, but GABHS has been isolated in symptomatic infants as young as 3 months.** It may present with the sudden onset of a sore throat, a fever as high as 104°F (40°C), erythematous tonsils with or without exudate, petechiae on the soft palate, and headache. Nausea, vomiting, and stomachache are often associated symptoms. Tender, anterior cervical adenopathy and a fine sandpaper-like rash may be noted on physical examination. Complications include acute otitis media, sinusitis, peritonsillar and retropharyngeal abscesses, acute glomerulonephritis, rheumatic fever, and suppurative cervical adenitis.

Evaluation

The parent should be asked about **associated symptoms** and whether the child has had **contact with anyone** at home or at school **with a sore throat, mononucleosis, strep throat, scarlet fever,** or **rheumatic fever.**

The **tonsils, pharynx, soft palate, skin, neck, lymph nodes, liver, spleen, and pulses** should be **examined,** and the patient's general appearance and overall **respiratory status** and **hydration status** should be assessed.

A **rapid strep test,** also known as a rapid antigen detection test, should be obtained if available for all patients with an inflamed throat on physical examination; and if the rapid strep test is negative, a throat culture for GABHS should be sent.

Treatment

The treatment for pharyngitis of any cause includes **acetaminophen and ibuprofen** for pain and fever (**avoid aspirin**), increased **fluids,** and the administration of **nonprescription lozenges** and gargle solutions to provide temporary pain relief. **Gargling with salt water** (1/4 to 1/2 tsp of salt in 8 oz of warm water) and drinking warm liquids may be soothing. In severe cases, especially with infectious mononucleosis, patients may need to be **hospitalized** for intravenous hydration and airway precautions. For infectious mononucleosis, short courses of corticosteroids reduce pain and swelling; however, their use should be considered only in select patients with marked tonsillar inflammation and impending airway compromise or other serious complications, such as hemolytic anemia. See Table 72-1 for the clinical findings useful in the diagnosis of streptococcal pharyngitis.

In patients with **GABHS** pharyngitis, the primary reason for treating with **antibiotics** is to **prevent rheumatic fever, which has not been**

TABLE 72-1 Clinical Findings Useful in the Diagnosis of Streptococcal Pharyngitis

Findings that Indicate Likely Viral Pharyngitis:

- Exposure to contacts with symptoms of upper respiratory tract infection
- Patient <2 years
- Cough, runny nose, or eye discharge predominate

Findings that Suggest Streptococcal Pharyngitis

- Exposure to contacts with strep throat, scarlet fever, or rheumatic fever
- Sore throat predominates
- History of fever, headache, and stomachache
- Inflamed throat on physical examination

Findings that Indicate Likely Streptococcal Pharyngitis:

- Palatal petechiae and tonsillar exudate
- Associated headache and abdominal pain
- Fine sandpaper-like rash over the torso and other parts of the body; strawberry tongue

described with group C or group G streptococcal pharyngitis. Antibiotic treatment for GABHS pharyngitis shortens the course of illness, decreases the incidence of suppurative complications, and prevents transmission to others. Penicillin V, 400,000 U, 250 mg for children, and 500 mg two to three times per day for adolescents and adults, is administered orally for 10 days. Amoxicillin is often used because of its palatability. For penicillin-allergic patients, use erythromycin, 40 mg/kg/day in two to four divided doses for 10 days. Other macrolides, including 5 days of azithromycin, clindamycin, and cephalosporins, are also effective against GABHS. Tetracycline, sulfonamides, and trimethoprim-sulfamethoxazole are ineffective in treating streptococcal infections. If poor compliance with oral medication is expected, benzathine penicillin G, 600,000 U for children <60 lb (27 kg); 1.2 million U for larger children and adults, should be administered in a single intramuscular dose (maximum dose, 1.2 million U). Following completion of 24 hours of antibiotics, the patient may return to school or child care. Good hand washing should be encouraged, and the patient should avoid sharing food and drink containers and towels. Empirical treatment of contacts is not recommended.

For isolated bacterial pharyngitis that is not caused by GABHS, antibiotic treatment is not required because rheumatic fever is not a complication and the effect of treatment is unknown or minimal. Groups C and G streptococci are very sensitive to penicillin and may be treated with this medication; however, effectiveness of treatment has not been studied. Bacterial pharyngitis caused by M. pneumoniae or C. pneumoniae is often associated with lower respiratory tract infection, which requires treatment.

Herpangina

Etiology

The etiologic agents of herpangina are viral: nonpolio enteroviruses, coxsackieviruses A and B, and echoviruses.

Clinical Features

Herpangina affects children of all ages. The typical clinical picture includes discrete, painful vesicular and ulcerative lesions on the tonsillar pillars, soft palate, uvula, and posterior pharynx; sore throat; poor appetite; and a fever as high as 105.8°F (41°C). Nausea, vomiting, and abdominal pain may be present. The course is usually self-limited and resolves within 1 week.

Evaluation

Herpangina can be differentiated from herpes simplex virus gingivostomatitis by the location of the ulcerative lesions. With herpangina, the lesions tend to be in the posterior pharynx. In herpes gingivostomatitis, the lesions are usually in the anterior oropharynx. Hydration status must be assessed.

Treatment

Herpangina should be treated with acetaminophen and ibuprofen for fever and pain. **Topical analgesics** may provide temporary relief. Some physicians prescribe a mixture of viscous lidocaine (2%), Maalox, and Benadryl liquid (often referred to as "Magic Mouthwash") in equal parts to be used topically. The patient should be given adequate **hydration** and **nutrition**. Severe cases, especially in young children, may require **hospitalization** for intravenous fluid administration.

Peritonsillar Cellulitis and Peritonsillar Abscess

Etiology

Peritonsillar **infections** may result from **acute tonsillar pharyngeal infection** or **obstruction and infection of Weber glands,** located in the superior pole of the tonsillar fossae. Peritonsillar **abscesses** are more commonly seen in **children >10 years.** Their causes are **polymicrobial,** involving either anaerobic or aerobic bacteria. The aerobic bacteria may include GABHS, α- and γ-hemolytic streptococci, group D streptococci, coagulase-negative staphylococci, and *Haemophilus influenzae.*

Clinical Features

The clinical features of peritonsillar cellulitis or abscess include **fever, dysphagia, voice changes** (e.g., "hot potato" or muffled voice), **trismus, and drooling. Unilateral tonsillar or peritonsillar swelling** (usually on the superior aspect of the tonsil), **deviation of the uvula** to the contralateral side, ipsilateral **cervical adenopathy,** and trismus may be seen on physical examination.

Dehydration, upper airway obstruction, or aspiration of ruptured abscess contents may occur.

Evaluation

Peritonsillar cellulitis that is not associated with the drainage of pus and **parapharyngeal abscess** that involves inflammation of the pharyngeal wall are in the differential diagnosis for peritonsillar abscess. The patient's **respiratory status and hydration status** should be assessed. The patient should be **encouraged to speak** so the examiner can assess the quality of the voice. The **pharyngeal wall and both tonsils** should be **thoroughly inspected for asymmetric swelling and** any **uvular deviation.** Avoid using a tongue blade if epiglottitis is suspected.

Treatment

A pediatric **otolaryngologist** should be consulted to confirm the diagnosis and, possibly, to perform a **needle aspiration** of the abscess. Needle aspiration should be performed initially in older children and adolescents. The contents of the abscess need not be cultured except in children who are immunocompromised.

Penicillin VK (15 to 40 mg/kg per day, divided every 6 to 8 hours for 10 to 14 days) should be started for **outpatient** management. **Aqueous penicillin G** (100,000 to 250,000 U/kg per day, divided, every 4 to 6 hours, with a maximum dose of 4.8 million U per 24 hours) should be given intravenously for **inpatient** management. If penicillin alone is not effective, a semisynthetic penicillin or clindamycin may be added. **Clindamycin** (25 to 40 mg/kg per day, divided, every 6 to 8 hours for 10 to 14 days) is used for patients who are **allergic to penicillin.**

Acetaminophen may be administered for fever and pain management. **Hydration** status should be carefully monitored. **Tonsillectomy** may be necessary in severe cases, in patients who are unresponsive to needle aspiration and antibiotics, and in patients with a history of recurrent peritonsillar abscesses.

Retropharyngeal Cellulitis and Retropharyngeal Abscess

Etiology

Retropharyngeal **infections** occur **in the potential space between the posterior pharyngeal wall and the prevertebral fascia.** They are believed to occur as a **complication of pharyngitis** but may also occur **following a foreign body or penetrating injury** to the posterior pharynx, and as an **extension of vertebral osteomyelitis.** Retropharyngeal abscesses most often occur in young children <4 years. The etiologic agents are **polymicrobial** and may include GABHS, anaerobic bacteria, *Staphylococcus aureus*, and *Klebsiella pneumoniae*.

Clinical Features

The clinical features of retropharyngeal cellulitis and retropharyngeal abscess include a **high fever, difficulty swallowing,** and a **severe sore throat.** The patient may **refuse to eat.**

Hyperextension of the neck; noisy, gurgling respirations or stridor; or meningismus (caused by irritation of the paravertebral ligaments) may be present. **Drooling** and **increased work of breathing** may be seen.

Complications include respiratory compromise, aspiration of the abscess contents, expansion along fascial planes to the mediastinum (resulting in mediastinitis), and erosion into major blood vessels.

Evaluation

The patient should be **assessed for drooling and difficulty breathing.** A bulge may be seen in the posterior pharyngeal wall. A **tongue blade** should be **used with caution** because the abscess may rupture if poked or digitally manipulated.

Treatment

An **otolaryngologist** should be consulted. A **semisynthetic penicillin** should be administered to cover penicillinase-producing *S. aureus.* **Clindamycin** (25 to 40 mg/kg per day, divided, every 6 to 8 hours for 10 to 14 days) is used for penicillin-allergic patients.

Cardiorespiratory monitoring is recommended because of the risk of airway compromise. **Acetaminophen** (with or without codeine) should be administered for pain; narcotics must be used with care because of the risk of airway obstruction.

EVALUATION OF SORE THROAT

Patient History

The following aspects of the history can provide important clues to the diagnosis:

- Concurrent upper respiratory tract symptoms (e.g., cough, runny nose) suggest a viral etiology.
- Thickened secretions suggest an infectious cause.
- Similar complaints in household and other close contacts suggest an infectious etiology.
- Seasonal variation and associated allergic symptoms, such as itchy eyes, suggest an allergic cause.
- Recurrence every 3 to 6 weeks: consider cyclic neutropenia or PFAPA.
- Bleeding with injections or easy bruisability may suggest a neoplastic process.
- Change in vocal quality suggests laryngitis but may also be the muffled voice heard with peritonsillar and retropharyngeal abscesses.
- Drooling or painful or difficult swallowing suggests the presence of ulcerative lesions or enlarged tissue.

Physical Examination

The following should be noted on physical examination:

- The patient's general appearance and any signs of drooling or difficulty breathing (e.g., nasal flaring, stridor).
- The patient's vital signs, including temperature.

- Mouth breathing or change in vocal quality.
- Tympanic membrane erythema or a middle ear effusion suggests acute otitis media, which often accompanies nasopharyngitis.
- Nasal mucosal erythema may suggest an infectious or allergic process.
- Oral vesicular eruptions, which suggest a viral cause (e.g., herpes simplex virus, enterovirus, coxsackievirus).
- Symmetric tonsillar hypertrophy may be seen in nasopharyngitis and pharyngitis.
- Unilateral tonsillar inflammation suggests peritonsillar cellulitis or abscess or the presence of a tumor.
- Tonsillar exudates may be seen in viral and bacterial infections.
- Palatal petechiae may be seen in strep throat and mononucleosis.
- Lymphadenopathy in the posterior cervical triangle is seen in mononucleosis.
- Tender anterior cervical adenopathy is typically seen in strep throat.
- Neck swelling and tenderness, and ill appearance should raise the suspicion for complications including lymph node abscess and Lemierre syndrome.

> **HINT:** When palpating potential intraoral/pharyngeal abscesses, use caution. Patients may aspirate contents of ruptured abscesses.

Laboratory Studies

A **rapid strep test** should be done. This test, which requires vigorous swabbing of the tonsillar pillars and the posterior pharynx, identifies the presence or absence of **GABHS carbohydrate** by specific antisera but does not detect group C and G streptococci. Avoid swabbing the uvula because doing so may result in dilution of the sample. The rapid strep test is **highly specific** and **sensitive.** False-negative results may occur if small numbers of streptococci are present. **Negative tests should always be confirmed by throat culture.** A positive test indicates that GABHS are present in the pharynx.

A **throat culture,** considered the **gold standard** for the diagnosis of strep throat, should be obtained. Untreated patients with strep throat may have positive cultures for several weeks to months. Notify the laboratory if *N. gonorrhoeae, C. diphtheriae,* or fungal infection is suspected, so that appropriate culture media is used.

A **complete blood cell count** may also be revealing. The white blood cell (WBC) count may be elevated in patients with peritonsillar abscesses, retropharyngeal abscesses, and other bacterial infections. Mild anemia and mild thrombocytopenia may be seen during viral illnesses. An **atypical lymphocytosis** making up 10% to 25% of the total WBC count is suggestive of infection with EBV.

EBV titers and **monospot tests** are useful for **confirming EBV infection.**

Diagnostic Modalities

A **lateral neck radiograph** should be obtained when the diagnosis of a **retropharyngeal abscess** is **suspected.** It is useful for assessing the airway caliber, the size of the adenoids and epiglottis, and ballooning of the hypopharynx. A retropharyngeal abscess appears as widening of the soft tissues immediately anterior to vertebral bodies C1-C4. Normally, the soft tissues measure less than half the width of the adjacent vertebral body. Air in the retropharynx or loss of the normal cervical lordosis should raise suspicion of a retropharyngeal abscess.

A **computed tomography scan of the neck** with contrast may be useful in determining the **surgical treatment** of retropharyngeal abscesses. It may also help **differentiate retropharyngeal cellulitis from retropharyngeal abscess.**

APPROACH TO THE PATIENT

First, **rule out life-threatening causes of sore throat** (e.g., epiglottitis, peritonsillar abscess, retropharyngeal abscess, diphtheria, severe tonsillar hypertrophy, Lemierre syndrome). Table 72-2 lists the symptoms associated with life-threatening causes of sore throat. **Oxygen** should be provided if **respiratory distress** is noted.

The patient should be examined for evidence of a **peritonsillar abscess or foreign body. If epiglottitis is suspected,** use of a **tongue blade should be avoided,** as should other invasive procedures (e.g., placement of an intravenous catheter, phlebotomy). The patient should be immediately referred to an **anesthesiologist,** a **critical care specialist,** and an **otolaryngologist.** If a retropharyngeal abscess is suspected, a **lateral neck radiograph** should be obtained.

Figure 72-1 outlines the approach to narrowing the differential diagnosis.

TABLE 72-2 Symptoms Associated with Life-Threatening Causes of Sore Throat
Ill appearance
Tachypnea
Respiratory retractions
Stridor
Drooling
Difficulty swallowing
Muffled, "hot potato" voice
Neck stiffness

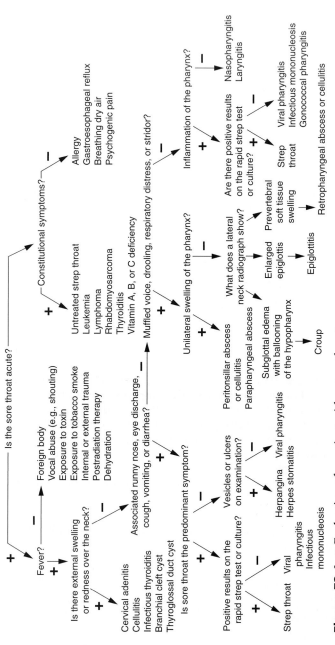

Figure 72-1 ■ Evaluation of a patient with a sore throat

Suggested Readings

American Academy of Pediatrics: Group A streptococcal infections. In *Red Book 2006: Report of the Committee on Infectious Diseases*, 27th ed. Edited by Pickering LK, Baker CJ, Long SS, et al. Elk Grove Village, Il, American Academy of Pediatrics, 2006, 610–620.

Brook I: Microbiology and management of peritonsillar, retropharyngeal, and parapharyngeal abscesses. *J Oral Maxillofac Surg* 62: 1545–1550, 2004.

Cabrera CE, Deutsch ES, Eppes S, et al.: Increased incidence of head and neck abscesses in children. *Otolaryngol Head Neck Surg* 136:176–181, 2007.

Feder HM Jr: Periodic fever, aphthous stomatitis, pharyngitis, adenitis: a clinical review of a new syndrome. *Curr Opin Pediatr* 12:253–256, 2000.

Gerber MA: Diagnosis and treatment of pharyngitis in children. *Pediatr Clin North Am* 52:729–747, 2005.

Zaoutis T, Klein JD: Enterovirus infections. *Pediatr Rev* 19(6):183–191, 1998.

73 | *Splenomegaly*
Nicholas Tsarouhas and Paula Agosto

INTRODUCTION

Splenomegaly may be evident in benign viral infections, serious systemic infections, hematologic diseases, neoplastic conditions, and metabolic disorders. Apparent splenomegaly may be caused by a normal-size spleen being pushed down by hyperinflated lungs. The terms "splenomegaly" and "hypersplenism" are not interchangeable. **Splenomegaly refers to an enlarged spleen,** whereas **hypersplenism refers to a hyperfunctioning spleen that results in a reduction in the number of circulating blood cells.** Hypersplenism usually results in splenomegaly but not always.

A palpable spleen tip is not necessarily pathologic. Approximately 3% of older adolescents and adults have **palpable spleens.** By adulthood, the normal spleen, which is located beneath the ninth and eleventh ribs, reaches dimensions of 12 cm long, 7 cm wide, and 3 cm thick. Careful examination of a calm patient and thoughtful consideration of the possible underlying pathophysiology is necessary to discern the cause of splenomegaly.

> **HINT:** Percussion can be used to evaluate splenic size. To delineate the lower "tip," the examiner starts in the area of tympany in the left anterior axillary line of the midabdomen and percusses upward toward the splenic dullness. The upper border is defined by starting in the left midaxillary line of the midthorax and percussing downward toward the splenic dullness.

DIFFERENTIAL DIAGNOSIS LIST

Infectious Causes
Viral Infection
 Benign infection
 Mononucleosis (Epstein-
  Barr virus [EBV] infection)
 Cytomegalovirus (CMV)
  infection
 AIDS
 Rubella

 Herpes
 Hepatitis B
Bacterial Infection
 Pneumonia
 Sepsis
 Endocarditis
 Brucellosis
 Tularemia
 Splenic abscess

Cat-scratch disease
Tuberculosis
Syphilis
Leptospirosis
Rocky Mountain spotted
fever (RMSF)
Ehrlichiosis
Other Infections
Malaria
Toxoplasmosis
Babesiosis
Histoplasmosis
Coccidioidomycosis
Trypanosomiasis

Neoplastic Causes

Leukemia
Lymphoma
Hemangioma
Hamartoma
Metastatic disease
(neuroblastoma)

Traumatic Causes

Laceration
Hematoma
Traumatic cyst

Metabolic or Genetic Causes

Lipid Metabolism Defects
Gaucher disease
Niemann-Pick disease
Gangliosidoses
Mucolipidoses
Metachromatic
leukodystrophy
Wolman disease
Mucopolysaccharidoses
Hurler syndrome
Hunter syndrome

Hematologic Causes

Red Blood Cell Membrane (RBC) Defects

Hereditary spherocytosis
Hereditary elliptocytosis
Hereditary stomatocytosis
RBC Enzyme Defects
Glucose-6-phosphate
dehydrogenase (G6PD)
deficiency
Pyruvate kinase deficiency
Hemoglobin Defects
Sickle cell disease (SCD)
Thalassemia
Extrinsic Hemolytic Anemias
Autoimmune hemolytic
anemia
Erythroblastosis fetalis

Congestive Causes

Congestive heart failure
Constrictive pericarditis
Intrinsic liver disease
Perisplenic anatomic
obstructions
Splenic vein thrombosis
Splenic artery aneurysm

Miscellaneous Causes

Serum sickness
Chronic granulomatous
disease
Juvenile rheumatoid arthritis
(JRA)
Systemic lupus erythematosus
(SLE)
Histiocytic Disorders
Langerhans cell histiocytosis
Hemophagocytic lympho-
histiocytosis
Malignant histiocytic
disorders
Beckwith-Wiedemann
syndrome
Amyloidosis
Sarcoidosis

DIFFERENTIAL DIAGNOSIS DISCUSSION

Benign Infection

Many benign infections, especially upper respiratory tract infections, can be associated with **mild, transient splenomegaly**. Adenovirus, coxsackievirus, and *Streptococcus* are commonly involved organisms.

Epstein-Barr Virus Infection (Infectious Mononucleosis)

Infectious mononucleosis is discussed in Chapter 50, "Lymphadenopathy."

Cytomegalovirus Infection

Epidemiology

CMV is ubiquitous, and **most people are infected with the virus by adulthood.** The source is body fluids, including blood, urine, breast milk, saliva, and feces. Transmission of CMV is both horizontal (**person to person**) and vertical (**mother to child**). CMV is the most common congenital viral infection.

Clinical Features

CMV infection manifests itself differently in different hosts:

- In **neonates**, intrauterine growth retardation, microcephaly, jaundice, hepatosplenomegaly, a petechial or purpuric rash, chorioretinitis, and neurologic symptoms may be seen.
- In **immunocompetent children or adults**, infection is most commonly asymptomatic; however, patients may develop fever, malaise, anorexia, pharyngitis, headache, myalgia, abdominal pain, and hepatosplenomegaly.
- In **immunocompromised children and adults**, retinitis, pneumonitis, and enteritis are the primary manifestations.

Evaluation

Diagnosis is best made by **isolation** of the organism in body fluids (or organs) by cell culture or polymerase chain reaction. **Serologic studies** are also available. A **computed tomography (CT) scan of the head** may demonstrate intracerebral calcifications in patients with congenital CMV infection.

Treatment

The immunocompetent host recovers completely in a few weeks with **supportive treatment**. Immunocompromised patients are commonly treated with **ganciclovir**.

Malaria

Etiology

Malaria, a disease transmitted by the *Anopheles* mosquito of the tropics and subtropics, is acquired when the host's erythrocytes are invaded by a **mosquito-borne parasite** of the genus *Plasmodium*. Four species of *Plasmodium* cause malaria: *P. falciparum*, *P. vivax*, *P. ovale*, and *P. malariae*. The incubation period is 1 to 2 weeks.

Clinical Features

Although constitutional symptoms are universal, the clinical presentation of malaria is often **dictated by the infecting species**. *P. vivax* and *P. ovale*, for example, are particularly associated with hypersplenism and splenic rupture.

Evaluation

Diagnosis is confirmed by **identification of the parasite** in the blood. Special stains and smears are required for optimal yield. Thick and thin blood films should be examined.

Treatment and Prevention

Treatment entails **antimicrobial therapy** (e.g., chloroquine) and **supportive** measures (e.g., management of fluid and electrolytes, RBC transfusions). Because resistance to chloroquine and other drugs is common, a multitude of **antibiotics** are used in the armamentarium against malaria (e.g., Atovaquone/proguanil, quinine, quinidine, primaquine, mefloquine, doxycycline, tetracycline, clindamycin) and may be necessary.

Control of the *Anopheles* mosquito population is important for prevention of malaria. **Chemoprophylaxis** with chloroquine, Atovaquone/proguanil, mefloquine, or doxycycline is recommended for travelers to endemic areas.

Babesiosis

Etiology

Like malaria, babesiosis is a **parasitic infection** of erythrocytes that is endemic in the coastal areas of the northeastern United States. The main reservoir of *Babesia* is the **white-footed mouse,** and the organism is transmitted by the *Ixodes scapularis* tick. The incubation period is 1 week to several months.

Clinical Features

Symptoms include fever, chills, sweats, malaise, myalgias, nausea, and vomiting. Jaundice, dark urine, and renal failure are also possible. The clinical presentations of **babesiosis and malaria are sometimes similar.**

Evaluation

Laboratory evaluation may demonstrate hemolytic anemia and elevation of liver enzymes. The diagnosis is confirmed by **blood smears** and **serologic studies.**

Treatment

Patients with moderate or severe illness are treated with **clindamycin and quinine,** or **atovaquone and azithromycin.**

Hematologic Disorders

Hereditary spherocytosis, G6PD deficiency, SCD, and thalassemia are discussed in Chapter 40, "Hemolysis."

Lymphomas

Lymphomas—non-Hodgkin lymphoma (NHL) and Hodgkin disease—are discussed in Chapter 50, "Lymphadenopathy."

Trauma

Mechanisms of injury to the spleen include motor vehicle accidents, bicycle accidents, and falls. Patients may complain of **diffuse or left upper quadrant pain.** The diagnosis is confirmed by **CT scan.**

Lacerations and hematomas are usually conservatively managed with **observation** and **supportive therapy.** Occasionally, **surgical splenectomy** is necessary. In rare cases, traumatic cysts are managed with aspiration, sclerosing, and surgery.

Gaucher Disease

Etiology

A **deficiency of β-glucosidase** leads to the pathologic accumulation of glucocerebroside in the reticuloendothelial system.

Clinical Features

Gaucher disease is categorized into three forms.

- **Type I, the "classic" type,** is one of the most common genetic disorders in Ashkenazi Jews. It may present at any age but usually presents in adolescence or adulthood. Its distinguishing feature is its lack of neurologic involvement.
- **Type II, the infantile form,** is characterized by slow or no achievement of developmental milestones, swallowing difficulties, and opisthotonos. Its progressive neurodegenerative course culminates in death within the first 2 years of life.
- **Type III, the juvenile form,** presents in infancy or childhood with behavioral changes, seizures, and extrapyramidal and cerebellar signs. With all three types, **splenomegaly is universal.**

Evaluation

A **bone marrow aspirate** demonstrating Gaucher cells engorged with glucocerebroside confirms the diagnosis.

Treatment

Splenectomy has been used to manage the hematologic consequences of hypersplenism. Cerezyme (Genzyme), given every 2 weeks, is effective in reversing the changes.

EVALUATION OF SPLENOMEGALY

Patient History

The following information is important to obtain:

- **Does the patient have a history of a recent upper respiratory tract infection?** Benign viral infections often result in mild splenomegaly.
- **What is the patient's travel history?** Constitutional symptoms, in the setting of travel to a tropical area, make malaria a likely diagnosis. These same symptoms, with a history of travel to the coastal north-eastern United States, suggest babesiosis.
- **Is there a history of tick exposure?** Ticks transmit the organisms responsible for babesiosis, RMSF, ehrlichiosis, and tularemia.
- **Is there a history of exposure to any animals?** Contact with cattle or other farm animals (as well as unpasteurized milk) could be the clue to brucellosis. Handling rabbits might point to tularemia as a diagnosis. Scratches from cats or kittens could lead to cat-scratch disease; toxoplasmosis is also commonly linked to interactions with cats. Leptospirosis may be transmitted through the urine of dogs, rats, or livestock.
- **Is the patient immunocompromised?** An immunocompromised host with splenomegaly and constitutional symptoms may have CMV infection.
- **Is there a history of weight loss?** Weight loss may be seen in patients with infectious mononucleosis, CMV infection, brucellosis, ehrlichiosis, malaria, or babesiosis. Oncologic processes, especially lymphoma and leukemia, must also be considered in this setting.
- **What is the patient's medication history?** Splenomegaly in a patient who developed a rash in response to ampicillin therapy makes mononucleosis a likely diagnosis. In patients with G6PD deficiency, exposure to medications with oxidant properties leads to hemolysis and splenomegaly. Splenomegaly in the setting of joint complaints and rash makes a drug-induced serum sickness a likely possibility.
- **Is there a history of trauma?** The spleen is the most commonly injured intra-abdominal organ.

Physical Examination

Physical findings often offer important clues to the diagnosis.

- **Growth retardation in a microcephalic neonate** should lead to an investigation for CMV.
- **Exudative pharyngitis** in combination with splenomegaly suggests mononucleosis.
- **Rash** of the palms and soles suggests RMSF or syphilis. The rash of RMSF is usually seen first on the wrists and ankles and may be maculopapular or petechial. A maculopapular rash is characteristic with both congenital and secondary syphilis. Bullous lesions are also common in congenital syphilis. A whole body rash with "iris" or "target" lesions suggests serum sickness. JRA and SLE also have characteristic rashes.
- **Jaundice** may be seen with many of the infectious processes but is more typical in the hemolytic diseases (e.g., G6PD deficiency, spherocytosis, autoimmune hemolytic anemia).
- **Adenopathy** in combination with splenomegaly most commonly points to mononucleosis, but lymphoma should also be considered. Axillary and cervical adenopathy are the two most common sites of lymph node enlargement in cat-scratch disease. Although the examination may demonstrate evidence of feline scratches, the classic papule is usually gone by the time the node manifests.
- **Abdominal pain** (either diffuse or localized to the left upper quadrant) should prompt an evaluation for a traumatic cause, such as a splenic laceration or hematoma. Furthermore, one of the complications of infectious mononucleosis is splenic rupture, which can present with acute abdominal pain. The presence of fever suggests a splenic abscess.

Laboratory Studies

The following studies may be appropriate:

- **"Monospot."** The mononucleosis rapid slide agglutination test for heterophil antibodies is a quick test for infectious mononucleosis, but false negatives are common in children <6 years.
- **EBV serologies.** The definitive way to diagnose both acute and past infection at any age is through the use of EBV serologies.
- **Complete blood count.** Atypical lymphocytosis is the hallmark finding of mononucleosis. Pancytopenia is common in sepsis, AIDS, ehrlichiosis, and oncologic processes. Thrombocytopenia is seen in RMSF and babesiosis. Evidence of a hemolytic anemia (e.g., sickled cells, target cells, schistocytes, spherocytes) should prompt consideration of the common hematologic disorders (SCD, thalassemia, G6PD deficiency, and spherocytosis), as well as certain infectious diseases (e.g., malaria, babesiosis).
- **Reticulocyte count.** Reticulocytosis is the confirmatory finding in hemolytic anemias.

- **Bilirubin level and liver enzymes.** Hyperbilirubinemia is found in both hemolytic anemias and intrinsic liver disease. An elevation in liver enzymes implicates the liver as a primary or secondary source of pathology. Common causes may be infectious, neoplastic, anatomic, metabolic, traumatic, or toxic.
- **Direct antibody test.** Autoimmune hemolytic anemias are usually antibody positive.
- **Routine blood smear.** Evidence of hemolysis is also evident on inspection of the peripheral blood smear. Additionally, infestations like malaria and babesiosis can often be readily identified on blood smears as long as the laboratory is made aware that these diseases are diagnostic possibilities.
- **Urinalysis (UA).** Hemoglobinuria is a common finding in hemolytic anemias. UA abnormalities are also seen with some metabolic disorders.

TREATMENT OF SPLENOMEGALY

Most of the diseases presenting with splenomegaly require supportive care and observation for complications.

- **Splenic rupture,** whether associated with mononucleosis or not, requires immediate surgical management.
- **Splenic abscess** is treated with intravenous antibiotics and sometimes surgical drainage.
- **Hemolytic anemias.** Patients with hemolytic anemias often require RBC transfusions until the hemolysis is either terminated or stable. Discontinuation of offending medications is indicated in patients with serum sickness and G6PD deficiency.

APPROACH TO THE PATIENT

- **In neonates with splenomegaly,** bacterial infection should be ruled out first. If no bacterial causes are isolated, a viral cause should be pursued aggressively. If infection is deemed unlikely, a hemolytic cause should be considered. If no hemolytic disorder can be identified, anatomic abnormalities of the spleen should be investigated.
- **In older infants and children with splenomegaly,** trauma is the first consideration. Infection and hemolysis are the next two possibilities to be considered. If these categories are eliminated and the patient has constitutional symptoms, an oncologic process is likely; rarely, a metabolic disorder also presents in this fashion.
- Regardless of age, in an **acutely ill patient** with splenomegaly and cardiomegaly, congestive heart failure is a likely diagnosis. In a nonacutely ill child, serum sickness should be considered if all other possibilities are ruled out.

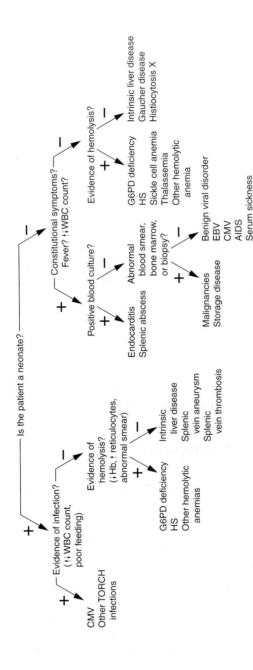

Figure 73-1 ■ **Approach to a nonacutely ill patient with splenomegaly**
CMV = cytomegalovirus; *EBV* = Epstein- Barr virus; *G6PD* = glucose-6-phosphate dehydrogenase; *Hb* = hemoglobin; *HS* = hereditary spherocytosis; *TORCH* = toxoplasmosis, other infections, rubella, cytomegalovirus, herpes simplex; *WBC* = white blood cell

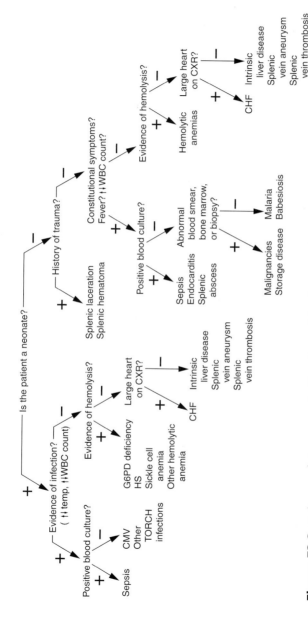

Figure 73-2 ■ Approach to an acutely ill patient with splenomegaly

CHF = congestive heart failure; *CMV* = cytomegalovirus; *CXR* = chest radiograph; *G6PD* = glucose-6-phosphate dehydrogenase; *HS* = hereditary spherocytosis; *TORCH* = toxoplasmosis, other infections, rubella, cytomegalovirus, herpes simplex; *WBC* = white blood cell

Figure 73-1 outlines the approach to nonacutely ill patients with splenomegaly. Figure 73-2 outlines the approach for acutely ill patients with splenomegaly.

Suggested Readings

American Academy of Pediatrics: Babesiosis. Brucellosis. Ehrlichiosis. Malaria. In *2006 Red Book: Report of the Committee on Infectious Diseases,* 27th ed. Edited by Pickering LK, Baker CJ, Long SS, et al. Elk Grove Village, Il, American Academy of Pediatrics, 2006, 223–224, 235–237, 281–284, 435–441.

Galanakis E, Bourantas KL, Leveidiotou S, et al.: Childhood brucellosis in north-western Greece. *Eur J Pediatr* 155:1–6, 1996.

Grover SA, Barkun AN, Sackett DL: Does this patient have splenomegaly? *JAMA* 270:2218–2221, 1993.

Khan SB, Alkan S, Pooley R: A 14-year old boy with splenomegaly. *Arch Pathol Lab Med* 124:1239–1240, 2000.

Scully RE (ed): Case records of the Massachusetts General Hospital. Weekly clinicopathological exercises. A two-year-old boy with thrombocytopenia, leukocytosis, and hepatosplenomegaly *N Engl J Med* 330:1739–1746, 1994.

Tamayo SG, Rickman LS, Mathews WC, et al.: Examiner dependence on physical diagnostic tests for the detection of splenomegaly: a prospective study with multiple observers. *J Gen Intern Med* 8:69–75, 1993.

Vane DW: Left upper quadrant masses in children. *Pediatr Rev* 13:25–31, 1992.

Woods M, Greenes D: A 16-year-old girl with epistaxis and hepatomegaly. *Curr Opin Pediatr* 7:733–739, 1995.

Syncope

William L. Border and Bradley S. Marino
Bernard J. Clark III (Third Edition)

INTRODUCTION

Syncope, a common complaint in children, refers to a **loss of consciousness**, usually lasting 1 to 2 minutes because of a **transient drop in cerebral perfusion pressure**. As many as 15% of children and adolescents have a syncopal event between 8 and 18 years of age. These episodes can cause significant anxiety in parents and caregivers, and they result in numerous visits to pediatricians and emergency rooms.

The most common form is **vasomotor, vasodepressor, or vasovagal syncope**, also known as **neurocardiogenic syncope**. More serious are the rarer **syncopal spells associated with heart disease**. This chapter focuses on outlining a systematic approach to those with a cardiovascular etiology.

DIFFERENTIAL DIAGNOSIS LIST 🔒⚷

Left Ventricular Outflow Tract Obstruction
Aortic stenosis
Subaortic stenosis
Hypertrophic cardiomyopathy

Arrhythmias
Ventricular tachycardia (VT)
Long QT syndrome (LQTS)

Bradyarrhythmias
  Sinus node dysfunction
  Conduction block

Other
Vasodepressor syncope
Primary pulmonary
  hypertension

DIFFERENTIAL DIAGNOSIS DISCUSSION

Cardiac syncope is the result of a **sudden decrease in cardiac output, leading to decreased cerebral perfusion and a loss of consciousness.** The differential diagnosis of cardiac syncope includes left ventricular outflow tract obstruction and arrhythmia.

Left Ventricular Outflow Tract Obstruction
Anatomic causes of left ventricular outflow tract obstruction can be considered as a single cause of cardiac syncope. All of these causes **limit cardiac output, especially during exercise,** and all have as part of the physical examination a **systolic ejection murmur.** In children with a

history of syncope and a significant ejection murmur, left ventricular outflow tract obstruction should be presumed and the patient referred to a **pediatric cardiologist**. Although the **chest radiograph or electrocardiogram (ECG)** may suggest left ventricular hypertrophy, echocardiography is the best method to identify and describe left ventricular outflow tract obstruction.

Treatment of symptomatic left ventricular outflow tract obstruction includes **balloon dilation or surgical valvotomy for aortic stenosis** and **surgical resection for subaortic stenosis**. After resection of subaortic stenosis, there is a small but finite rate of recurrence despite successful initial resection. **Hypertrophic cardiomyopathy** can be managed by the use of **β-receptor antagonists** (i.e., propranolol) or **calcium channel antagonists** or with **surgical resection** (myotomy and myomectomy).

Limited participation in competitive sports, especially those that result in isometric exercise such as football, wrestling, and heavy weight lifting, may be required in patients with unrepaired and, in some cases, repaired left ventricular outflow tract obstruction. Decisions regarding participation in sports should be made in consultation with a pediatric cardiologist.

Ventricular Tachycardia

Patients with VT can present with a history of **palpitation, chest pain, or syncope**. VT presents as a wide **QRS tachycardia** (QRS interval >100 milliseconds [ms]) with a rate of **120 to 240 beats per minute.**

VT can be a **medical emergency** because this rhythm can rapidly **deteriorate into ventricular fibrillation**. For patients who appear hemodynamically stable, an attempt at **intravenous access** and **pharmacologic conversion to sinus rhythm** should be attempted. For patients who are not hemodynamically stable or who present with mental status changes, **cardioversion** is the treatment of choice.

The presence of VT may be idiopathic or may result from congenital or acquired heart disease resulting in ventricular dilation or hypertrophy, right ventricular dysplasia, anomalous left coronary artery from the pulmonary artery, a suture line in the myocardium, electrolyte imbalance, or drug ingestion. Emergent evaluation of VT should include **assessment and correction of electrolyte disturbances** including hypocalcemia, hypokalemia, and/or hypomagnesemia. In adolescents, a toxicology screen should be sent because **illegal drug abuse (e.g., cocaine)** may result in ventricular arrhythmia. New-onset VT can be caused by myocardial damage secondary to a process resulting in myocarditis. Patients who have undergone corrective **open heart surgery** for congenital heart disease, **especially tetralogy of Fallot,** are at risk for ventricular arrhythmias. Other causes of VT include long QT syndrome or prolonged corrected

QT interval from other causes. Patients with a suspected history of VT require evaluation by a **pediatric cardiologist.**

Long QT Syndrome

In patients with a **history of syncope** and a **family history of sudden death,** it is essential to rule out LQTS as the cause of syncope. The corrected QT interval (QTc) is calculated from the surface ECG by measuring the **QT interval in seconds from the onset of the Q wave to the end of the T wave and dividing this interval by the square root of the R-R interval in seconds.** The corrected QTc interval is independent of heart rate and outside the infant period has an **upper normal limit of 450 ms.** When the patient's heart rate is <60 beats per minute, no QT interval correction is necessary.

Children with **LQTS** may have **life-threatening paroxysmal episodes of VT,** specifically, a form of polymorphic VT known as torsade de pointes. If a child is found to have a prolonged QTc, the **entire family,** including all first-degree relatives, **should be screened** because several inherited forms of this disease exist. Evaluation includes a **12-lead ECG,** looking specifically at the QTc interval, and **Holter monitoring** to measure the QTc at several time points at a variety of heart rates and to assess for occult ventricular arrhythmia. Often **exercise testing** is used to calculate changes in the QTc during exercise. In normal patients, the QTc remains constant or shortens slightly during exercise. In patients with LQTS, the QTc may lengthen during exercise.

Bradyarrhythmias

Symptomatic bradycardia caused by sick sinus syndrome or the onset of late, complete heart block can cause cardiac syncope. This is most commonly seen in children who have undergone **cardiac surgery.** Patients with **transposition of the great arteries who have undergone an atrial switch procedure** (Mustard or Senning procedure) or patients who have had a Fontan palliation have a high incidence of both **automatic atrial tachycardia and sick sinus syndrome.** Patients who have had **ventricular septal defect closure** or who have L-transposition of the great arteries (ventricular inversion) may suffer from late complete heart block. These patients are typically cared for by a cardiologist and have routine annual follow-up examinations that include **24-hour Holter monitoring** to evaluate for these arrhythmias. Symptomatic bradycardia in patients with congenital heart disease from sinus node dysfunction or conduction block after surgical palliation may require pacemaker placement. Syncope may also result from bradycardia caused by **second-degree heart** block (Mobitz Type II), in which several atrial beats are not conducted to the ventricle, or complete heart block resulting from **inflammatory/infectious diseases** such as rheumatic fever, myocarditis, Lyme disease, or endocarditis.

Neurocardiogenic Syncope

Neurocardiogenic syncope is the **most common cause of cardiac syncope in childhood.** It is included here as a cardiac cause of syncope because its pathophysiology includes an **inappropriately low heart rate and/or blood pressure,** typically triggered during a time of **decreased ventricular filling.** In this condition, an extended period in the upright position, dehydration, a vagal trigger, or external stimuli such as pain or emotional upset increases vagal tone leading to a slowed heart race, peripheral vasodilation, and decreased cerebral perfusion pressure. The child with recurrent episodes is frequently referred for cardiac evaluation.

Cardiac evaluation includes a **detailed history, cardiac examination, and a 12-lead ECG.** An **echocardiogram** may be ordered if abnormalities are noted on the ECG or cardiovascular examination. Typically, this is sufficient to rule out a serious cardiac cause. Rarely, in cases where the mechanism of syncope is believed to be **neurocardiogenic** but symptoms are atypical, a **tilt-table test** may be ordered. In this test the child or adolescent is placed on a table and tilted to 70° degrees while being monitored by ECG and an automated blood pressure monitor. This creates an artificial orthostatic stress that often provokes a drop in heart rate and/or blood pressure, which is diagnostic. Patients with a **positive tilt-table test** (i.e., those with **neurocardiogenic syncope**) are encouraged to **increase their intake of fluids.** If syncope persists, treatment with a **mineralocorticoid** may be initiated to help expand the intravascular blood volume.

EVALUATION OF CARDIAC SYNCOPE

Patient History

In patients who present with syncope as a chief complaint, questions regarding the history should be directed toward **defining the circumstances** under which the child fainted.

- Were there **definable triggers** to account for the event such as a long period of standing, dehydration, or an emotional or vagal trigger?
- Did the child have **palpitations** prior to syncope?
- Is there a **family history** of syncope, arrhythmias, or sudden cardiac events?

In suspected cases of vasodepressor syncope, a **detailed history of diet** is important, specifically, how much on average the child drinks in a day.

Physical Examination Findings

The physical examination should be directed toward cardiac evaluation to help rule out cardiac syncope:

- Is there a significant systolic murmur?
- Are the heart tones normal?
- Is there a gallop rhythm suggestive of cardiac dysfunction?
- In younger children, is there evidence of hepatomegaly?

Laboratory Studies

It is suggested that **every child with syncope should have an ECG.** This test is readily available and reliable. An ECG can help delineate those children with a prolonged QTc that can be life threatening. Placement of a **Holter monitor or event recorder** should be performed in any child suspected of an **arrhythmia** as the cause of syncope. This includes the child with a history of palpitations, a history of an irregular heartbeat following syncope, or in the child with syncope during exercise. Any patient with **syncope and a significant murmur** should have an **echocardiogram.**

APPROACH TO THE PATIENT

The most common cause of syncope in children is **neurocardiogenic syncope.** The child with symptoms consistent with neurocardiogenic syncope should have a screening ECG but does not need further evaluation unless syncope is recurrent. In a patient without symptoms consistent with neurocardiogenic syncope, an **ECG** should be performed **to assess the QTc.** If an arrhythmia is thought to be responsible for a syncopal episode, then **Holter monitoring** or an **event monitor** should be placed to attempt to document a ventricular arrhythmia as the potential cause. The child with **recurrent syncope and a positive family history of sudden death** should have an evaluation by a **pediatric cardiologist** for LQTS. Finally, in a patient with syncope, especially if it occurs **during exercise,** or in a child with a **significant murmur,** evaluation by a **pediatric cardiologist** is indicated and an **echocardiogram** should be performed.

Suggested Readings

Bush DM: Evaluating cardiovascular presentations: what does an electrocardiogram have to offer? *Pediatr Ann* 34(11):892–824, 2005.

Cadman CS: Medical therapy of neurocardiogenic syncope. *Cardiol Clin* 19(2):203–213, v, 2001.

Lewis DA, Dhala A: Syncope in the pediatric patient: the cardiologist's perspective. *Pediatr Clin North Am* 46(2):205–219, 1999.

McLeod KA: Dysautonomia and neurocardiogenic syncope. *Curr Opin Cardiol* 16(2):92–96, 2001.

Strieper MJ: Distinguishing benign syncope from life-threatening cardiac causes of syncope. *Semin Pediatr Neurol* 12(1):32–38, 2005.

75

Tachycardia

Mitchell I. Cohen
Bernard J. Clark (Third Edition)

INTRODUCTION

Tachycardia can be defined as a **ventricular rate in excess of the age-related normal range**. Table 75-1 describes the upper limits of normal.

- **Sinus tachycardia** is caused by abnormalities of the sinus node (or normal sinus node responses to physiologic alterations).
- **Supraventricular tachycardia (SVT)** is caused by abnormalities originating above the ventricle.
- **Ventricular tachycardia (VT)** is caused by abnormalities originating below the bundle of His.

DIFFERENTIAL DIAGNOSIS LIST

Sinus Tachycardia

Noncardiac Causes
  Exercise
  Fever
  Anemia
  Hyperthyroidism
  Excessive catecholamines—
    stress, pheochromocytoma
  Arteriovenous malformation
    (AVM)
  Drugs—therapeutic, illicit
  Seizures
Cardiac Causes
  Congestive heart failure
  Myocardial dysfunction
  Congenital heart disease
  Cardiac tamponade
  Sick sinus syndrome

Supraventricular Tachycardia

Abnormal (Nonsinus) Focus of Automaticity
  Automatic (ectopic) atrial
    tachycardia
  Multifocal atrial
    tachycardia
  Junctional ectopic
    tachycardia
Accessory Route of Electrical Conduction (Re-Entrant Mechanism)
  Atrial flutter
  Atrioventricular nodal
    re-entrant tachycardia
  Atrioventricular
    reciprocating tachycardia
  Permanent junctional
    reciprocating tachycardia

Ventricular Rhythm Disturbance

  VT
  Ventricular fibrillation
  Accelerated idioventricular
    rhythm
  Torsades de pointes—long QT
    syndrome, electrolyte distur-
    bance, drug toxicity
  Structural heart defects

TABLE 75-1 Upper Limit of Normal for Heart Rate	
Age (Years)	Upper Limit of Normal for Heart Rate (beats/min)
<1	180
1–3	150
4–6	130
7–10	110
>10	100

DIFFERENTIAL DIAGNOSIS DISCUSSION

Sinus Tachycardia

Etiology

Sinus tachycardia occurs when the **normal pacemaker, the sinoatrial cells, respond either normally or abnormally to an alteration in physiologic conditions.** Sinus tachycardia occurs as a normal response to increased physiologic demands (e.g., exercise, fever, anemia) and as a normal response to certain pathologic changes (e.g., hyperthyroidism, pheochromocytoma, AVM). Various medications and drugs of abuse can elevate the resting sinus rate (Table 75-2), especially decongestants, caffeine, and β-adrenergic agonists. The normal physiologic response to increased metabolic demands is to **increase cardiac output,** either by **increasing the stroke volume or the heart rate (or both).** During infancy,

TABLE 75-2 Drugs Associated with Rapid Heart Rates
Prescription Drugs
β-adrenergic agonists (e.g., albuterol)
Methylxanthines (e.g., theophylline)
Tricyclic antidepressants (e.g., imipramine)
Nonsedating histamines (e.g., terfenadine)
Over-the-Counter Drugs
Decongestants (e.g., pseudoephedrine)
Diet aids (e.g., phenylpropanolamine)
Inhaled bronchodilators (e.g., albuterol)
Caffeine-containing products
Drugs of Abuse
Nicotine
Cocaine
Amphetamines
Alcohol
Marijuana
LSD
Phencyclidine
Amyl nitrate

the heart is less able to increase stroke volume; therefore, the cardiac output is primarily augmented by an increase in heart rate.

- **Cardiac causes** for sinus tachycardia include any condition that depresses myocardial function (e.g., myocarditis, pericarditis, endocarditis).
- **Noninfectious causes** include congestive heart failure from large left-to-right shunts (Qp:Qs >2:1), atrioventricular valve regurgitation, or left ventricular outflow tract obstruction (aortic stenosis or coarctation of the aorta).
- **The sinus node may be injured by certain surgeries** (e.g., Mustard, Senning, or Fontan operations), resulting in sick sinus syndrome (tachycardia-bradycardia syndrome).

Clinical Features

Patients with sinus tachycardia may be asymptomatic or minimally symptomatic with complaints of **palpitations, chest pain, dyspnea, or lightheadedness.** Rarely, a patient presents with cool extremities as a result of a low cardiac output. Symptoms often **depend on the age of the patient and the duration of the tachycardia.**

Evaluation

A **12-lead electrocardiogram (ECG)** should be obtained to determine the correct P-wave axis. During sinus tachycardia, the P-wave axis is 0° to 90° and the QRS complex is narrow, unless there is a preexisting intraventricular conduction delay (e.g., bundle branch block). There is typically a "warm-up and cool-down" period that lasts a few minutes.

A **complete blood cell count, glucose level, thyroid tests, and 24-hour urine catecholamine studies** may be indicated. Often, observing the patient on a monitor for a short period of time helps make the diagnosis.

Treatment

Treatment of nonphysiologic sinus tachycardia is geared toward **correction of the underlying abnormality,** such as infection, anemia, or hyperthyroidism.

Supraventricular Tachycardia

> **HINT:** There are generally two epidemiologic SVT peaks: infancy and adolescence.

Etiology

Although SVT occurs in anatomically normal hearts, it is usually the result of either an **abnormal focus of automaticity** or an **accessory route** of electrical conduction, which results in a re-entrant circuit within the atrium or to the ventricles.

■ **Ectopic atrial tachycardia** is an automatic tachycardia identified on an ECG by an abnormal P-wave axis or different morphologic P wave. It can be difficult to distinguish ectopic atrial tachycardia from sinus tachycardia when the ectopic focus is in the high right atrium (near the sinus node) and has a normal P-wave axis. The tachycardia typically has a "warm-up and cool-down" phase.

■ **Atrial flutter** is caused by one or more re-entrant circuits within the atrium and does not require the atrioventricular node or ventricle to sustain itself. Atrial flutter is frequently seen in patients after the Mustard/Senning operation for D-transposition of the great arteries or following the Fontan operation for single-ventricle heart disease.

■ **Atrioventricular nodal re-entrant tachycardia** is most common in adolescents and young adults.

■ **Atrioventricular reciprocating tachycardia** is the most common type of SVT seen in children. It is caused by an abnormal accessory pathway that bypasses normal atrioventricular node conduction. There are generally two types—an accessory pathway that allows antegrade conduction to the ventricle, bypassing the normal atrioventricular node (Wolff-Parkinson-White syndrome), or an accessory pathway that allows only retrograde conduction and is "concealed" on the resting ECG. Wolff-Parkinson-White syndrome is often seen in patients with Ebstein anomaly of the tricuspid valve. In a significant number of infants with Wolff-Parkinson-White syndrome, the condition resolves without treatment within the first few years of life.

Clinical Features

Patients with SVT may be minimally symptomatic, complaining of **palpitations, chest pain, dyspnea, or lightheadedness.** Symptoms often depend on the age of the patient and the duration of the tachycardia. Patients who have been in SVT for **more than 24 to 48 hours** may have **cool extremities and pallor,** suggesting low cardiac output. Patients with **Wolff-Parkinson-White syndrome** may have **atrial fibrillation** with rapid conduction down an accessory pathway, resulting in **ventricular fibrillation and sudden death.**

On admission, the patient's **heart rate, blood pressure, and intravascular status** should be assessed. A **12-lead ECG and rhythm strip** should be obtained. It is important to answer the following questions: Is the **RR interval** regular? Can **P waves** be identified, and if so, what is the relationship to the QRS complex? How does this ECG differ from the patient's **baseline ECG**? If P waves cannot be seen, a transesophageal recording may be helpful to identify P waves and their association with ventricular beats.

- **Automatic (ectopic) atrial tachycardia.** The P wave morphology, the PR interval, or both may be different from the baseline sinus rhythm. The atrial rate is usually 100 to 240 beats/minute, and atrioventricular block can occur during the tachycardia.
- **Atrial flutter.** In general, the rate in atrial flutter is 150 to 400 beats/minute, with the ventricular rate a multiple of the atrial rate, based on variable atrioventricular block. Classic "sawtoothed" flutter waves are typically seen in the inferior leads (II, III, and aVF) in children with structurally normal hearts. This may not be apparent in children after the Fontan operation, in which the flutter cycle lengths are longer.
- **Wolff-Parkinson-White syndrome** appears on the resting ECG as a short PR interval accompanied by a "delta wave" (i.e., slurring of the initial component of the QRS complex, as a result of ventricular pre-excitation).

> **HINT:** If the patient complains of palpitations, but no documented rhythm disturbance is seen on the 12-lead ECG, 24-hour ambulatory Holter monitoring, transtelephonic recordings, or exercise testing may be helpful.

Treatment

Acute conversion of SVT is indicated for all initial events, symptomatic episodes, and whenever the patient shows signs of hemodynamic compromise.

- **Vagal maneuvers.** Mainstays of nondrug therapy include performing a Valsalva maneuver, standing the patient on his head, or inducing the diving reflex by placing ice on the patient's face.
- **Adenosine.** Adenosine causes a profound but short-lived increase in the atrioventricular nodal refractory period. Adenosine may be given as a rapid intravenous bolus (50 to 300 µg/kg, to a maximum dose of 12 mg) while a 12-lead ECG is continuously running.
- **Direct current (DC) cardioversion.** If the patient is hemodynamically compromised, synchronized DC cardioversion (0.5 to 1 joule/kg) is the most effective means of terminating SVT.
- **Transesophageal or transvenous overdrive atrial pacing** can also be effective in acute situations. These procedures should be attempted only by an experienced cardiologist.
- **Verapamil** should be avoided as acute treatment of SVT in children <3 years because of its vasodilating and negative inotropic effects.

In older children it may be used, but intravenous calcium chloride and isoproterenol should be readily available.

> **HINT:** Adenosine or vagal maneuvers may be therapeutic as well as diagnostic, in that flutter waves or ventricular pre-excitation can occasionally be seen in the first few posttachycardia beats as the atrioventricular node is blocked.

Treatment of **chronic SVT** (e.g., atrioventricular reciprocating tachycardia, atrioventricular nodal re-entrant tachycardia) entails the use of **agents that alter refractoriness** of an integral component of the circuit.

- **Digoxin** is given initially for atrioventricular nodal re-entrant tachycardia caused by a concealed accessory pathway. The risk of increasing antegrade conduction through an accessory pathway makes the use of this drug in patients with Wolff-Parkinson-White syndrome controversial.
- **β-Blockers** (e.g., propranolol, atenolol, nadolol) should be the first-line agent in patients with pre-excitation syndromes. Side effects of the β-blockers include fatigue, bronchospasm, hypoglycemia, and/or exercise intolerance.
- **Procainamide, flecainide, sotalol, and amiodarone** are alternative second-line agents in the treatment of SVT. Careful attention to myocardial performance, proarrhythmia, and hepatic and thyroid dysfunction should be carefully monitored.
- **Radiofrequency catheter ablation** can be performed safely in children (>4 years) who have SVT refractory to single-line medications or side effects associated with medications (e.g., increased bronchospasm in a patient with asthma who is being treated with a β-blocker). Patients with potentially rapidly conducting accessory pathways should be considered for an ablation, even in the absence of a history of SVT.

Ventricular Tachycardia

Etiology

A premature ventricular contraction (PVC) is defined as a **single ventricular beat that arises earlier than the sinus beat with a full compensatory pause**. A consecutive pair of PVCs is a **couplet; three or more PVCs are defined as VT**. PVCs may be further classified as **monomorphic or polymorphic** and occur in either a **bigeminal, trigeminal, or quadrigeminal pattern**.

TABLE 75-3 Structural Heart Disease Associated with Tachycardia

Defect	Type of Tachycardia
Congenital heart Disease	
Mitral valve prolapse	SVT, VT
Aortic valve stenosis or regurgitation	VT
Ebstein anomaly of the tricuspid valve	SVT (WPW) commonly, VT less commonly
Tetralogy of Fallot	VT
Mustard/Senning repair of D-TGA	SVT (particularly atrial flutter)
Fontan repair of single ventricle	SVT (particularly atrial flutter)
Cardiomyopathy	
Hypertrophic cardiomyopathy	SVT, VT
Dilated cardiomyopathy	SVT, VT
Arrhythmogenic right ventricular dysplasia	VT (monomorphic, left bundle branch block)
Miscellaneous Causes	
Eisenmenger complex (pulmonary vascular disease and pulmonary hypertension)	VT
Cardiac tumor (atrial myxoma, rhabdomyosarcoma)	SVT, VT (depending on tumor site)

D-TGA = D-transposition of the great arteries; SVT = supraventricular tachycardia; VT = ventricular tachycardia; WPW = Wolff-Parkinson-White syndrome.

- **Isolated finding.** VT can be an isolated finding in children with otherwise normal hearts and is usually monomorphic and suppressed with exercise.
- **Structural heart defects.** VT can be associated with structural heart defects (Table 75-3) and is often inducible with exercise and other catecholamine stimulation.
- **Torsades de pointes ("twisting of the point")** is a variant of polymorphic VT in which the QRS morphology changes over time. Torsades de pointes can be associated with any of the long QT forms (Table 75-4).
- **Ventricular fibrillation** is rare in the pediatric population and characterized by rapid, bizarre, chaotic QRS complexes without any effective cardiac output. Ventricular fibrillation may be seen in children with the long QT syndrome or cardiomyopathy, after cardiac surgery, or rarely in association with atrial fibrillation and antegrade accessory pathway conduction (Wolff-Parkinson-White syndrome).

Clinical Features

Symptoms generally depend on the **age of the patient** and **the rate and duration of the VT.** Patients may present with **simple palpitations, signs of low cardiac output, shock, or "sudden death."**

TABLE 75-4 Causes of Prolonged QT Interval

Congenital

Hereditary
Jervell-Lange-Nielsen syndrome: long QT interval, stress-induced syncope,
  congenital nerve deafness, autosomal recessive inheritance
Romano-Ward syndrome: long QT interval, stress-induced syncope, autosomal
  dominant inheritance (usually incomplete penetrance)
Brugada syndrome
Right ventricular dysplasia
Sporadic

Acquired

Electrolyte abnormalities
Hypocalcemia
Hypomagnesemia
Metabolic disturbances
  Malnutrition
  Liquid protein diets
Drugs
  Phenothiazines (e.g., haloperidol)
  Tricyclic antidepressants (e.g., imipramine)
  Nonsedating antihistamines (e.g., terfenadine)
  Class Ia antiarrhythmic agents (e.g., quinidine)
  Class III antiarrhythmic agents (e.g., amiodarone)
Central nervous system trauma
Cardiac abnormalities
  Ischemia
  Mitral valve prolapse
  Myocarditis
Intraventricular conduction abnormalities
  Bundle branch blocks

Evaluation

A **complete history and physical examination** should be performed, with particular attention to the patient's **vital signs** and any underlying structural heart disease. Always determine the **corrected QT interval** and take a detailed **family history** regarding **sudden death, history of congenital heart disease, and deafness** (some syndromes are associated with long QT and deafness).

A **12-lead ECG** should be obtained to determine QRS duration, morphology, axis, and ventriculoatrial relationship. If a **prior ECG is** available, the **two should be compared.** A tachycardia originating below the bundle of His typically has a wide QRS complex, with a different QRS axis from that seen in patients in sinus rhythm. Atrioventricular dissociation may be present. The ventricular rate is typically 100 to 350 beats/minute. Accelerated idioventricular rhythm ("slow VT") has the same ECG characteristics as VT, with a slower rate (80 to 120 beats/minute).

If the 12-lead ECG reveals only single monomorphic PVCs, **ambulatory Holter recordings or transtelephonic monitors** may help determine if the patient is having VT. An **exercise stress test** in older children and adolescents can determine the response to exercise; idiopathic VT is usually suppressed with exercise.

Consultation with a **cardiologist** is indicated for all patients suspected of having ventricular arrhythmias.

Treatment

Treatment for VT, like that for SVT, is **based on the underlying mechanism.**

- **Asymptomatic VT.** In patients who have structurally normal hearts, normal QT intervals, and asymptomatic slow VT suppressed by exercise, no treatment may be indicated. These patients should be followed periodically with noninvasive monitoring.
- **Acute, symptomatic VT.** Therapy with lidocaine (1 mg/kg administered as an intravenous push, followed by an infusion at a rate of 20 to 50 μg/kg per minute, assuming normal renal function) is indicated for these patients. If the patient is known to have long QT syndrome (or clinical suspicion is strong for this disorder), intravenous magnesium sulfate (30 to 50 mg/kg for children, 1 to 2 g for adults) can be given over 1 minute. Lidocaine and phenytoin may also be used. Overdrive transvenous pacing may also be needed. Amiodarone and other medicines known to prolong the QT interval should be avoided.
- **VT with hemodynamic compromise.** If the patient has hemodynamically compromising VT, synchronized cardioversion with 1 to 2 joules/kg (adult: 100 to 400 joules) should be used, and cardiopulmonary resuscitation should be initiated. Ventricular fibrillation should be treated with emergent electrical asynchronous defibrillation and initiation of advanced cardiac life support.
- **Chronic, symptomatic VT.** Chronic treatment of patients with long QT syndrome is with β-blockers, the only medication demonstrated to decrease the mortality rate associated with this syndrome. Patients with structural heart disease or symptomatic or exercise-induced VT are generally treated after an electrophysiology study. Medications typically used, alone or in combination, include mexiletine, phenytoin, β-blockers, and amiodarone. Radiofrequency ablation can also be performed, and some patients may warrant implantation of an internal cardiac defibrillator.

Suggested Readings

Batra AS, Hohn AR: Consultation with the specialist: palpitations, syncope, and sudden cardiac death in children: who's at risk? *Pediatr Rev* 24:269–275, 2003.

Campbell RM, Strieper MJ, Frias PA, et al.: Survey of current practice of pediatric electrophysiologists for asymptomatic Wolff-Parkinson-White syndrome. *Pediatrics* 111:e245–e247, 2003.

Hegenbarth MA; Committee on Drugs: Preparing for pediatric emergencies: drugs to consider. *Pediatrics* 121:433–443, 2008.

Reynolds JL, Pickoff AS: Accelerated ventricular rhythm in children: a review and report of a case with congenital heart disease. *Pediatr Cardiol* 22: 23–28, 2001.

Tingelstad J: Consultation with the specialist: cardiac dysrhythmias. *Pediatr Rev* 22(3):91–94, 2001.

76 *Thermal Injury*

Andrew Hashikawa and Marc H. Gorelick

INTRODUCTION

Thermal injury in children can involve not only the **skin** but also the **respiratory, circulatory, immune,** and **central nervous systems.** Successful treatment of pediatric thermal injuries requires comprehensive assessment and management. Management of burn injury is dictated by **assessment of burn severity,** determined by the mechanism, depth, and extent of injury.

DIFFERENTIAL DIAGNOSIS LIST

Thermal causes—direct flame burns, contact burns, scald burns

Chemical causes
Electrical causes
Radiation

DIFFERENTIAL DIAGNOSIS DISCUSSION

Thermal Burns

Thermal burns are the **most common type of burns** affecting children. They may result from contact with **hot liquids** (scalds), **hot surfaces,** or **flames.** Scald burns tend to be more extensive but more superficial than contact burns. Flame injuries are most often associated with inhalation injuries.

Chemical Burns

Chemical burns are caused by contact with **corrosive substances.** Contact with **acids** causes **coagulation necrosis,** whereas contact with **alkali** causes **liquefaction necrosis.** Alkali burns are typically deeper and more severe than acid burns. Chemical burns require **extensive irrigation** with water or saline to remove the corrosive agent and prevent further injury.

Electrical Burns

Electrical injury results from contact with a source of electrical current or from arcing of current near the body.

Electrical injury typically produces a **depressed entry wound** and an **exit wound** that appears "blown out." With high-voltage currents (>1,000 V), the extent of the underlying deep tissue damage is typically far in excess of that suggested by the appearance of the cutaneous burn. Both low- and high-voltage currents can cause **cardiac arrhythmias,** even in the absence of visible burns.

Patients exposed to significant electrical current should have an **electrocardiogram** to monitor for arrhythmia.

> **HINT:** Alternating current (AC) is usually considered more dangerous than direct current. AC, found in most households, rapidly changes direction every second, typically 60 cycles/second. When in contact with a rapidly alternating electrical current, the child's muscles may not relax and allow the child to let go, causing increased contact time and injury.

Radiation Burns

The most common type of radiation burn in children is **sunburn.** Sunburn is typically **first degree** or, rarely, **superficial second degree.**

EVALUATION OF THERMAL INJURY

Patient History

The following information should be ascertained:

- Mechanism of injury
- Duration of exposure
- If the cause of injury was fire, whether the fire occurred in a closed space
- History of loss of consciousness
- Tetanus immunization status

Physical Examination

> **HINT:** Always consider the possibility of an intentionally inflicted injury. The following features may be cause for concern: inconsistent or implausible explanation (remember to relate the reported mechanism with the developmental age of the child); the presence of other abuse risk factors; burns to typically protected areas (e.g., the dorsum of the hand or back of the neck); burns in a "stocking-glove" distribution, particularly in the absence of splash marks; burns to the buttocks or genitalia; or multiple cigarette burns.

Burns are classified according to their **depth and extent** (Table 76-1). Depth of injury is assessed on the basis of the clinical findings and is

TABLE 76-1 Classification of Burns

Type of Burn	Affected Skin Layer	Appearance
First degree	Epidermis	Erythema, hypersensitivity
Second degree		
Superficial	Upper (papillary) dermis	Erythema, blistering intact hairs, exquisite pain
Deep	Deep (reticular) dermis	Skin may be white or mottled and nonblanching, or blistered and moist; pain may or may not be present; hairs easily pulled
Third degree	Entire dermis	Dry, white, or charred skin; leathery appearance, painless, no hair
Fourth degree	Subcutaneous tissue	Same as third degree; may have exposed muscle and bone

classified as **superficial** (first degree), **partial thickness** (superficial second degree), or **full thickness** (deep second degree, third degree, and fourth degree). Initially, the percentage of body surface area (BSA) involved with partial- and full-thickness burns should be estimated using the "**rule of nines**" (Table 76-2). After the patient is stabilized, a more detailed assessment of the extent of burns is made using a modified **Lund and Browder chart**.

The patient should be assessed for signs of **inhalation injury** (Table 76-3). Significant inhalation injury may exist in the absence of any surface burns; therefore, a high index of suspicion should be maintained in the face of a suggestive history (e.g., fire in a closed space).

HINT: The presence of signs of pulmonary injury early in the course is a poor prognostic indicator.

TABLE 76-2 "Rule of Nines"

Body Part	Percentage of BSA		
	Infant	Child	Adolescent/Adult
Head	18%	13%	9%
Anterior trunk	18%	18%	18%
Posterior trunk	18%	18%	18%
Upper extremity (each)	9%	9%	9%
Lower extremity (each)	14%	16%	18%
Genitalia	1%	1%	1%

For small burns, a rough estimate of the affected BSA can be made by comparing the burn with the size of the child's palm (which represents approximately 1% of the BSA). *BSA* = body surface area.

TABLE 76-3 Signs of Inhalation Injury

Pulmonary	Central Nervous System	Skin
Tachypnea	Confusion	Facial burns
Stridor	Dizziness	Singed nasal hairs
Hoarseness	Headache	Cyanosis
Rales	Hallucinations	Cherry-red color
Wheezing	Restlessness	
Cough	Coma	
Retractions	Seizures	
Nasal flaring		
Carbonaceous sputum		

> **HINT:** Frank shock is uncommon in the first 30 to 60 minutes after a burn. Its presence should prompt a search for other causes of shock (e.g., abdominal trauma with occult blood loss, spinal cord injury).

Laboratory Studies

For children with minor burns, no laboratory studies are routinely needed. The following may be helpful in specific circumstances:

- **Arterial blood gases.** Arterial blood gas measurements must be interpreted with caution; normal arterial blood gases are not reassuring in the presence of clinical findings. The arterial oxygen tension (PaO_2) and the calculated oxygen saturation are unaffected, even by significant carbon monoxide (CO) poisoning. Metabolic acidosis in a patient with inhalation injury suggests the possibility of cyanide toxicity.
- **Carboxyhemoglobin level.** An elevated carboxyhemoglobin level helps in making the diagnosis of CO poisoning, but a normal level does not exclude it, especially if there is a delay in measuring the level.
- **Blood work.** A complete blood count and blood type and cross-match may be indicated for patients with concomitant trauma or extensive burns.
- **Electrolytes, blood urea nitrogen, creatinine, and serum creatine kinase.** Baseline electrolytes, blood urea nitrogen, and creatinine may be helpful if large fluid shifts are expected for extensive burns. A serum creatine kinase level should be considered for patients with electrical injury to assess the extent of deep tissue injury and rhabdomyolysis.

Diagnostic Modalities

A chest radiograph is not helpful in the initial assessment of smoke inhalation because findings are usually delayed by 24 to 36 hours. Diagnosis should be based on **clinical assessment.**

TREATMENT OF THERMAL INJURY

The appropriate treatment depends on the severity of the injury. The American Burn Association classifies burns as **major** (requires burn center referral), **moderate** (requires inpatient treatment), or **minor** (requires outpatient treatment). Table 76-4 lists the American Burn Association criteria for burn severity and disposition.

Emergency Management of Major Burns

- **First, an airway must be secured.** Concomitant trauma is common in burn patients, and cervical spine immobilization should be maintained if injury is suspected. Because rapid edema formation can make airway management difficult, intubation should be considered early in patients with evidence of significant thermal injury to the upper airway.
- **Hyperbaric oxygen therapy** should be considered if any of the following are present: a carboxyhemoglobin level >30%, neurologic symptoms (confusion and disorientation, focal deficit, history of loss of consciousness), or cardiac disturbance.
- Consider **presumptive therapy with sodium thiosulfate** (25% solution), 1.65 mL/kg given intravenously over 30 to 60 minutes, to counteract cyanide toxicity.
- **Burns covering a large surface area cause substantial fluid losses and shifts, necessitating special fluid management,** with smaller children requiring relatively greater amounts of fluid (Figure 76-1). Lactated

TABLE 76-4 Burn Severity and Disposition (American Burn Association Criteria)

Major Burns: Burn Center Referral

Partial-thickness burns affecting >10% of the BSA in children <10 years
Partial-thickness burns affecting >20% of the BSA in children ≥10 years
Full-thickness burns affecting >5% of the BSA
Burns involving the face, eyes, ears, hands, feet, genitalia, perineum, or major joints that may result in functional or cosmetic impairment
Associated inhalation injury
Significant chemical burns
Electrical injury
Burns complicated by underlying illness or major trauma

Moderate Burns: Inpatient Treatment

Partial-thickness burns affecting 10%–20% of the BSA in older child
Partial-thickness burns affecting 5%–10% of the BSA in younger child
Full-thickness burns affecting 2%–5% of the BSA

Minor Burns: Outpatient Treatment

Partial-thickness burns affecting <5% of the BSA
Full-thickness burns affecting <2% of the BSA (may still require surgical referral)

BSA = body surface area.

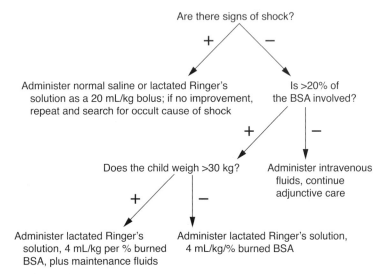

Are there signs of shock?

+ / −

Administer normal saline or lactated Ringer's solution as a 20 mL/kg bolus; if no improvement, repeat and search for occult cause of shock

Is >20% of the BSA involved?

+ / −

Does the child weigh >30 kg?

Administer intravenous fluids, continue adjunctive care

+ / −

Administer lactated Ringer's solution, 4 mL/kg per % burned BSA, plus maintenance fluids

Administer lactated Ringer's solution, 4 mL/kg/% burned BSA

Figure 76-1 ■ Fluid replacement in a patient with major burns
BSA = body surface area

Ringer's is recommended for fluid resuscitation during the first 24 hours. The amounts given in Figure 76-1 are totals for the first 24 hours: 50% of the total volume is administered over the first 8 hours after the occurrence of the burn, and the remaining 50% is administered over the subsequent 16 hours.

> **HINT:** Add maintenance fluids as well as dextrose for children <5 years or 30 kg. Monitor fluid status by maintaining urine output of at least 1 mL/kg per hour.

- **Adjunctive care** of the patient with major burns includes the removal of all clothing from the burn areas. Adherent molten material (e.g., tar, metal) should be cooled but left in place. All burns should be irrigated with water or saline solution. Chemical burns require copious irrigation (15 to 30 minutes) with water; a small child may be placed in a sink for this purpose. Following irrigation, the burns should be covered with saline-soaked gauze or a dry sterile sheet if the burns are extensive.
- **Analgesics** (e.g., morphine 0.05 to 0.1 mg/kg intravenously, meperidine 1 mg/kg intravenously) should be administered early. Tetanus immunoprophylaxis should be administered as needed. Steroids and prophylactic antibiotics should be avoided. Nasogastric decompression

and placement of an indwelling bladder catheter are needed for seriously injured patients.

- **Definitive wound management** should be undertaken only in consultation with the burn surgeon who will assume care of the child.

Emergency Management of Minor Burns

- **An open dressing** should be applied to small burns or burns in hard-to-dress areas. Burns should be washed with mild soap and water, and an antibacterial ointment (e.g., bacitracin polymyxin B) should be applied. No covering is needed. The wound should be washed at home and ointment reapplied two to three times daily until healed.

- **A closed dressing** is used for most burns in children. The clothing should be removed from the area, and the burn should be irrigated with water or saline solution. Chemical burns should be irrigated for 15 to 30 minutes. Analgesia (oral acetaminophen with codeine for small burns, intravenous morphine or meperidine for larger burns) should be provided, and then the burn should be washed again with mild soap and water and rinsed with saline solution. Loose or clearly nonviable tissue should be débrided with forceps. Intact blisters should be left undisturbed; ruptured bullae should be unroofed and debrided.

- Several **gauze dressings** are available, either plain or treated (e.g., Adaptic, Xeroform, Vaseline, Aquaphor). Silver sulfadiazine (1%) cream is applied to the wound surface or to the underside of the dressing, in a layer approximately 2 to 3 mm thick. Silver sulfadiazine should not be used for facial burns. The entire wound surface is covered with the dressing, and then an outer absorbent dressing or roller gauze is applied.

- Synthetic occlusive dressings (e.g., Biobrane) are increasingly being used by surgeons within the first 6 to 12 hours to decrease eschar formation, limit number of dressing changes, and expedite healing time.

- If the child has a second- or third-degree burn and her tetanus immunization status is not up to date, **tetanus immunoprophylaxis** should be administered.

The burn should be rechecked in 24 to 48 hours to assess for healing and signs of infection. Home dressing changes should be performed once or twice daily until healed, usually for 10 to 14 days. An analgesic (e.g., acetaminophen with codeine) should be provided for the first few days.

HINT: Consider hospitalization or referral when there are concerns about loss of function (e.g., burns over the hands or joints), cosmetic results (e.g., large facial burns), or the risk of poor compliance with the treatment regimen. Final results depend largely on meticulous burn care.

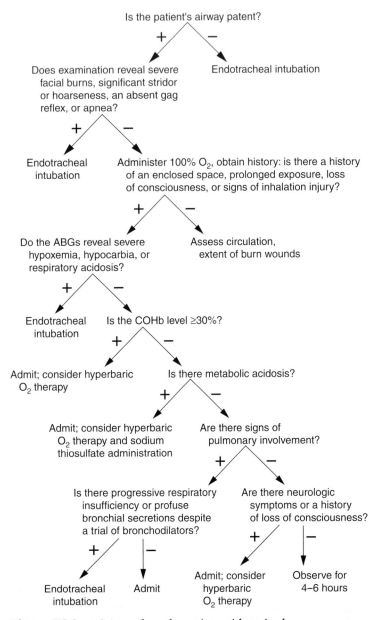

Figure 76-2 ▪ **Approach to the patient with major burns**
ABGs = arterial blood gases; *COHb* = carboxyhemoglobin;
O_2 = oxygen

APPROACH TO THE PATIENT (FIGURE 76-2)

Suggested Readings

Baxter CR, Waeckerle JF: Emergency treatment of burn injury. *Ann Emerg Med* 17:1305–1315, 1988.

Finkelstein JL, Schwartz SB, Madden MR, et al.: Pediatric burns: an overview. *Pediatr Clin North Am* 39:1145–1163, 1992.

Monafo WW: Initial management of burns. *New Engl J Med* 335: 1581–1586, 1996.

Morgan ED, Bledsoe SC, Barker J: Ambulatory management of burns. *Am Fam Physician* 62: 2015–2026, 2029–2030, 2032, 2000.

Reed JL, Pomerantz WJ: Emergency management of pediatric burns. *Pediatr Emerg Care* 21: 118–129, 2005.

Schonfeld N: Outpatient management of burns in children. *Pediatr Emerg Care* 6:249–253, 1990.

Thom SR: Smoke inhalation. *Emerg Med Clin North Am* 7:371–387, 1989.

Tibble PM, Perrotta PL: Treatment of carbon monoxide poisoning: a critical review of human outcome studies comparing normobaric oxygen with hyperbaric oxygen. *Ann Emerg Med* 24:269–276, 1994.

Urinary Frequency and Polyuria

Matthew Sampson
Seth L. Schulman (Third Edition)

INTRODUCTION

A perceived increase in urination is a common concern that a pediatrician may be asked to evaluate. A key task is to determine whether true polyuria is present. **Polyuria,** defined formally as urine output >2,000 mL/1.73m^2 over 24 hours, is usually caused by excessive fluid intake, a lack of release of antidiuretic hormone (ADH), tubular insensitivity to ADH, or an osmotic diuresis. **Urinary frequency** not associated with polyuria is a common finding in children most typically caused by urinary tract infection (UTI), pollakiuria (frequent daytime urination), or chemical irritation.

DIFFERENTIAL DIAGNOSIS LIST

Infectious Causes
Pyelonephritis
Meningoencephalitis
Congenital cytomegalovirus
and toxoplasmosis

Toxic Causes
Furosemide
Phenytoin
Demeclocycline
Amphotericin B
Vinblastine
Cisplatin
Lithium

Metabolic or Genetic Causes
Inherited nephrogenic diabetes
insipidus
Sickle cell disease (SCD)
Fanconi syndrome
(e.g., cystinosis)
Polycystic kidney disease
Familial juvenile
nephronophthisis

Bartter syndrome
DIDMOAD (diabetes
insipidus, diabetes mellitus,
optic atrophy, and deafness)
syndrome
Laurence-Moon-Biedl syndrome

Psychosocial Causes
Primary polydipsia

Miscellaneous Causes
Diabetes mellitus
Idiopathic central diabetes
insipidus
Hand-Schüller-Christian disease
Sarcoidosis
Sjögren syndrome
Postobstructive diuresis

Neoplastic Causes
Craniopharyngioma
Meningioma
Glioma
Metastasis—lymphoma,
leukemia

Traumatic Causes

Severe head trauma
Hypophysectomy

Congenital or Vascular Causes

Obstructive uropathy
Cerebral hemorrhage

Urinary Frequency

Cystitis
Urethritis
Constipation
Pollakiuria
Hypercalciuria
Neuropathic bladder

DIFFERENTIAL DIAGNOSIS DISCUSSION

Central Diabetes Insipidus

Etiology

Central diabetes insipidus is urinary loss of water caused by impairment of vasopressin (ADH) production in the central nervous system (CNS) and may be **idiopathic, acquired,** or **inherited.** Approximately a third of affected infants and children have the idiopathic (primary) form. Secondary causes include trauma, tumors (especially craniopharyngioma), hemorrhage, CNS infection, hypoxia, and Langerhans cell histiocytosis. The autosomal dominant form of central diabetes insipidus is rare.

Clinical Features

Children present with a **sudden onset of polyuria, nocturia, and polydipsia with a predilection for cold water.** Hypernatremia and dehydration do not occur if the thirst mechanism is intact and there is ample access to water. There are no specific abnormal physical findings in primary central diabetes insipidus.

Evaluation

Laboratory studies reveal a consistently **low urine osmolality,** but in the absence of dehydration it is difficult to distinguish central diabetes insipidus from nephrogenic diabetes insipidus and psychogenic polydipsia. A **water-deprivation study** is **diagnostic** for central diabetes insipidus when the serum osmolality is increased and the urine osmolality and the plasma vasopressin concentration remain decreased in the face of strict withholding of water. A brisk response to the administration of exogenous antidiuretic hormone is expected.

Radiographic imaging of the head is necessary to exclude secondary causes. In both primary and secondary forms, the **hyperintense signal of the posterior lobe of the pituitary** seen on T1-weighted images on **magnetic resonance imaging (MRI)** is **absent.**

Treatment

Treatment consists of replacement therapy with **desmopressin acetate,** a synthetic analogue of vasopressin administered either intranasally or orally. The dose is adjusted to the patient's needs. Hyponatremia can develop if the patient drinks inappropriately while on therapy. **Specific treatment** is recommended **for secondary causes.**

Inherited Nephrogenic Diabetes Insipidus

Etiology

Nephrogenic diabetes insipidus (NDI) is characterized by an **inability of the kidney to concentrate urine** because of insensitivity of the distal nephron to arginine vasopressin. NDI is most often found to be an acquired condition, secondary to drug ingestion (lithium, tetracycline) or systemic illness like sickle-cell disease or trait. Rarely, NDI is caused by a primary genetic mutation in the vasopressin V2 receptor or water channel protein aquaporin 2.

Clinical Features

Infants initially present with **dehydration, lethargy,** poor weight gain, or **unexplained fever.** Symptoms may be severe during concomitant episodes of gastroenteritis. **Older children** have **polydipsia** and **polyuria** with **failure to thrive,** possibly secondary to the preference of water over calorie-containing formula and foods. Recurrent episodes of dehydration and the resulting deleterious effects of rapid rehydration may affect psychomotor development.

Evaluation

A dehydrated infant with polyuria accompanied by hypernatremia is suggestive of inherited NDI. The diagnosis is **confirmed** by the presence of **hyposmolality of the urine** and the **lack of response to exogenous vasopressin** during periods of dehydration. The dehydration may need to be induced by a **water-deprivation study.** Fluids should not be restricted at home in an attempt to make the diagnosis. Serum levels of vasopressin are often normal or only slightly elevated. A **family history** of NDI is often sufficient to avoid performing this study. It is **imperative to exclude medications and systemic conditions** (e.g., sickle cell anemia, tubulointerstitial diseases) that cause an acquired form of NDI.

Treatment

Treatment consists of providing **sufficient free water** to prevent complications associated with dehydration. **Restricting sodium intake** may reduce urine output. **Thiazide diuretics** decrease extravascular volume and increase proximal tubular sodium reabsorption, reducing urine output. **Amiloride** and **nonsteroidal anti-inflammatory drugs,** particularly indomethacin, are also beneficial.

Primary Polydipsia

Etiology

Primary polydipsia is **water ingestion greater than** that **necessary** to maintain water balance. It may be the result of **behavioral abnormalities** (psychogenic polydipsia or compulsive water drinking) or **physiologic abnormalities** of the hypothalamus affecting the thirst mechanism (neurogenic polydipsia).

Clinical Features

It is **difficult to distinguish primary polydipsia from diabetes insipidus.** Symptoms are similar to that seen in diabetes insipidus, although there may not be nocturia or the desire for iced water. Because excess free water is ingested, the patient should not be dehydrated.

Evaluation

Patients with primary polydipsia may have serum sodium concentrations slightly below normal. A **water-deprivation study** may be necessary to differentiate this condition from diabetes insipidus. A thorough **neurologic and psychologic examination** is recommended before labeling primary polydipsia as psychogenic in origin.

> **HINT:** In patients with primary polydipsia, the water-deprivation study may not allow maximal urinary concentrating ability secondary to "washout" of the medullary concentration gradient. These patients must be watched carefully during the study to avoid the possibility of surreptitious water ingestion, which will confound the results.

Treatment

Psychiatric counseling aimed at gradual weaning of water intake is recommended if it appears the polydipsia and polyuria are interfering with the patient's ability to function.

Urinary Tract Infection

UTI is a common disease in all stages of childhood that is important to identify because of potential long-term complications of renal scarring, hypertension and end-stage renal failure. Older children presenting with UTI may have the classic complaints of dysuria, frequency, or suprapubic, flank, or abdominal pain. In contrast, younger children, especially infants, are often well appearing with only fever as a presenting symptom (see discussion of occult UTI in Chapter 33, "Fever").

The **definitive diagnosis** of a UTI is via a positive **urine culture.** This should be done via either a midstream clean catch urine in a toilet-trained child or via bladder catheterization or suprapubic aspiration in younger children. A positive urine culture is usually defined as $>10^5$ colony-forming units (CFUs) of a single pathogen from a clean catch urine, $>10^4$ CFU from a catheter, or >100 CFU from a suprapubic aspiration. While waiting the 24 to 48 hours for a urine culture result to return, rapid tests can be used to decide whether to initiate antibiotics. **Urine dipstick** for leukocytes and nitrites has moderately good sensitivity and specificity and performs similarly to standard laboratory urinalysis. Tests with higher accuracy include **enhanced urinalysis** demonstrating ≥ 10 white blood cells/mm^3 or a positive Gram stain on uncentrifuged urine.

Empirical treatment of a UTI while waiting for culture results can either be done as an inpatient or outpatient. Strict criteria for admission would include age <2 months, inability to tolerate oral medication or maintain adequate hydration, inability to assure outpatient support or follow up, or previous failure to respond to outpatient therapy.

The majority of UTIs are caused by **Gram negatives** such as *Escherichia coli*; 5% to 10% of UTIs are caused by Gram-positive bacteria. Increasing bacterial resistance to amoxicillin and other antibiotics has been observed, and empirical therapy may be guided by knowledge of local resistance patterns. Appropriate choices might include trimethoprim-sulfamethoxazole or cephalosporins such as cefdinir or cefixime. Quinolones are effective and safe in pediatric patients with complex medical conditions or multidrug resistance. Once culture results are available, the antibiotic regimen can be tailored to the specific sensitivity pattern.

After diagnosis of a UTI in a young child, a further workup of urinary tract anatomy may be indicated including tests such as renal ultrasound, voiding cystourethrogram (VCUG), or dimercaptosuccinic acid (DMSA) scan. Ultrasound and VCUG are recommended to identify anatomic causes such as **vesicoureteral reflux** that are associated with UTI. However, controversy exists about the specific role for these tests as well as the benefit of long-term antibiotic prophylaxis for reflux.

Pollakiuria

Etiology

Pollakiuria, or the **sudden onset of increased urinary frequency,** may be related to stress and is seen most commonly in children 4 to 6 years of age.

Clinical Features

Children with pollakiuria present with **extraordinary urinary frequency,** voiding in low volumes as often as 15 times an hour during the day. Incontinence is absent, and affected children usually sleep through the night without awakening or wetting the bed.

Evaluation

Urinalysis and **urine culture** are recommended to exclude occult renal disease, diabetes mellitus, and UTI. A thorough **history** of potential **factors leading to stress** (e.g., marital discord, recent move, family illness) should be obtained.

Treatment

Reassurance and **relaxation techniques** are usually recommended in this self-limited condition.

EVALUATION OF POLYURIA AND URINARY FREQUENCY

Patient History

Key associated complaints include **polydipsia, nocturia, incontinence, enuresis, urgency,** and **dysuria.** Symptoms associated with tumors of the CNS, such as **headache** or **visual disturbances,** may be present. The patient may have a **family history** of nephrogenic diabetes insipidus. Any past **history of neurosurgery, malignancy, systemic illness, dehydration, or UTI** should be recorded, along with any **medications** recently taken. Finally, a **social history** with emphasis on stress factors should be obtained.

Physical Examination

Clinical evidence of dehydration may be present, especially in infants, if the urine output exceeds the fluids ingested. Growth parameters suggesting **failure to thrive** are seen in patients with nephrogenic diabetes insipidus or renal insufficiency. **Ophthalmologic and neurologic examinations** must be performed to seek findings suggestive of an intracranial mass.

Laboratory Studies

- **Urinalysis, urine culture,** and **serum chemistries** (including a serum creatinine concentration) should be performed to exclude diabetes mellitus, most renal conditions, and UTI. A low urine specific gravity should be expected in diabetes insipidus and primary polydipsia. Hypernatremia may be noted in diabetes insipidus if dehydration is

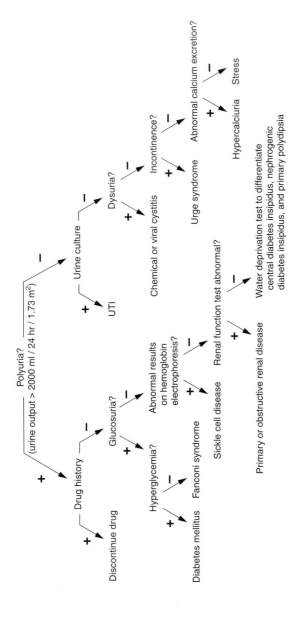

Figure 77-1 ■ Algorithm for the evaluation of polyuria and increased urinary frequency

CBC = complete blood count; *ECG* = electrocardiogram; *EEG* = electroencephalogram; *EMG* = electromyelogram; *ENG* = electronystagmogram; *MRI* = magnetic resonance imaging; *NCV* = nerve conduction velocity; *UTI* = urinary tract infection present. Hemoglobin electrophoresis should be considered if SCD is suspected.

- **Renal ultrasound** may be performed to exclude renal parenchymal disorders and obstructive uropathy. Some degree of hydronephrosis may be seen caused by high-output states.

- A **water-deprivation study** may be necessary to distinguish central diabetes insipidus, nephrogenic diabetes insipidus, and primary polydipsia.

TREATMENT OF POLYURIA AND URINARY FREQUENCY

In general, polyuria does not require treatment prior to diagnosis except when hypernatremic dehydration is present. Patients with **diabetes insipidus** have hypernatremia on the basis of free water losses and require **replacement with low-sodium solutions** (except in the case of intravascular depletion). It is important to recognize that ongoing losses occur; typical calculations for maintenance fluids will be inappropriately low and urine output must be taken into account. Frequent **serum electrolyte determinations, body weight measurements, vital signs,** and **strict intake and output measurements** are necessary to judge the efficacy of treatment.

APPROACH TO THE PATIENT WITH POLYURIA OR URINARY FREQUENCY (FIGURE 77-1)

Suggested Readings

Alon U, Warady BA, Hellerstein S: Hypercalciuria in the frequency-dysuria syndrome of childhood. *J Pediatr* 116:103–105, 1990.

Baylis PH, Cheetham T: Diabetes insipidus. *Arch Dis Child* 79:84–89, 1998.

Benchimol C: Nephrogenic diabetes insipidus. *Pediatr Rev* 17:145–146, 1996.

Horev Z, Cohen AH: Compulsive water drinking in infants and young children. *Clin Pediatr* 33:209–213, 1994.

Leung AKC, Robson WLM, Halperin ML: Polyuria in childhood. *Clin Pediatr* 30:634–640, 1991.

Zoubek J, Bloom DA, Sedman AB: Extraordinary urinary frequency. *Pediatrics* 85:1112–1114, 1990.

INTRODUCTION

Decreased urine output can be caused by either a **decrease in urine production (oliguria)** or an **obstruction to urinary flow.** Oliguria is defined as a urine output <0.5 mL/kg per hour in a child or adolescent and <1.0 mL/kg per hour in a neonate. Decreased urine output may result from prerenal, intrarenal, or postrenal factors. Oliguria may occur as the result of an **acute process** or an **acute exacerbation** of an unrecognized chronic renal disease.

DIFFERENTIAL DIAGNOSIS LIST

Prerenal

Decreased Intravascular Volume
  Dehydration (typically caused by gastrointestinal losses)
  Hemorrhage
  Inadequate fluid intake
  Sepsis (with capillary leak)
***Ineffective* Intravascular Blood Volume ("Edematous States")**
  Hypoalbuminemia/ decreased oncotic pressure
  Nephrotic syndrome
  Hepatic dysfunction
Impaired cardiovascular status
  Congestive heart failure
  Sepsis (with peripheral vasodilation and/or cardiac depression)

Intrarenal

Glomerular Causes
  Primary glomerulonephritis (e.g., acute postinfectious, membranoproliferative)

Secondary GN associated with systemic disease (e.g., lupus nephritis)
Tubulointerstitial
  Acute tubular necrosis (ATN)
  Prolonged prerenal azotemia or ischemia
  Medications
  Toxins
  Pigment deposition— myoglobin or hemoglobin
  Acute interstitial nephritis (drugs, infections)
Vascular
  Hemolytic uremic syndrome
  Renal venous or arterial thrombosis

Postrenal

Congenital or Anatomic
  Congenital obstructive uropathies (e.g., posterior urethral valves)
  Urinary stone
  Trauma
  Abdominal mass

Functional
  Acute urinary retention
  Neurogenic bladder

Other
  Syndrome of inappropriate
  antidiuretic hormone
  (meningitis, pneumonia)

DIFFERENTIAL DIAGNOSIS DISCUSSION

Dehydration

Dehydration is the **most common cause** of **oliguria** in the pediatric population. The causes, clinical features, and evaluation are discussed in detail in Chapter 25, "Dehydration." Treatment is directed toward restoring intravascular volume. If dehydration is mild, **oral rehydration** may be attempted. If the patient cannot tolerate oral fluids, or if the dehydration is more severe, initial **fluid resuscitation with normal saline** should be performed, followed by oral or intravenous rehydration. In most patients, urine output improves within a few hours when these simple measures are used.

> **HINT:** Because kidney function is preserved, prerenal azotemia is rapidly reversible if the underlying cause is corrected (e.g., restoring intravascular volume in a dehydrated patient). Intrarenal causes are not usually readily reversible.

Acute Postinfectious Glomerulonephritis

See Chapter 39, "Hematuria."

Acute Tubular Necrosis

Etiology

ATN is the **final common pathway of a number of renal insults,** including **prolonged prerenal ischemia, sepsis, toxicity,** and **pigment deposition.** ATN is a relatively common occurrence in severely ill patients in intensive care units; these patients often have multiple causes for the ATN (e.g., sepsis with hypotension plus aminoglycoside therapy).

Clinical Features

ATN traditionally has three phases:

- **Oliguric phase.** The oliguric phase may last days or several weeks. The hallmarks of this phase are decreased urine output and loss of renal concentrating ability, resulting in an elevated urine sodium level and a decreased urine specific gravity. Hypertension may be present, as with other forms of acute renal failure.

- **Diuretic phase.** In the diuretic phase, urine output increases dramatically; urine sodium and water losses may be significant.
- **Recovery phase.** In the recovery phase, urine output returns to a normal rate and concentrating ability returns.

Evaluation

The evaluation of patients with ATN is twofold: **assessing the clinical status** (including the volume and electrolyte status) and **determining the underlying cause,** which may not be immediately apparent.

- **Pertinent questions** focus on prior medication use (especially antimicrobials such as aminoglycosides and amphotericin B), recent radiocontrast dye studies, and toxin exposures (such as lead). Patients with hemoglobinuria or myoglobinuria may have a history of trauma, muscle pain, or pallor. Because prolonged ischemia from any prerenal cause can result in ATN, patients should be queried about recent gastrointestinal or blood losses.
- **Urinalysis** in patients with ATN typically shows a low specific gravity and variable degrees of hematuria or proteinuria. The urine sodium level in the oliguric phase is usually elevated (>40 mEq/L). Specific tests as directed by the history (e.g., antibiotic levels and serum creatine kinase levels) may also be indicated.

Treatment

Treatment of ATN is similar to that of other causes of acute renal failure. A significant number of patients with ATN, especially those with life-threatening conditions such as septic shock, require **dialysis.** ATN is not rapidly reversible because tubular damage has occurred. However, a significant number of pediatric patients, even those with prolonged oliguria, may recover all or partial renal function.

Hemolytic Uremic Syndrome

Hemolytic uremic syndrome is a syndrome of **microangiopathic hemolytic anemia, thrombocytopenia,** and **renal failure.** There are two main categories: **diarrheal-associated** (D+ or "typical") and **nondiarrheal-associated** (D− or "atypical"). Most cases of hemolytic uremic syndrome fall into the first category.

Etiology

D+ hemolytic-uremic syndrome results from infection with Shiga-toxin-producing *Escherichia coli*, usually the strain O157:H7. Other infectious agents are also implicated in this form of hemolytic uremic syndrome, including *Salmonella* and *Shigella* species. Infection usually results from **ingestion of contaminated foods,** especially ground beef, or from **person-to-person contact.**

Clinical Features

Patients with D+ hemolytic uremic syndrome present with a **history of diarrhea, often bloody. Oliguria** often becomes evident as the diarrhea subsides. Patients also develop **pallor** and occasionally a **petechial rash. Hypertension** is common.

Hemolytic uremic syndrome can affect organs other than the kidney and gastrointestinal tract. Patients may have associated **central nervous system (CNS) symptoms** (e.g., irritability, lethargy, and coma), **pancreatic dysfunction** (resulting in hyperglycemia), and **cardiomyopathy** (resulting in congestive heart failure).

> **HINT:** With the advent of improved supportive care for patients with renal failure, CNS complications have become the leading cause of mortality in patients with hemolytic uremic syndrome.

Evaluation

Evaluation of hemolytic uremic syndrome includes a careful **history** to determine exposure to contaminated foods or ill contacts.

Physical examination is directed toward **assessing volume status** as well as **neurologic status.**

Laboratory tests include serum electrolytes, blood urea nitrogen (BUN) and creatinine levels, a glucose level, liver function tests and pancreatic enzyme measurements, urinalysis, and a complete blood count (CBC) with careful examination of the smear for evidence of schistocytes and fragmented red blood cells (RBCs). Proteinuria, hematuria, and cellular casts are common urinalysis findings.

Treatment

Treatment of D+ hemolytic uremic syndrome is **largely supportive.** Establishing the diagnosis early in the course of disease is essential to avoid complications (e.g., volume overload). As with other forms of renal failure, specific treatments for electrolyte abnormalities may be required. **Transfusions of packed RBCs** are given only if the hemoglobin level is <6 g/dL and should be administered slowly to avoid hypertension. **Platelet transfusions** should be avoided unless active bleeding is present. As many as 50% of patients with hemolytic uremic syndrome require **dialysis. Consultation with a pediatric nephrologist** early in the course of disease is strongly advised.

Posterior Urethral Valves

Etiology

Posterior urethral valves (PUV) are the **most common cause of obstructive uropathy in infant boys.** The condition is caused by an **abnormality in** urethral development that results in the formation of mucosal folds, which act as valves, obstructing the outflow of urine.

Clinical Features

Patients usually present in the **first year of life** with **oliguria, poor intermittent urinary stream,** and a **distended bladder.** With the widespread use of screening antenatal ultrasounds, a significant number of patients are now identified **in utero,** by the finding of **bilateral hydronephrosis** with or without oligohydramnios. **Older patients** occasionally present with **urinary tract infection** (UTI) and a history of **poor urinary stream.** A **urinary concentrating defect is common** in this disorder, resulting in renal water and salt wasting. Patients with a history of severe oligohydramnios may have **pulmonary hypoplasia** and **respiratory distress.**

Evaluation

Specific evaluation of suspected PUV includes a **renal ultrasound** to confirm obstruction and hydronephrosis, and a **voiding cystourethrogram. Serum electrolytes** and **creatinine** should also be measured. A serum creatinine level obtained within the first 24 hours following birth is not useful because it largely reflects maternal renal function.

Urinalysis and **urine culture** should be obtained to assess for UTI.

Treatment

A **pediatric urologist** should be consulted if PUV is suspected. Initial treatment consists of placement of a **Foley catheter** to facilitate bladder drainage. Following bladder decompression, it is important to **monitor serum electrolytes and volume status closely.** Because of renal concentrating defects and a postobstructive diuresis, hypernatremia or hyponatremia, hyperkalemia, and metabolic acidosis may ensue. Once the electrolyte abnormalities are normalized, definitive **valve ablation** can be performed (often in the first week of life). Despite surgical correction of the obstruction, patients with PUV are at **risk for progression to chronic renal failure.** Therefore, **referral to a pediatric nephrologist** is recommended for patients with evidence of renal insufficiency or metabolic acidosis.

EVALUATION OF DECREASED URINE OUTPUT

Patient History

The history should be directed toward assessing the onset and severity of the oliguria, as well as determining possible causes, and includes assessment of the following:

- Fluid intake and losses (e.g., diarrhea, vomiting, and blood loss)
- History of poor feeding, pallor, cyanosis, or difficulty with exertion (may suggest underlying cardiac disease)
- History of poor growth, recent weight loss, polyuria, fatigue or "unexplained" anemia (may suggest chronic kidney disease)
- Associated symptoms, such as macroscopic hematuria or flank pain (may suggest pyelonephritis, urolithiasis, or renal vein thrombosis)
- Toxin exposures (e.g., lead and mercury) and recent medication use (e.g., nonsteroidal anti-inflammatory agents)
- Recent illnesses and environmental exposures (e.g., recent skin or pharyngeal infection or exposure to undercooked meat)
- Results of prenatal ultrasounds (if obtained)

Physical Examination

Physical examination findings vary depending on the underlying cause:

- Dry mucous membranes, sunken eyes, poor skin turgor, and tachycardia suggest dehydration.
- Hypotension and poor perfusion are seen in patients with septic shock or cardiac dysfunction.
- A third heart sound (S_3) cardiac gallop may be noted if significant volume overload is present.
- Edema and hypertension are common in patients with acute renal failure secondary to glomerular disease.
- Joint symptoms and rashes may be present in patients with systemic lupus erythematosus or vasculitic diseases.
- Patients with rhabdomyolysis have diffuse muscle tenderness, especially in the larger muscle groups of the legs and arms.
- Abdominal masses may signal an obstructing malignancy.

> **HINT:** A very distended, obstructed bladder may be mistaken for an abdominal mass.

Laboratory Studies

Initial laboratory studies in any patient with oliguria include the following:

- A **serum electrolyte panel** and **BUN** and **creatinine levels** should be obtained first. If abnormal renal function is noted, calcium, phosphorus, and uric acid should also be assayed. A BUN-to-creatinine ratio >20 is suggestive of prerenal disease.
- A **urinalysis** with microscopy is obligatory.

- A **CBC** is indicated in almost all instances of acute renal failure except in certain cases, such as medication-induced acute urinary retention.
- **Urine sodium level and fractional excretion of sodium.** Measuring the urine sodium level is useful in helping determine whether the disorder is prerenal or renal in origin. A urine sodium level <20 mEq/L suggests a prerenal cause, whereas one >40 mEq/L suggests an intrinsic cause. Intermediate values of urine sodium are not diagnostic. Alternatively, a formal calculation of the fractional excretion of sodium (FENa) can be made:

$$\text{FENa} = (\text{Urine sodium/Plasma sodium}) \times (\text{Plasma creatinine/} \\ \text{Urine creatinine}) \times 100$$

A FENa <1% suggests a prerenal cause, and values >2% suggest an intrinsic cause.

> **HINT:** Urinary sodium and FENa are not reliable for diagnostic purposes if diuretics were administered in the previous 24 hours.

> **HINT:** Measurement of BUN-to-creatinine ratio and urine sodium/FENa are not useful in distinguishing among the *prerenal* etiologies because the physiologic response (sodium and water retention) is the same whether the patient has decreased intravascular volume (e.g., dehydration) or ineffective intravascular volume (e.g., congestive heart failure). The key to managing prerenal azotemia is an accurate *clinical* assessment of the patient's overall volume status, so that the appropriate therapy (e.g., fluid administration in dehydration versus diuretics in congestive heart failure) can be instituted.

- **Additional laboratory studies** are ordered according to the suspected cause of the renal failure, and they include laboratory investigation for past or current infection, drug levels, urine myoglobin, or serum creatine phosphokinase levels (if rhabdomyolysis suspected). Complement levels (C3, C4) and serologies, including antinuclear antibodies and antineutrophil cytoplasmic antibodies, should be considered in all patients with suspected glomerulonephritis.

Diagnostic Modalities

A **renal ultrasound** is indicated in all cases of suspected obstruction and most cases of acute renal failure (especially if unexplained). Additional **radiographic studies** are indicated based on the suspected cause of the acute renal failure. A **renal biopsy** may be necessary to diagnose certain forms of glomerulonephritis and for patients with unexplained renal failure.

TREATMENT OF DECREASED URINE OUTPUT

The initial treatment for acute renal failure from any cause is directed toward the potentially life-threatening complications of volume depletion or overload, electrolyte imbalances, and hypertension.

- **Volume depletion is treated with normal saline,** 20 mL/kg administered as an intravenous bolus over 20 to 30 minutes and may be repeated up to two times until the patient's vital signs (heart rate and/or blood pressure) have stabilized and the patient has urinated.

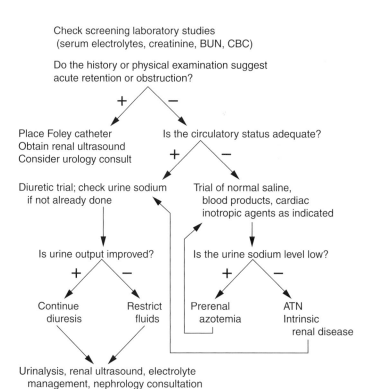

Figure 78-1 ■ Management of the patient with decreased urine output
ATN = acute tubular necrosis; *BUN* = blood urea nitrogen; *CBC* = complete blood cell count

Rehydration can then be completed with oral or intravenous fluids. Packed RBC transfusions or cardiac inotropic agents are given if the clinical situation dictates. Normal saline should not be administered to patients with *ineffective* intravascular volume unless they also have clinical evidence of volume depletion.

■ **Patients unresponsive to fluid administration or those who are overtly edematous may be given a diuretic challenge.** Intravenous furosemide (2 mg/kg per dose) is given as a onetime dose. If a response is seen, the dose may be repeated every 3 to 4 hours. If no response is seen, additional doses are of no benefit and may cause ototoxic and nephrotoxic side effects.

■ **Patients with persistent oliguria should be fluid restricted** to insensible losses (25% to 30% of maintenance requirements given as 5% to 10% dextrose in water) plus urine output (replaced milliliter for milliliter with a quarter to a half normal saline).

■ **Specific therapies for electrolyte disturbances** are outlined in Chapter 32, "Electrolyte Disturbances."

HINT: If intravascular volume has been restored and minimal or no urine output is observed, other diagnoses should be considered, such as ATN. Continuing to administer fluid to such patients will be of no benefit and could precipitate volume overload.

APPROACH TO THE PATIENT (FIGURE 78-1)

Suggested Readings

Andreoli SP: Acute renal failure. *Curr Opin Pediatr* 14:183–188, 2002.
Klahr S, Miller SB: Acute oliguria. *N Engl J Med* 338:671–675, 1998.

DIFFERENTIAL DIAGNOSIS LIST

Premenarchal Patients

Infectious Causes
  Infectious vulvovaginitis
  Genital herpes
  Condyloma acuminatum
Toxic Causes
  Exogenous estrogens
Neoplastic Causes
  Sarcoma botryoides
  Adenocarcinoma of the
    cervix or vagina
  Estrogen production from
    an ovarian cyst or
    neoplasm
  Hemangioma
Traumatic Causes
  Accidental trauma
  Sexual abuse
  Foreign body
Congenital or Vascular Causes
  Urethral prolapse
Miscellaneous Causes
  Vulvar skin disorders
  Neonatal withdrawal
    bleeding
  Precocious puberty
  McCune-Albright syndrome

  Cervicitis
  Pelvic inflammatory disease
Neoplastic Causes
Traumatic Causes
  Accidental trauma
  Sexual abuse
  Foreign body
Metabolic or Genetic Causes
  Hyperthyroidism or
    hypothyroidism
  Hyperprolactinemia
Gynecologic Causes
  Dysfunctional uterine
    bleeding
  Abortion—threatened,
    incomplete, complete,
    or missed
  Ectopic pregnancy
  Polycystic ovarian disease
Hematologic Causes
  Idiopathic thrombocy-
    topenic purpura
  von Willebrand disease
Miscellaneous Causes
  Chronic systemic illness
    (e.g., liver disease, connec-
    tive tissue disorder)

Postmenarchal Patients

Infectious Causes
  Infectious vulvovaginitis

DIFFERENTIAL DIAGNOSIS DISCUSSION

Vulvovaginitis

Vulvovaginitis is discussed in detail in Chapter 80, "Vaginal Discharge (Vulvovaginitis)." Bleeding, when present, is usually **minimal,** although a **blood-tinged discharge** is common in severe cases. *Shigella* and group A β-hemolytic streptococci are the most common causes of a bloody vaginal discharge associated with vulvovaginitis.

Vulvar Hemangiomas

Etiology

Bleeding can result following trauma to a vulvar hemangioma. Vulvar hemangiomas are common and generally **disappear as the child ages.**

Clinical Features

Patients usually present with **painless bleeding** and a **history of vulvar hemangiomas.** The bleeding is usually self-limited; however, heavy bleeding can be seen with cavernous hemangiomas. Careful examination of the external genitalia identifies the source of bleeding. Vaginoscopy is not required if bleeding is limited to the external genitalia.

Treatment

When bleeding does not respond to **pressure, surgical ligation** may be required.

Trauma

Incidence and Etiology

Genital trauma is a **serious** and common cause of vaginal bleeding. The incidence is highest in children between 4 and 12 years of age. Most genital trauma results from a **straddle injury** (e.g., a child landing on the center bar of a bicycle), but **sexual abuse, accidental penetration, sudden abduction** of the lower extremities, and **pelvic fractures** must also be considered.

Clinical Features and Evaluation

- **In patients with straddle injuries** (a type of blunt trauma), a small ecchymotic area or a large vulvar hematoma may be noted. Hematomas are tender, tense, and rounded swellings that may enlarge if bleeding continues. Lacerations of the hymen or vagina may occur in association with straddle injuries; however, their presence should alert the physician to other possible sources of trauma.
- **Accidental penetration with pens and other small objects** is common in 2- to 4-year-olds. Lacerations can be superficial or deep and can extend to the peritoneal cavity. Isolated injuries to the hymen alone are rare, and careful examination of the vagina is mandatory.
- **Lacerations of the vagina can also occur as a result of sudden abduction of the legs,** as in gymnastics or water skiing. These injuries can be difficult to distinguish from injuries sustained secondary to sexual abuse. The paucity of other injuries helps distinguish these injuries from sexual abuse.

- **In patients with pelvic fractures,** injuries to the urinary system are more common than are vaginal lacerations. However, in complex fractures, lacerations of the vagina can be extensive, accounting for a significant loss of blood. A thorough examination is mandatory, including evaluation of the urinary system and rectum.

If bleeding is noted from the vagina, direct pressure should be applied to the area followed by vaginoscopy under anesthesia.

Treatment

- **Superficial abrasions and lacerations** of the vulva, if not actively bleeding, may be cleaned and left to heal.
- **Small vulvar hematomas** that are not expanding may be managed conservatively with ice packs and pressure.
- **Large or expanding hematomas** should be managed surgically with evacuation and ligation of bleeding vessels. At times, it may prove difficult to locate actively bleeding vessels. A vaginal packing should be placed in this instance and removed after several hours. Perioperative antibiotics are required.

Foreign Body

Foreign bodies placed into the vagina account for 5% of gynecologic visits in childhood. Most children **will not remember or admit** to placing an object in the vagina. The incidence is highest in children between 2 and 4 years of age. **Rolled toilet tissue** is one of the most common findings.

Clinical Features

The child presents with a history of a **foul-smelling, often bloody, vaginal discharge.** The vaginal bleeding is usually **bright red, scant, and intermittent.** A strong odor may be the most bothersome symptom.

Evaluation

On physical examination, the vagina is **erythematous** and a **foul-smelling discharge** is present. A **large foreign body may be easily palpated on rectal examination.** Smaller items (e.g., toilet tissue) may not be discerned.

Radiographic studies are of little use because most foreign bodies are not radiopaque.

Treatment

Vaginoscopy may aid in the diagnosis and removal. However, small items may be removed with **saline irrigation alone. General anesthesia** is frequently required for **removal of larger objects. Antibiotic therapy** is recommended before removing foreign bodies that may have been **in place ≥1 week.**

Urethral Prolapse

Etiology

Prolapse is thought to result from **increased abdominal pressure,** which could be caused by coughing or constipation. Some children are predisposed to prolapse secondary to a weakness of collagen.

Clinical Features

A **small hemorrhagic, friable mass surrounding the urethra** is the most common presentation. The bleeding associated with prolapse of the urethra is usually **painless** (because the urethra and vagina are so close in proximity, urethral bleeding may be thought to be from the vagina). The average age at diagnosis is 5 years.

The lesion can easily be **confused with condyloma acuminatum.** If the diagnosis is in question, **3% acetic acid** may be applied; condyloma acuminatum has an **acetowhite appearance.**

Treatment

If voiding is not inhibited, **local therapy** (i.e., with topical estrogen and sitz baths) may be all that is needed. The prolapse usually **resolves after 4 weeks** of therapy.

If **urine retention or necrosis** is present, **surgical removal and catheterization** are necessary.

Vulvar Skin Disorders

Most vulvar skin conditions involve the labia majora and labia minora and do not extend to the vagina or perianal area. **Seborrhea, psoriasis, and eczema** are the most common diagnoses. These lesions tend to be **pruritic.** The constant **scratching with subsequent infection** can lead to a bloody discharge similar to that seen in vaginitis.

Neonatal Withdrawal Bleeding

Withdrawal of maternal estrogen after delivery causes **physiologic bleeding** in a small percentage of **newborns.** The bleeding is limited and usually **resolves within 1 week.** The parents may notice an increased blood-tinged discharge. **No treatment** is necessary unless bleeding persists for **>10 days.** At that point, a thorough examination should be performed.

Dysfunctional Uterine Bleeding

Dysfunctional uterine bleeding is defined as **any abnormal bleeding** from the uterus that is **not caused by structural abnormalities.** The average menstrual cycle has a mean interval of 28 days, with a mean duration of 4 days. The average blood loss is 30 mL/cycle, with an upper normal limit of 80 mL. A **menstrual cycle with an interval of ≤ 21 days, length >7 days,** or blood loss of **>80 mL is abnormal.**

Etiology

Anovulation, most commonly caused by an **immature hypothalamic-pituitary axis,** is responsible for >75% of cases of dysfunctional uterine bleeding. Without ovulation, and the resulting formation of the corpus luteum, there is no cyclic or monthly production of progesterone. The cyclic production and withdrawal of progesterone results in a normal period. Anovulation causes continuous estrogenic stimulation of the endometrium, resulting in a thick, unstable endometrium that sheds irregularly. Hypothalamic-pituitary axis immaturity can last for as many as **18 months after menarche.** McDonough and Ganett found that 55% to 82% of cycles in adolescents between menarche and 2 years after menarche were anovulatory. These percentages decreased with time.

Anovulation may also be caused by obesity, hyperthyroidism, hypothyroidism, hyperadrenalism, hyperprolactinemia, diabetes mellitus, polycystic ovarian syndrome, chronic systemic illness, substance abuse, eating disorders, physical or emotional stress, and excessive exercise.

Clinical Features

The presentation is highly variable ranging from amenorrhea to heavy irregular vaginal bleeding. Typically, a patient may experience several months of **amenorrhea followed by heavy bleeding.** The bleeding may last for weeks and be associated with cramping. Additionally, heavy menstrual bleeding with passage of clots may lead to significant pelvic pain.

Evaluation

Dysfunctional uterine bleeding is a **diagnosis of exclusion.** Organic lesions, pregnancy, and coagulation disorders must be ruled out. The history and physical examination should emphasize the **common and life-threatening conditions** in the differential, with **coagulation defects** and **complications of pregnancy** leading the list. If a patient is obese, hirsute, or displays signs of insulin resistance such as acanthosis nigricans, **polycystic ovarian syndrome** should be considered.

Studies helpful in the diagnosis include **serum thyroid-stimulating hormone, fasting prolactin, follicle-stimulating hormone, luteinizing hormone, free testosterone, dehydroepiandrosterone sulfate, androstenedione, and 17-hydroxyprogesterone levels.**

Treatment

Management of dysfunctional uterine bleeding in an adolescent **depends on the severity** of the bleeding, with the emphasis placed on stopping the bleeding and preventing recurrent episodes (Table 79-1).

- **Patients with mild bleeding** (i.e., bleeding at 20- to 60-day intervals without anemia) should be advised that the situation usually resolves after 1 to 2 years with maturation of the hypothalamic-pituitary axis

TABLE 79-1 Treatment of Dysfunctional Uterine Bleeding

Mild Dysfunctional Uterine Bleeding

Reassurance
Menstrual calendar
Oral contraceptives

Severe or Recurrent Dysfunctional Uterine Bleeding Without Anemia

Medroxyprogesterone acetate, 10 mg for 14 days each month
Norethindrone, 5–10 mg for 14 days each month
Oral contraceptives

Acute Anovulatory Bleeding in a Stable Patient

Oral contraceptives (35–50 mcg; one pill every 6 hours until bleeding stops)
After bleeding stops, taper oral contraceptives:
   One pill every 8 hours for 3 days
   Then one pill every 12 hours for 3 days
   Then one pill every day to complete 21 days
   Continue on oral contraceptives for 3–6 months

Acute or Heavy Bleeding Associated with Anemia or Hypotension

Hospitalization
Transfusion if unstable
Intravenous conjugated estrogen (25 mg every 4–6 hours) until bleeding stops
Begin monophasic combined oral contraceptives (35–50 mcg):
   One pill every 6 hours for 3 days
   Then one pill every 8 hours for 3 days
   Then one pill every 12 hours for 3 days
   Then one pill every day to complete 21 days
   Continue on oral contraceptives for 3–6 months

and subsequent ovulation. If the patient has mild dysfunctional uterine bleeding and desires some form of contraception, a monophasic oral contraceptive may be prescribed that will provide the added benefit of regular menstrual cycles.

■ **For patients with severe or recurrent dysfunctional uterine bleeding associated with anemia,** hormonal therapy is indicated. **Monophasic combined oral contraceptive pills are appropriate first-line treatment even if the patient is not sexually active.** Otherwise, progestational agents can be administered (see Table 79-1). Therapy should be continued for 6 to 8 months and then discontinued. Most patients have spontaneous maturation of the hypothalamus-pituitary axis with onset of regular menses after cessation of therapy. If patients continue to have irregular bleeding after stopping therapy, they must be reevaluated.

■ **An acute episode of bleeding in a stable patient** may be treated with a 35 to 50 μg combined oral contraceptive (see Table 79-1). If the bleeding does not stop within 5 days, another cause for the bleeding, such as a coagulation disorder, must be considered. When the bleeding slows, the pills may be tapered as described in Table 79-1. The patient should be maintained on the pills for at least 3 months, or longer if sexually active.

- **Patients who have undergone heavy bleeding leading to hypovolemia or anemia** should be hospitalized for therapy and coagulation studies. Intravenous conjugated estrogens are given every 4 to 6 hours until the bleeding stops, usually 24 to 48 hours after initiating therapy. Once the bleeding has stopped, the patient may be started on oral contraceptives (see Table 79-1). Dilation and curettage is to be avoided in adolescents; however, when medical therapy fails, it may be necessary for diagnostic purposes. Along with dilation and curettage, hysteroscopy may be helpful in making a diagnosis.

Pregnancy

Bleeding **in early pregnancy is common.** In most cases, it is scant and has little clinical significance. However, bleeding may be a sign of **ectopic pregnancy, which is life threatening.** Therefore, **pregnancy must be ruled out in all adolescent patients with bleeding,** regardless of the history. Figure 79-1 illustrates the approach to a patient with a positive

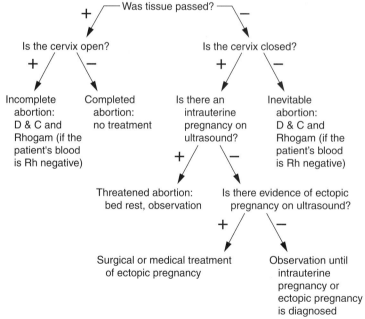

Figure 79-1 ■ Evaluation of a patient with a positive pregnancy test and vaginal bleeding
D & C = dilation and curettage

pregnancy test and vaginal bleeding. A **gynecologic consultation is mandatory** in patients who have bleeding in pregnancy.

EVALUATION OF VAGINAL BLEEDING

Patient History

The history is always helpful when evaluating children with vaginal bleeding. The physician must be aware, however, that much **information may be intentionally withheld** by both the patient and the parent. Children generally do not provide information regarding foreign bodies, manipulation, or sexual abuse. Likewise, parents do not often admit to sexual abuse. Whenever a child presents with vaginal bleeding, regardless of the history, other **indications of abuse must be sought** (see Chapter 69, "Sexual Abuse").

Physical Examination

A careful and thorough physical and gynecologic examination is mandatory. Consultation with a **gynecologist or adolescent medicine specialist** is essential.

APPROACH TO THE PATIENT

Figure 79-2 depicts the approach to a premenarchal girl with vaginal bleeding.

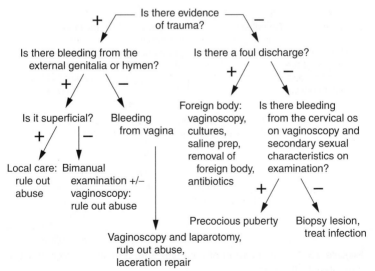

Figure 79-2 ■ Evaluation of a premenarchal girl with vaginal bleeding

Suggested Readings

Altchek A: Common problems in pediatric gynecology. *Compr Ther* 10:19–28, 1984.

Behrman RE, Kliegman RM, Nelson WE, et al.: *Nelson Textbook of Pediatrics*, 14th ed. Philadelphia, WB Saunders, 1992.

Carpenter SE, Rock JA: *Pediatric and Adolescent Gynecology*. Philadelphia, Lippincott-Raven, 1992.

Emans JH, Goldstein DP: *Pediatric and Adolescent Gynecology*. Boston, Little, Brown, 1990.

Grossman M, Dieckmann RA: *Pediatric Emergency Medicine*. Philadelphia, JB Lippincott, 1991.

Hertweck SP: Dysfunctional uterine bleeding. *Obstet Gynecol Clin North Am* 19:129–149, 1992.

Reece RM: *Manual of Emergency Pediatrics*. Philadelphia, WB Saunders, 1992.

Taber BZ: *Manual of Gynecologic and Obstetric Emergencies*, 2nd ed. Philadelphia, WB Saunders, 1984.

80 Vaginal Discharge (Vulvovaginitis)

Erin Rebele and Jenell Coleman
Courtney Schreiber (Third Edition)

INTRODUCTION

Vulvovaginitis, a common problem for both pediatric and adolescent patients, is an entity consisting of **vaginal and vulvar irritation** associated with **vaginal discharge**. **A lack of estrogen,** which protects and toughens the skin in the genital region, renders **premenarchal girls particularly susceptible** to vulvovaginitis. **Poor hygiene,** a common problem in young girls, also contributes to the problem. Some causes of vulvovaginitis are more prevalent in adolescents (e.g., *Candida* vulvovaginitis).

DIFFERENTIAL DIAGNOSIS LIST

Infectious Causes

Bacterial Infection
 Group A β-hemolytic
  streptococci
 Staphylococcus aureus
 Gardnerella vaginalis
 Streptococcus pneumoniae
 Neisseria gonorrhoeae,
  Neisseria meningitidis
 Chlamydia trachomatis
 Shigella flexneri
 Yersinia enterocolitica
 Haemophilus influenzae

Fungal Infection
 Candida albicans
 Candida glabrata

Parasitic Infection
 Trichomonas vaginalis
 Enterobius vermicularis
  (pinworm)

Viral Infection
 Herpes simplex virus (HSV)

Neoplastic Causes

Sarcoma botryoides

Traumatic Causes

Sexual abuse
Local irritants—bubble bath,
 harsh soaps, tight-fitting
 clothes, nylon underwear,
 allergy to laundry detergent
 or fabric softener

Congenital or Vascular Causes

Hemangioma
Ectopic ureter

Miscellaneous Causes

Nonspecific vulvovaginitis
Foreign body
Physiologic leukorrhea of the
 adolescent
Predisposing diseases—
 diabetes mellitus, immuno-
 suppression
Systemic illness—roseola,
 varicella, scarlet fever,
 Stevens-Johnson syndrome,
 Kawasaki syndrome

Dermatologic disorder—
seborrhea, eczema, psoriasis,
lichen sclerosis et atrophicus

Physiologic discharge of the
newborn
Urethral prolapse

DIFFERENTIAL DIAGNOSIS DISCUSSION

Group A β-Hemolytic Streptococcal Infection

Group A β-hemolytic streptococci can cause vulvovaginitis that may be
associated with a **bloody vaginal discharge**. The vulvovaginitis typically
develops **7 to 10 days after an upper respiratory tract infection or sore
throat**. Examination reveals a **beefy red vulvar erythema**. Diagnosis is
via **vaginal culture**. Treatment is with penicillin VK, 125 to 250 mg four
times daily for 10 days, or amoxicillin.

Bacterial Vaginosis

Etiology

Bacterial vaginosis results from the **overgrowth of normal bacteria**
including anaerobes, G. vaginalis, and Mycoplasma hominis. This overgrowth results from the imbalance between normal lactobacillus and
anaerobes, which could be precipitated by changes in alkalization by
sex or douches, for example. The significance of G. vaginalis infection
or bacterial vaginosis in children is uncertain, but one should consider
the possibility of sexual abuse.

Clinical Features

The patient may complain of a **vaginal discharge or a "fishy" odor after
coitus or menses**, and a **gray or yellow, thin, homogeneous discharge** is
noted on physical examination.

Evaluation

Using Amsel's criteria, patients must have three of the following four
criteria to make the diagnosis:

- Thin, homogeneous discharge
- Clue cells seen on a saline preparation (>20% of all epithelial cells)
- A positive "whiff" test (a fishy odor noted before or after discharge
  is mixed with potassium hydroxide [KOH] stain)
- Vaginal secretions with a pH ≥4.5

Treatment

Treatment of bacterial vaginosis is with **metronidazole, 500 mg orally
twice daily for 7 days; metronidazole vaginal gel 0.75%, one applicator**

(5 g) intravaginal at bedtime for 5 days; clindamycin **cream 2%,** one applicator (5 g) intravaginal at bedtime for 7 days; or **clindamycin,** 300 mg orally twice daily for 7 days.

Gonorrhea

N. gonorrhoeae infection is discussed in Chapter 70, "Sexually Transmitted Diseases."

Chlamydia

C. trachomatis infection is discussed in Chapter 70, "Sexually Transmitted Diseases."

Shigella Vulvovaginitis

Etiology

S. flexneri is most often responsible for this inflammation, which is **rare in children.**

Clinical Features and Evaluation

A **mucopurulent vaginal discharge** is seen; it is **bloody** in 40% to 50% of patients. Fewer than 25% of patients have associated **diarrhea.** **Vaginal culture** reveals the organism.

Treatment

The infection is treated with **trimethoprim** and **sulfamethoxazole,** twice daily for 7 days.

Candida Vulvovaginitis

Etiology

The most common pathogen is *C. albicans.* However, in difficult to treat cases, *C. glabrata* should be suspected. The disorder is **more common in adolescents** than in prepubescent girls.

Predisposing factors include diabetes mellitus, recent antibiotic or steroid use, immunosuppression, pregnancy, use of oral contraceptives, and tight-fitting clothes.

Clinical Features and Evaluation

- Patients usually present complaining of intense **vulvovaginal itching, thick white discharge,** and **external dysuria.** On examination, vulvar and perianal **erythema,** inflammation, and excoriations may be visible. White satellite candidal plaques are sometimes noted, and thick "cottage cheese" discharge is often present. A KOH smear revealing hyphae and budding yeast confirms the diagnosis of *C. albicans. C. glabrata,* alternatively, may not be visible by KOH microscopy.

Treatment

- **In prepubescent girls** an antifungal cream (e.g., miconazole, clotrimazole, nystatin) should be applied to the external genitalia. The applicator should not be used to avoid trauma to the hymen. If this is not successful, intravaginal nystatin liquid or gentle insertion of a vaginal suppository that has been cut in half may be prescribed. A topical steroid cream may be used to alleviate the inflammation.
- **Adolescents** should be treated with an antifungal medication (e.g., miconazole or terconazole) given as a cream or vaginal suppositories for a 3- to 7-day course. Oral fluconazole is available in a onetime dose; however, symptomatic relief may take up to 72 hours.

Trichomoniasis

Etiology

This infection is caused by *T. vaginalis,* a protozoan. Premenarchal girls are generally resistant to this organism because of their lack of estrogen. However, perinatal transmission can persist for up to 1 year.

Clinical Features

Some patients are **asymptomatic,** but the classic complaint is of a **gray, yellow, or green foul-smelling vaginal discharge** and **vaginal irritation.** The patient may note **postcoital spotting.**

Evaluation

Vulvar erythema may be seen on physical examination. Copious, **green frothy discharge** is noted in the vaginal vault. A **"strawberry red" cervix caused by punctuate hemorrhage on the surface** is classically described but uncommonly seen. A **saline preparation** often reveals the **flagellated protozoa** as well as a **heavy polymorphonuclear infiltrate.** For definitive diagnosis, a culture may be sent. Because trichomoniasis is transmitted sexually, the patient should be **tested for gonorrhea and chlamydia** and **counseled about testing for HIV, hepatitis, and syphilis.**

Treatment

Trichomonas is a **sexually acquired pathogen;** therefore children infected with *T. vaginalis* should be **referred to agencies** familiar with evaluating children who have been **sexually abused.**

In sexually active adolescents, the preferred treatment is metronidazole in a single oral dose (2 g). Sexual partners must also be treated and abstinence encourage until both partners are treated.

Enterobius Vermicularis Infestation (Pinworms)

Clinical Features

A typical history includes **perianal and vulvar itching,** especially at night.

Evaluation

Perianal excoriations and an **erythematous vulvar area** are seen on physical examination. Parents should be **asked to examine the child's anus at night using a flashlight**; it may be possible to see the worms. Cellophane tape applied to the child's anus in the morning may reveal characteristic eggs.

Treatment

Pinworm infestation is treated with **one dose of mebendazole** (100 mg), **repeated in 2 weeks.** Consideration should be given to **treating family members.**

Herpes Simplex Virus

Etiology

Precise time of infection with HSV can be difficult to discern. Because of long latency, infection at time of childbirth may become apparent several years after delivery. Type 2 is more commonly associated with sexual transmission. **Sexual abuse must be considered.**

Evaluation

Symptoms such as **dysuria, genital erythema,** and **edema** are the most common complaints. The child might also experience generalized symptoms such as fatigue, adenopathy, and fever. Examination findings include clusters of vesicles. Viral culture is important because other viruses may cause mucosal ulcers, such as coxsackievirus.

Treatment

Treatment is mostly **symptomatic.** Care must be taken to ensure that the child is voiding appropriately because the edema and pain can cause urinary retention requiring Foley catheterization. Soaking in a warm bath may ease the pain of urination. Acyclovir may be used to shorten the duration of symptoms and quicken the resolution of lesions.

Nonspecific Vulvovaginitis

Etiology

Nonspecific vulvovaginitis accounts for 25% to 70% of all cases of pediatric vulvovaginitis and is caused by an **alteration in the vaginal flora.** The most common cause of this alteration is **poor perineal hygiene.**

Clinical Features

Nonspecific vulvovaginitis is characterized by **vaginal discharge, odor, vulvar and vaginal irritation, and dysuria.**

Evaluation

The history should include the following questions:

- After a bowel movement or urination, does the child wipe her perineum from back to front?
- Does the child urinate with her knees together?
- Is the child exposed to local irritants such as harsh soaps, bubble bath, and shampoos?
- Does she wash her hair in the bathtub?
- Is the child's laundry washed with hypoallergenic soap?
- Is fabric softener (a possible local irritant) used?
- Does the child wear tight clothes (e.g., tights and leotards)?
- Does the child wear white cotton underwear and use white, unscented toilet paper?

Physical examination usually reveals **vulvar erythema** and **inflammation.** A vaginal discharge may or may not be present. A saline wet mount reveals predominantly white blood cells (WBCs) and bacteria. A KOH smear reveals no evidence of mycotic infection. If local measures fail, vaginal yeast and bacterial cultures should be sent. Typically in patients with nonspecific vulvovaginitis, the culture reveals normal vaginal flora.

Treatment

Application of **1% hydrocortisone cream, A & D ointment, or Desitin cream** may be soothing. Patients may also take **sitz baths three times a day** (Aveeno oatmeal or baking soda may be added to the bath). The vulva should be **gently patted dry** or may be dried using a **hair dryer on the cool setting.**

If symptoms do not improve with local measures and a **predominant organism** is present on vaginal culture, an **appropriate antibiotic** can be prescribed. If no predominant organism is identified by culture, and vulvovaginitis does not respond to local measures, **empirical antibiotic** treatment may be tried (e.g., amoxicillin, amoxicillin-clavulanate, or cephalexin for 7 to 10 days).

Prevention entails **improved perineal hygiene,** including correct voiding and wiping technique, and **avoidance of bubble baths, harsh soaps, and tight clothes.** The child should wear **white cotton underwear.**

Physiologic Leukorrhea

Etiology and Clinical Features

Physiologic leukorrhea, caused by **desquamation of epithelial cells under the influence of estrogen,** is classically described as **white, mucoid, and without odor.** It is seen in **newborns** (secondary to maternal estrogens) **and adolescents.** Sometimes it is noted months prior to the first menses.

Evaluation and Treatment

Physical examination reveals **copious white, mucoid vaginal secretions without an odor.** Saline and KOH preparations reveal epithelial cells, but no yeast, *Trichomonas*, or WBCs. **No treatment** is necessary.

Lichen Sclerosis

Etiology and Clinical Features

Lichen sclerosis is characterized by **vulvar pruritus** and **irritation.** The cause is unknown. Patients also often complain of vaginal discharge, constipation (secondary to tenesmus), and dysuria. Chronic ulcerations and inflammation may result in areas of **ecchymosis** and **secondary infection** of the vulva.

Evaluation

The diagnosis is generally made by the classic appearance of **whitened papules and plaques on the vulva and perineum** in a characteristic **"figure eight" or "hourglass" distribution** around the anus and introitus. Small ivory areas join to form raised patches. Some areas may contain yellow plugs in the centers. The lesion is classically described as wrinkled tissue paper. In some patients, this disorder may be difficult to distinguish from vitiligo. A **vulvar biopsy** may be necessary.

Treatment

The patient should be **referred to a dermatologist or gynecologist familiar with this condition.** Instruction in **improving perineal hygiene, including use of ointments** (e.g., A & D ointment, Desitin) and **avoidance of harsh soaps.** is appropriate. **Topical steroid creams** may be of benefit.

Foreign Body

Vaginal foreign bodies are discussed in Chapter 79, "Vaginal Bleeding."

EVALUATION OF VAGINAL DISCHARGE

Physiologic discharge varies throughout a female patient's life. As an infant, maternal estrogens primarily influence the infant's physiology; therefore her hymen is pale and thickened, and she may have a white discharge, similar to that of puberty. Withdrawal of these hormones may cause a pink or bloody discharge. After the maternal hormones clear, vaginal discharge is rare. At puberty, with the surge in hormones, the hymen again becomes pale and thicker. The vaginal mucosa produces physiologic leukorrhea.

Physical Examination

A **pelvic examination must be done slowly,** and the physician should tell the child that she or he will not hurt her. The physician must be prepared to abandon the examination if it is too painful or traumatic for the child. The examination should be tailored to the severity of the child's symptoms and her age; severe symptoms require a more thorough examination.

The child may be positioned in the "frog leg" position, the lithotomy position (with the aid of stirrups), or the knee-chest position. The knee-chest position often causes gaping of the hymen, allowing visualization of the vagina and the cervix.

The physician should start by examining the external genitalia, paying particular attention to the presence or absence of genital lesions and vulvar inflammation. Having the patient cough may elicit vaginal discharge.

A rectoabdominal examination is useful for detecting an intravaginal foreign body or a pelvic mass, and for expressing vaginal discharge.

The hymen should be examined for signs of trauma or tears and the presence of a perforation. If a hymenal opening cannot be visualized, placing gentle traction on the labia majora while depressing the perineum generally causes the hymenal opening to open, enabling visualization of the lower vagina.

Visualization of the upper vagina and cervix in a premenarchal girl can be accomplished by using one of the following methods:

- Using a pediatric otoscope, cystoscope, or vaginoscope after applying a local anesthetic (e.g., 2% viscous lidocaine) to the vulva and hymen
- Using a narrow vaginal speculum

> **HINT:** When vulvovaginitis is recurrent or bloody, vaginoscopy is required to rule out a foreign body or tumor.

Laboratory Studies

Microscopic Examination

If vaginal discharge is present, microscopic examination of the discharge is indicated. If discharge is not present at the introitus, a moistened cotton swab is gently inserted into the vagina to collect a specimen. Care should be taken to avoid touching the hymen, which can cause discomfort. The pH of the discharge is assessed first followed by transfer of the swab into a test tube containing two to three drops of sterile saline. Preparation of saline and KOH slides are as follows:

- Saline (wet) preparation. Touch the saturated swab containing the specimen on a glass slide and cover with a glass cover slip. Examine the slide under a microscope for the presence of *T. vaginalis*, bacteria, WBCs, red blood cells, and clue cells.

- **KOH preparation.** Touch the swab to a small amount of 10% KOH on a glass slide. Swirl to mix the contents and perform the "whiff test." Cover the slide with a glass cover slip and examine it under a microscope for hyphae and budding yeast.

In some circumstances, it may be appropriate to obtain the following microbial studies:

- **Vaginal culture.** A bacterial vaginal culture may identify a predominant pathologic organism in premenarchal girls with nonspecific vulvovaginitis. Recurrent vulvovaginal yeast infections should be evaluated with a yeast culture.
- **N. gonorrhoeae or C. trachomatis** nucleic acid amplification techniques (**NAATs**). Several assays are available. The specimen can be obtained from a urine sample or the endocervical canal (in postmenarchal girls). In sexual abuse evaluations, some authorities recommend sequential testing (i.e., NAAT followed by culture in positive tests). Sequential testing yields fewer false-negative and false-positive results compared with either culture or NAAT alone.
- **Viral culture.** If an ulcer lesion is noted, a swab may aid in the diagnosis.

Suggested Readings

Carpenter SE, Rock JA: *Pediatric and Adolescent Gynecology.* Philadelphia, Lippincott-Raven, 1992.

Emans JH, Goldstein DP: *Pediatric and Adolescent Gynecology.* Boston, Little, Brown, 1990.

Shapiro RA, Schubert CJ, Siegel RM: *Neisseria gonorrhea* infections in girls younger than 12 years of age evaluated for vaginitis. *Pediatrics* 104(6):e72, 1999.

Sweet RL, Gibbs RS: *Infectious Disease of the Female Genital Tract,* 3rd ed. Baltimore, Williams & Wilkins, 1995.

Taber BZ: *Manual of Gynecologic and Obstetric Emergencies,* 2nd ed. Philadelphia, WB Saunders, 1984.

INTRODUCTION

Dizziness is caused by a **distortion in spatial orientation.** The primary sensory modalities of vision, vestibular function, joint position sense, touch-pressure sense, and hearing are normally rapidly integrated by the central nervous system (CNS) into a composite sensation, keeping one aware of the body's position in space. Incorrect or insufficient sensory information or an error in integration of the perceptions produces distorted orientation, which in turn causes dizziness.

Vertigo is a sensation of spinning or rotation. Milder forms may be described as producing a rocking sensation or vague lightheadedness. Patients may describe the room spinning around them, rather than a sense that they are moving. Usually vertigo is of sudden onset and associated with loss of balance, nausea, and nystagmus. It may also be associated with diaphoresis and pallor. The sensation can be terrifying to small children.

Vertigo can be caused by a disorder of the CNS, where primary sensory input is integrated, or peripherally, in sensory nerve dysfunction of the vestibular system.

DIFFERENTIAL DIAGNOSIS LIST 🔓

Peripheral Vertigo
Vestibular neuronitis
Labyrinthitis
Benign paroxysmal positional
  vertigo (BPPV)
Ménière disease
Medications
Head trauma

Central Vertigo
Benign paroxysmal vertigo
  (BPV)

Migraine
Seizure
Other

Presyncope

Disequilibrium

DIFFERENTIAL DIAGNOSIS DISCUSSION

Historical points to document include the **course** (acute versus recurrent versus chronic), **precipitating events** (position change, trauma, infection), association with **alteration of hearing** (tinnitus or hearing impairment), **drug exposure, cardiovascular disease,** and **family history of migraine.**

Peripheral Vertigo

Etiology and Clinical Features

Up to 85% of vertigo in children has a peripheral cause. Historical points that help identify peripheral vertigo are an episodic or acute course, improvement with visual fixation or holding head still, accompanying hearing complaints, and absence of other complaints worrisome for cranial nerve dysfunction (e.g., difficulty swallowing, double vision, drooling).

- **Vestibular neuronitis.** This common disorder can occur several days after an upper respiratory tract infection, most often in adolescents. There is no associated hearing loss. Vestibular neuronitis is a self-limited, postinfectious neuropathy, and symptoms generally resolve in 7 to 14 days.
- **Labyrinthitis** is a common inflammatory cause of vertigo. This also follows preceding infection, but hearing impairment is present. Furthermore, patients are often younger than in vestibular neuronitis (preschool to school age). There is a positional component because vertigo worsens with movement. The course is self-limited with resolution after several days. **Acute suppurative labyrinthitis** is caused by extension of otitis media or mastoiditis. Chronic otitis media can lead to the development of cholesteatoma, which in turn can cause labyrinth damage.
- **BPPV** is a rare disorder in children, although it is described in adolescents. Dislodged otoliths cause aberrant vestibular input in the setting of head movement. As such, affected patients experience vertigo only with a change in head position. Symptoms are usually recurrent, with each attack lasting several weeks.
- **Ménière disease** is rare in children. It is characterized by recurring bouts of tinnitus, vertigo, and hearing loss.
- **Medications** that enter the CNS can cause ataxia, incoordination, and abnormal vestibular function, but vertigo is an unusual symptom in anticonvulsant and neuroleptic toxicity. Other drugs, especially aminoglycosides, can produce vertigo as a result of toxic damage to the peripheral vestibular apparatus.
- **Head trauma** may be followed by persistent vertigo. Vertigo caused by trauma-induced perilymphatic fistula is most likely to occur suddenly, and it is accompanied by hearing loss. This diagnosis should be particularly considered in cases of barotrauma. When isolated posttraumatic vertigo without hearing loss occurs, it is more likely caused by dislocation of the otoliths from the macula (see BPPV). Labyrinthine concussion can cause severe and persistent vertigo. This presents with a tendency to fall to the ipsilateral side, and symptoms often last up to 6 weeks.

Treatment

Treatment of peripheral vertigo is symptomatic. Administration of meclizine and diazepam or lorazepam may provide relief in some children; adolescents may respond to transdermal scopolamine. Note that chronic vertigo usually self-resolves as the result of central compensation for the impaired peripheral signaling. Long-term use of symptomatic medication may impair or delay this compensation, and it may even prevent permanent recovery. Ondansetron and phenothiazines can be used to treat nausea and vomiting. Antibiotics are used to treat acute suppurative labyrinthitis.

Central Vertigo

Etiology and Clinical Features

Historical points that help localize central vertigo are complaints suggesting additional cranial nerve dysfunction (e.g., double vision, difficulty swallowing, drooling, abnormal facial sensation), improvement with visual fixation removed (e.g., closing eyes), and lack of improvement with holding the head still.

- **BPV** is a common cause of vertiginous attacks, occurring mostly in toddlers and early-school-age children. Patients report sudden onset of severe vertigo lasting only seconds, less often minutes, in duration. In younger children this may manifest primarily as crying or falling over. Although nystagmus may be reported, it is often not noticed by observers. Pallor and diaphoresis may be prominent. Symptoms quickly resolve on their own with no postictal findings or residual impairments. Many consider BPV a migraine precursor. Although there is no associated headache, patients are more likely to have a family history of migraine and to develop migraines later in life. (Note that BPV is unrelated to BPPV, described earlier.)
- **Migraines** can occur in older children and adolescents, with a vertiginous component, and episodes lasting minutes to hours. These episodes are usually associated with a strong family history.
- **Seizures.** Vertigo may rarely present as the only manifestation of a seizure, although generally there is some alteration in consciousness. Careful questioning often reveals confusional attacks and automatisms or other symptoms of partial complex seizures when vertigo is caused by epilepsy.
- **Other causes.** Other rare causes of central vertigo include stroke (lateral medullary syndrome of Wallenberg, with accompanying Horner syndrome), cerebellopontine angle tumors, neurofibromatosis type II, and demyelinating disease affecting the posterior fossa (e.g., multiple sclerosis).

Treatment

BPV rarely requires treatment because spells are brief and self-resolve. Migraine prophylaxis (e.g., cyproheptadine, topiramate) can be used in patients with frequent episodes suggesting migraine. Treatment focuses on management of the underlying cause in patients with other types of central vertigo (e.g., seizure disorder).

Presyncope

Symptoms of faintness, giddiness, or lightheadedness include **dimness of vision, "roaring" in the ears,** and **diaphoresis** with recovery on assuming a recumbent position. If symptoms are of **short duration and sudden onset,** the symptoms are most likely of **cardiovascular origin.** If symptoms persist, one must consider **hypoglycemia, hyperventilation,** or a **mood disturbance** (e.g., depression, anxiety).

Disequilibrium

Disequilibrium is **loss of balance** without an abnormal sensation in the head. Disequilibrium can be caused by cerebellar, peripheral nervous system, or bilateral vestibular lesions.

EVALUATION OF VERTIGO (DIZZINESS)

Patient History

An effort should be made to clarify the types of dizziness by asking the following questions:

- Was the onset of symptoms acute, recurrent, or chronic?
- Were there any precipitating events (e.g., changes in position, motion, trauma, infection)?
- What is the quality of the dizziness? For older children, it may be helpful to ask, "Describe what you feel without using the word 'dizzy.'" For younger children it may be helpful to offer suggestions— like a spinning top or a swing (suggesting true vertigo), or like feeling very sleepy or confused (suggesting lightheadedness).
- Are there any associated symptoms? Hearing loss, ear pain, or tinnitus suggests inner ear or eighth cranial nerve dysfunction, whereas nausea and vomiting indicate a peripheral vestibular apparatus disorder.
- Is there a family history of cardiovascular disease, drug exposure, or a family history of migraine or ataxia?

Physical Examination

- **Ear examination.** One should look for perforations, infection, hemorrhage, or mass lesions. Blowing air into the external ear canal produces vertigo in patients with a fistula of the round or oval window of the labyrinth.

- **Neurologic examination**
  - **Oculovestibular and cranial nerve testing.** Vestibular testing should include assessment for the presence of nystagmus, changes in visual fixation, or other evidence of cranial nerve dysfunction. Many normal children have "end gaze" (or physiologic) nystagmus with far lateral gaze in either direction. However, abnormal nystagmus includes spontaneous or induced nystagmus within a normal range of vision. Unidirectional, horizontal, or rotary nystagmus suggests a peripheral cause of vertigo. Vertical, irregular, and variable nystagmus suggests a central cause. Accompanying hearing loss suggests a peripheral cause. Older children may be asked to march in place; in the presence of a peripheral lesion of the vestibular system, the child may rotate toward the ipsilateral side.
  - **Cerebellar testing.** Cerebellar testing can help clarify if there is a central component to nystagmus. Romberg testing evaluates proprioception, which might contribute to a sense of imbalance.
  - **Other.** Although the neurologic examination should focus on vestibular and cerebellar function, a complete examination is needed to screen for other abnormalities. Evidence of decreased sensation, mild hemiparesis, or other neurologic deficits may indicate an underlying central lesion.
- **Orthostatic blood pressure.** Blood pressure should be recorded while lying, sitting, and standing to assess for possible orthostatic hypotension.
- **Valsalva maneuver.** The patient should be asked to squat for 30 seconds and then to stand up and strain against a closed glottis. The examiner should note whether this maneuver provokes symptoms (suggesting vasovagal syncope or near fainting).
- **Rapid deep breathing.** Reproduction of symptoms via rapid deep breathing or within 3 minutes suggests hyperventilation syndrome.
- **Hallpike maneuver.** The examiner guides the patient's head backward from a seated position to laying supine with head past the edge of the table, so that it is hanging 45° to one side. Vertigo with nystagmus indicates benign paroxysmal positional vertigo, with the nystagmus worst when the affected ear is turned down.

Laboratory Studies

Laboratory testing is guided by the presenting signs and symptoms. A **complete blood cell count and electrolyte analysis,** including glucose, blood urea nitrogen, and creatinine levels, may be obtained. **Anemia** may cause presyncopal lightheadedness. **Renal failure, hyperglycemia, and hypoglycemia** are also associated with vertigo.

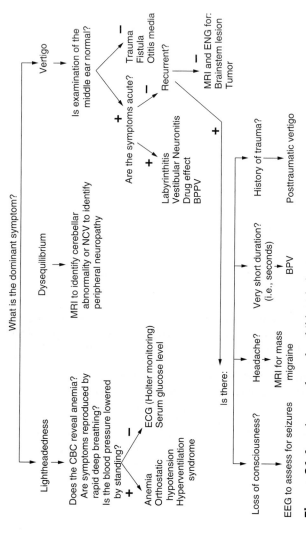

Figure 81-1 ■ Approach to the child with dizziness or vertigo

BPV = benign paroxysmal vertigo; *CBC* = complete blood count; *ECG* = electrocardiogram; *ENG* = electronystagmogram; *MRI* = magnetic resonance imaging; *NCV* = nerve conduction velocity

Approach to The Patient (Figure 81-1)

- Magnetic resonance imaging is indicated if there is prolonged vertigo or additional neurologic signs. One should look for evidence of a tumor or hemorrhage into the cerebellum, brainstem, or labyrinth.
- Electroencephalography is indicated when vertigo is associated with alterations of consciousness.
- Audiography is indicated when there is evidence of hearing loss, ear pain, or tinnitus.
- Electronystagmography allows one to distinguish central vertigo from peripheral vertigo.

Suggested Readings

Casselbrant ML, Mandel EM: Balance disorders in children. *Neurol Clin* 23:807–829, 2005.

Drigo P, Carli G, Laverda AM: Benign paroxysmal vertigo of childhood. *Brain Dev* 23(1):38–41, 2001.

Fenichel M: *Clinical Pediatric Neurology—A Signs and Symptoms Approach*, 5th ed. Philadelphia, Elsevier Saunders, 2005, 347–351.

Golz A, Netzer A, Angel-Yeger B, et al.: Effects of middle ear effusion on the vestibular system in children. *Otolaryngol Head Neck Surg* 119(6):695–699, 1998.

MacGregor DL. Vertigo. *Pediatr Rev* 23:10–16, 2002.

Ravid S, Bienkowski R, Eviatar A: A simplified diagnostic approach to dizziness in children. *Pediatr Neurol* 29:317, 2000.

Russell G, Abu-Arafeh I: Paroxysmal vertigo in children—an epidemiological study. *Int J Pediatr Otorhinolaryngol* 49(Suppl 1):S105–S107, 1999.

INTRODUCTION

Vomiting is the expulsion of stomach contents through the mouth. In children, vomiting is one of the **most common presenting symptoms of upper gastrointestinal disease.** The degree of emesis can vary from forceful, projectile vomiting to effortless regurgitation, to unseen rumination.

DIFFERENTIAL DIAGNOSIS LIST

Infectious Causes

Sepsis
Meningitis
Urinary tract infection
Parasitic infection—giardiasis, ascariasis
Helicobacter pylori gastritis
Otitis media
Gastroenteritis—viral, bacterial
Hepatitis A, B, or C
Bordetella pertussis infection
Pneumonia
Sinusitis
Streptoccocal pharyngitis

Toxic Causes

Drugs—aspirin, ipecac, theophylline, digoxin, opiates, anticonvulsants, barbiturates
Metals—iron, lead
Caustic ingestions
Alcohol

Neoplastic Causes

Intracranial mass lesions

Traumatic Causes

Duodenal hematoma
Pancreatic trauma

Congenital, Anatomic, or Vascular Causes

Esophageal stricture, web, ring, or atresia
Hypertrophic pyloric stenosis
Gastric web or duplication
Duodenal atresia
Malrotation
Intestinal duplication
Hirschsprung disease
Imperforate anus
Superior mesenteric artery syndrome

Metabolic or Genetic Causes

Galactosemia
Hereditary fructose intolerance
Other inborn errors of metabolism—amino acid or organic acid disorders, urea cycle defects, fatty acid oxidation disorders
Diabetes
Adrenal insufficiency

Inflammatory Causes

Cholecystitis or cholelithiasis
Eosinophilic enteritis

Inflammatory bowel disease
Appendicitis
Necrotizing enterocolitis
Peritonitis
Celiac disease
Peptic ulcer
Pancreatitis

Gastrointestinal Causes

Gastroesophageal reflux disease (GERD)
Eosinophilic esophagitis
Achalasia
Pseudo-obstruction
Obstruction—intussusception, volvulus, incarcerated hernia
Foreign body
Gastric and intestinal bezoars

Psychosocial Causes

Rumination

Bulimia
Psychogenic vomiting
Overfeeding

Functional Causes

"Cyclic vomiting" syndrome
Gastroparesis

Miscellaneous Causes

Pregnancy
Central nervous system (CNS) disorders—hydrocephalus, pseudotumor cerebri, migraine, motion sickness, seizure
Renal disorders—ureteropelvic junction obstruction, obstructive uropathy, nephrolithiasis, glomerulonephritis, renal tubular acidosis

DIFFERENTIAL DIAGNOSIS DISCUSSION

Helicobacter pylori Infection

In older children and adults, *H. pylori* (a Gram-negative, urease-producing bacterium) is the **major cause of gastric and duodenal ulcers.** Although the infection rate increases with age, children are susceptible; approximately 15% of children undergoing gastric biopsy via endoscopy are infected.

H. pylori appears to promote disease via several mechanisms: production of urease and ammonia, adhesion to the gastric mucosa, and proteolysis of gastric mucus. All of these mechanisms result in disruption of the gastric epithelium.

Clinical Features

Complaints commonly center around **epigastric abdominal pain, vomiting, heartburn,** and **regurgitation.** Hematemesis can also occur.

Evaluation

Currently, **upper endoscopy with biopsy** is the gold standard for the diagnosis of *H. pylori* infection. **Serum antibodies** to *H. pylori* can be detected; however, this test carries a poor specificity because previously infected individuals may remain serum antibody positive, despite lacking clinical evidence of gastritis. A recently developed noninvasive **urea breath test** may supplant the need for upper endoscopy.

Treatment

Many treatment strategies are reported in the literature, but no single therapy is 100% effective in the eradication of *H. pylori*. Currently, the recommended treatment consists of a combination of a **drug to suppress acid production** (e.g., omeprazole), **clarithromycin,** and **either metronidazole or amoxicillin.** In the past, the treatment of choice was a combination of bismuth subsalicylate and antibiotics (amoxicillin and metronidazole).

Gastroesophageal Reflux Disease

Etiology

Gastroesophageal reflux is the movement of stomach contents into the esophagus, past the lower esophageal sphincter. It is commonly caused by a **delay in gastric emptying** or transient **relaxation of the lower esophageal sphincter.**

Clinical Features

Many **newborns manifest inconsequential regurgitation after meals;** this condition typically resolves by 3 to 6 months of age. In the usual presentation of GE reflux, frequent small mouthfuls of stomach contents are **regurgitated in an effortless manner.** No active emesis is observed. This phenomenon is frequently referred to as "spitting" or "wet burps." Other symptoms, such as **heartburn, chest or epigastric pain, dysphagia, water brash** (a sour taste in mouth), or **globus** (the sensation that something is stuck in the throat), may be present.

In more **pathologic cases,** GERD is associated with more severe symptoms, such as **recurrent wheezing or coughing, recurrent pneumonia** from aspiration, or **apparent life-threatening episodes.** Many times, concomitant **esophagitis** (manifested as irritability in infants) can occur. In many cases, no obvious spitting is seen, but studies clearly document gastroesophageal reflux.

Recently, an increasing number of children with symptoms of GERD were identified with **eosinophilic esophagitis** (EE). The presentation of EE is often very similar to GERD; however, these patients fail to respond adequately to antireflux medications. The disease is caused by **food allergy** and characterized by a severe isolated histologic esophageal eosinophilia despite aggressive acid suppression therapy.

Complications associated with GERD include **hematemesis, aspiration,** and **failure to thrive.**

Evaluation

GERD is primarily a clinical diagnosis, but several diagnostic tests can aid in the evaluation:

- Contrast studies (upper gastrointestinal series) provide information regarding the upper intestinal anatomy.
- Upper endoscopy is useful in assessing the degree of reflux and the presence of complications (e.g., esophagitis) and for reaching a definitive diagnosis in children.
- Radiographic nuclear scintiscans (milk scans) provide information regarding gastric emptying and possible aspiration.
- 24-hour pH probe is useful when attempting to correlate acid reflux with atypical symptoms such as cough, hoarseness, or bronchospasm.

Treatment

Conservative treatment includes **improved positioning** (upright and prone with head elevated 45°) after eating and while sleeping; feeding infants **thickened food;** and **eliminating spicy foods** and foods containing **caffeine** and **peppermint.**

The mainstay of medical treatment consists of **gastric acid suppression** and the use of **intestinal prokinetic agents** (e.g., metoclopramide). **Acid-blocking medications** (e.g., ranitidine, famotidine) are effective for preventing heartburn and for healing esophagitis. Proton pump inhibitors (PPIs) can be used for children with refractory disease. Antacids can be substituted; however, large doses must be given and the duration of action is short.

Eosinophilic Esophagitis

Etiology

EE is an **allergic (autoimmune) esophageal disorder** based on a **clinico-pathologic diagnosis** that includes the presence of a large number of tissue eosinophils isolated to the esophagus.

Clinical Features

In children, EE presents with symptoms similar to those seen with GERD. These symptoms include **vomiting, regurgitation, epigastric pain, poor feeding, and failure to thrive.** Older children commonly manifest symptoms of **heartburn, water brash, nausea, and dysphagia.** It is not uncommon for adolescents to complain of **difficulty swallowing solid foods** or have **intermittent food impactions.**

Evaluation

- **Upper endoscopy with biopsy** is required to make the diagnosis. More than 15 esophageal eosinophils must be present per high power microscopic field. GERD must be ruled out.
- Currently, there are no other useful **noninvasive tests** that can be performed.

> **HINT:** Because patients with GERD can also manifest esophageal eosinophils, patients suspected of having EE should be treated with a PPI prior to performing upper endoscopy.

> **HINT:** EE should be strongly considered whenever a patient presents with an unexplained esophageal food impaction.

Treatment

There are several treatment options for patients with EE. Treatments include **dilation for esophageal strictures, dietary management, and pharmacologic therapy. Dietary restriction** or elimination should be considered in all children with EE. Because of the difficulty in identifying the causative foods, referral to a pediatric allergist or gastroenterologist is often required. Effective medications include **corticosteroids and PPIs.** Swallowed topical corticosteroids act to reduce esophageal inflammation; however, when the medication is discontinued, the disease almost always recurs. **Acid blockade** is helpful in controlling secondary acid reflux; however, it should not be a primary therapy for EE.

Achalasia

Etiology

Achalasia is caused by an abnormality in the smooth muscle ganglion cells of the esophagus, which produces incomplete relaxation of the lower esophageal sphincter and poor esophageal motility. The **esophagus can become extremely dilated,** serving as a **reservoir for food,** which can be **vomited hours or days after ingestion.**

Clinical Features

Achalasia rarely develops before the **teenage years** and occurs in fewer than 1 in 10,000 individuals. **Vomiting and dysphagia** are the cardinal symptoms. Patients are typically "slow" eaters and complain of food and liquids "sticking in the throat."

Choking, coughing, gagging, and **aspiration pneumonias** typically occur in **infants** and **young children** with achalasia.

Evaluation

Although the presence of an air-fluid level in the mediastinum on the chest radiograph suggests the diagnosis of achalasia, the diagnosis is usually made using an upper gastrointestinal series or esophageal manometry:

- An **upper gastrointestinal series** reveals a dilated esophagus with a narrow, beak-like appearance at the level of the lower esophageal sphincter.
- **Esophageal manometry** reveals abnormal function of the esophageal smooth muscle.

Treatment

Balloon dilation of the lower esophageal sphincter is the usual treatment. Unfortunately, **symptoms often recur** and repeat dilations are typically necessary. Other treatments include **esophageal myotomy** and the injection of **botulinum toxin** into the distal esophageal mucosal wall.

Hypertrophic Pyloric Stenosis

Etiology

Hypertrophic pyloric stenosis is the most common **congenital abnormality** of children. It is caused by hypertrophy and hyperplasia of the smooth muscle that surrounds the gastric pylorus. The hypertrophy causes the **mucosal** and **submucosal tissue** to **protrude into the pyloric channel.**

Clinical Features

The incidence of pyloric stenosis is approximately 1 in 1,000; symptoms usually begin between 4 and 7 weeks of age.

Progressive, forceful, nonbilious vomiting is the first sign of pyloric stenosis in infants. **Dehydration, weight loss,** and **failure to thrive** can develop. If the diagnosis is not made and the vomiting continues, infants develop a serious hypochloremic **metabolic alkalosis;** an associated **jaundice** occurs in as many as 5% of infants.

Evaluation

Physical examination may reveal a palpable **"olive"** in the right upper quadrant; however, in most cases, the physical examination is of no benefit. Currently, **abdominal ultrasound** (demonstrating a thickened pyloric channel muscle layer) is the diagnostic test of choice. An upper gastrointestinal series demonstrates an elongated **"double tract"** of barium along the pyloric channel.

Treatment

Infants with severe dehydration and alkalosis require **fluid resuscitation.** Once the patient is stabilized, **pyloromyotomy** can be performed to correct the defect.

Malrotation

Etiology

Intestinal malrotation is **failure** of the **fetal midgut to rotate to its normal position.** The associated shortened mesenteric ligament (ligament of Treitz) may result in twisting and torsion of the intestine and its blood supply, resulting in **intestinal obstruction** and **ischemic bowel.**

Clinical Features

Most affected infants present with **signs and symptoms of intestinal obstruction,** including bile-stained emesis, abdominal pain, and borborygmi; however, the symptoms can be delayed for many years.

Older children present with **intermittent vomiting** and **abdominal pain;** rarely, malabsorption and diarrhea are seen.

Evaluation

Radiographic contrast studies of the upper gastrointestinal tract demonstrate the positioning of the ligament of Treitz. Whenever the position of this ligament is in question, contrast should be allowed to flow into the jejunum, ileum, and cecum to define the intestinal rotation.

Treatment

Surgery is indicated to prevent the complications of malrotation, which include small bowel obstruction and midgut volvulus.

Esophageal Atresia

Etiology

Esophageal atresia occurs when the **esophagus ends as a blind tube** as a result of malformation of the tracheoesophageal septum during embryologic development. Although many forms of esophageal atresia can occur, the most common include **proximal esophageal atresia with a distal tracheoesophageal fistula** (>80% of patients), **isolated esophageal atresia** (10% of patients), and **pure tracheoesophageal fistula** (<5% of patients).

Clinical Features

Esophageal atresia is almost always **diagnosed within hours of birth.** Most commonly, the infant **coughs, chokes,** and **vomits** all liquids immediately. Occasionally, **aspiration pneumonia** develops.

Evaluation

The condition can be diagnosed quickly by passing a **nasogastric tube;** if the tube meets resistance at 3 to 5 inches, esophageal atresia is suspected. A plain **chest radiograph** confirms the presence of a blind esophageal pouch. Pure tracheoesophageal fistulas (H-type) may be missed because the esophagus is intact. **Radiographic contrast studies** can be performed; however, very small amounts of a water-soluble contrast material should be used to prevent pulmonary edema and respiratory distress.

Treatment

Initial conservative therapy includes **upright positioning,** frequent **nasopharyngeal suctioning,** and **intravenous fluids.** The infant should be placed on **nothing per mouth status.**

Surgical correction is performed to reconnect the esophagus to the gastric cavity and to repair any associated fistulas. Occasionally, reconnection of the esophagus and stomach is not possible, and **colonic interposition** (i.e., using a portion of colon to connect the distal esophagus to the stomach) is required.

Patients often require long-term **antireflux medical therapy** secondary to poor esophageal motility.

Bezoars

Etiology

Bezoars are accumulations of exogenous matter in the stomach or small intestine. The various types include **trichobezoars** (hair balls), **phytobezoars** (food balls), **lactobezoars** (milk or formula in infants), and **foreign body bezoars.**

> **HINT:** Although lactobezoars usually occur in infants, the other types of bezoars most commonly occur in developmentally delayed individuals between 10 and 19 years of age. Bezoars are often seen in institutionalized children.

Clinical Features

Children typically present with **vomiting, abdominal distention, pain, severe halitosis,** and **weight loss,** and they may have a history of **pica. Patchy baldness** is often a clue to the presence of a trichobezoar. Commonly, an **abdominal mass** can be palpated in the epigastrium or left upper quadrant.

Evaluation

Plain radiographs and **radiographic contrast studies** may demonstrate the mass; however, **upper endoscopy** is the most useful test because it may be both diagnostic and therapeutic. Children with documented bezoars should be evaluated for **pica, iron-deficiency anemia,** and **lead toxicity.**

Treatment

Lactobezoars respond to **withholding oral feeding** for 48 hours. Trichobezoars require **surgical removal.** The removal of all other bezoars may be attempted **endoscopically;** however, in many cases, surgical removal is necessary.

Cholecystitis

Etiology

Cholecystitis, **inflammation of the gallbladder**, is caused by bile stasis within the gallbladder. The causes of bile stasis in children include **cholelithiasis (most common), congenital ductal anomalies, external compression of the bile duct,** and **trauma.**

Clinical Features

The history typically reveals **right upper quadrant pain** radiating to the back, **jaundice, rigors,** and **fever. Nausea and vomiting** occur after eating. Symptoms usually develop rapidly; however, the patient may have mild symptoms for several years.

Evaluation

Murphy sign (a palpable tender mass located between the ninth and tenth ribs) can often be appreciated.

Hyperbilirubinemia, an **elevated γ-glutamyl transpeptidase** level, and **leukocytosis** may suggest cholecystitis.

Although **abdominal plain radiographs** can detect the calcified stones, **abdominal ultrasound** is warranted to detect a thickened gallbladder wall, dilated ducts, or an obstructing stone. Occasionally, **cholescintigraphy** is indicated to show abnormal filling of bile into the gallbladder (the administration of cholecystokinin can help reproduce clinical symptoms).

Treatment

Conservative therapy includes hospitalization for the administration of **intravenous fluids** and **antibiotics** (for patients with a high fever or clinical deterioration) and the **cessation of eating.** In some patients with acalculous cholecystitis, conservative therapy is all that is required for the resolution of symptoms; however, in most patients (and all of those with cholelithiasis), the accepted treatment is **cholecystectomy.**

Central Nervous System Disorder

Irritation of the brainstem vomiting center by brain tumors, congenital cysts, hydrocephalus, or infections can cause severe vomiting; a **neurologic cause should always be considered in a child with vomiting.**

The vomiting commonly occurs in the **early morning** and is associated with **headaches.** Other signs and symptoms include **changes in the child's personality, fatigue, ataxia, diplopia, nystagmus, papilledema, head tilt,** and **loss of vision.**

Ureteropelvic Junction Obstruction

Etiology

An unusual but important cause of vomiting in children is ureteropelvic junction obstruction, a morphologic **abnormality** of the **ureteropelvic junction** that causes obstruction or restriction of urinary outflow and subsequent hydronephrosis.

Clinical Features

Children frequently present with **right- or left-sided abdominal pain and vomiting.** The pain is often **intermittent,** which makes the diagnosis difficult. Occasionally, patients also have **hematuria** or signs of a **urinary tract infection.**

Evaluation

Abdominal ultrasound usually permits diagnosis; however, because the kidneys may appear normal between episodes, the ultrasound should be performed when the child is experiencing symptoms. In rare cases, an **intravenous pyelogram** is indicated.

Treatment

Surgical correction is required.

Bulimia

Etiology

A **psychogenic cause** of vomiting should be considered in adolescents, especially adolescent girls, who otherwise appear well and have no other cause for their vomiting.

Clinical Features and Evaluation

A **careful history** should be taken, looking for evidence of **anorexia, bulimia,** or **laxative and ipecac abuse.** Questions should be designed to elicit information regarding diet, eating habits, self-worth, exercise, changes in menses, purging, and medication use. The diagnostic criteria for bulimia include repeated episodes of **binge eating,** regular episodes of **self-induced vomiting,** a persistently **poor self-image** (e.g., of being overweight), and a **lack of control of eating during meals.**

The **nails, teeth, and gums** should be examined for evidence of nutritional inadequacies. **Laboratory studies** may reveal electrolyte abnormalities (as a result of persistent vomiting) and provide an overview of the patient's nutritional health (e.g., albumin, calcium, phosphorus, iron stores). An **electrocardiogram** may be abnormal in severely affected patients.

Treatment

The prevention of acute life-threatening complications (e.g., dehydration, cardiac abnormalities, electrolyte disturbances) is the primary concern. Patients should be referred to a qualified **psychotherapist** who has expertise in the management of eating disorders.

EVALUATION OF VOMITING

Patient History

The following questions may provide insight into the cause of the vomiting:

- **Does the patient have a fever?** Fever implies infection.
- **Does the patient have a history of pica?** Pica implies bezoar.
- **Does the patient complain of heartburn, globus, water brash, or epigastric pain related to meals?** Think GERD and esophagitis.
- **If the child is an infant, does he have an unusual odor?** Unusual odors may be a sign of a metabolic disorder.
- **When does the vomiting occur?** Frequent vomiting in the morning can be a sign of pregnancy or a neurologic disorder.
- **How old is the patient?** Some causes of vomiting are more prevalent in certain age groups (Table 82-1).
- **Is the vomitus bilious or bloody?** Bile-stained vomitus points to an anatomic problem (e.g., intestinal volvulus, intussusception, incarcerated hernia).

Physical Examination

The following should be noted during physical examination:

- **Head and neck**—abnormal teeth, reflux, bulging fontanelle, hydrocephalus
- **Abdomen**—right upper quadrant mass, signs of gallbladder disease, epigastric pain (suggests pancreatitis, gastritis, or esophagitis), right upper quadrant pain (suggests liver disease), borborygmi (suggests possible intestinal obstruction)

TABLE 82-1	Common Causes of Vomiting by Age
Infant	Anatomic obstruction, metabolic disorder, infection, GERD, overfeeding, bezoar
Toddler	Infection, medication, GERD, intussusception, foreign body, bezoar, malrotation
Child	GERD, cyclic vomiting, malrotation, infection
Adolescent	Pregnancy, bulimia, infection, ulcer, malrotation, celiac disease, pseudo-obstruction, drug abuse, pancreatitis, GERD, cyclic vomiting

GERD = gastroesophageal reflux disease.

- **Rectum**—heme-positive stools (suggest mucosal disease)
- **Neurologic examination**—cranial nerve abnormalities, gait abnormalities (suggest CNS disease)

Laboratory Studies

The following studies may be appropriate:

- **Complete blood count with differential**—eosinophilia suggests eosinophilic enteritis or allergic disease
- **Erythrocyte sedimentation rate (ESR)**—an abnormal ESR suggests inflammation, possibly of the intestine
- **Chemistry panel**—increased alanine aminotransferase, γ-glutamyl transpeptidase, or bilirubin levels suggest gallbladder or liver disease
- **Amylase and lipase levels**—increased amylase or pancreatic lipase levels suggest pancreatitis
- **Antiendomysial and tissue transglutaminase antibodies**—elevation suggests celiac disease
- **Stool sample**—occult blood suggests intestinal mucosal disease

Diagnostic Modalities

The following diagnostic modalities may be appropriate:

- **Contrast radiographic studies** are integral in the diagnosis of intestinal anatomic abnormalities.
- **Endoscopy** may be the most important tool for the definitive diagnosis of many esophageal, gastric, and duodenal disorders.
- A **barium enema** identifies distal obstructions.
- **Abdominal ultrasound** is useful in the evaluation of liver and gallbladder disorders, pyloric stenosis, pancreatitis, and kidney disease.
- An **abdominal computed tomography (CT) scan** defines the anatomy of the abdominal cavity (when used with both enteral and intravenous contrast). In most patients, CT provides a more specific image than ultrasound.

Suggested Readings

Behrman RE, Kliegman RM, Jensen HB: *Textbook of Pediatrics*, 16th ed. Philadelphia, WB Saunders, 2000.

Fleisher GR, Ludwig S, Henretig FM, et al.: *Textbook of Pediatric Emergency Medicine*, 4th ed. Baltimore, Williams & Wilkins, 2000.

Furuta GT, Liacouras CA, Collins MH, et al.: Eosinophilic esophagitis in children and adults: a systematic review and consensus recommendation for diagnosis and treatment. *Gastroenterology* 133: 1342–1363, 2007.

Li BK, Sunku BK: Vomiting and nausea. In *Pediatric Gastrointestinal and Liver Diseases: Pathophysiology/Diagnosis/Management*, 3rd ed. Edited by Wyllie R, Hyams JS. Elsevier, Philadelphia, 2006, 127–150.

Polin RA, Ditmar MF: *Pediatric Secrets*, 4th ed. Philadelphia, Hanley & Belfus, 2005.

Sadow KB, Atabaki SM, Johns CM, et al.: Bilious emesis in the pediatric emergency department: etiology and outcome. *Clin Pediatr* 41(7):475–479, 2002.

Sondheimer JM: Vomiting. In *Pediatric Gastrointestinal Disease*, 4th ed. Edited by Walker WA, Goulet O, Kleinman RE, et al. Hamilton, On, BC Decker, 2004, 203–209.

GASTRIC DECONTAMINATION

Administration of **activated charcoal** is the preferred method of gastric decontamination. **Whole bowel irrigation and gastric lavage** play a much lesser role in the management of the poisoned patient but may still be of benefit in selected patients. **Syrup of ipecac** is not recommended for most poisonings.

Activated Charcoal

Indications and Contraindications

Activated charcoal is indicated for all ingestions if administration can occur within 1 hour of ingestion, unless specifically contraindicated. **Contraindications** include the following:

- Compromised, unprotected airway (aspiration risk)
- Gastrointestinal bleeding or perforation
- Caustic ingestions (charcoal impedes endoscopic visualization)
- Aliphatic hydrocarbon ingestion (may promote vomiting and aspiration)

> **HINT: Not all substances bind to activated charcoal (Table 83-1).**

Administration

The **dose is 1 g/kg, up to 100 g total** of activated charcoal. Mixing the charcoal with **flavored syrups** and putting it in a covered cup with a straw facilitates oral administration. **Nasogastric intubation** is required in patients with altered mental status and in alert but uncooperative patients.

Complications

Complications of activated charcoal use include **vomiting** and **aspiration**, **constipation or obstipation**, **desorption of poison** from charcoal, and **late**

TABLE 83-1 Agents with Limited or Uncertain Binding to Activated Charcoal

Iron	Caustics*
Lithium	NaOH
Heavy metals	KOH
Arsenic	HCl
Mercury	H_2SO_4
Lead	Low-molecular-weight compounds
Thallium	Cyanide
Alcohols	Pesticides
Methanol	Organophosphates
Ethanol	Carbamates
Isopropanol	
Ethylene glycol	
Hydrocarbons	
Kerosene	
Gasoline	
Mineral seal oil	

*Administration of activated charcoal may also impede further management.

absorption in patients with delayed gastrointestinal motility (e.g., those taking drugs with anticholinergic properties). **Death** has occurred in a child who aspirated activated charcoal mixed with a magnesium cathartic.

Whole Bowel Irrigation

Whole bowel irrigation involves **copious irrigation of the gastrointestinal tract,** via nasogastric tube, to force the poisons rapidly through the bowel before significant absorption can occur. The solution used, polyethylene glycol 3500 MW iso-osmotic bowel solution (**GoLYTELY**), causes no significant fluid or electrolyte loss in the gut.

Indications and Contraindications

Potential indications, to date, have been limited to **agents that do not adsorb well to charcoal** or that have the potential for absorption distally in the gastrointestinal tract, such as **iron, heavy metals, lithium,** and **sustained-release products** (e.g., many antiarrhythmics, theophylline). Other drugs may be amenable to whole bowel irrigation as an adjunct to activated charcoal administration, e.g. ingested patch medications. In addition, whole bowel irrigation is used to **treat body packers** (people who ingest large numbers of packets of cocaine or heroin wrapped in latex condoms). Whole bowel irrigation is **contraindicated in patients with evidence of ileus or bowel perforation.**

Administration

GoLYTELY is administered at a dose of **500 mL/hour in young children** and at a dose of **up to 2 L/hour in adolescents and adults,** usually via nasogastric tube. The patient should be sitting up during treatment.

The **endpoint** for stopping whole bowel irrigation is a **clear rectal effluent** and **recovery from poisoning.**

Complications

The major complications reported from whole bowel irrigation are **vomiting** and **abdominal pain.**

Gastric Lavage

Gastric lavage removes 10% to 25% of ingested toxin when performed within 30 to 60 minutes of ingestion.

Indications and Contraindications

Gastric lavage may **not be useful >1 hour after ingestion** unless the ingested poison delays gastric emptying. It has been shown to improve outcome in patients who are comatose and receive gastric lavage **within 60 minutes.** In other patients, the potential risks of gastric lavage must be weighed heavily against its benefit.

Gastric lavage should be reserved for the **critically ill poisoning patient** or a patient who is likely to undergo rapid decompensation. In addition, **patients who ingest large amounts of a strong acid** (e.g., toilet bowl cleaner) should receive gastric lavage via a small flexible nasogastric tube. **Patients who ingest liquid medicines** may benefit from nasogastric lavage if it is performed within 30 to 60 minutes.

Gastric lavage **should not be performed in patients with airway compromise before endotracheal intubation.** Other **contraindications** include the **ingestion of caustic alkaline substances** or small amounts of **acids or hydrocarbons, abnormal esophageal anatomy,** and **bleeding diatheses.**

Administration

Gastric lavage requires the placement of a **large-bore (24 to 36 French) orogastric tube** followed by **repeated infusion and withdrawal** of room temperature **normal saline** in 50- to 200-mL aliquots. Before lavage, one must **ensure a protected airway:** Position the patient on the left side with the head below the feet, and determine correct gastric tube position.

Complications

Complications include **vomiting** with pulmonary aspiration, **gastric or esophageal perforation, hypopharyngeal and airway trauma with bleeding, laryngospasm,** and **accidental tracheal intubation** with inadvertent pulmonary lavage.

Syrup of Ipecac

Syrup of ipecac, derived from the ipecacuanha plant, causes vomiting by **direct gastric irritation** and through a direct central effect at the chemotactic trigger zone in the medulla. Up to 93% of patients who receive ipecac vomit within 30 to 60 minutes.

Indications and Contraindications

Indications are now limited to patients <30 to 90 minutes after ingestion who are at substantial risk of toxicity, do not have a contraindication to ipecac administration, who will be delayed beyond 1 hour before receiving emergency care, and for whom syrup of ipecac will not delay or adversely affect definitive treatment. Except for rural residents, these guidelines severely limit the potential use of syrup of ipecac, and the American Academy of Pediatrics no longer recommends routine prescribing of syrup of ipecac as part of well child care.

Contraindications to ipecac use consist of altered mental status (lethargy, coma, seizures—either existing or impending) and ingestion of caustic substances, aliphatic hydrocarbons, or drugs with a high likelihood of rapid serious effects (e.g., cyclic antidepressants, antiarrhythmics, clonidine, isoniazid, lithium, alcohol). In addition, patients who have already spontaneously vomited will not receive any further benefit from syrup of ipecac administration.

Administration

Dose is based on age: for children 6 months to 1 year of age, give 10 mL (2 tsp); 1 to 12 years, 15 mL (1 Tbsp); and >12 years, 30 mL (2 Tbsp). Give the child 10 mL/kg of water, up to 240 mL (8 ounces), after administering the syrup of ipecac. Repeat the dose if no vomiting occurs within 30 minutes.

Complications

Complications include excessive vomiting, Mallory-Weiss tears, pneumomediastinum, and delayed delivery of activated charcoal. Chronic use of syrup of ipecac or inadvertent administration of the much more concentrated extract of ipecac has caused myocardial and neuromuscular toxicity.

Cathartics

Indications and Contraindications

Cathartics have no demonstrated efficacy in poisoning treatment. Coadministration of cathartic with activated charcoal in patients >12 years of age may prevent obstipation. Cathartics are contraindicated in patients with bowel perforation, ileus, or diarrhea.

Administration

Cathartics should only be given as a single dose when administered with activated charcoal; multiple doses of cathartics should be avoided except as outlined in the section on elimination enhancement. If a cathartic is given, sorbitol **35%** is the preferred agent because it has a rapid onset of catharsis. The **dose of sorbitol 35% is 1 g/kg** (3 mL/kg).

Complications

Complications include **electrolyte imbalance** and **dehydration.** Sorbitol also increases the likelihood of **vomiting** when given with activated charcoal. **Death** has occurred in several patients who received four to six doses of sorbitol over 24 hours.

ELIMINATION ENHANCEMENT

Extracorporeal clearance of toxin can be achieved by administering multiple-dose activated charcoal or by alkaline diuresis, hemodialysis, or charcoal hemoperfusion.

Multiple-Dose Activated Charcoal

Multiple doses of activated charcoal **increase the clearance of theophylline, carbamazepine, phenytoin, phenobarbital,** and some **cyclic antidepressants.** The dose is **1 g/kg with cathartic initially, followed by 0.5 to 1 g/kg of activated charcoal without cathartic every 4 hours** until the patient has nontoxic blood levels, has shown clinical improvement, and has passed charcoal-laden stool.

Alkaline Diuresis

Alkaline diuresis can **enhance the excretion of weak acids,** especially **salicylates** and **phenobarbital** (but not other barbiturates). This procedure promotes conversion of these drugs to their ionized form within the proximal renal tubule and prevents distal tubular resorption (ion trapping). **Sodium bicarbonate** is given **intravenously** until a urine pH >7.0 is achieved. Care must be taken to **avoid fluid overload, hypernatremia, hypokalemia, hypocalcemia,** and **hypomagnesemia** during alkaline diuresis.

Hemodialysis

Hemodialysis can **remove toxins with low molecular weight** (200 d), **low plasma protein binding,** and **low tissue binding** as expressed by the volume of distribution (Vd):

Vd (L/kg) = Dose absorbed (mg/kg/Plasma concentration (mg/L)

Hemodialysis is most effective for drugs with a Vd <1 L/kg (Table 83–2).

Hemoperfusion

Hemoperfusion **diverts the patient's circulation** through a charcoal filter where the toxin binds to an activated charcoal cartridge. Charcoal

TABLE 83-2 Toxins Removed by Hemodialysis

Toxin	Measured Level Suggestive of Need for Hemodialysis*
Acetaminophen	>1,000 µg/mL in conjunction with antidote
Arsenic	Only with coexistent renal failure
Bromide	>150 mg/dL and severe symptoms
Ethanol	500 mg/dL
Ethylene glycol†	25 mg/dL
Isopropanol	400 mg/dL
Lithium	4 mEq/L in acute overdose
	As needed for severe symptoms in chronic overdose
Methanol	25 mg/dL
Salicylates	100–120 mg/dL in acute overdose
	60–80 mg/dL in chronic overdose
Theophylline	80–100 µg/mL in acute overdose
	60–80 µg/mL in chronic overdose

*The decision to perform hemodialysis should be based on physical findings as well as drug levels. A repeat measure should be obtained when the drug level is elevated to ensure that a laboratory error has not occurred. In addition, units of measurement should be checked before instituting hemodialysis.
†Administration of fomepizole may allow for management of higher levels of ethylene glycol without hemodialysis.

hemoperfusion is technically more difficult and less available than hemodialysis. Furthermore, ingestions of theophylline and phenobarbital, the drugs most amenable to removal with hemoperfusion, are now more typically managed using multiple-dose activated charcoal or hemodialysis.

> **HINT:** Fewer than 1% of all pediatric poisoning patients require hemodialysis or hemoperfusion.

APPROACH TO THE POISONED PATIENT

Stabilization

Airway, breathing, circulation, and disability (ABCD) must be assessed in order, and compromise in any of these areas requires prompt attention. Complete exposure of the patient occurs as part of the rapid assessment. Vital signs, including temperature, continuous monitoring of the heart rate, respiratory rate, blood pressure, and pulse oximetry, should be initiated. Supplemental oxygen in an inspired concentration of 100% should be administered.

Administration of Substrates and Antidotes

Dextrose and Thiamine

The glucose level should be determined in any poisoned child with a depressed level of consciousness, using a rapid reagent strip. Hypoglycemia

TABLE 83-3 Agents Causing Hypoglycemia in Overdosed Children
Ethanol
Salicylates
Oral hypoglycemic agents
Propranolol
Insulin

suggests certain ingestants (Table 83-3) and requires correction with **0.5 to 1 g/kg dextrose** administered as an **intravenous bolus followed by a 6 to 8 mg/kg per minute dextrose infusion**. Thiamine (**100 mg** intramuscularly or intravenously) should precede dextrose infusion in a patient who is suspected to be **alcoholic**.

> **HINT:** Hypoglycemia is the one metabolic abnormality that can cause focal neurologic findings.

Naloxone

Naloxone (**2 mg** intravenously, intramuscularly, or via endotracheal tube) **reverses coma caused by opiates**. It may also help some patients who have ingested clonidine. It should be given to **any child** with a **depressed level of consciousness** because it has **few adverse effects** in this setting and may prevent the need for aggressive intervention, such as endotracheal intubation. Response to naloxone occurs within 1 to 2 minutes of administration. After 30 minutes, the naloxone has worn off and resedation may occur. **Repeated naloxone administration or continuous intravenous naloxone infusion** is often required to prevent further depressed mental status.

> **HINT:** Children who have ingested **codeine, dextromethorphan, propoxyphene, pentazocine, butorphanol, synthetic fentanyl derivatives, LAAM (long-acting acetyl morphine), or methadone** may require up to 10 mg of naloxone to fully reverse the narcotic effects.

Flumazenil

Flumazenil is a benzodiazepine antagonist that has **reversed lethargy and coma** in adult benzodiazepine overdose patients. Flumazenil **may cause seizures** in a patient who has also ingested cyclic antidepressants or in a patient with a seizure disorder controlled by benzodiazepines, and it **may cause cardiac arrhythmias** in a poisoned patient who has also ingested chloral hydrate. Other side effects include **vomiting** and **anxiety**. Flumazenil administration **may help differentiate benzodiazepine overdose from other causes of coma** in children.

Given its potential risks, flumazenil should only be given to children with severe symptoms of benzodiazepine ingestion and only if no signs of significant cyclic antidepressant overdose are present and only if the patient does not have a seizure disorder. The currently recommended dose is 0.01 mg/kg over 1 minute up to 0.5 mg per dose and a total maximum amount of drug administered of 1 mg. Response occurs within 1 minute in most cases. Resedation may occur.

Physostigmine

Physostigmine, a cholinesterase inhibitor, reverses the central anticholinergic effects of severe agitation and seizures caused by antihistamines (e.g., diphenhydramine, doxylamine, scopolamine), certain plants (jimson weed, deadly nightshade, henbane), antiparkinsonian medications, dilating eyedrops, and skeletal muscle relaxants. Physostigmine administration has preceded asystole and death in patients who ingested cyclic antidepressants and should be avoided in these patients and in patients with asthma, gastrointestinal obstruction, or genitourinary obstruction. The dose of physostigmine for children is 0.5 to 1 mg, given intravenously, slowly over 5 minutes, with atropine immediately available for administration should cholinergic symptoms develop. Response to physostigmine occurs within minutes, and beneficial effects may persist longer than expected based on physostigmine's half-life of 60 minutes.

> **HINT:** Given the risks of physostigmine, it should be reserved for patients with a clear central anticholinergic syndrome who display hyperthermia, seizures, or severe agitation and only if no evidence exists of cyclic antidepressant toxicity.

Pyridoxine (Vitamin B$_6$)

Pyridoxine stops seizures caused by ingestion of isoniazid by reversing γ-aminobutyric acid (GABA) depletion. The dose is 3 to 5 g or the equivalent dose of isoniazid ingested. This dose is much larger than the therapeutic dose and requires the administration of multiple vials of pyridoxine.

> **HINT:** If you anticipate that it will be necessary to reverse seizures from an isoniazid ingestion, call the pharmacy and inform them so that they can obtain an adequate supply of pyridoxine.

Antidotes

Table 83-4 lists the most commonly used antidotes. Those who are unfamiliar with the use of antidotes should consult with a regional poison control center or medical toxicologist before attempting administration.

TABLE 83-4 Common Poisons and Antidotes

Poison	Antidote	Administration
Acetaminophen	N-Acetylcysteine	Loading dose 140 mg/kg, then 17 doses at 70 mg/kg/dose. Dilute 20% solution to 5%–10% with juice or soda to improve palatability OR IV NAC (Acetadote) given as 150 mg/kg over 1 hr, then 50 mg/kg over 4 hr and finally 100 mg/kg over 16 hr; use recommended pediatric concentration in young children.
Anticholinergics	Physostigmine	See text.
Benzodiazepines	Flumazenil	See text.
β-Adrenergic antagonists	Glucagon	1–10 mg bolus, followed by 3–6 mg/hr.
Calcium channel blockers	Glucagon	As for β-adrenergic antagonists.
	Calcium gluconate 10%	0.3–0.6 mL/kg (8–16 mEq calcium/kg).
	Insulin	Insulin bolus 1 IU/kg followed by infusion of 0.5–1 IU/kg given concomitantly with 0.25 g/kg bolus dextrose followed by D10W+ ½ NS of and 20 mEq/L of potassium at 0.8 times maintenance with close monitoring of glucose and potassium.
Carbon monoxide	Hyperbaric oxygen Sodium thiosulfate 25%*	See cyanide.
Cyanide	Sodium nitrate 3%	Dose depends on hemoglobin (see cyanide antidote kit package insert). Do not exceed recommended dosage. Do not give to patients suffering from concomitant carbon monoxide exposure.
	Sodium thiosulfate 25%	Dose depends on hemoglobin (see cyanide antidote kit package insert).
Digitalis	Digitalis Fab fragments	Calculate dose based on level or dose ingested or 10 vials if acute overdose, 5 vials if chronic overdose.
Ethylene glycol	Ethanol	0.6 g/kg load over 1 hr followed by 100 mg/kg/hr infusion.
	OR Fomepizole	15 mg/kg loading dose, then 10 mg/kg every 12 hr for four doses followed by 15 mg/kg every 12 hr until ethylene glycol level <25 mg/dL. Give fomepizole every 4 hr during hemodialysis.
	Pyridoxine	2 mg/kg.
	Thiamine	0.5 mg/kg.
Methanol	Ethanol	As for ethylene glycol.
	OR Fomepizole	As for ethylene glycol.
	Folate	1 mg/kg every 4 hr.

(Continued)

TABLE 83-4 Common Poisons and Antidotes *(continued)*

Poison	Antidote	Administration
Iron	Deferoxamine	5–15 mg/kg/hr IV infusion.
Isoniazid	Pyridoxine	3–5 g IV or dose equal to grams of isoniazid ingested.
Lead	Lead level 45–69 μg/dL	
	Dimercaptosuccinic acid	10 mg/kg PO three times daily for 5 days, then twice daily for
	OR	14 days (may be useful at lower levels).
	Calcium NaEDTA	50–75 mg/kg/day divided, every 6 hr either IM or by slow IV infusion (IV use not FDA approved).
	Lead level ≥70 μg/dL	
	Calcium NaEDTA and	Administer as described earlier.
	British antilewisite (BAL)	3–5 mg/kg IM every 4 hr for 5 days.
	d-Penicillamine	10 mg/kg/day for 1 wk increasing to 30 mg/kg/day as tolerated, only if unacceptable adverse reactions to dimercaptosuccinic acid or calcium NaEDTA.
Methemoglobinemia	Methylene blue 1%	1–2 mg/kg (0.1–0.2 mL/kg).
Opiates	Naloxone	2 mg IV, ETT, IM; repeat as needed.
Organophosphates	Atropine	0.1–0.5 mg/kg initial dose with additional doses as needed to counteract bronchorrhea.
	Pralidoxime	25–50 mg/kg (up to 1 g); for severe cases, consider 10–15 mg/kg/hr infusion.
Phenothiazines (dystonia)	Diphenhydramine	1–2 mg/kg IM or IV.
	Benztropine	1–2 mg/kg IM or IV.

D10W = 10% aqueous dextrose solution; *ETT* = endotracheal tube; *FDA* = Food and Drug Administration; *IM* = intramuscularly; *IV* = intravenously; *NaEDTA* = sodium ethylenediaminetetraacetic acid; *NS* = normal saline; *PO* = orally.
*Consider for possible cyanide inhalation if the patient suffers from smoke inhalation.

HINT: Antidotes help in approximately 3% of poisonings.

Decontamination

Gastric decontamination should be carried out as described in the previous section. External decontamination of the patient requires **removal**

of any clothing and copious irrigation of the skin and eyes with room-temperature normal saline solution.

> **HINT:** External decontamination of some poisoned patients (e.g., those who have ingested pesticide) may place health care providers at risk. Universal precautions should be used.

Supportive Care

The patient's clinical course is altered by administration of specific antidotes in only 3% of toxic exposures. Good outcome for the remainder of patients depends on adherence to general principles of toxicology and good general medical care, primarily rapid assessment and intervention to maintain airway, breathing, and circulation.

> **HINT:** Institution of supportive care is most important to the successful resuscitation of the poisoned patient.

Identification of the Toxin

Presumptive Diagnosis

Presumptive diagnosis of the type of agent causing poison symptoms can guide treatment until a definitive diagnosis is made. Many times the exact toxin is known from the outset by the history. However, with very ill children, the first history is often not the best, and one must look for specific clues on physical examination. Combinations of physical findings ("toxidromes") indicate specific classes of drugs with effects on vital signs, pupillary response, neurologic status, breath and body odors, and skin changes (Tables 83-5 and 83-6).

> **HINT:** The history and physical examination can provide valuable clues to the possible ingestant even when the patient does not display all the components of a toxidrome.

Bedside Tests

Bedside tests give additional information as to the poison ingested but require definitive laboratory studies for confirmation. Rapid glucose reagent stick detects the presence of hypoglycemia (see Table 83-3 for a list of the common toxic causes of hypoglycemia in children).

TABLE 83-5 Common Toxidromes in Children

Agent		Toxidrome
Opiates	VS:	Hypothermia, bradypnea, bradycardia, hypotension
	CNS:	Flaccid coma
	Pupils:	Miotic to pinpoint
	Other:	Extraocular paralysis, delayed GI motility
Sedatives	VS:	Hypothermia, bradypnea, bradycardia, hypotension
	CNS:	Coma, often prolonged or cyclical; nystagmus
	Pupils:	Miotic (early barbiturate)
		Dilated (late barbiturate, glutethimide)
	Other:	Delayed GI motility
Ethanol	VS:	Hypothermia, bradypnea, bradycardia
	CNS:	Coma, nystagmus
	Pupils:	Miotic
	Skin:	Flushed
	Odor:	Sickly sweet breath odor
	Other:	Hypoglycemia, increased osmolal gap
Anticholinergic agents	VS:	Hyperthermia, tachycardia, hypertension
	CNS:	Agitation, delirium, seizures
	Pupils:	Mydriatic
	Skin:	Flushed, dry, warm
	Other:	Decreased GI motility, urine retention, cardiac tachyarrhythmias
Sympathomimetic agents	VS:	Hyperthermia, tachycardia, hypertension (bradycardia if pure α-adrenergic)
	CNS:	Agitation, delirium, seizures
	Pupils:	Mydriatic
	Skin:	Diaphoretic, cool and clammy
	Other:	Increased GI motility, piloerection
Cholinergic agents	VS:	Bradycardia or tachycardia, hypotension, tachypnea with bronchospasm
	CNS:	Coma, seizures
	Pupils:	Miotic
	Skin:	Diaphoretic
	Other:	Muscle fasciculation, weakness, paralysis, salivation, lacrimation, vomiting, urinary and fecal incontinence
Serotonin syndrome	VS:	Hyperpyrexia, tachycardia, hypertension
	CNS:	Agitation, coma
	Pupils:	Mydriatic
	Skin:	Diaphoretic
	Other:	Lower extremity rigidity, myoclonus, hyperreflexia

Note: Toxidromes represent a collection of clinical findings often associated with poisoning by a specific class of drugs. However, a poisoned child may not display all physical findings commonly associated with a specific drug or may have findings not usually associated with a specific drug. Toxidromes by themselves cannot be used to exclude or confirm ingestion of a particular drug.
CNS = central nervous system; *GI* = gastrointestinal; *VS* = vascular system.
(Adapted from Henretig FM, Shannon M: Toxicologic emergencies. In *Textbook of Pediatric Emergency Medicine,* 3rd ed. Baltimore, Williams & Wilkins, 1993, 750, and Mofenson HC, Greensher J: The unknown poison. *Pediatrics* 54:446, 1974.)

TABLE 83-6 Common Causes of Toxidromes in Children

Opiates
  Cough syrups (dextromethorphan)
  Codeine
  Methadone (child of a heroin addict)
Sedatives
  Benzodiazepines
  Barbiturates
  Gamma-hydroxybutyrate (GHB)
Anticholinergic agents
  Antihistamines
  Antidepressant drugs*
  Antipsychotic drugs*
  Plants (jimsonweed, Amanita muscaria mushrooms, henbane, Atropa
    belladonna)
  Skeletal muscle relaxants (cyclobenzaprine)
Sympathomimetic agents
  Decongestants (pure α-adrenergic drugs)
  Cocaine
  Amphetamines
Cholinergic agents
  Pesticides (organophosphate, carbamate)
  Mushrooms
Serotonin syndrome
  Serotonin specific reuptake inhibitors
  Monoamine oxidase inhibitors

*Drug effects may not be primarily anticholinergic.

- The **ketone square on the urine dipstick** turns purple in the presence of acetoacetic acid (nitroprusside reaction). Urinary ketones are commonly seen after ingestion of salicylates and isopropanol.
- **Discordance between patient appearance and pulse oximetry** may suggest the presence of carboxyhemoglobin or methemoglobinemia (pulse oximetry reading appears higher than expected or normal in the presence of cyanosis). This impression should be confirmed by direct measurement of carboxyhemoglobin or methemoglobin on a venous or arterial blood sample.

Laboratory Studies

Initial studies in symptomatic poisoned patients may include **arterial or venous blood gases, electrolytes** with calculation of the anion gap (Table 83-7), **serum glucose, blood urea nitrogen (BUN) and creatinine levels,** and **serum osmolarity** by the freezing point depression method with calculation of the osmolar gap:

$$\text{Osmolar gap} = \text{Measured osmolarity} - [(2 \times \text{Na}) + \text{BUN}/2.8 + \text{Glucose}/18]$$

Normally, the osmolar gap is <10 mOsm. An **elevated osmolar gap suggests** the presence of alcohols (e.g., ethanol, methanol, isopropanol, ethylene glycol).

TABLE 83-7 Poisons Causing an Abnormal Anion Gap

Increased anion gap with metabolic acidosis
    Carbon monoxide*
    Cyanide
    Ethanol*
    Ethylene glycol*
    Iron*
    Isoniazid
    Methanol*
    Salicylates*
    Theophylline*
Decreased anion gap
    Bromide
    Lithium*
    Hypermagnesemia*
    Hypercalcemia*

Anion gap $= Na^+ - (Cl^- + CO_2^-)$
*Specific levels rapidly available.

> **HINT:** A normal osmolar gap does not exclude the potential for serious ethylene glycol poisoning.

Specific drug levels are useful when the poison shows a dose-dependent toxicity, when treatment with an antidote is contemplated, or when a specific intervention, such as extracorporeal removal, is helpful (Table 83-8).

The **comprehensive drug screen ("tox screen") has limited usefulness** in the management of the poisoned child. **False-positive** and **false-negative drug screens** can lead to misinterpretation of the patient's signs and symptoms. **Toxicologic screening may be warranted to confirm the diagnosis of poisoning** as opposed to other conditions such as central nervous system (CNS) infection or trauma, **or if intentional ingestion or child abuse is suspected.**

> **HINT:** Results of comprehensive drug screens typically take 6 to 24 hours and rarely change immediate management of the patient.

> **HINT:** Testing in the poisoned patient should progress from less specific to more specific, with emphasis on clearly identifying the presence of toxins that require antidotes or other specific procedures to prevent morbidity or mortality.

TABLE 83-8 Helpful Specific Drug Levels

Drug	Time to Peak Blood Level (Hours Postingestion)	Potential Intervention
Acetaminophen	4	N-Acetylcysteine administration
Carbamazepine	2–4[*†]	—
Carboxyhemoglobin	Immediate	Hyperbaric oxygen therapy
Digoxin	2–4	Fab (digoxin antibody) fragment
Ethanol	1/2–1[†]	—
Ethylene glycol	0.5–1	Ethanol infusion OR fomepizole and hemodialysis
Iron	2–4	Deferoxamine administration
Isopropanol	0.5–1[†]	—
Lead	5 wk[*]	Chelation and environmental abatement
Lithium	2–4	Hemodialysis
Methanol	0.5–1	Ethanol infusion OR fomepizole and hemodialysis
Methemoglobinemia	Immediate	Methylene blue administration
Phenobarbital	2–4	Alkaline diuresis, multiple-dose activated charcoal
Phenytoin	1–2[*]	Multiple-dose activated charcoal
Salicylates	6–12[*]	Alkaline diuresis, multiple-dose activated charcoal, hemodialysis
Theophylline	1–36[*]	Multiple-dose activated charcoal, whole bowel irrigation, charcoal hemoperfusion, hemodialysis

(Adapted from Weisman RS, Howland MA, Verebey K: The toxicology laboratory. In *Goldfrank's Toxicologic Emergencies*, 5th ed. Edited by Goldfrank LR, Flomenbaum NE, Lewin NA, et al. East Norwalk, Ct, Appleton Lange, 1994, 105.)

[*]Repeated measurement of levels is necessary because of significant variation in time to reach to peak level.

[†]The peak level is predictive of toxicity and clinical course.

Diagnostic Modalities

A 12-lead electrocardiogram (ECG) is an important adjunct in identifying seriously poisoned children. Strict attention should be paid to rhythm, QRS interval, and QT interval. Prolongation of the QRS interval (i.e., longer than 0.10 msec) or the QT interval indicates an increased risk of ventricular arrhythmias and commonly suggests ingestion of cyclic antidepressants, selected antipsychotics, quinidine, and type IA antidysrhythmic agents. Bradycardia with atrioventricular block suggests ingestion of digitalis-like agents, β-adrenergic blockers, and calcium channel blockers.

■ **An abdominal radiograph** allows detection of some toxic agents (e.g., iron, calcium salts, potassium salts, heavy metals [lead], chlorinated hydrocarbons).

> **HINT:** The absence of radiopaque pills or fragments does not exclude the possibility of ingestion if the film is taken after the substance (e.g., iron) has been absorbed.

Suggested Readings

Flomenbaum NE, Goldfrank LR, Hoffman RS, et al.: *Goldfrank's Toxicologic Emergencies*, 8th ed. New York, McGraw-Hill, 2006.

Olson KR (ed): *Poisoning & Drug Overdose*, 4th ed. New York, McGraw-Hill, 2004.

Shannon MW, Borron SW, Burns MJ: *Haddad and Winchester's Clinical Management of Poisoning and Drug Overdose*, 4th ed. Philadelphia, Saunders Elsevier, 2007.

PART four

Cardiology Laboratory

84

Cardiology Laboratory
Timothy M. Hoffman

BLOOD PRESSURE MEASUREMENT

Accurate measurement of the blood pressure depends on **selection of an appropriate cuff size** of a sphygmomanometer. By convention, an appropriate cuff size is a cuff with an inflatable bladder width that is at least 40% of the arm circumference at a point midway between the olecranon and the acromion. For a cuff to be optimal for an arm, the cuff bladder length should cover 80% to 100% of the circumference of the arm. Such a requirement demands that the bladder width-to-length ratio be at least 1:2. If the cuff size is too small, the blood pressure will be overestimated, and if it is too large, the blood pressure will be underestimated.

Auscultation of the diastolic component of the blood pressure exhibits **two end points, Korotkoff phases IV and V,** respectively. **In children, Korotkoff phase IV** (i.e., the point of diminution or muffling of the Korotkoff sound) is generally considered a **more accurate representation** of the diastolic pressure. Korotkoff phase V (i.e., the disappearance of the Korotkoff sounds) should be **considered the diastolic end point if it falls within 6 mm Hg of Korotkoff phase IV.**

Pulsus Paradoxus

Pulsus paradoxus, a **decrease of >10 mm Hg in the systolic blood pressure during inspiration,** may be associated with **cardiac tamponade** (e.g., as a result of pericardial effusion), **constrictive pericarditis,** or **severe respiratory compromise** (e.g., asthma exacerbation).

> **HINT:** Pulsus paradoxus must not be confused with pulsus alternans (i.e., a decrease in the systolic pressure on alternate contractions that indicates left ventricular failure).

Using a sphygmomanometer, the cuff is **inflated until the pressure is 20 mm Hg above the systolic pressure.** The bladder is then **slowly deflated until the Korotkoff phase I sound is heard** independent of the respiratory cycle—this is the first data point. The slow deflation of the bladder is **continued until the Korotkoff phase I sound is noted throughout the respiratory cycle** (during inspiration *and* expiration)—the second data point. The difference between the points is considered the reduction in systolic pressure during inspiration and is abnormal (pulsus paradoxus) if it is >10 mm Hg. Figure 84-1 depicts pulsus paradoxus schematically.

HYPEROXIA TEST

The hyperoxia test can be useful for **differentiating cardiac and pulmonary causes of cyanosis,** and it is **one of the first evaluations** performed when confronted **with a cyanotic newborn.** Cyanosis usually becomes apparent at a mean capillary concentration of 3 to 4 g/dL of deoxygenated hemoglobin, a concentration that corresponds to an oxygen saturation of 70% to 80%.

In infants with **cyanotic heart disease and hypoxemia,** the **arterial oxygen tension** (PaO_2) is generally **<50 mm Hg** on 100% oxygen in patients who have transposition of the great arteries (TGA) or a lesion with restrictive pulmonary blood flow (tricuspid atresia with pulmonary stenosis or atresia, pulmonary atresia or critical pulmonary stenosis with intact ventricular septum, or tetralogy of Fallot). In an infant with **cardiac cyanosis** and a complete mixing lesion without restrictive pulmonary blood flow (truncus arteriosus, total anomalous pulmonary venous return, single ventricle, hypoplastic left heart syndrome, TGA with ventricular septal defect, tricuspid atresia without pulmonary stenosis or atresia), the **PaO_2 does not increase beyond 150 mm Hg** in response to the administration of 100% oxygen. In an infant with a **pulmonary cause** for the cyanosis, administration of **100% oxygen increases the PaO_2** to a level significantly **>150 mm Hg.** In patients with **congenital heart disease,** this phenomenon is attributable to **right-to-left shunting** (i.e., the mixing of deoxygenated blood and oxygenated blood within the circulatory system). Right-to-left shunting may be either **intracardiac or extracardiac** (intrapulmonary shunting from ventilation-perfusion mismatch) (see later section on agitated saline contrast echocardiography).

ELECTROCARDIOGRAPHY

The electrocardiogram (ECG) provides data concerning the following:

- Rate
- Rhythm
- Axes
- Intervals
- Hypertrophy
- Wave changes (Q waves and ST/T waves)

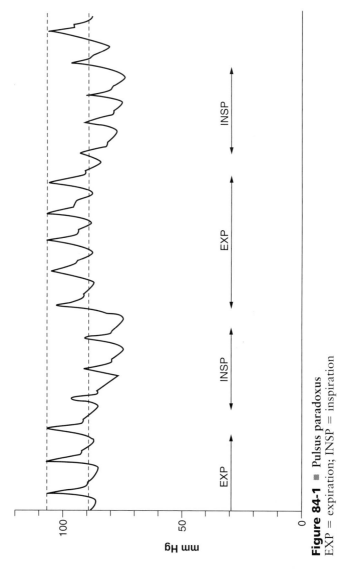

Figure 84-1 ■ Pulsus paradoxus
EXP = expiration; INSP = inspiration
(Modified with permission from Park MK: *Pediatric Cardiology for Practitioners*, 3rd ed. St. Louis, Mosby-Year Book, 1996, 15.)

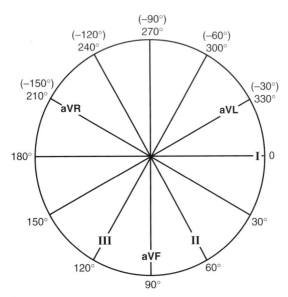

Figure 84-2 ■ Hexaxial reference system (frontal axis)
The shaded area represents the normal axis

Rate

The heart rate is determined accurately by **dividing 60 by the RR interval** (measured in seconds). For example, if the RR interval is 0.4 second (10 small boxes), the heart rate is 60 divided by 0.4, or 150 beats/minute.

Rhythm

Rhythm diagnosis is beyond the scope of this chapter.

Axes

The frontal axis should be determined for the **P, QRS, and T waves from the limb leads** (I, II, III, aVR, aVL, aVF). The **hexaxial reference system** (Figure 84-2) is usually used. The **normal** axes generally fall between 0° and 90°.

The specific axis is **equal to the direction of the largest positive force on depolarization.** A cursory way to determine the frontal axis is to **note the complex that is isoelectric** and **locate the two planes perpendicular** to it. The **perpendicular plane with the greatest positive deflection** is indicative of the axis.

P-Wave Axis

The location of the P-wave axis **determines the origin of an atrial-derived rhythm:**

- 0° to 90° = high right atrial rhythm (normal sinus rhythm)
- 90° to 180° = high left atrial rhythm (ectopic atrial rhythm)
- 180° to 270° = low left atrial rhythm (ectopic atrial rhythm)
- 270° to 0° = low right atrial rhythm (ectopic atrial rhythm)

> **HINT:** Classic "mirror image" dextrocardia is associated with a P-wave axis of 90° to 180° in conjunction with high amplitude forces in the right chest leads and low voltage in the left chest leads (i.e., lead V_{4R} has a greater amplitude than lead V_4).

QRS Axis

The QRS axis value is **age specific** (Table 84-1) but **may correlate with congenital heart disease** in certain clinical settings. For example, a northwest axis or left axis deviation (−30° to −120°) may correlate with an endocardial cushion defect or tricuspid atresia. Left axis deviation is always abnormal in a newborn.

T-Wave Axis

The T-wave axis helps **determine strain associated with ventricular hypertrophy.** A T-wave axis that is **90° different from the QRS** axis suggests a strain pattern.

Intervals (Figure 84-3)

Standard calculated intervals include the **PR, QRS, and corrected QT** intervals. The **normal heart rate, PR interval, and QRS duration vary with age** (Table 84-2).

TABLE 84-1 Age-Specific QRS Axis Values

Age	Mean (Degrees)	Range (Degrees)
<1 day	135	60–180
1–7 days	125	60–180
8–30 days	110	0–180
1–3 months	80	20–120
3–6 months	65	20–100
6–12 months	65	0–120
1–3 years	55	0–100
3–5 years	60	0–80
5–8 years	65	340–100
8–12 years	65	0–120
12–16 years	65	340–100

Adapted with permission from Liebman J, Plonsey R, Gillette PC: *Pediatric Electrocardiography.* Baltimore, Williams & Wilkins, 1982, 90.

Figure 84-3 ■ A normal electrocardiogram showing waveforms and intervals
The standard paper speed is 25 mm/second; therefore, a single 1-mm box equals 0.04 second, and a large (5-mm) box equals 0.20 second

PR Interval

First-degree atrioventricular block is characterized by a **PR interval that is greater than the standard** range for age. A short PR interval associated with a **delta wave** is indicative of **Wolff-Parkinson-White syndrome.**

QRS Interval

The QRS duration represents the **intraventricular conduction time** and is normally <0.09 second (in children <4 years) or 0.1 second (in children <4 years). A QRS duration **greater than normal is identified as a bundle branch block:**

TABLE 84-2 Normal Heart Rate, PR Interval, and QRS Duration for Age

Age	Heart Rate (beats/min) Mean	Range	PR Interval in Lead II (sec) Mean	Range	QRS Duration (sec) Mean	Range
<1 day	126	95–155	0.106	0.082–0.138	0.05	0.025–0.069
1–7 days	135	100–180	0.107	0.079–0.130	0.05	0.025–0.068
8–30 days	160	120–190	0.100	0.075–0.128	0.053	0.026–0.075
1–3 months	147	95–200	0.098	0.075–0.126	0.052	0.027–0.069
3–6 months	139	114–170	0.105	0.078–0.137	0.053	0.028–0.075
6–12 months	130	95–170	0.105	0.077–0.138	0.055	0.03–0.070
1–3 years	121	95–150	0.113	0.090–0.140	0.056	0.032–0.070
3–5 years	98	70–130	0.119	0.092–0.150	0.058	0.03–0.069
5–8 years	86	65–120	0.124	0.094–0.155	0.059	0.035–0.075
8–12 years	86	65–120	0.129	0.093–0.165	0.062	0.038–0.079
12–16 years	86	65–120	0.135	0.098–0.169	0.065	0.040–0.081

Adapted with permission from Liebman J, Plonsey R, Gillette PC: *Pediatric Electrocardiography.* Baltimore, Williams & Wilkins, 1982, 96–97, and Cassels DE, Ziegler RF: *Electrocardiography in Infants and Children.* Philadelphia, WB Saunders, 1966, 100.

■ **Left bundle branch block**
Criteria:

1. Left axis deviation for the patient's age.
2. QRS duration longer than the upper limit of normal for the patient's age.
3. Loss of Q waves in I, V5, and V6.
4. The slurred QRS complex is directed to the left and posteriorly
   a. Slurred and wide R waves in I, aVL, V5, and V6.
   b. Wide S waves in V1 and V2.
5. ST depression and T wave inversion in V4 through V6 are common.
6. QRS voltages may be greater than normal because of the asynchrony of depolarization of each ventricle. One should not make a diagnosis of ventricular hypertrophy when left bundle branch block is present.

■ **Right bundle branch block** is diagnosed when there is a wide S wave in leads I and V_6, right axis deviation, and an M-shaped (RSR′ pattern) QRS complex in lead V_1.
Criteria:

1. Right axis deviation, at least for terminal portion of QRS (QRSt). Initial part of QRS (QRSi) is unchanged.
2. QRS duration longer than the upper limit of normal for the patient's age.
3. Terminal slurring of the QRS complex directed to the right and usually, but not always, anteriorly.
   a. Wide and slurred S in I, V5, and V6.
   b. Terminal, slurred R′ in a VR and the RPLs (V4R, V1, and V2).

4. ST depression and T wave inversion are common in adults with right bundle branch block but not in children.
5. Asynchrony of the normally opposing electromotive force of each ventricle may result in a greater manifest potential for both ventricles. Therefore, the diagnosis of ventricular hypertrophy is insecure when either right or left bundle branch block is present.

■ **Left anterior hemiblock** can be diagnosed in the setting of left axis deviation associated with right bundle branch block.

Left posterior hemiblock is manifested by marked right axis deviation and normal QRS duration. It is extremely rare in children.

QT Interval
The QT measurement is **corrected for heart rate** using this formula:

$$QTc = \frac{\text{measured QT (seconds)}}{\sqrt{\text{RR interval (seconds)}}}$$

The accepted normal QTc interval is **<0.45 second for infants <6 months, and <0.44 second for children.**

Hypertrophy

Right Atrial Hypertrophy
Right atrial hypertrophy is shown on ECG when there is a **peaked P wave >3.0 mm in any lead.** This pattern is present most often in lead II and occasionally in V1 and V2.

Left Atrial Hypertrophy
A **P wave with a notched contour** and a duration of **<0.08 second in lead II** is diagnostic of left atrial hypertrophy. Alternatively, a **biphasic P wave in lead V_1 or V_{3R} with a terminal inverted portion** that measures 1 × 1 mm is diagnostic.

Right Ventricular Hypertrophy
Table 84-3 summarizes the normal measurements of R and S waves in leads V_1 and V_6 by age. Right ventricular hypertrophy can be diagnosed if any one of the following is seen:

■ An R wave in lead V_1 >98th percentile for age
■ An S wave in lead V_6 >98th percentile for age
■ An upright T wave in lead V_1 in a patient >4 days
■ Pure qR in leads V_{3R} or V_1
■ An RSR′ pattern in leads V_{3R} or V_1, in which the R′ portion is 15 mm greater than the R wave (in a child <1 year) or 10 mm greater than the R wave (in a child >1 year)

TABLE 84-3 Normal Range of Values (5th–95th Percentile) for R and S Waves in Leads V_1 and V_6

Age	Lead V_1		Lead V_6	
	R Wave (mm)	S Wave (mm)	R Wave (mm)	S Wave (mm)
<1 day	7.0–20.0	2.5–27.0	2.3–7.0	1.6–10.3
1–7 days	9.0–27.4	4.6–18.8	2.2–13.1	0.8–9.9
8–30 days	4.2–19.8	2.5–12.8	1.7–20.5	0.6–9.0
1–3 months	3.6–17.9	2.0–17.4	3.6–12.9	0.8–5.8
3–6 months	6.1–16.7	2.1–11.8	5.0–15.8	0.6–4.9
6–12 months	4.0–16.0	1.9–14.4	5.5–17.6	0.7–3.3
1–3 years	3.6–15.0	2.2–20.5	5.0–17.5	0.6–3.4
3–5 years	2.6–15.6	5.0–24.8	5.4–20.6	0.6–2.4
5–8 years	2.6–13.5	5.3–21.0	7.9–20.5	0.6–2.9
8–12 years	3.6–11.3	4.8–22.3	8.4–19.2	0.6–2.8
12–16 years	2.1–11.1	5.5–22.3	7.9–17.4	0.7–3.1

Adapted with permission from Liebman J, Plonsey R, Gillette PC: *Pediatric Electrocardiography.* Baltimore, Williams & Wilkins, 1982, 84–85.

Left Ventricular Hypertrophy

Left ventricular hypertrophy can be diagnosed if any one of the following is seen:

- An R wave in lead V_6 >98th percentile for age
- A narrow Q wave in lead V_5 or V_6 >4 mm
- An R wave in lead V_1 <5th percentile for age
- An S wave in lead V_1 >98th percentile for age

Wave Changes

- **ST segment elevation** >2 mm in the precordial leads may indicate pericarditis, myocardial injury, ischemia, infarction, or digitalis effect.
- **Tall peaked T waves** may be seen in patients with hyperkalemia.
- **Flat T waves** can occur in children with myocarditis, hypokalemia, or hypothyroidism.

CHEST RADIOGRAPH

When examining a chest radiograph, one must comment on the **cardiac size, organ situs, and the pulmonary vascular markings** (i.e., normal, increased, or decreased).

Cardiac Size

Cardiac size is determined by **estimating the cardiothoracic ratio.** The ratio is calculated by **dividing the largest diameter of the heart by the largest internal diameter of the thorax.** If the result is >0.5, **cardiomegaly** is present.

A

B

Figure 84-4 ■ Normal cardiac silhouette (A) Anteroposterior view. (B) Lateral view. [AO = aorta; C = clavicle; D = diaphragm; E = esophagus; IVC = inferior vena cava; LA = left atrium; LV = left ventricle; P = pulmonary outflow tract; RA = right atrium; RV = right ventricle; S = sternum; SVC = superior vena cava; T = trachea.]

(Modified with permission from Sapire DW: Understanding and Diagnosing Pediatric Heart Disease. East Norwalk, Ct, Appleton & Lange, 1991, 64.)

Organ Situs

Figure 84-4 depicts the normal cardiac silhouette in the anteroposterior and lateral views.

Pulmonary Vascular Markings

Pulmonary vascular markings **reflect the appearance of the pulmonary arteries and veins** on a chest radiograph **over the lung fields**.

These markings can be **increased in states of excessive pulmonary arterial flow** (e.g., ventricular septal defect, atrial septal defect, patent ductus arteriosus [PDA]), as well as in states characterized by **excessive pulmonary venous flow** (e.g., congestive heart failure, conditions characterized by pulmonary edema or pulmonary venous obstruction). On the radiograph, **increased pulmonary vasculature is noted when cephalization occurs and the vascular shadows extend across more than two thirds of the lung field.**

Decreased pulmonary vasculature markings are manifested radiographically as **hyperlucency of the lung field** and a **paucity of pulmonary vasculature,** as seen in patients with **tetralogy of Fallot.**

> **HINT:** The following signs, seen on the anteroposterior projection, offer clues to the diagnosis:

- A **"boot-shaped" heart** is often seen in newborns with tetralogy of Fallot.
- An **"egg on a string"** is noted in newborns with a narrow mediastinum owing to absence of a large thymus and is associated with TGA.
- A **"snowman sign"** is also associated with supracardiac total anomalous pulmonary venous return. The left vertical vein, innominate vein, and the superior vena cava form the superior aspect of the "snowman."

ECHOCARDIOGRAPHY

In pediatric patients, echocardiography is **performed in a stepwise fashion** to obtain **subcostal views, apical four-chamber views, parasternal views, and suprasternal views** (Figure 84-5).

M-mode Echocardiography

A parasternal short axis view using M-mode echocardiography reveals a **cross section of the left ventricle,** and therefore it can be used to **estimate cardiac dimensions.** Most commonly it is used to obtain a **shortening fraction** (SF) calculated in the following manner:

$$SF = \frac{\text{LV end-diastolic dimension} - \text{end-systolic dimension}}{\text{LV end-diastolic dimension}} \times 100$$

The **normal value** for the SF is generally considered to be **28% to 40%,** independent of age. SF is commonly used in pediatrics to assess left ventricular systolic performance.

A. Subcostal views

B. Apical views

Figure 84-5 ▪ Echocardiographic series
The *numbers* represent different planes along a sweep of the echocardiographic beam. (*A*) Subcostal views. (*B*) Apical views. (*Continued*)

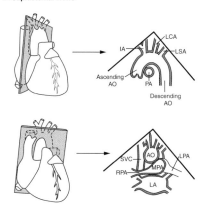

Figure 84-5 ■ *(continued)* Echocardiographic series
(C) Parasternal views. (D) Suprasternal views. [AO = aorta; AV =
aortic valve; IA = innominate artery; LA = left atrium; LCA = left
coronary artery; LPA = left pulmonary artery; LSA = left subclavian
artery; LV = left ventricle; MPA = middle pulmonary artery; MV =
mitral valve; PA = pulmonary artery; PM = papillary muscle; PV =
pulmonary valve; RA = right atrium; RCA = right coronary artery;
RPA = right pulmonary artery; RV = right ventricle; RVOT = right
ventricular outflow tract; SVC = superior vena cava]
*(Modified with permission from Park MK: Pediatric Cardiology for Practitioners, 3rd ed.
St. Louis, Mosby-Year Book, 1996, 70–73.)*

> **HINT:** A more accurate manner in which to assess left ventricular perform-
> ance is by performing an ejection fraction (EF). The normal values for
> EF are 54% to 75%. Estimates of EF use volume measurements calcu-
> lated in the following manner:
>
> $$EF = \frac{LV\ End-Diastolic\ Dimension\ -\ End-Systolic\ Dimension}{LV\ End-Diastolic\ Volume} \times 100$$

Doppler Echocardiography

Doppler echocardiography detects a **frequency shift** that reflects the **direction and velocity of blood flow.** Doppler echocardiography is used to detect **valvular insufficiency or stenosis and abnormal vasculature flow patterns.** The Bernoulli equation is used to assess gradients or pressure estimates depending on the flow pattern sampled. The equation can be simplified to the following:

> ΔP (pressure difference across an obstructed orifice) $= 4 \times V_2$ (velocity distal to the obstruction)^2. For example, if one is measuring Doppler flow across the aortic valve and V_2 is 3 m/second, using the modified Bernoulli equation would estimate the pressure gradient to be 4×3^2, which equals 36 mm Hg.

Agitated Saline Contrast Echocardiography

Agitation of saline produces 10- to 100-μ-diameter microbubbles that are absorbed by transit in the capillary bed. If a patient has a suspected right-to-left shunt (either extracardiac [intrapulmonary] or intracardiac) that cannot be detected by standard echocardiographic techniques, agitated saline contrast echocardiography may be helpful. The presence of microbubbles in the left heart after venous injection of agitated saline confirms the presence of right-to-left shunting.

- The site of injection to answer specific questions must be carefully planned. For example, investigation of a potential left superior vena cava drainage pattern would be best served with an intravenous saline injection in the left upper extremity.
- Extracardiac (intrapulmonary) shunts (i.e., pulmonary arteriovenous malformations) are marked by microbubbles appearing in the left side of the heart three to four cardiac cycles after injection.
- Intracardiac shunts (i.e., atrial septal defect) are marked by microbubbles appearing in the left side of the heart almost immediately after their injection into the right side of the heart.

Figure 84-6 ▪ Normal pressures (systolic over diastolic, in mm Hg), mean pressures, and oxygen saturations for children
The data are based on information compiled from healthy patients between 2 months and 20 years of age. [*AO* = aorta; *IVC* = inferior vena cava; *LA* = left atrium; *LV* = left ventricle; *PA* = pulmonary artery; *PV* = pulmonary vein; *RA* = right atrium; *RV* = right ventricle; *SVC* = superior vena cava]

CARDIAC CATHETERIZATION

Cardiac catheterization allows **sampling of oximetric and hemodynamic data.** Figure 84-6 depicts the normal pressures and oxygen saturations for children. Cardiac catheterization, an **invasive procedure,** is often used in **conjunction with angiography** to confirm the **diagnosis and physiology** of certain **acquired and congenital heart diseases.** The technique also has **therapeutic applications,** such as PDA coil embolization, coil embolization of aortopulmonary collaterals, pulmonary artery angioplasty and stent placement, and balloon valvuloplasty of semilunar valvular stenosis.

Shunts

Data obtained from cardiac catheterization can be used to calculate the degree and direction of an intracardiac or extracardiac shunt. The calculation is based on the **Fick principle,** using oxygen as the indicator.

The **oxygen content is equal to the dissolved oxygen** (which is usually negligible) **plus the oxygen capacity** [hemoglobin (g/dL) $\times$ 1.36 mL O_2/dL $\times$ 10] **multiplied by the oxygen saturation** (as a percentage).

Flow (Q) is the **oxygen consumption divided by the arteriovenous oxygen content difference:**

$$Qp = \frac{Vo_2}{PV-PA} \quad Qs = \frac{Vo_2}{AO-MV}, \text{ where}$$

Qp = pulmonary flow
Qs = systemic flow
Vo_2 = oxygen consumption per unit time
PV = pulmonary venous oxygen content
PA = pulmonary arterial oxygen content
MV = mixed venous oxygen content
AO = aortic oxygen content

To calculate the **amount of a shunt,** one needs to **calculate the effective pulmonary blood flow** (Qp eff):

$$Qp \text{ eff} = \frac{Vo_2}{PV-MV}$$

A **left-to-right shunt** is the **pulmonary flow less the effective pulmonary flow** (Qp − Qp eff), and a **right-to-left shunt** is the **systemic flow less the effective pulmonary flow** (Qs − Qp eff).

Resistance

Systemic and pulmonary vascular resistance can also be calculated using **catheterization data.** This calculation is based on **Ohm's law** (essentially, the pressure change across the vascular bed divided by flow equals resistance):

$$Rp = \frac{PA - LA}{Q_p} \quad Rs = \frac{AO - RA}{Q_s}, \text{ where}$$

Rs = systemic resistance
Rp = pulmonary resistance
AO = mean aortic pressure
RA = mean right atrial pressure
PA = mean pulmonary artery pressure
LA = mean left atrial pressure

A **pulmonary resistance (Rp)** of $\leq$**2.5 Wood units** is considered within the **normal** range; however, no vascular bed is rigid, and **variations in flow can affect the result** obtained.

chapter

85

Surgical Glossary

Joseph J. Zorc
Aaron E. Carroll and Nahush A. Mokadam (Third Edition)

aortopexy—procedure in which the aorta is approximated to the anterior thoracic wall; for the treatment of tracheomalacia.

Bishop-Koop procedure—resection of a dilated loop of bowel proximal to meconium obstruction, with end-to-side anastomosis between the proximal bowel and obstructed loop, combined with end ileostomy; for the treatment of meconium ileus.

bladder augmentation—procedure in which a portion of the intraabdominal gastrointestinal tract is used to increase the volume of the bladder.

Blalock-Taussig shunt—procedure in which the subclavian artery is anastomosed to the pulmonary artery; for the temporary treatment of tetralogy of Fallot.

Boix-Ochoa procedure—restoration of the intraabdominal esophageal length, repair of the esophageal hiatus, fixation of the esophagus to the hiatus, and restoration of the angle of His; for the treatment of incompetent lower esophageal sphincter.

chordee correction—procedure in which the corpus spongiosum is moved ventrally and the corpus cavernosa are approximated dorsally; for the treatment of chordee (abnormal penile curvature associated with epispadias or hypospadias).

Clatworthy mesocaval shunt—division of the common iliac veins and side-to-end anastomosis of the inferior mesenteric vein to the left renal vein; for the treatment of portal hypertension.

Cohen procedure—trigonal reimplantation of the ureter; for the treatment of vesicoureteral reflux.

colonic conduit diversion—procedure involving two stages: (1) a loop diversion using a colonic segment, and (2) an end-to-side anastomosis of the colonic segment to the gastrointestinal tract.

colonic interposition—replacement of the esophagus with a colonic segment; for treatment of esophageal atresia or stricture when gastric mobilization is not feasible.

diaphragmatic plication—surgical shortening of the diaphragm (abdominal, transthoracic, or bilateral); for the treatment of diaphragmatic eventration.

distal splenorenal shunt—see **Warren shunt**.

Drapanas mesocaval shunt—prosthetic graft implantation from the inferior mesenteric vein to the inferior vena cava; for the treatment of portal hypertension.

Duckett transverse preputial island flap—technique in which a flap of foreskin is used to elongate the urethra; for the treatment of hypospadias.

Duhamel procedure—resection of the aganglionic colon above the dentate line with stable anastomosis to the rectal stump, normally performed in children 6 to 12 months of age for the treatment of Hirschsprung disease (see **Martin modification**).

end-to-side portocaval shunt—procedure in which the portal vein is divided and anastomosed to the inferior vena cava; for the treatment of portal hypertension.

esophagectomy—resection of the esophagus, with gastric pull-up and anastomosis with the cervical esophagus; for the treatment of esophageal atresia or stricture.

Fontan procedure—procedure in which a graft is created to connect the pulmonary artery to the right atrium; for the treatment of hyperplastic right heart syndrome.

Glenn shunt—shunt from the superior vena cava to the pulmonary artery; for the treatment of tricuspid atresia or stenosis.

gridiron incision—see **McBurney incision**.

Hegman procedure—surgical release of the tarsal, metatarsal, and intertarsal ligaments; for the treatment of metatarsus adductus.

Heller myotomy—myotomy of the anterior lower esophagus (always accompanied by a Thal fundoplication); for the treatment of achalasia.

ileal loop diversion—resection and implantation of ureters into an isolated ileal segment, with an ileal stoma and primary anastomosis of ileum to cecum.

ileal ureter—ileal interposition between the renal pelvis and bladder when the ureteral length is insufficient for anastomosis; for the treatment of urinary obstruction.

ileocecal conduit diversion—bilateral ureteral diversion and anastomosis to an isolated ileocecal segment and cecostomy with primary anastomosis of ileum to the right colon.

Jatene procedure—arterial retransposition; for the treatment of transposition of the great vessels.

J-pouch—creation of an ileal reservoir in the distal ileum using a J-shaped configuration; used following colectomy.

Kasai procedure—resection of atretic extrahepatic bile ducts and gallbladder with Roux-en-Y anastomosis of the jejunum to the remaining common hepatic duct; for the treatment of biliary atresia or other extrahepatic obstruction.

Kimura procedure (parasitized cecal patch)—a multistep operation in which (1) a side-to-side anastomosis is made with a portion of the distal ileum and the right colon, and (2) an ileoanal pull-through is performed; for the treatment of Hirschsprung disease.

King operation—resection of the knee with placement of a Küntscher rod to fix the femur to the tibia, followed by a Syme amputation for the treatment of proximal focal femoral deficiency.

Koch pouch diversion—procedure involving bilateral ureteral diversion with anastomosis to a neobladder formed from an isolated ileal segment, combined with an ileal stoma and primary anastomosis of ileum to ileum.

Ladd operation—restoration of intestinal anatomy from a malrotated state; for the treatment of intestinal malrotation.

Lanz incision—abdominal incision made in the left iliac fossa; for colostomy formation.

left hepatectomy—resection of the left hepatic lobe (medial and lateral segments).

MAGPI (meatal advancement and glanduloplasty) procedure—distal advancement of the urethral meatus and granuloplasty; for the treatment of hypospadias.

Mainz pouch diversion—procedure involving bilateral ureteral division with anastomosis to a neobladder formed from isolated cecum and terminal ileum; combined with an ileal stoma and primary anastomosis of the ileum to the right colon.

Martin modification (of Duhamel procedure)—right and transverse colectomy with ileoanal pull-through and side-to-side anastomosis of the remaining left colon to the ileum; procedure preserves some absorptive capacity of the large bowel; for the treatment of total colonic Hirschsprung disease.

McBurney (gridiron) incision—abdominal incision from the anterior superior iliac spine to the umbilicus; used for appendectomy.

Mikulicz procedure—diverting enterostomy performed proximal to the meconium obstruction without resection; for the treatment of meconium ileus.

mini-Pena procedure—anterior sagittal anorectoplasty; for the treatment of anterior rectoperianal fistula (boys) or rectal-fourchette fistula (girls).

Mitrofanoff technique—modification of neobladder diversion procedures, in which vascularized appendix is used to create the stoma.

Mustardé procedure—correction, using simple mattress sutures, of a prominent ear with normal or absent antihelical folds.

Mustard technique—redirection of blood through an atrial septal defect using a pericardial pathway; for the treatment of transposition of the great vessels; because of associated increased turbulence, this technique is not widely used today.

Nissen fundoplication—technique involving a 360° wrap of the gastric fundus around the gastroesophageal junction; for the treatment of incompetent lower esophageal sphincter; patient is rendered unable to vomit or belch.

Norwood procedure—three-stage palliative procedure including (1) atrial septectomy, transection, and ligation of the pulmonary artery, "neoaorta" formation using the proximal pulmonary artery, and creation of a synthetic porto-aortal shunt; (2) creation of a Glenn shunt; and (3) performance of a modified Fontan procedure; for the treatment of hypoplastic left heart syndrome.

onlay island flap—technique in which a flap of foreskin is used to elongate the urethra; for the treatment of hypospadias.

orchidopexy—testicular pull-down and attachment; for the treatment of undescended testis.

orthoplasty—surgical correction of excessive penile curvature.

parasitized cecal patch—see **Kimura procedure**.

Pena procedure—posterior sagittal anorectoplasty performed in children 1 to 6 months of age; for the treatment of imperforate anus.

Pfannenstiel incision—an abdominal incision used to gain access to the lower abdomen and bring pelvic organs within reach without dividing muscular tissue.

pharyngoplasty—elevation of the posterior pharyngeal wall following a primary cleft palate repair (to narrow the pharyngeal space); for the treatment of velopharyngeal incompetence.

Potts shunt—anastomosis of the descending aorta to the pulmonary artery for the permanent treatment of tetralogy of Fallot.

proximal splenorenal shunt—end-to-side anastomosis of the splenic vein to the left renal vein with splenectomy; for the treatment of portal hypertension.

pyeloplasty—resection of an atretic ureter with primary anastomosis to the renal pelvis; for the treatment of ureteropelvic junction obstruction.

Ramstedt operation—relaxation of the pyloric sphincter; for the treatment of pyloric stenosis.

Rashkind procedure—balloon atrial septostomy; for the treatment of palliation of the great vessels.

Rastelli repair—technique involving the closure of a ventricular septal defect with a patch and the creation of a conduit from the distal pulmonary artery to the right ventricle; for the treatment of transposition of the great vessels.

Ravitch procedure—procedure involving (1) creation of osteotomies between the manubrium and costal cartilages, (2) a greenstick fracture of the manubrium, and (3) the temporary insertion (for 6 to 12 months) of a stabilizing bar; for the treatment of pectus excavatum or pectus carinatum.

right colon pouch—procedure involving bilateral ureteral division with anastomosis to a neobladder (formed from an isolated segment of the right colon), combined with an ileal stoma and primary anastomosis of the ileum to the transverse colon.

right hepatectomy—resection of the right hepatic lobes (anterior and posterior segments).

rooftop (bilateral subcostal) incision—abdominal incision used to access the liver and portal structures.

Roux-en-Y anastomosis—division of the jejunum distal to the ligament of Treitz with end-to-side anastomosis of the duodenum to the distal jejunum and anastomosis of the proximal jejunum (typically) to the bile duct.

Santulli-Blanc enterostomy—modification of the Bishop-Koop procedure that involves the resection of a distal dilated bowel segment with side-to-end anastomosis to the proximal enterostomy; for the treatment of meconium ileus.

Senning procedure (venous switch)—technique involving intraatrial redirection of venous return so that systemic caval return is shunted through the mitral valve to the left ventricle and pulmonary return is brought through the tricuspid valve to the right ventricle; for the treatment of transposition of the great vessels.

side-to-side portocaval shunt—procedure in which the portal vein is anastomosed to the inferior vena cava; for the treatment of portal hypertension.

side-to-side splenorenal shunt—side-to-side anastomosis of the splenic vein to the left renal vein; for the treatment of portal hypertension.

Sistrunk operation—complete excision of a thyroglossal duct cyst.

Soave procedure—technique involving endorectal pull-through; for the correction of rectal resection.

S-pouch—creation of an ileal reservoir in the distal ileum using an S-shape configuration following colectomy.

Stamm gastrostomy—placement of an open gastrostomy tube; the opening is designed to close spontaneously on removal of the tube.

Sting procedure—subureteric Teflon injection; for the endoscopic correction of vesicoureteral reflux.

Sugiura procedure—technique that involves lower esophageal transection and primary anastomosis, devascularization of the lower esophagus and stomach, and splenectomy; for the treatment of esophageal varices.

Swenson procedure—resection of the posterior rectal wall to the dentate line (aganglionic region); for the treatment of Hirschsprung disease; technically difficult and rarely performed.

Syme amputation—amputation of the foot, calculated to bring the end of the stump above the opposite knee at maturity; for the treatment of proximal focal femoral deficiency.

Thal procedure—procedure involving a 180° anterior wrap of the gastric fundus around the gastroesophageal junction, preserving the patient's ability to vomit and belch; for the treatment of incompetent lower esophageal sphincter.

Thiersch operation—procedure in which a distal rectal segment that has prolapsed is approximated to the external sphincter muscle; for the treatment of rectal prolapse.

trisegmentectomy—resection of the right hepatic lobe and the quadrate lobe of the liver (right posterior segment, right anterior segment, and medial segment).

ureteropyelostomy—partial resection and side-to-side anastomosis of a partially duplicated ureter.

uretocalycostomy—technique for the treatment of urinary obstruction involving division of the ureter (distal to the obstruction) and intrarenal anastomosis to the most dependent renal calyx; when the renal pelvis is insufficient for anastomosis, the lower pole of the kidney is resected.

vaginal switch operation—procedure in which the vagina is separated from the urinary tract; for treatment of duplicated vagina.

Van Ness procedure—rotational 180° osteotomy of the femur in which the foot and ankle are brought to the level of the opposite knee; for prosthetic attachment for the treatment of femoral deficiency.

venous switch—see **Senning procedure.**

ventricular shunt procedure—procedure in which a Silastic catheter is positioned in a lateral ventricle and tunneled subcutaneously to drain into the central venous system or peritoneal cavity; for the treatment of hydrocephalus.

Warren (distal splenorenal) shunt—procedure in which the splenic vein is anastomosed to the left renal vein; for the treatment of portal hypertension.

Waterston aortopulmonary anastomosis—procedure involving anastomosis of the ascending aorta and the right pulmonary artery; for the temporary treatment of tetralogy of Fallot.

Whipple procedure—resection of the pancreatic head, duodenum, and gallbladder with gastrojejunostomy, hepatojejunostomy, and pancreaticojejunostomy.

4p syndrome—characterized by a round face, prominent nasal tip, polydactyly, and scoliosis.

5p syndrome—characterized by macrocephaly; small mandible; long, thin fingers; short, big toes; and anorectal and renal anomalies.

13q syndrome—typically involves malformations of the brain, heart, kidneys, and digits; usually lethal.

Aagenaes syndrome—hereditary (autosomal-recessive transmission); characterized by recurrent intrahepatic cholestasis, with lymphedema.

Aarskog syndrome—x-linked recessive disorder characterized by short stature and musculoskeletal and genital anomalies of unknown etiology. Physical features include short stature (90%), hypertelorism, small nose with anteverted nares, broad philtrum and nasal bridge, abnormal auricles and widow's peak, brachyclinodactyly (80%), broad feet with bulbous toes (75%), simian crease (70%), ptosis (50%), syndactyly (60%), "shawl" scrotum (80%), cryptorchidism (75%), inguinal hernia (60%), hyperopic astigmatism, large corneas, ophthalmoplegia, strabismus, delayed puberty, mild pectus excavatum, prominent umbilicus. Radiographs show delayed bone age.

abetalipoproteinemia—recessive transmission; characterized by progressive cerebellar ataxia and pigmentary degeneration of the retina (starts with malabsorption of fat and progresses to ataxia); absent or reduced lipoproteins and low carotene, vitamin A, and cholesterol levels; and acanthocytosis (spiny projections on red blood cells).

acanthosis nigricans (Lawrence-Seip syndrome)—characterized by hyperpigmented lichenoid plaques in the neck and axilla; may be associated with insulin resistance.

acrodermatitis enteropathica—autosomal-recessive transmission; characterized by zinc deficiency, vesicobullous and eczematous skin lesions in the perioral and perineal areas, cheeks, knees, and elbows; photophobia, conjunctivitis and corneal dystrophy; chronic diarrhea; glossitis; nail dystrophy; growth retardation; and superinfections and *Candida* infections.

Adie syndrome—characterized by a large pupil with little or no reaction to light; pupil may react to accommodation; patients have hyperreflexia.

agenesis of corpus callosum—cause unknown (rarely, X-linked recessive); absence of the major tracts connecting the right and left hemispheres is usually associated with hydrocephalus, seizures, developmental delay, abnormal head size, and hypertelorism.

Alagille syndrome (arteriohepatic dysplasia)—characterized by paucity or absence of intrahepatic bile ducts with progressive destruction of bile ducts; patients have a broad forehead, deep-set eyes that are widely spaced and underdeveloped, a small, pointed mandible, cardiac lesions, vertebral arch defects, and changes in the renal tubules and interstitium.

Albers-Schönberg disease (osteopetrosis tarda, marble bone disease)—most cases are autosomal dominant, a few are autosomal recessive; patients are prone to fractures and have mild anemia and craniofacial disproportion; radiologic changes include increased cortical bone density, longitudinal and transverse dense striations at the ends of the long bones, lucent and dense bands in the vertebrae, and thickening at the base of the skull.

Albright syndrome—see **McCune-Albright syndrome.**

Alexander disease—unknown pathogenesis; characterized by megaloencephaly in infants, dementia, spasticity, and ataxia; may cause seizures in younger children; patients become mute, immobile, and dependent; hyaline eosinophilic inclusions occur in the footplates of astrocytes in subpial and subependymal regions.

Alport syndrome—several forms are hereditary male-to-male autosomal dominant, and an X-linked form also exists; characterized by neurosensory deafness and progressive renal failure.

Anderson disease (glycogen storage disease, type IV)—caused by a defect in the glycogen branching enzyme 1, 4-α-glucan branching enzyme; characterized by hepatomegaly and failure to thrive in the first few months, progressing to liver cirrhosis and splenomegaly.

Apert syndrome (acrocephalosyndactyly)—autosomal dominant; characterized by high and flat frontal bones, underdevelopment of the middle third of the face, hypertelorism and proptosis; a narrow, high, arched palate; a short, beaked nose; and syndactyly of the toes and digits.

arthrogryposis multiplex congenita—characterized by fixed contractures of the middle joints; present at birth.

Asperger syndrome—a developmental disorder on the higher functioning end of the autism spectrum. These patients, often viewed as brilliant, eccentric, and physically awkward, fail to develop relationships with peers, have repetitive and stereotyped behaviors, usually with hand movements. See www.aspergersyndrome.org.

Bart syndrome—autosomal dominant; congenital aplasia of the skin; characterized by nail defects and recurrent blistering of the skin and mucous membranes.

Bartter syndrome—hypertrophy of the juxtaglomerular apparatus; characterized by hypokalemic alkalosis, hypochloremia, and hyper-aldosteronism; patients have normal blood pressure but the renin level is elevated; may lead to mental retardation and small stature.

Beckwith-Wiedemann syndrome—characterized by hypoglycemia, macrosomia, and visceromegaly; patients have umbilical anomalies and renal medullary dysplasia.

Behçet syndrome—unknown cause; involves relapsing iridocyclitis and recurrent oral and genital ulcerations; 50% of patients have arthritis.

blind loop syndrome—stasis of small intestine, usually secondary to incomplete bowel obstruction or a problem of intestinal motility.

Bloch-Sulzberger syndrome (incontinentia pigmenti)—characterized by mental retardation; a third of patients have seizures and ocular malformations.

Bloom syndrome—autosomal recessive; characterized by erythema and telangiectasia in a butterfly distribution, photosensitivity, and dwarfism.

Blount disease (tibia vara)—characterized by irregularity of the medial aspect of the tibial metaphysis adjacent to the epiphysis; bowing starts as angulation at the metaphysis.

blue diaper syndrome—defective tryptophan absorption; characterized by bluish stains on the diapers, digestive disturbances, fever, and visual difficulties.

Brill disease (Brill-Zinsser disease)—repeat episode of typhus; caused by a *Rickettsia* infection.

bronchiolitis obliterans—begins with necrotizing pneumonia secondary to viral infection (e.g., adenovirus, influenza, measles); tuberculosis; or inhalation of fumes, talcum powder, or zinc; and involves the obstruction of small bronchi and bronchioles by fibrous tissue.

Byler disease—autosomal-recessive familial cholestasis; characterized by hepatomegaly, pruritus, splenomegaly, elevated bile acids, and gallstones.

Caroli disease—autosomal recessive; cystic dilation of the intrahepatic bile ducts; characterized by recurrent bouts of cholangitis and biliary abscesses secondary to bile stasis and gallstones.

cat's eye syndrome—autosomal dominant; characterized by ocular coloboma, down-slanting eyes, congenital heart disease, and anal atresia.

Charcot-Marie-Tooth disease (peroneal muscular atrophy)—most common cause of chronic peripheral neuropathy; characterized by foot drop, high-arch foot; patients may have stocking-glove sensory loss.

Chédiak-Higashi syndrome—autosomal-recessive disorder; involves partial oculocutaneous albinism, increased susceptibility to infection, lack of natural killer cells, and large lysosome-like granules in many tissues; patients have splenomegaly, hypersplenism, hepatomegaly, lymphadenopathy, nystagmus photophobia, and peripheral neuropathy.

Coat disease—telangiectasia of retinal vessels, with subretinal exudate.

Cobb syndrome—intraspinous vascular anomaly and port-wine stains.

Cockayne syndrome—autosomal recessive; characterized by dwarfism, mental retardation, birdlike facies, premature senility, and photosensitivity.

Cornelia de Lange syndrome—prenatal growth retardation; characterized by microcephaly, hirsutism, anteverted nares, down-turned mouth, mental retardation, and congenital heart defects.

cri du chat syndrome—characterized by growth retardation, mental deficiency, hypotonia, microcephaly, round "moon face," hypertelorism, epicanthal folds, and down-slanting palpebral fissures.

Crigler-Najjar syndrome (congenital nonhemolytic unconjugated hyperbilirubinemia)—type 1 is recessive; a deficiency of uridine diphosphate (UDP) glucuronyl transferase causes a rapid increase in the unconjugated bilirubin level on the first day of life; no hemolysis occurs and patients have no conjugation activity; type 2 is autosomal dominant and characterized by variable penetrance and partial activity of UDP glucuronyl transferase.

Cronkhite-Canada syndrome—diffuse intestinal polyps involving large and small intestine; characterized by alopecia, brown skin lesions, and onychatrophia; patients have diarrhea and protein-losing enteropathy.

Crouzon syndrome (craniofacial dysostosis)—autosomal dominant with a range of expressivity; characterized by exophthalmos, hypertelorism, and hypoplasia of maxilla; patients have oral cavity anomalies and premature closure of the external auditory meatus.

cyclic neutropenia—syndrome involving lack of granulocyte macrophage colony-stimulating factor; characterized by fever, mouth lesions, cervical adenitis, and gastroenteritis occurring every 3 to 6 weeks; neutrophil count may be zero.

de Toni-Fanconi-Debré acute syndrome—fatal; infantile myopathy with renal dysfunction; involves abnormal mitochondria and lipid and glycogen accumulation; patient has weak cry, poor muscle tone, poor suck, and lactic acidosis.

De Sanctis-Cacchione syndrome—autosomal recessive; characterized by xeroderma pigmentosum with mental retardation, dwarfism, and hypogonadism; skin is unable to repair itself after exposure to ultraviolet light; patients may have erythema, scaling bullae, crusting telangiectasia keratoses, photophobia, corneal opacities, and tumors of the eyelids.

Diamond-Blackfan syndrome (congenital hypoplastic anemia)—failure of erythropoiesis; characterized by macrocytic anemia; patients have anemia, pallor, and weakness, no hepatomegaly, elevated fetal hemoglobin, and defect in abduction with retraction of the eye on adduction.

DiGeorge syndrome—thymic hypoplasia with hypocalcemia; patients have tetany, abnormal facies, congenital heart disease, and increased incidence of infection.

Dubin-Johnson syndrome—autosomal recessive; characterized by elevated conjugated bilirubin, large amounts of coproporphyrin I in urine, and deposits of melaninlike pigment in hepatocellular lysosomes.

Dubowitz syndrome—Children with this syndrome nearly always have a history of intrauterine growth retardation involving both low birthweight and reduced length. Primary microcephaly. Facial characteristics include triangular face; small receding chin; and broad and sometimes flat nasal bridge. As the child matures, the nasal bridge appears less wide and often becomes prominent, producing a continuous line with the forehead when viewed in profile. Tip of nose is frequently wide, rounded, or prominent; hypertelorism; shortened palpebral fissure that may be slanted; ptosis; sloping and high forehead; scanty hair and eyebrows; ear abnormalities.

Eagle-Barrett syndrome (prune-belly syndrome)—characterized by deficiency of the abdominal musculature, dilation and dysplasia of the urinary tract, cryptorchidism, dilation of the posterior urethra, and a hypoplastic or absent prostate.

ectodermal dysplasia—characterized by the poor development, or absence, of teeth, nails, hair, and sweat glands; patients have hyperextensible skin, hypermobile joints, and easy bruisability.

Eisenmenger syndrome—characterized by ventricular septal defect with pulmonary hypertension.

Fabry disease—X-linked lipid storage disease; involves a defect of the ceramide trihexoside α-galactosidase; characterized by tingling and burning in the hands and feet; small red maculopapular lesions on the buttocks, inguinal area, fingernails, and lips; and an inability to perspire; patients have proteinuria, progressing to renal failure.

Farber syndrome—autosomal recessive; involves a deficiency of acid ceramidase; characterized by hoarseness; painful, swollen joints; and palpable nodules over affected joints and pressure points.

fetal alcohol syndrome—characterized by a small body, head, and maxillary bone; abnormal palpebral fissures; epicanthal folds; cardiac septal defect; delayed development; and mental deficiency.

fetal hydantoin syndrome—characterized by hypoplasia of the midface, low nasal bridge, ocular hypertelorism, cupid bow upper lip; patients experience slow growth, may have mental retardation, cleft lip, and cardiac malformation.

Friedreich ataxia—mostly autosomal recessive; appears in late childhood or in adolescence; involves progressive cerebellar and spinal cord dysfunction; patients have high-arched foot, hammer toes, and cardiac failure.

fructose intolerance, hereditary—autosomal recessive; involves deficiency of fructose-1-phosphate aldolase or fructose 1,6-diphosphatase; characterized by vomiting, diarrhea, hypoglycemic seizures, and jaundice.

Gardner syndrome—characterized by multiple gastrointestinal polyps with malignant transformation, skin cysts, and multiple osteoma.

Gaucher disease—abnormal storage of glucosylceramide in the reticuloendothelial system; three types: (1) adult, or chronic, (2) acute neuropathic, or infantile, (3) subacute neuropathic, or juvenile; characterized by splenomegaly, hepatomegaly, delayed development, strabismus, swallowing difficulties, laryngeal spasm, opisthotonos, and bone pain.

Gianotti-Crosti syndrome—papular acrodermatitis and hepatitis B virus infection; usually benign and self-limited.

Gilles de la Tourette syndrome—dominant trait with partial penetrance; characterized by multiple tics (e.g., blinking, twitching, grimacing) and involvement of muscles of swallowing and respiration; patient may exhibit swearing behavior and may have learning disabilities.

Glanzmann disease—autosomal recessive; involves defective primary platelet aggregation (size and survival of platelets is normal).

Goldenhar syndrome—characterized by oculoauriculovertebral dysplasia and mandibular hypoplasia; patients have a hypoplastic zygomatic arch; malformed, displaced pinnae, and hearing loss.

Goltz syndrome—focal dermal hypoplasia; herniations of fat through thinned dermis produce tan papillomas associated with other skin defects and skeletal anomalies (e.g., syndactyly, polydactyly, spinal defects); patients also have colobomas, strabismus, and nystagmus.

Gradenigo syndrome—acquired palsy of the abducens nerve and pain in the trigeminal nerve distribution, usually occurs after otitis media; produces diplopia, ocular and facial pain, photophobia, and lacrimation.

Hand-Schüller-Christian disease—see histiocytosis X.

Hartnup disease—autosomal recessive defect in transport of monoamine monocarboxylic amino acids by intestinal mucosa and renal tubules; characterized by photosensitivity and a pellagralike skin rash; patients may have cerebellar ataxia.

histiocytosis X—See Langerhans cell histiocytosis

Hunter syndrome (mucopolysaccharidosis II)—X-linked recessive; characterized by an accumulation of heparan sulfate and dermatan sulfate, and enzyme deficiency of l-iduronate sulfatase.

Hurler syndrome (mucopolysaccharidosis IH)—autosomal recessive; characterized by an accumulation of heparan sulfate and dermatan sulfate, and enzyme deficiency of α-L-iduronidase.

hyper-immunoglobulin E (IgE)—characterized by recurrent deep tissue and skin staphylococcal infections; patients have eosinophilia and IgE levels that are 10 times greater than normal.

incontinentia pigmenti—see **Bloch-Sulzberger syndrome.**

Jeune thoracic dystrophy—characterized by respiratory distress, short limbs, and polydactyly; may progress to renal insufficiency.

Job syndrome—characterized by severe staphylococcal infections, chronic skin disease, and cold abscesses; patients may have elevated immunoglobulin E.

Kallmann syndrome—familial; characterized by isolated gonadotropin deficiency and anosmia.

Kartagener syndrome—characterized by sinusitis, bronchiectasis, and immotile cilia.

Kasabach-Merritt syndrome—characterized by hemangioma and consumption coagulopathy, platelet trapping, and microangiopathic hemolytic anemia.

Kleine-Levin syndrome—characterized by unusual hunger, somnolence, and motor restlessness.

Klinefelter syndrome—XXY karyotype; characterized by seminiferous tubule dysgenesis, testicular atrophy, eunuchoid habitus, and gynecomastia.

Klippel-Feil syndrome—characterized by a short neck, limited neck motion, and low occipital hairline.

Krabbe leukodystrophy—autosomal recessive; characterized by cerebroside lipidosis and lack of myelin in white matter; usually presents by 1 year of age; patients have hyperreflexia, rigidity, swallowing difficulties, lack of development.

Langerhans cell histiocytosis—(reticuloendotheliosis) formerly called eosinophilic granuloma, Hand-Schüller-Christian disease, or Letterer-Siwe disease; patients may have a few solitary bone lesions or seborrheic dermatitis of scalp, lymphadenopathy, hepatosplenomegaly, tooth loss, exophthalmos, or pulmonary infiltrates.

Larsen syndrome—usually autosomal dominant; characterized by hyperlaxity, multiple dislocations, and skin hyperlaxity .

Laurence-Moon-Biedl syndrome—characterized by retinitis pigmentosa, polydactyly, obesity, and hypogonadism.

Lennox-Gastaut syndrome (childhood epileptic encephalopathy)—characterized by severe seizures, mental retardation, and characteristic electroencephalography pattern (i.e., generalized bilaterally synchronous sharp wave and slow wave complexes); patients have seizures starting in infancy; condition is difficult to treat; mental retardation is common.

Lesch-Nyhan syndrome—X-linked recessive disorder; characterized by a defect in purine metabolism; patients have hyperuricemia as a result of diminished or absent hypoxanthine guanine phosphoribosyl transferase activity, choreoathetosis, compulsive self-mutilation, mental retardation, and growth failure.

Letterer-Siwe disease—component of histiocytosis X; characterized by acute disseminated histiocytosis; patients have seborrheic-looking skin lesions, bone lesions, gingival lesions, and liver and lung infiltrates.

Lowe syndrome (oculocerebral dystrophy)—X-linked recessive; patients have congenital cataracts, glaucoma, hypotonia, hyperreflexia, severe mental retardation, rickets, osteopenia, pathologic fractures, aminoaciduria, and organic aciduria.

Maffucci syndrome—multiple enchondromata and hemangioma of the bone and overlying skin; patients have short stature, skeletal deformities, scoliosis, and limb disproportion.

Marfan syndrome—connective tissue disorder characterized by ectopia lentis; dilation of the aorta; long, thin extremities; pectus excavatum or carinatum; scoliosis; and pneumothorax.

McCune-Albright syndrome—polyostotic fibrous dysplasia; characterized by prominent skin discoloration with ragged edges; patients may have precocious puberty, hyperthyroidism, gigantism, headaches, epilepsy, and mental deficiency.

MELAS syndrome—*m*itochondrial *e*ncephalopathy, *l*actic *a*cidosis, and *s*trokelike episodes; causes seizures, alternating hemiparesis, hemianopsia, or cortical blindness; patients have lactic acidosis, spongy degeneration of the brain, sensorineural hearing loss, and short stature.

Menkes syndrome—X-linked recessive; patients have short scalp hair, hypopigmentation, hypothermia, growth failure, skeletal defects, arterial aneurysms, seizures, and progressive central nervous system failure.

Möbius syndrome—characterized by cranial nerve defects and a hypoplastic tongue or digits.

Morquio syndrome (mucopolysaccharidosis)—characterized by severe skeletal deformities, pectus carinatum, kyphoscoliosis, short neck, hypoplasia of the odontoid processes, C1 and C2 dislocation, neurosensory deafness, and aortic insufficiency.

multiple cartilaginous exostosis—characterized by bony projections near the ends of the tubular bones and ribs, scapula, vertebral bodies, and iliac crest; the exostoses become calcified and cause skeletal deformities; appears after 3 years of age.

nail-patella syndrome—autosomal dominant; characterized by dystrophic and hypoplastic nails, hypoplastic patellae and iliac horns, and malformed radial heads; may lead to nephrotic syndrome and renal failure.

Niemann-Pick disease—four types; storage of sphingomyelin and cholesterol causes hepatomegaly; patients are normal at birth but experience delayed development; 50% have a macular cherry red spot.

Noonan syndrome—normal karyotype; syndrome is characterized by cardiac lesions (atrial septal defect or pulmonic stenosis); facial changes (palpebral slant, broad flat nose); webbed neck; short stature; a high arched palate; and malformed ears.

Osler-Weber-Rendu syndrome—hereditary hemorrhagic telangiectasia; patients have telangiectasia in the skin, respiratory tract mucosa, lips, nails, conjunctiva, and nasal and oral mucosae.

Parinaud syndrome—characterized by weakness of upward gaze, poor convergence and accommodation, refractive nystagmus with upward gaze, and pupillary changes.

Patau syndrome—see **trisomy 13.**

Pelizaeus-Merzbacher disease—characterized by dancing eye movements, delayed motor development and spasticity, small head, poor head control, and possible optic atrophy and seizures.

Peutz-Jeghers syndrome—autosomal dominant; patients have bluish black macules around the mouth and intestinal polyposis in the small bowel.

Pickwickian syndrome—characterized by obesity and hypoventilation syndrome; patients may have respiratory arrest, restless sleep.

Pierre Robin syndrome—characterized by severe micrognathia, glossoptosis, and cleft palate.

Poland syndrome—characterized by a unilateral hypoplastic pectoral muscle with ipsilateral upper limb deficiency, syndactyly, and a defect of the subclavian artery.

Prader-Willi syndrome—characterized by hypotonia, hypomentia, hypogonadism, obesity, narrow bifrontal diameter, and hypotonia; patients may have a deletion in chromosome 15.

progeria—characterized by premature aging, severe growth failure, atherosclerosis, alopecia, and dystrophic nails.

prune-belly syndrome—see **Eagle-Barrett syndrome.**

Rieger syndrome—sporadic autosomal dominant; characterized by microcornea with opacity, iris hypoplasia, anterior synechiae, hypodontia, and maxillary hypoplasia.

Riley-Day syndrome—familial dysautonomia; affects sensory and autonomic functions; patients have poor feeding, aspiration, no tears, high threshold to pain, markedly decreased reflexes, smooth tongue and impaired taste, and erratic blood pressure and temperature.

Rotor syndrome—autosomal recessive; characterized by elevated conjugated bilirubin, elevated coproporphyrin I and coproporphyrin in urine, and normal liver biopsies.

Rubinstein-Taybi syndrome—characterized by broad thumbs and toes, short stature, mental retardation, beaked nose, hypoplastic mandible, and congenital heart defect.

Russell-Silver dwarf syndrome—characterized by intrauterine growth retardation, subnormal growth velocity, triangular facies, clinodactyly, simian creases, and genitourinary malformations.

Sandhoff GM$_2$-gangliosidosis type II—characterized by deficient hexosaminidase activity leading to cherry red spot in macula, failure to develop motor skills, blindness, weakness, and seizures.

Sanfilippo type A syndrome (mucopolysaccharidosis IIIA)—autosomal recessive; characterized by accumulation of heparan sulfate, dermatan sulfate, and sulfatidase.

Sanfilippo type B syndrome (mucopolysaccharidosis IIIA)—autosomal recessive; characterized by accumulation of heparan sulfate, dermatan sulfate, and α-N-acetylglucosaminidase.

Scheie syndrome (mucopolysaccharidosis IS)—autosomal recessive; characterized by accumulation of heparan sulfate and dermatan sulfate, and an enzyme defect affecting α-L-iduronidase.

scimitar syndrome—characterized by hypoplasia of the right lung with systemic arterial supply, anomalous right pulmonary vein, and dextroposition of heart.

Seckel syndrome—characterized by intrauterine growth retardation, microcephaly, sharp facial features with underdeveloped chin, and mental retardation.

Shwachman syndrome—characterized by pancreatic dysfunction, short stature, bone marrow dysfunction, and skeletal abnormalities.

silo filler disease—acute pneumonitis caused by inhalation of nitrogen dioxide; patients have chills, fever, cough, dyspnea, and cyanosis; associated with a high mortality rate.

Smith-Lemli-Opitz syndrome—characterized by short stature, microcephaly, ptosis, anteverted nares, micrognathia, syndactyly, cryptorchidism, and mental retardation.

Sotos syndrome—characterized by cerebral gigantism, large head and ears, prominent mandible, mental retardation, and poor coordination.

Stickler syndrome—autosomal dominant; characterized by high myopia, cataract formation, and retinal detachment.

Sturge-Weber syndrome—characterized by a port-wine stain on the face at the first branch of the trigeminal nerve; patients have seizures and mental retardation.

Swyer-James syndrome—characterized by unilateral hyperlucent lung following bronchiolitis obliterans.

Tourette syndrome—see **Gilles de la Tourette syndrome.**

Treacher Collins syndrome—autosomal dominant with incomplete penetration; characterized by mandibulofacial dysostosis; patients have hypoplastic mandible; hypoplastic zygomatic arches; antimongoloid slant to eyes; deformities of the pinna; and a high arched palate with or without cleft palate.

trisomy 9—characterized by deep-set eyes, bulbous nasal tip, an anxious facial expression, and cleft lip.

trisomy 13 (Patau syndrome)—characterized by cleft lip, microphthalmia, postaxial polydactyly, and cardiovascular anomalies.

trisomy 18—characterized by a small face, high nasal bridge, short palpebral fissures, micrognathia, small mouth, overriding fingers, and hypoplastic nails; patients have mental retardation and intrauterine growth retardation.

tuberous sclerosis—characterized by epiloia; patients have seizures, mental deficiency, adenoma sebaceum foci of intracranial calcification, hypopigmented macules, ash leaf spots, connective tissue nevi (shagreen spots), adenoma sebaceum, and angiofibroma.

Turcot syndrome—characterized by adenomatous colonic polyposis associated with malignant brain tumors, especially glioblastomas.

Turner syndrome—characterized by gonadal dysplasia (streak gonads stem from XO karyotype), short stature, sexual infantilism, atypical facies, low hairline, webbed neck, congenital lymphedema of the extremities, coarctation of the aorta, and increased carrying angle.

Usher syndrome—autosomal recessive; characterized by retinitis pigmentosa, cataracts, and sensorineural deafness.

vanishing testes syndrome—characterized by bilateral gonadal failure with normal external male genitalia, normal 46,XY karyotype, absent testes, and no male puberty.

VATER syndrome—syndrome involving *v*ertebral defects, *a*nal atresia, *t*racheo*e*sophageal atresia, *r*adial dysplasia, *r*enal dysplasia, and congenital heart defect.

Vogt-Koyanagi-Harada syndrome—characterized by vitiligo, uveitis, dysacousia, and aseptic meningitis.

von Gierke disease (type 1 glycogenosis)—glucose-6-phosphate dehydrogenase is absent in the liver, kidney, and intestinal mucosa; characterized by hypoglycemia under stress (e.g., fasting), hepatomegaly, and seizures.

von Hippel–Landau disease—autosomal dominant (linked to chromosome 3); characterized by hemangioblastoma of the cerebellum and retina; patients have cystic cerebellar neoplasm with increased intracranial pressure.

Waardenburg syndrome—autosomal dominant; characterized by white forelock, heterochromic irides, displacement of the inner canthi, broad nasal root, and confluent eyebrows.

Wegener granulomatosis—necrotizing granulomatous vasculitis of the arteries and veins; involves airways, lungs, and kidneys with resultant rhinorrhea, nasal ulceration, hemoptysis, and cough; patients have hematuria caused by necrotizing vasculitis.

Werner syndrome—autosomal recessive; characterized by short stature, juvenile cataracts, hypogonadism, gray hair in second decade.

Williams syndrome—characterized by mental retardation, hypoplastic nails, periorbital fullness, supravalvular aortic stenosis, growth delay, and stellate iris.

Wilson-Mikity syndrome—characterized by pulmonary immaturity; occurs in premature infants; patients have slow onset of respiratory distress, retractions, and apnea; may clear in several weeks.

Wiskott-Aldrich syndrome—characterized by thrombocytopenia, severe eczema, and recurrent skin infections.

Wolff-Parkinson-White syndrome—characterized by a short PR interval and slow upstroke of the QRS-delta wave; usually occurs in patients with a normal heart but also may occur in patients with Ebstein anomaly and cardiomyopathy.

Wolman disease—fatal condition characterized by primary xanthomatosis, adrenal insufficiency, vomiting, failure to thrive, steatorrhea, hepatomegaly, and adrenal calcification.

Zellweger syndrome—cerebrohepatorenal syndrome; characterized by hepatic fibrosis and cirrhosis; patients have seizures, mental retardation, hypotonia, glaucoma, congenital stippled epiphyses, and cysts of the renal cortex.

Zollinger-Ellison syndrome—characterized by islet cell tumors that produce duodenal and jejunal ulcers; patients have high gastrin levels and excessive acid secretion.

Index

Page numbers followed by *t* refer to tables; page numbers in *italic* refer to figures.